General Principles of Tumor Immunotherapy

General Principles of Tumor Immunotherapy

Basic and Clinical Applications of Tumor Immunology

Edited by

Howard L. Kaufman
The Tumor Immunology Laboratory,
Division of Surgical Oncology,
Columbia University,
New York, NY

and

Jedd D. Wolchok
Department of Medicine,
Memorial Sloan-Kettering Cancer Center,
Weill Medical College of Cornell University,
New York, NY

Springer

A C.I.P. Catalogue record for this book is available from the Library of Congress.

ISBN 978-1-4020-6086-1 (HB)
ISBN 978-1-4020-6087-8 (e-book)

Published by Springer,
P.O. Box 17, 3300 AA Dordrecht, The Netherlands.

www.springer.com

Printed on acid-free paper

TABLE OF CONTENTS

LIST OF CONTRIBUTORS

Scott I. Abrams Laboratory of Tumor Immunology and Biology Center for Cancer Research, National Cancer Institute National Institutes of Health, Bethesda, MD

Sylvia Adams NYU Cancer Institute Tumor Vaccine Center, New York University School of Medicine New York, NY

James P. Allison Howard Hughes Medical Institute, Department of Immunology, Memorial Sloan-Kettering Cancer Center, New York, NY

Nina Bhardwaj NYU Cancer Institute, Tumor Vaccine Center, New York University School of Medicine, New York, NY

Michael R. Bishop Experimental Transplantation and Immunology Branch, Center for Cancer Research, National Cancer Institute, National Institutes of Health, Bethesda, MD

Timothy M. Clay Duke University Medical Center, Durham, NC

Adam D. Cohen Department of Medicine, Memorial Sloan-Kettering Cancer Center, Weill Medical College of Cornell University, New York, NY

Gail DeRaffele The Tumor Immunology Laboratory, Division of Surgical Oncology, Columbia University, New York, NY

Madhav V. Dhodapkar Laboratory of Tumor Immunology and Immunotherapy, The Rockefeller University and Hematology Service, Memorial Sloan Kettering Cancer Center, New York, NY

Mary L. Disis Center for Translational Medicine in Women's Health, Tumor Vaccine Group, University of Washington Seattle, WA

Leisha A. Emens Department of Oncology, Johns Hopkins University School of Medicine, Sidney Kimmel Comprehensive Cancer Center, Baltimore, MD

Mark B. Faries Sonya Valley Ghidossi Vaccine Laboratory of the Roy E. Coats Research Laboratories of the John Wayne Cancer Institute at Saint John's Health Center, Santa Monica, CA

Jarett Feldman Laboratory of Tumor Immunology and Biology, Center for Cancer Research, National Cancer Institute, National Institutes of Health Bethesda, MD

Soldano Ferrone Hillman Cancer Research Institute, University of Pittsburgh, Pittsburgh, PA

Douglas W. Grosenbach Laboratory of Tumor Immunology and Biology, Center for Cancer Research, National Cancer Institute, National Institutes of Health, Bethesda, MD

Alan N. Houghton Swim Across America Laboratory, Memorial Sloan-Kettering Cancer Center, New York, NY

Robert R. Jenq Memorial Sloan-Kettering Cancer Center, Weill Medical School and Graduate School of Cornell University, New York, NY

Joseph G. Jurcic Memorial Sloan-Kettering Cancer Center, Weill Medical School and Graduate School of Cornell University, New York, NY

Howard L. Kaufman The Tumor Immunology Laboratory, Division of Surgical Oncology, Columbia University, New York, NY

John M. Kirkwood Departments of Medicine and Dermatology, University of Pittsburgh School of Medicine, Melanoma and Skin Cancer Program, University of Pittsburgh Cancer Institute, Pittsburgh, PA

Keith L. Knutson Department of Immunology, Mayo Clinic, Rochester, MN

Richard A. Lake National Research Centre for Asbestos-related Diseases, UWA, Department of Medicine, Sir Charles Gairdner Hospital Perth, Western Australia

Irma Larma National Research Centre for Asbestos-related Diseases, UWA, Department of Medicine, Sir Charles Gairdner Hospital Perth, Western Australia

Philip O. Livingston Laboratory of Tumor Vaccinology, Department of Medicine, Memorial Sloan-Kettering Cancer Center, New York, NY

H. Kim Lyerly Duke Comprehensive Cancer Center, Durham, NC

Michael A. Morse Duke University Medical Center, Durham, NC

Donald L. Morton Sonya Valley Ghidossi Vaccine Laboratory of the Roy E. Coats Research Laboratories of the John Wayne Cancer Institute Melanoma Program at Saint John's Health Center, Santa Monica, CA

Stergios J. Moschos The University of Pittsburgh Cancer Institute, Melanoma Center, Hillman Cancer Center, Pittsburgh, PA

Deborah A. Mulford Memorial Sloan-Kettering Cancer Center, Weill Medical School and Graduate School of Cornell University, New York, NY

David W. O'Neill NYU Cancer Institute, Tumor Vaccine Center, New York University School of Medicine, New York, NY

Karl S. Peggs Howard Hughes Medical Institute Department of Immunology, Memorial Sloan-Kettering Cancer Center, New York, NY

Miguel-Angel Perales Department of Medicine Memorial Sloan-Kettering Cancer Center, Weill Medical School and Graduate School of Cornell University, New York, NY

Christian A. Petrulio The Tumor Immunology Laboratory, Division of Surgical Oncology, Columbia University, New York, NY

Sergio A. Quezada Howard Hughes Medical Institute, Department of Immunology Memorial Sloan-Kettering Cancer Center, New York, NY

Christoph Rader Experimental Transplantation and Immunology Branch, Center for Cancer Research, National Cancer Institute, National Institutes of Health Bethesda, MD

Govind Ragupathi Laboratory of Tumor Vaccinology, Department of Medicine Memorial Sloan-Kettering Cancer Center, New York, NY

Yvonne M. Saenger Memorial Sloan-Kettering Cancer Center, Weill Medical School and Graduate School of Cornell University, New York, NY

David A. Scheinberg Memorial Sloan-Kettering Cancer Center, Weill Medical School and Graduate School of Cornell University, New York, NY

Jeffrey Schlom Laboratory of Tumor Immunology and Biology, Center for Cancer Research, National Cancer Institute, National Institutes of Health, Bethesda, MD

Barbara Seliger Institute of Medical Immunology, Martin Luther University Halle, Germany

Robbert G. van der Most National Research Centre for Asbestos-related Diseases, UWA, Department of Medicine, Sir Charles Gairdner Hospital Perth, Western Australia

Jeffrey S. Weber Donald A. Adam Comprehensive Melanoma Research Center, H. Lee Moffitt Cancer Center and Research Institute, Tampa, FL

Theresa L. Whiteside University of Pittsburgh Cancer Institute, Departments of Pathology, Immunology and Otolaryngology, University of Pittsburgh School of Medicine, Pittsburgh, PA

Jedd D. Wolchok Department of Medicine, Memorial Sloan-Kettering Cancer Center, Weill Medical College of Cornell University, New York, NY

Raymond M. Wong Department of Molecular Microbiology and Immunology and Medicine, Keck School of Medicine, University of Southern California, Los Angeles, CA

Cassian Yee Program in Immunology, Clinical Research Division, Fred Hutchinson Cancer Research Center, University of Washington, Seattle, WA

INTRODUCTION

As stated so elegantly by Dr. Alan Houghton in Chapter 1 of ***General Principles of Tumor Immunotherapy: Basic and Clinical Applications of Tumor Immunology,*** the connection between infection and tumor immunity has been recognized for millennia. However, it is only in the last few decades that the molecular and cellular basis for tumor immunotherapy been elucidated. The promise for manipulating the immune system to fight cancer is enormous given the fine specificity of immune responses and the ability to develop memory responses allowing long term protection from recurrent disease. The practical application of tumor immunotherapy, however, has lagged behind the promise. This is partly due to our incomplete understanding of how the host immune system interacts with tumor cells and partly due to the slow nature of clinical and translational research. Nonetheless, a clearer understanding of the complex host-tumor interactions coupled with new insight from two decades of productive clinical trial activity provides new enthusiasm for the use of tumor immunotherapy in the armamentarium of therapeutic strategies for patients with cancer.

General Principles of Tumor Immunotherapy: Basic and Clinical Applications of Tumor Immunology seeks to bring together the most current information related to how the immune system recognizes and eradicates cancer with a particular focus on the application of tumor immunotherapy in the clinic. This volume is organized into four sections designed to focus on particular aspects of tumor immunotherapy. In Part I the basic principles upon which tumor recognition and rejection are based will be discussed and includes chapters on the identification of tumor antigens, the mechanisms used to present tumor antigens to the immune system, features of the innate and adaptive immune systems as they relate to tumor immunology and an examination of the tumor microenvironment as it relates to host-tumor interactions. In Part II a highly focused discussion of the various active vaccine strategies that have been brought forward over the last decade is presented. In Part III we focus on the role of passive immunotherapy in cancer treatment. Finally, in Part IV we discuss some of the current clinical applications of immunotherapy and provide a provocative discussion on the future of combination therapy utilizing immunotherapy and more standard cancer therapeutics. These chapters have been authored by world class tumor immunologists and clinical investigators dedicated to pursuing the potential of tumor immunotherapy.

There are many people to thank when writing a book such as this. First, we want to thank all of our authors who so willingly agreed to contribute to this endeavor. The final product speaks for itself. We also want to express our sincerest gratitude to Dr. Alan Houghton, who not only provided one of the most comprehensive and insightful reviews of the history of tumor immunotherapy, but also provided significant inspiration in the pursuit of writing this book. Finally we want to thank Melania Ruiz and the folks at Springer for their encouragement, patience, and dedication to excellence. Our hope is that this volume will be a useful guide to those scientists and physicians who seek to understand the current status of tumor immunotherapy and the basic biology that supports its use as a cancer therapeutic. We also hope that this book will help motivate the students of tumor immunology and immunotherapy to keep working in this important and exciting field.

Howard L. Kaufman, MD
Jedd D. Wolchok, MD, PhD

PART 1

GENERAL PRINCIPLES OF TUMOR IMMUNOLOGY

CHAPTER 1

A PERSPECTIVE ON CANCER IMMUNOLOGY AND IMMUNOTHERAPY

ALAN N. HOUGHTON
Swim Across America Laboratory
Memorial Sloan-Kettering Cancer Center
1275 York Ave, New York, NY 10021

Abbreviations: MHC, major histocompatibility complex TLR, toll-like receptor TNF, Tumor necrosis factor

INTRODUCTION

The origins of cancer immunology are deeply rooted in the treatment of tumors. References to a relationship between tumor treatment and infection can be found in Chinese scripts dating back over a millennium. It is quite possible that immunologic treatments for cancer predate these ancient descriptions, perhaps into prehistory. Western European accounts of hemorrhagic necrosis of tumors and regressions following infection and high fevers are more than 300 years old. European medical texts describe treatment of tumors with materials coated with infectious pathogens, such as covering tumors with bandages or blankets that had contacted infected sores, and injecting pus from purulent wounds into tumors. However, these early narratives all suffered from the imprecise definition of "tumors" and a lack of pathologic classification. Were these lumps really cancer, or was there some other cause for the swellings that appeared to respond to these manipulations?

This short commentary presents an admittedly selective and personal view of the development of modern cancer immunology and immunotherapy, with all the inherent biases of an individual's own perspective (Table 1). The author apologizes for any omissions, which are a consequence of the restrictions of a short narrative.

H.L. Kaufman and J.D. Wolchok (eds.), General Principles of Tumor Immunotherapy, 3–15.

Table 1.

Historical events relevant to modern cancer immunology[†]

Investigator(s)	Year(s)	Discovery or Theory
Louis Pasteur	1859	Microbes, refuting spontaneous generation
Robert Koch*	1876	Microbial basis of disease (anthrax, tuberculosis)
Ilya Metchnikoff*	1883	Cellular theory of immunity (phagocytes)
Emil von Behring* & Shibasaburo Kitasato	1890	Discovery of antibodies (antitoxins)
William B. Coley	1891	Treatment of human cancer with bacteria and bacterial filtrates
Paul Ehrlich*	1897–1901	"Side chain" theory of antibody specificity "Horror autotoxicus"
Karl Landsteiner*	1901	Serologic discovery of blood groups
Carl Jensen & Leo Loeb	1901–1908	Studies of transplantable tumors in mice
Emil von Dungern & Ludwik Hirszfeld	1910	Heritability of blood group antigens
Clarence Little	1914	Genetic basis for rejection of transplantable tumors
Leonell Strong & Clarence Little	1915–1920	Establishment of inbred strains of mice
Peter Gorer	1936	Serological identification of erythrocyte II antigen which determined injection of tumor transplants
George Snell* & Peter Gorer	1948	Discovery of histocompatibility antigens as the basis for transplantation rejection
Richmond Prehn & Joan Main	1957	Immune rejection of transplanted syngeneic chemically-induced tumors
Lewis Thomas & McFarlane Burnet	1959	The theory of immune surveillance of cancer
H.B. Hewitt	1976	Lack of demonstrable immunogenicity of spontaneous tumors
George Koehler* & Caesar Milstein*	1975	Monoclonal antibodies
Lloyd Old & colleagues	1975	Discovery of TNF
Robert North	1981	The role of suppressor T cells in limiting tumor immunity
Thierry Boon	1983	Rejection of poorly immunogenic spontaneous tumors after immunization with mutagenized tumors

*Nobel laureates;
[†] References for discoveries are found in the text.

Infections and Cancer Therapy

The foundations of modern cancer immunology arise out of the science of microbiology, a biologic discipline arguably dated to 1859 with the defining experiments of Louis Pasteur showing that "spontaneous generation" was actually a consequence of airborne microorganisms. In 1879, Pasteur went on to demonstrate that injection of chickens with avirulent cholera bacilli produced resistance to subsequent challenge with infectious bacteria. These experiments provided the first reported experimental demonstrations of the protective effects of a vaccine. However, vaccination had been long practiced in ancient Chinese and other Asian cultures, using inoculation or scarification with cowpox to produce immunity against smallpox. More recently, Europeans had begun widespread vaccination triggered by the single case observation of the Englishman Edward Jenner in 1798 [1], who vaccinated a young boy with cowpox and then demonstrated protection to a subsequent challenge with smallpox (this would certainly be considered an unethical experiment today).

Pasteur's discoveries together with the painstaking characterizations of bacteria and bacterial infection by Robert Koch in Germany established the Germ Theory of Disease and the embryonic discipline of immunology by the end of the 19th century. Immunology quickly splintered into the "humoralists" (immunity dominated by soluble anti-toxins, or antibodies, in the blood) led by Emil Adolf von Behring (who discovered antibodies with Shibasaburo Kitasato) and Koch versus the "cellularists" (immunity controlled by phagocytes) of Ilya Metchnikoff and Pasteur working in Paris. Interestingly, this split coincided with the Franco-Prussian War. For the first half of the 20th century, the "humoralists" dominated the field of immunology, but immunologists would be gradually reunited into the current consensus view of the complex and intimate interrelatedness of the innate and adaptive immune systems that describes immunity (although some might argue that the T cell "cellularists" have dominated the last 20 years). Even today, microbiology and immunology remain integrally intertwined fields.

During these fomenting, formative early years following the birth of microbiology and immunology, William B. Coley, a young 28-year old New York surgeon and recent graduate of Harvard Medical School, had become deeply affected by the death of one of his first patients. She was an 18-year old woman, and close friend of John D. Rockefeller, Jr., who rapidly progressed and died from metastatic "round cell" sarcoma, after Coley had performed a heart wrenching amputation of her forearm. This death was to have profound and long-lasting consequences on cancer research and cancer immunology. John D. Rockefeller, Jr. (affectionately called "Junior" by his family) was deeply affected. He developed a long-standing interest in cancer research and treatment, providing major support from his family's philanthropy to catalyze the specialization of cancer treatment and the field of cancer research, and more broadly to biomedical research in general.

Coley was transformed by the death. He turned to clinical case records, with input by one of his mentors, Professor William Tillinghast Bull, to search for some hint of treatments that might prevent recurrence and spread of sarcoma. Poring over more than 100 records, he came across a single clue, the case history of a young man with "round cell" sarcoma of the neck who had developed severe erysipelas following incomplete surgical resection of multiple recurrences by Dr. Bull. Remarkably, the young man had survived both the cancer and infection, with no further recurrence of tumor years later. Coley spent weeks tracking down the German immigrant in the sprawling, chaotic tenements in the multicultural lower east side of Manhattan in 1888 to confirm the cure from recurrent soft tissue sarcoma, which was usually lethal. This single observation sparked Coley's obsessive interest in the relationship between infection and cancer over the next 48 years. The story of how Coley entered the field of cancer immunotherapy highlights the importance of the remarkable N = 1 case history in scientific discovery, a lesson for clinicians and laboratory researchers alike.

By 1891, Coley had acquired bacterial cultures from the Koch laboratory, and began to inject live *Micrococcus (Streptococcus) pyogenes* organisms (the pathogen of erysipelas) into tumors, a dangerous endeavor in the pre-antibiotic era. The first patient he treated, with tumors in the neck and tonsils, developed severe rigors and high fever after inoculations, but survived to experience tumor hemorrhagic necrosis and had no further recurrence over at least 10 years. Another 17 patients were treated, with additional regressions reported [2, 3]. Coley was not alone in treating patients with bacterial cultures at the time; a Dr. Busch in Germany concurrently was using the same approach. Busch did not receive the broad recognition that Coley did for this work, probably in part because Coley was much more effective in publishing and reporting results to the medical and academic communities.

Recognizing that live bacteria posed a great risk to patients, patients' families and hospital staff, Coley turned to cell-free filtrates of mixed bacteria cultures of *Micrococcus pyogenes* and *Serratia marcescens* (called *Bacillus prodigiosus* at that time), which he termed "mixed bacterial vaccines" (but were popularly, if unfortunately, called Coley's toxins). Between 1891 and 1936 when he died, Coley treated hundreds of patients, and mixed bacterial vaccines produced by Parke-Davis were marketed to physicians and surgeons.

Nevertheless, Coley's work became increasingly contentious, in part instigated by the renowned cancer pathologist James Ewing, who questioned the validity of cancer diagnoses in responding patients (in fact suggesting that if patients responded, they must not have cancer!). Coley was an outstanding surgeon, with remarkable clinical instincts and some scientific intuition, but he was not a card-carrying scientist who had undergone rigorous scientific training required to conduct carefully controlled, meticulously documented experiments. First radiation therapy and then chemotherapy stole the spotlight, relegating immunological therapies of cancer to the category of unconventional cancer treatments.

Now it is realized that Coley's legacy is far-reaching, in part because of his doggedness, persisting over many decades, and the case records that he dutifully reported periodically in the academic literature. His daughter, Helen Coley Nauts, gets much of the credit for keeping the embers of cancer immunotherapy alive through the middle-late part of the 20th century in the face of extreme skepticism. Her tenacious lifelong campaign publicized the cases of Coley, rebuffed often vicious attacks of his critics although she did not carry the academic credentials necessary to carry the arguments, and directly and indirectly recruited experienced scientists to tackle the murky minefield of cancer immunology. Now that immunotherapies have entered the mainstream of cancer therapies, many of us who have studied the work of Coley consider him "the founder of modern cancer immunotherapy."

Over time, the observations of Coley have been put on firmer scientific footing, with the unraveling of the underlying mechanisms of the innate immune system's response to bacterial products. An important steppingstone was revealing the role of bacterial endotoxin, and specifically its active component lipopolysaccharide (the lipid A component), in triggering post inflammatory mediators to induce hemorrhagic necrosis of tumors [4–9]. Moreover, the discovery of tumor necrosis factor (TNF), produced by the host in response to bacteria, was the pivotal event that produced a more fundamental understanding of how host inflammatory molecules mediated tumor hemorrhagic necrosis [10]. Cancer immunology was beginning to enter the molecular age. TNF produced by innate immune cells, particularly macrophages (the phagocytes of Metchnikoff), in response to bacterial products was in fact sufficient to induce the tumor hemorrhagic necrosis observed with bacterial inoculation into tumors, providing a molecular footing for the linkage between infection and cancer immunity.

The crucial role of the innate immune system in driving adaptive immune responses, specifically to generate the remarkable specificities of T cells and antibodies, is being now rapidly dissected, following the prescient predictions of Charles Janeway in 1989 [11]. Identification of pattern recognition receptors for molecules of pathogens, such as toll-like receptors (TLRs) that signal upon binding bacterial cell wall ligands (e.g., TLR-4 for lipopolysaccharide), RNA and DNA of bacteria and viruses, and bacterial lipopeptides, now provides a firm basis for understanding how cellular signals from innate immune cells mediate the profound inflammatory effects of microbial products.

The Historical Relationship of Cancer Immunology, Transplantation Immunology and Histocompatibility

Most young investigators do not realize that the discipline of transplantation immunology and the discovery of the role of major histocompatibility molecules have their origins in tumor immunology [12]. The stage was initially set at the turn-of-the-century by Paul Ehrlich with his "side chain" theory of immune recognition to explain the enormous specificities of antibodies [13, 14]. Using the power of antibodies, Karl Landsteiner defined the blood group antigens A and B in 1901 [15], followed 10 years later by Emil von Dungern and Ludwik Hirszfeld revealing the heritability of ABO blood groups [16]. Thus, antibodies could be used to follow inherited traits, providing the best tools for studying Mendelian inheritance in those days.

At the same time, Carl Jensen and Leo Loeb, along with many other investigators, were describing rejection of transplanted rodent tumors after transfer from the host of origin to an unrelated host of the same species. A remarkable finding, at least at the time, was that transplantation of tumors back into the original host or to closely related hosts (e.g., siblings) did not lead to rejection. Paul Ehrlich had also stumbled on to this immunological barrier to self, coining the term "horror autotoxicus" based on his inability to raise antisera against autologous blood cells in goats [17, 18].

Clarence Little, in his Ph.D. thesis work at Harvard, came to the conclusion based on his experimental work that there was a hereditary basis for rejection of transplanted tumors, controlled by Mendelian inheritance and involving multiple genes [19]. However, the findings were limited because the only genetic trait measured was resistance to transplantation of tumors, a variable assay that was not very discriminating. Thus, there were no effective methods or tools to identify individual loci that determined resistance to transplanted tumors. Subsequently, Little and Leonell Strong were guided by these observations to initiate the generation of inbred strains of mice [20]. Little went on to become the founder of the Jackson Laboratory, the famous repository and research laboratory for the genetics of inbred strains of mice.

Meanwhile, the experiments of Landsteiner on defining blood group antigens had spawned attempts to use antibodies raised against tumors to map the complex heritability of resistance to tumor transplants. Research into the genetics of tumor transplantation resistance was an increasingly active area of research, culminating during the 1930s and 1940s in unrealistic optimism for unraveling the mechanisms of cancer resistance and for future cancer immunotherapy. These views were partly a consequence of the successes of vaccines and serum therapy for prevention and treatment of infectious diseases. However, there was still little understanding of the genetic loci that determined tumor resistance following transplantation. It took a collaboration between an immunologist and a mouse geneticist to solve the problem.

In a laboratory at Guy's Hospital in London in the 1930s, the serologist Peter Gorer was intensely studying tumor antigens in the context of the genetics of transplantation rejection. After completing M.D. degree studies at Guy's, Gorer had received guidance from a mentor, the extraordinary but eccentric geneticist J.B.S. Haldane[1], to explore the unknown factors responsible for rejection of tumor transplants. Haldane and Gorer felt that there might be a link to blood group antigens because rejection of transplanted tumors appeared to mimic destruction of blood cells following incompatible blood transfusions. Transfusion reactions were known by that time to be caused by antibodies in the blood. Applying the exquisite discriminatory powers of antibodies, Gorer injected cancer cells from one mouse into another to raise antisera, and then analyzed the specificity of the antibodies against different tumors, relating antibody reactivity to whether tumors were rejected or not in different mouse recipients. He was using the sera to follow the heritability of resistance versus acceptance of transplanted tumors, with only color of the mouse and serology to follow the genetics.

In these experiments, Gorer defined "antigen II" in 1936 and went on to show that antibodies to this "blood group" antigen segregated with tumor resistance [21–24].

---

[1]Haldane had a giant intellect, and a great sense of humor. At the end of his life, while dying of colorectal cancer, in the hospital he wrote the following short poem:

"Cancer's a Funny Thing:
I wish I had the voice of Homer
To sing of rectal carcinoma,
Which kills a lot more chaps, in fact,
Then were bumped off when Troy was sacked..."

This was the first identification of a histocompatibility antigen. The discovery was the beginning of understanding tumor resistance in these mouse experiments, but more importantly of immunity against tissue transplants from one individual to another individual of a species (allografts). The real quantum leap in understanding the genetics came when Gorer spent a year in the lab of George Snell at Jackson Laboratory in Maine.

Snell, a Ph.D. trained in genetics, had been deeply influenced by Clarence Little. After joining Jackson Laboratory, Snell continued Little's work to generate and characterize inbred strains of mice, which required years, even decades, of extensive cross-breeding and backcrossing. One of Snell's great contributions was the creation of "coisogenic" mouse strains (today called congenic) that differ only at a single genetic locus. By the mid-1940s, Snell had created a series of mouse strains that linked resistance or acceptance of tumor transplants to other readily identified, visible phenotypic traits that were genetically determined. He wanted to understand the genetics of transplantation resistance to tumors described by Little. In particular, he was focusing on several strains, which through breeding he had co-segregated resistance to tumor transplants with a linked genetic trait called "fused tail" (which Snell called the *Fu* locus, caused by fusion of the tail vertebrae and characterized by a tail shaped like a twisted rope).

In 1946, Little met Gorer at a conference in Italy. Impressed by Gorer's serologic studies of tumor transplantation resistance, he invited Gorer to come to Jackson Laboratory as a visiting investigator. After Gorer arrived in Maine, Snell and Gorer, completely unaware of each other's results, compared notes and were astonished at the relationship of their findings. Perhaps they had independently come across the same genetic system that determined resistance to transplanted tumors. Setting up a collaboration, Gorer serologically typed mice for genetic segregation of resistance to transplanted tumors by measuring expression of antigen II, using Snell's crosses of tumor-resistant *Fu* mice (specifically, [*Fu* mice x tumor-susceptible inbred strains] F1 mice). The well-characterized mouse strains combined with serologic typing (a less variable assay) revealed the remarkable finding that the major genetic system determining both rejection of transplanted tumors and expression of antigen II was either the identical locus or closely linked loci. In 1948, Gorer and Snell published their earthshaking paper reporting that antigen II and Fu were closely linked to the same genetic locus, which they called *H2* (combining the terms histocompatibility and antigen II) [25]. This report was the birth announcement of transplantation immunology and more importantly the major histocompatibility (MHC) complex, whose products determine transplant rejection, selection and specificity of T cells, susceptibility to disease, and much more.

These findings revealed that some previous assumptions about immunological resistance to tumors had been built on a house of cards. It was quickly realized that researchers had been measuring allogeneic immunity (defined by genetic disparities between individuals of the same species) determined largely by these newly discovered polymorphic gene products of the MHC loci. All of these previous tumor transplantation experiments could be criticized for measuring tissue transplantation rejection, not specific tumor rejection. Today, more than 800 alleles of MHC I genes and 600 alleles of MHC II genes have been identified in humans [26]. As a side story, the long-lived debate between antibodies and cellular immunity lived on after this discovery, although at a more genteel level. Gorer remained a major proponent throughout his scientific life for antibodies as the mediators of rejection of both allografts and tumors, in contrast to Peter Medawar who argued the dominant role of cellular immunity.

Studies of Transplantable Tumors in Syngeneic Mice

The realization that transplantation resistance between genetically non-identical individuals could be determined by genes in the MHC complex quickly brought into question the whole concept of "cancer immunity". Most researchers grew extremely skeptical of the notion of immune rejection of cancer by the host. Quietly, reports in the early 1950s by Ludwig Gross, using the AKR leukemia, and Edward Foley, using transplantable methylcholanthrene-induced tumors, suggested that genetically identical (syngeneic) adult mice might be resistant to transfer of syngeneic leukemia and sarcoma cells [27, 28], but these experiments were not convincing.

It was the careful and thorough study of methylcholanthrene-induced sarcomas by Prehn and Main that set the field back on course, by showing definitive and specific rejection of tumors in syngeneic mice [29]. The most notable message of these experiments was that immunity was generally specific for each individual tumor, leading to minimal rejection of unrelated tumors and no rejection of normal tissues. These experiments thus defined the tumor-specific transplantation antigens, also called tumor-specific antigens or unique antigens [30]. How specific were these tumor-specific transplantation antigens? In follow-up experiments, unique antigens were individually distinct for 25 independently derived carcinogen-induced tumors [31]. Nevertheless, careful analysis of the Prehn and Main data reveals that immunization with one tumor not only generates strong immunity against that same tumor, but also weak cross-reactive immunity against unrelated syngeneic tumors. This conclusion infers that weakly immunogenic tumor antigens are shared by tumors. The field of tumor immunology was again on the rise, with tentative but reproducible experimental models. With the report of Prehn and Main, and confirmation of their results by multiple laboratories, Lewis Thomas and McFarlane Burnet were emboldened to independently propose a theory of "immune surveillance of cancer", speculating that, in fact, the immune system might be capable of destroying incipient malignancies, which implies that many or most de novo cancers never become clinically apparent [32, 33].

But the history of cancer immunology has never been a straight path. Rather, the story is better characterized by a series of switch-back trails used to climb a mountain, with upwards steps frequently punctuated by sharp downturns. Cancer immunity was again called on the question by a report from Hewitt and colleagues in 1976 showing a lack of immunogenicity of spontaneously arising tumors [34]. Just as the field of tumor immunology was beginning to pick itself up again,

Hewitt was in fact arguing that any tumor that demonstrates immunogenicity is an "artifact", stating that only "non-immunogenic" spontaneous tumors were relevant to human cancers. Furthermore, the concept of cancer immune surveillance became moribund following experiments by Stutman showing that athymic nude mice did not have increased susceptibility to tumors induced by methylcholanthrene [35,36]. The fundamental notion of cancer immunity was again in deep trouble.

This pessimistic view of cancer immunity was gradually refuted by many experimental observations. For instance, Boon and colleagues showed that so-called "non-immunogenic" spontaneous tumors could be mutagenized to generate immunogenic variants that, most importantly, produced immunity also against the non-mutagenized, previously "non-immunogenic" parental tumor [37]. More importantly, studies by Robert North and colleagues in a series of elegant experiments showed the relevance of "suppressor" T cells (nowadays termed regulatory T cells) in quelling immune responses to tumors, providing a mechanism for lack of tumor immunogenicity [38–43].

The past 15 years have witnessed a resurgence of experimental support for immune surveillance against cancer, pointing to the flaws of observations based in nude mice (which have high levels of natural killer cells and other innate immune cells) (reviewed in [44]). Finally, the field entered the molecular era of immunology with the identification of antigen structures and the sequences of genes encoding both mouse and human tumor antigens that are recognized by the host immune system [45–48]. These discoveries have provided tools to move the field rapidly forward. So much has happened in the last 20 years that our historical narrative that will stop at this point, allowing future commentaries to reflect on these recent events.

Concluding Comments

Effective immunotherapy of cancer will come from: (i) better biologic understanding of the components of the immune system and how they fit together and (ii) improved understanding of malignant transformation and cancer progression, leading to insights into how cancers escape the immune system. We have much to learn. One also must be aware of the ups and downs in the field - much like the stock market, the expectations and hype that sometimes surround new reports of immunotherapy lead to inevitable disappointments and downswings. Yet, if one takes a longer perspective of the last 25 years, or more remarkably the >110 years since Coley's first clinical experiments, the field has made enormous progress. Immunologic treatments are now routine parts of cancer therapy, including interferon-alfa, interleukin-2, monoclonal antibodies and BCG. Vaccines against hepatitis and human papilloma virus have the potential to prevent certain forms of cancer. Following allogeneic hematopoietic stem cell transplants for leukemias, and perhaps lymphomas, the host's immune system is crucial for cures through graft-versus-leukemia effects.

Nevertheless, we still have limited insights into how the innate and adaptive immune systems fit together to control or reject cancer, or alternatively to suppress potential immune and inflammatory responses to cancer. Adaptive immune responses (T cells and antibodies) can potentially recognize unique antigens, which probably represent mutations in most cases. Although responses to these tumor-specific antigens can be particularly potent, as revealed by tumor transplantation experiments with transplanted chemically-induced tumors, we have little understanding of how the immune system recognizes these unique antigens, how frequently are mutations recognized, and what types of mutations are most immunogenic. Furthermore, is the biology of these chemically-induced tumors (induced by massive doses of mutagens, presumably generating thousands if not millions of mutations) relevant to most human cancers? In addition, how well does the immune system recognize those specific mutations that are important for the pathogenesis of cancer? Another caveat is that most experimental systems have used transplantable tumors, which do not recapitulate the physiology of the different stages of an endogenously emerging and progressive tumor in the host. At this time, for practical reasons, most experimental antigen-targeted immunotherapies are directed at shared antigens, such as differentiation antigens, overexpressed antigens, and germ cells/cancer-testes antigens. These shared antigens bring up crucial issues about overcoming immune ignorance or tolerance, and the relationship of immunity to cancer versus the risk of autoimmunity, an area where our understanding is still relatively unsophisticated [49].

Finally, big questions emerge about whether evolutionary adaptation of the immune system over a billion years was in part driven by the necessity of increasingly complex multicellular organisms to control endogenous aberrant cells, such as transformed cells. Certainly, the evidence is very strong that the immune system was driven and shaped by requirements of evolving metazoa to fight off foreign pathogens. However, if the evolution of the immune system was also shaped to destroy incipient transformed cells or to control progression of malignant cells in the host, this finding would have profound implications for the long-standing paradigm of the immune system's role in recognizing self versus nonself. What does one do with normal symbiotic bacteria in the bowel? Are they self or nonself? These symbiotes provide crucial functions for the development and homeostasis of the immune system [50], and yet they can also kill the host if epithelial barriers are breached and the immune system suppressed.

These ideas brings up the notion that our immune system might not just distinguish "us versus them" (i.e., host versus exogenous pathogens), to serve a defensive barrier for invaders from outside. Rather, the immune system might be a much more subtle and complex organ (actually, rather than an "organ", it is more a closely interactive and somewhat redundant confederation of diverse cell types and molecules). The system recognizes and responds to potentially hazardous situations for the host, whether they be infection from nonself pathogens, foreign bodies, tissue damage from trauma, or malignancy – a paradigm we term distinguishing "self versus altered self", and that Polly Matzinger has described as responding to "danger" [51, 52].

REFERENCES

1. Jenner, E., 1801. *An inquiry into the causes and effects of the Variolae Vacciniae, a disease discovered in some of the western counties of England, particularly Gloucestershire, and known by the name of the cow-pox*, Third edition, D.N. Shury, London.
2. Coley, W. B., 1893, The treatment of malignant tumors by repeated inoculations of erysipelas with a report of ten original cases, *Am. J. Med. Sci.* 105:487–511.
3. Hall, S. S., 1997. *A Commotion in the Blood. Life, Death and the Immune System*, Henry Holt & Co., New York.
4. Gratia, A. and Linz, R., 1931, Le phénomène de Schwartzman dans le sarcome du Cobaye, *CR Séances Soc. Biol. Ses. Fil.* 108:427–428.
5. Shear, M. J., Turner, F. C., Perrault, A. and Shovelton, T., 1943, Chemical treatment of tumors. V. Isolation of the hemorrhage-producing fraction from *Serratia marcescens* (*Bacillus prodigiosus*) culture filtrate, *J. Natl. Cancer Inst.* 4:81–97.
6. Shear, M. J., 1944, Chemical treatment of tumors. IX. Reactions of mice with primary subcutaneous tumors to injection of a hemorrhage-producing bacterial polysaccharide, *J. Natl. Cancer Inst.* 4:461–476.
7. Algire, G. H., Legallais, F. Y. and Anderson, B. F., 1952, Vascular reactions of normal and malignant tissues in vivo. V. Role of hypertension in action of bacterial polysaccharide on tumors, *J. Nat. Cancer Inst.* 12:1279–1295.
8. Nowotny, A., 1969, Molecular aspects of endotoxic reactions, *Bacteriol. Rev.* 33:72–98.
9. Parr, I., Wheeler, E. and Alexander, P., 1973, Similarities of the antitumor actions of endotoxin, lipid A and double-stranded RNA, *Br. J. Cancer.* 27:370–389.
10. Carswell, E. A., Old, L. J., Kassel, R. L., Green, S., Fiore, N. and Williamson, B., 1975, An endotoxin-induced serum factor that causes necrosis of tumors, *Proc. Natl. Acad. Sci. U. S. A.* 72:3666–3670.
11. Janeway, C. A., Jr., 1989, Approaching the asymptote? Evolution and revolution in immunology, *Cold Spring Harb. Symp. Quant. Biol.* 54 Pt 1:1–13.
12. Amos, D. B., 1986, Recollections of Dr. Peter Gorer, *Immunogenetics.* 24:341–344.
13. Ehrlich, P., 1897, Die Wertbestimmung des Diphterieheilserums und deren theoretische Grundlagen, *Klinische Jahrbucher.* 6:299–326.
14. Ehrlich, P., 1906. *Collected Studies on Immunity*, John Wiley & Sons, New York.
15. Landsteiner, K., 1901, Ueber Agglutinationserscheinungen normalen menschlichen Blutes, *Wein Klin. Wochenschr.* 14:1132–1134.
16. von Dungern, E. and Hirszfeld, L., 1911, Ueber gruppenspezifische Strukturen des Blutes III., *Zeitschrift für Immunologische Forschung.* 8:526–562.
17. Ehrlich, P. and Morgenroth, J., 1901, Ueber haemolysin, *Berliner Klin. Wochenschr.* 38:569.
18. Ehrlich, P. and Morgenroth, J., 1957. *On haemolysins: Third and fifth communications*, Pergamon Press, London.
19. Little, C. C., 1914, A possible Mendelian explanation for a type of an inheritance apparently non-Mendelian in nature, *Science.* 40:904–906.
20. Little, C. C., 1941. *The genetics of tumor transplantation*, Dover, New York.
21. Gorer, P. A., 1937a, Further studies on antigenetic differences in mouse erythrocytes, *J. Pathol. Bacteriol.* 44:31–36.
22. Gorer, P. A., 1937b, The genetic and antigenetic basis of tumour transplantation, *J. Pathol. Bacteriol.* 44:691–697.
23. Gorer, P. A., 1938, The antigenic basis of tumour transplantation, *J. Pathol. Bacteriol.* 44:231–252.
24. Gorer, P. A., 1959, The immunogenetics of cancer, *Jaarb. K. Ned. Bot. Ve.* 9:90–97.
25. Gorer, P. A., Lyman, S. and Snell, G. D., 1948, Studies on the genetic and antigenic basis of tumor transplantation: linkage between a histocompatibility gene and "fused" in mice, *Proc. Royal Soc. London Ser. B.* 135:499–505.
26. Robinson, J., Waller, M. J., Parham, P., de Groot, N., Bontrop, R., Kennedy, L. J., Stoehr, P. and Marsh, S. G., 2003, IMGT/HLA and IMGT/MHC: sequence databases for the study of the major histocompatibility complex, *Nucleic Acids Res.* 31:311–314.

27. Gross, L., 1950, Susceptibility of suckling-infant, and resistance of adult, mice of the C3H and of the C57 lines to inoculation with AKR leukemia, *Cancer*. 3:1073–1087.
28. Foley, E. J., 1953, Antigenic properties of methylcholanthrene-induced tumors in mice of the strain of origin, *Cancer Res*. 13:835–837.
29. Prehn, R. T. and Main, J. M., 1957, Immunity to methylcholanthrene-induced sarcomas, *J. Natl. Cancer Inst*. 18:769–778.
30. Klein, G., 2001, The strange road to the tumor-specific transplantation antigens (TSTAs), *Cancer Immunity*. 1:6.
31. Basombrio, M. A., 1970, Search for common antigenicities among twenty-five sarcomas induced by methylcholanthrene, *Cancer Res*. 30:2458–2462.
32. Burnet, F., 1970, The concept of immunological surveillance, *Prog. Exp. Tumor Res*. 13:1–27.
33. Thomas, L., 1982, On immunosurveillance in human cancer, *Yale J. Biol. Med*. 55:329–333.
34. Hewitt, H. B., Blake, E. R. and Walder, A. S., 1976, A critique of the evidence for active host defense against cancer, based on personal studies of 27 murine tumours of spontaneous origin, *Br. J. Cancer*. 33:241–259.
35. Stutman, O., 1974, Tumor development after 3-methylcholanthrene in immunologically deficient athymic-nude mice, *Science*. 183:534–536.
36. Stutman, O., 1975, Immunodepression and malignancy, *Adv Cancer Res*. 22:261–422.
37. Pel, A. V., Vessiere, F. and Boon, T., 1983, Protection against two spontaneous mouse leukemias conferred by immunogenic variants obtained by mutagenesis, *J. Exp. Med*. 157:1992–2000.
38. Dye, E. S. and North, R. J., 1981, T cell-mediated immunosuppression as an obstacle to adoptive immunotherapy of the P815 mastocytoma and its metastases, *J. Exp. Med*. 154:1033–1042.
39. North, R. J., 1982, Cyclophosphamide-facilitated adoptive immunotherapy of an established tumor depends on elimination of tumor-induced suppressor T cells, *J. Exp. Med*. 155:1063–1074.
40. Mills, C. D. and North, R. J., 1983, Expression of passively transferred immunity against an established tumor depends on generation of cytolytic T cells in recipient. Inhibition by suppressor T cells, *J. Exp. Med*. 157:1448–1460.
41. Bursuker, I. and North, R. J., 1984, Generation and decay of the immune response to a progressive fibrosarcoma. II. Failure to demonstrate postexcision immunity after the onset of T cell-mediated suppression of immunity, *J. Exp. Med*. 159:1312–1321.
42. North, R. J. and Bursuker, I., 1984, Generation and decay of the immune response to a progressive fibrosarcoma. I. Ly-1+2- suppressor T cells down-regulate the generation of Ly-1-2+ effector T cells, *J. Exp. Mede*. 159:1295–1311.
43. Bursuker, I. and North, R. J., 1985, Suppression of generation of concomitant antitumor immunity by passively transferred suppressor T cells from tumor-bearing donors, *Cancer Immunology & Immunotherapy*. 19:215–218.
44. Dunn, G. P., Old, L. J. and Schreiber, R. D., 2004, The immunobiology of cancer immunosurveillance and immunoediting, *Immunity*. 21:137–148.
45. Pukel, C. S., Lloyd, K. O., Travassos, L. R., Dippold, W. G., Oettgen, H. F. and Old, L. J., 1982, GD3, a prominent ganglioside of human melanoma. Detection and characterisation by mouse monoclonal antibody, *J. Exp. Med*. 155:1133–1147.
46. De Plaen, E., Lurquin, C., Van Pel, A., Mariame, B., Szikora, J. P., Wolfel, T., Sibille, C., Chomez, P. and Boon, T., 1988, Immunogenic (tum-) variants of mouse tumor P815: cloning of the gene of tum-antigen P91A and identification of the tum- mutation, *Proc. Natl. Acad. Sci. U. S. A*. 85:2274–2278.
47. Vijayasaradhi, S., Bouchard, B. and Houghton, A. N., 1990, The melanoma antigen gp75 is the human homologue of the mouse b (brown) locus gene product, *J. Exp. Med*. 171:1375–1380.
48. van der Bruggen, P., Traversari, C., Chomez, P., Lurquin, C., De Plaen, E., Van den Eynde, B., Knuth, A. and Boon, T., 1991, A gene encoding an antigen recognized by cytolytic T lymphocytes on a human melanoma, *Science*. 254:1643–1647.
49. Bowne, W. B., Srinivasan, R., Wolchok, J. D., Hawkins, W. G., Blachere, N. E., Dyall, R., Lewis, J. J. and Houghton, A. N., 1999, Coupling and uncoupling of tumor immunity and autoimmunity, *J. Exp. Med*. 190:1717–1722.

50. Mazmanian, S. K., Liu, C. H., Tzianabos, A. O. and Kasper, D. L., 2005, An immunomodulatory molecule of symbiotic bacteria directs maturation of the host immune system, *Cell.* 122:107–118.
51. Houghton, A. N., 1994, Cancer antigens: Immune recognition of self and altered self, *J. Exp. Med.* 180:1–4.
52. Matzinger, P., 1994, Tolerance, danger, and the extended family, *Ann. Rev. Immunol.* 12:991–1045.

CHAPTER 2

TUMOR ANTIGENS

MICHAEL A. MORSE[1,*], TIMOTHY M. CLAY[2], AND H. KIM LYERLY[3]

[1]*Associate Professor of Medicine Duke University Medical Center*
[2]*Associate Professor of Surgery Duke University Medical Center*
[3]*George Barth Geller Professor of Research in Cancer Director, Duke Comprehensive Cancer Center*

INTRODUCTION

The concept of specific immunotherapy depends on the notion that tumors may be specifically targeted by immune effectors such as T cells and antibodies that distinguish distinct differences between normal tissues and tumors. This is in contrast to the concept of non-specific immunotherapy which is mediated by effectors such as NK cells that kill tumor in a non-antigen dependent fashion. Tumor antigens are protein, peptide, or carbohydrate molecules that the immune system uses to distinguish tumor cells from normal cells. While target antigens in the form of surface proteins or carbohydrates that may be recognized by antibodies had been well accepted for quite some time, it was not until observations on the MHC-restricted killing of tumor cells by cytolytic T cells, that attempts were made to clone the genes that encoded the antigens recognized by the T cells. In 1991, the first human tumor antigen recognized by T cells, called MAGE-1, was first discovered [1]. The ensuing years saw an explosion in the number of tumor antigens described and an even greater growth in the number of immunogenic peptide epitopes present within these antigenic molecules. These have now been catalogued in recent, excellent reviews [2] or published on websites (http://www.cancerimmunity.org/peptidedatabase/differentiation.htm). To

*Associate Professor of Medicine Division of Medical Oncology Box 3233 Duke University Medical Center Durham, NC 27710 michael.morse@duke.edu

H.L. Kaufman and J.D. Wolchok (eds.), General Principles of Tumor Immunotherapy, 17–31.

create some order to the long list of varied antigens, it is helpful to group them according to their expression patterns (for example, cancer-testis antigens found predominantly in tumors or germ cells or differentiation antigens, found predominantly during fetal development in normal tissues) and we will discuss them in this order. Nonetheless, the purpose of this chapter is not to recapitulate the information collected in these publications, but to briefly describe the categories of tumor antigens, explain their relevance to cancer immunotherapy strategies, and to discuss how tumor antigens are discovered. Also, while some tumor antigens may be recognized by T cells or antibodies, we will focus on the antigens recognized by T cells, the primary immune effector for destroying tumor cells.

HOW TUMOR ANTIGENS ARE RECOGNIZED BY T CELLS?

Unlike antibodies which directly recognize three-dimensional molecular patterns, T cells recognize their epitopes when presented in the context of MHC molecules. Therefore, T cell epitopes must be processed, generally by the immunoproteosome, within the target cell, transported into the lumen of the endoplasmic reticulum (ER) via the transporter associated with antigen processing (TAP), loaded onto newly synthesized MHC molecules, and trafficked to the cell surface before they can be recognized. CD8+ T receptors recognize 9 amino-acid peptides presented within MHC class I (HLA A,B,C, in humans) molecules and CD4+ T cell receptors recognize longer peptide fragments within MHC Class II (HLA–DR, DP, DQ). While this need to recognize antigen within the context of MHC may seem to be a drawback at first, in fact, it allows for T cell recognition of epitopes derived from virtually any protein, whether typically cell surface-expressed or not. Also, it permits exquisite sensitivity to even single amino acid changes in proteins so that it is possible T cells might respond to mutated proteins but not their normal counterparts. Despite this exquisite discriminant ability, there is a sufficient capacity for cross reactivity that the number of T cell receptors randomly generated can recognize the vastly larger number of possible epitopes. Of course, T cells auto-reactive to self antigens are usually deleted in the thymus. This is not a relevant issue for T cells that recognize antigens unique to tumors, so called tumor-specific antigens (for example, tumors driven by viral infection such as EBV associated lymphoproliferative disorders or cervical cancer or for tumors expressing antigens created by translocations such as the bcr-abl rearrangement in chronic myelogenous leukemia), but represents a potential hurdle for T cells recognizing self antigens, so called tumor associated antigens. Again, it is likely that T cells that have cross reactivity for self antigens but have low enough affinity to avoid thymic deletion, possess the ability to recognize tumors bearing self antigens. It is also usually the case that the self antigens are expressed differently by tumor compared with normal tissues (for example, someantigens such as carcinoembryonic antigen (CEA) are expressed predominantly during fetal development and in only minimal quantities in adult tissues). An important decision for cancer vaccine strategies then becomes choosing antigens that are distinctly expressed and are targets of existent peripherally circulating T cells.

WHAT MAKES A TUMOR ANTIGEN?

For a protein to be considered a tumor antigen, several features must be present. Of course, the gene must be transcribed and some attempt at protein production must occur. This does not necessarily mean that the protein must be expressed to any great degree such that it may be difficult to detect by immunohistochemistry. The protein must contain epitopes that can fit within MHC molecules and be recognized by T cell receptors. Nonetheless, it is not always the case that the T cell epitope is a simple peptide fragment of the full length protein. T cell epitopes may be generated by splicing aberrations leading to cryptic epitopes encoded by nonspliced introns, alternative open reading frames, or post-translational modification or splicing. For example, an alternative open reading frame of the human macrophage colony-stimulating factor gene is independently translated and codes for an antigenic peptide recognized by tumor-infiltrating CD8+ T lymphocytes in renal cell carcinoma [3]. A splicing variant of survivin called survivin-2B retains a portion of intron 2 and encodes an immunogenic peptide in the context of HLA A24 [4]. Hanada [5] described a nine amino acid fibroblast growth factor peptide (FGF-5) generated by protein splicing that could be recognized by T cells cloned from lymphocytes infiltrating a renal cell carcinoma. This type of splicing had not been previously reported in humans. Another unusual antigen was discovered to be translated from an antisense transcript [6]. These unusual situations demonstrate that peptides recognized by T cells cannot always be predicted from the amino acid sequence of the antigen. Most importantly, the protein must be processed and presented within MHC molecules on the cell surface. Some proteins may not have epitopes that fit efficiently within MHC molecules and some may not reach the processing machinery at all or may be degraded before presentation [7].

TUMOR ANTIGEN DISCOVERY

The initial method for discovery of tumor antigen genes involved the use of CD8+ CTL clones that lyse an autologous tumor cell line to probe target cells transfected with tumor genetic material to detect which gene leads to sensitivity to lysis by the CTL clone. In the case of MAGE-1, a cosmid library was prepared with the DNA of a tumor cell line subclone (MZ2-MEL) and this was then transfected into an antigen-loss variant MZ2-MEL.2.2 [8]. To identify the immunogenic peptide epitopes, the fragments of gene MAGE-1 that transfered the sensitivity to lysis of the CTL clone were tested until a nonapeptide was identified that conferred HLA A1-restricted recognition by the CTL [9]. This method, screening cDNA libraries with CTL clones, has been a very fruitful way to identify tumor antigens, but is very complex and labor intensive. Once the nature of peptide-MHC interactions was better understood, it became possible to elute peptides from MHC molecules and to identify them by HPLC [10]. Once more information about the binding requirements for peptides within the MHC peptide binding pockets became available, it was possible to identify potential peptide epitopes by use of algorithms that incorporate definitions of peptide binding motifs for multiple HLA class I and class II alleles [11]. It is well established that class I peptides should be at least 8–10 amino acids long, and certain amino acids are preferred at the anchor positions (position 2 or 3). Peptides that bind to HLA-A2 generally contain an L or M at position 2 and a V or L at position 9 or 10. The HLA class II molecule binding pocket allows more promiscuity, but also seems to require several anchor positions. Once a series of peptides is chosen based on these algorithms, they can be tested for their binding affinity to cells expressing the MHC molecule of interest. The use of patient sera to screen tumor cell cDNA expression libraries, a technique that has been designated SEREX (serological analysis of gene expression) has also resulted in the identification of antigens that are expressed on a variety of tumor types. It is then necessary to determine if the protein targets of the patient antibodies also contain T cell epitopes. Regardless of how discovered, for a candidate epitope to be established as immunogenic requires testing its binding affinity to MHC molecules, studying the elicited responses using various T cell populations derived from a large group of HLA-matched patients, and confirming that the T cells recognize the native target cells *in vivo* by demonstrating that T cells specific for them can lyse tumors expressing the antigen that harbors the epitope.

ALTERED PEPTIDE LIGANDS

It has been frequently observed that peptides identified by MHC binding algorithms do not always stimulate the most potent T cell responses. It is hypothesized that this may be due to low binding affinity to the MHC molecules and low T cell affinity for them. Typically, CTL induction is related to the relative HLA binding affinity [12]. Binding affinity may be improved by altering peptides at the anchor residues as described above. For example, substitutions at the anchor positions of three peptides derived from the melanoma-associated antigen gp100 enhanced HLA binding and immunogenicity relative to the parental sequence [13]. Substitutions can also be made at secondary anchor positions with an improvement in immunogenicity as was demonstrated for a HER2/neu analog [14]. Caution should be taken whenever changes to the peptide sequence are made. For example, an altered peptide ligand hTERT699T-707, designed to increase HLA-A1-binding affinity of the hTERT699-707 peptide, did not activate CTL that recognized endogenously processed hTERT [15].

The other type of modification strategy involves amino acid substitutions at positions other than the main HLA anchors of the peptide which results in heteroclitic analog epitopes. These modifications seem to enhance T cell stimulation by increased binding of the peptide-HLA complex to the TCR [16]. An heteroclitic analog of the HLA-A2 restricted, CEA-derived CAP1 peptide (called CAP1-6D), although it does not increase the HLA-A2 binding affinity of the peptide, does stimulate wild-type specific CTL [17]. Fong [18] and colleagues administered CAP1-6D loaded Flt3-ligand mobilized dendritic cells and observed a high frequency CAP-1 specific T cell responses detected by tetramers.

CANCER-TESTIS ANTIGENS

The first T cell tumor antigens discovered and the most frequently targeted in clinical trials of cancer vaccines, cancer-testis (CT) antigens (or germ cell antigens) were so-called because they were thought to be expressed only in tumors and spermatocytes and spermatogonia of the testis and the placenta. There have been 44 gene or gene families identified, many of which are located on the X chromosome. In general, it is not known what their normal function is, although some potential functions in migration/motility have been suggested for CAGE -1 and SSX [19,20]. Their limited expression in normal tissue and the fact that the testis generally does not express class I or II molecules and is thus priveleged from immune surveillance, allows CT antigens to be targeted with reduced risk of autoimmune disease. This limited expression is due to the fact that CT antigens are proteins that represent reactivation of genes in tumors that are usually silent in adult tissues [21]. This reactivation may occur by hypomethylation of the CpG island in the cancer testis gene promoter [22]. This has led to suggestions that greater expression of these antigens could be achieved by use of demethylating agents such as 5-aza-2'-deoxycytidine [23]. It should also be noted that despite the generally limited expression, in fact, some of the CT genes are tissue restricted while others are more ubiquitous [24]. For example, 10/43 CT genes were tissue-restricted (mRNA detected in 2 or fewer non-gametogenic tissues), 9/43 CT genes were differentially expressed (mRNA detected in 3-6 non-gametogenic tissues), and 5/43 CT genes were ubiquitously expressed.

The list of CT antigens includes the MAGE, BAGE, and GAGE families, NY-ESO-1/LAGE/ CAMEL, SSX-2, TRAG-3, CT9 and CT10 (see reference 24 for a complete list). Class I and in some cases, class II restricted peptide epitopes of all these antigens have been reported. At least one of these antigens has been identified in melanoma, myeloma, lung carcinoma, head and neck cancer, esophageal cancer, superficial and infiltrating bladder carcinoma, prostate, colorectal and breast carcinomas, cholangiocarcinoma, hepatocellular carcinoma, and sarcoma [24–33]. Some tumors express a broad array of CT antigens while others have a limited range of expression [24]. For example bladder and non-small cell lung cancer, and melanoma have detectable mRNA for more than half of the described CT genes, whereas breast and prostate cancers express more than 30% of the CT genes, and a minority of renal and colon cancers express even 20% of the CT genes. Nonetheless, with more sophisticated methods such as RT-PCR, more frequent expression of CT antigens has been observed in colon cancers [34]. Although all the CT antigens have been found to be targets for antigen-specific T cells *in vitro*, not all reproducibly activate *in vivo* immune responses. For example, Chianese-Bullock, et al.[35] observed that only a subset of melanoma antigens were immunogenic when administered as part of a cancer vaccine. Overall, 14/29 cancer testis gene families that are tissue (or testis)-restricted have been shown to induce a cellular and/or humoral immune response in humans [24].

Because the MAGE family has been extensively studied (reviewed in 36), we will elaborate on it further. The MAGE family proteins are related by sharing the MAGE homology domain. There are 3 subgroups of acidic MAGEs, termed A, B, and C, and one basic subgroup, MAGE-D (including Necdin and Restin). As with other cancer-testis antigens, MAGE gene activation may occur due to promoter demethylation. The promoter of the MAGE-A1 gene contains regulatory sequences that are sites for Ets transcription factor binding. If an important CpG site is methylated, the Ets transcription factor cannot bind and expression of MAGE-1 is inhibited, whereas demethylation at this site allows transcription to proceed. Numerous HLA restricted epitopes of the various MAGE antigens have been described and have been used in clinical trials. For example, we tested an immunization strategy using dendritic cell derived dexosomes loaded with MAGE-A3, -A4, and -A10 [37]. Chianese-Bullock, et al. [35] targeted Mage A1 and A10 in their peptide vaccine strategy. The availability of class II epitopes has permitted their incorporation into vaccines. For example, we [37] included the MAGE-3DPO4 peptide in an attempt to activate CD4+ T cell help. CD4+ T cell immune responses have been detected in patients immunized with MAGE protein [38]. As described above, cancer testis antigens in general and MAGE antigens in particular are expressed by many tumors although not always the same antigen. Thus one goal would be to find an epitope that is in common across many of the MAGE antigens to permit targeting a large number of tumors. Graff-Dubois, et al.[39] described a heteroclitic peptide (p248V9) that corresponds to two HLA-A*0201-restricted, cross-recognized epitopes, derived from MAGE-A2, -A3, -A4, -A6, -A10, -A12 (p248G9) and MAGE-A1 (p248D9). CTL stimulated by this peptide could recognize each of the MAGE-A antigens and kill MAGE-A-expressing tumor cells.

NY-ESO-1, initially identified by antibodies present in patient sera, was ultimately found to contain T cell epitopes [40]. HLA A2 epitopes that have been identified include NY-ESO-$1_{157-167}$, NY-ESO-$1_{157-165}$ and NY-ESO-$1_{155-163}$ but NY-ESO-$1_{157-165}$ may be the naturally processed antigen. An HLA-A31 restrictred epitope has also been identified which recognizes a peptide derived from translation of an alternative open reading frame of the NY-ESO-1 transcript [41]. This represents a novel and somewhat unexpected observation, but additional examples where a single transcript encodes two protein products have now been described. The alternative open reading frame of LAGE-1 (a gene that encodes an antigen closely related to NY-ESO-1 with 94% nucleotide and 87% amino acid homology) was recently found to contain multiple promiscuous HLA-DR-restricted epitopes recognized by tumor antigen-specific CD4+ T cells [29].

DIFFERENTIATION ANTIGENS

Differentiation antigens are generally expressed early in development of normal tissues and may be re-expressed in tumors that arise from these normal tissues. Most of the antigens were originally described in melanomas and melanocytes (tyrosinase, gp100, TRP-1, and MART-1/Melan-A) but others have been well described in other malignancies (CEA, Epcam, PSA). While the function of these molecules may be poorly described, their relative overexpression in tumors suggests they can serve as targets of immunotherapies with a reduced, but not a completely eliminated, risk of auto-immunity. We have worked extensively to understand targeting of CEA and will elaborate on it further as a model tumor antigen. The CEA family includes CEA, CEA cell adhesion molecule 1, CEA cell adhesion molecule 6, meconium antigen, and Tex [43]. CEA appears to be involved in adhesion but may also interact with other molecules important for cellular transformation. CEA is normally expressed during oncofetal development, but is overexpressed in virtually 100% of colorectal cancers, 70% of non–small-cell lung cancers, and approximately 50% of breast cancers [43]. The only normal tissue expression is low-level expression in gastrointestinal epithelium. A number of T cell epitopes that can be recognized in the context of HLA-A2, -A3, and -A24 have been described and these epitopes can be used as immunogens to activate T cell responses against CEA. The best described epitope is the HLA A2 restricted epitope called CAP-1 that has been further modified to create the CAP1(6D) peptide with enhanced recognition by the T-cell receptor [42]. HLA class II epitopes restricted by HLA-DR1 and HLA-DR4 have also been described. Importantly, HLA restricted peptide epitopes have been found to be expressed by tumors as evidenced by the ability to identify them bound to HLA molecules of tumor cells [43]. CEA has been a frequent target of cancer vaccines in the form of peptides, full length protein, mRNA loaded dendritic cells, plasmid DNA, and viral vectors. Others [44] and we [45] have recently reported immune responses specific for CEA in cancer patients immunized with viral vectors encoding CEA or dendritic cells infected with these vectors.

The family of melanocyte differentiation antigens (MART-1, TRP-1, -2, gp100, and tyrosinase), while expressed in normal skin melanocytes and pigmented retinal epithelial cells, are found amongst tumors only in melanomas. Epitopes restricted by HLA-A2 have been the most extensively developed. Two native immunodominant HLA-A2-restricted MART-1_{26-35} and MART-1_{27-35} peptides have been reported to induce a CTL response *in vitro* and *in vivo* [46,47]. Nonetheless, the magnitude of the response is low, possibly due to low affinity of binding to MHC class-I [48]. Immunogenicity of the peptide was improved by substituting one or two amino acids [49,50]. The MART- 1_{26-35} A27L peptide analogue (ELAGIGILTV), in which the parental immunodominant peptide (MART- 1_{26-35}) is modified by replacing the alanine with leucine (A27L), demonstrated better immunogenicity in vitro and in vivo than did the parental sequence (EAAGIGILTV) [49],[51]. Peptides restricted by HLA B*3501 and B45 have also been described. HLA-DP restricted (class II) epitopes of MART-1 have been demonstrated to activate specific immune responses in patients with melanoma [52].

The native HLA-A2-restricted immunodominant epitope of gp100 (gp100 (209–217)) has been modified by a substitution of methionine for threonine at position 2 to yield (gp100(209-2M)). This modified peptide, binds HLA-A2 with an approximately 9-fold greater affinity and has an approximately 7-fold slower dissociation rate at physiological temperature than the native peptide and it is more immunogenic *in vitro* and *in vivo*. Peptides restricted by HLA-A3, -A24, and B*3501 have also been described.

The human tyrosinase gene codes for two distinct antigens that are recognized by HLA-A*0201-restricted CTLs. For one of them, tyrosinase peptide 368–376, the sequence identified by mass spectrometry in melanoma cell eluates differs from the gene-encoded sequence as a result of posttranslational modification of amino acid residue 370 (asparagine to aspartic acid) and is called $tyrosinase_{368--376}$ (370D). Peptides restricted by HLA-A1, -A24, B44 and B*3501 have also been described. Recent clinical trials have used MART-1, gp100, and tyrosinase epitopes as part of vaccine strategies and immune responses have been observed [53–55].

BROADLY EXPRESSED ANTIGENS

These antigens have been described in many tumors and may be expressed to a lesser degree in normal tissues. Some could also be called "universal" antigens because they are of interest for the possibility that they may be expressed in all tumors and could therefore be part of a vaccine strategy with wide applicability. The list of these antigens includes AFP, HER2/neu, livin, survivin, hTERT, MUC-1, PSMA, p53, and WT1.

Telomerase (hTERT) is a reverse transcriptase which adds a repeated sequence onto the ends of newly replicated chromosomes thus stabilizing the chromosomes during replication and conferring cellular immortality. It thus allows pre-cancerous cells to proliferate continuously and become immortal and is found expressed in many malignancies thus suggesting the possibility that it can act as a widely expressed tumor antigen. Telomerase can act as a tumor antigen as demonstrated by the ability of hTERT-specific CD8+ T cells in patients with metastatic prostate cancer to lyse hTERT-expressing targets [56]. Zanetti and colleagues perfomed a series of experiments (reviewed in 57) to identify two HLA-A2-restrcited peptides derived from hTERT, ^{540}ILAKFLHWL^{548} and ^{865}RLVDDFLLV^{873}, since termed p540 and p865, which bind tightly to HLA-A2, activate specific CTL in HLA-A2 transgenic mice, and they showed that that CTL specific for p540 and p865 kill HLA-A2^{+}human breast, colon, prostate, and melanoma cell lines. Because of concern that high affinity T cells against hTERT, a self antigen, might be deleted in humans, they evaluated a series of low affinity peptides and then altered them to place a tyrosine (Y) in position 1 to enhance binding to HLA-A2. One of these peptides pY572 (the analogue of wild-type p572) was able to activate CTL that could recognize the wild type peptide from the blood of 5/8 patients with prostate cancer. The wild type peptide could generate a specific CTL response in one out of seven individuals only. In order to rule out a risk of autoimmunity, they showed that CTL against the p572 did not lyse CD34+ hematopoietic cells. An HLA-A1-restricted epitope (hTERT$_{325-333}$) has been identified that could induce intermediate-to low-avidity CTLs that recognized endogenously processed hTERT [15].

Survivin, a member of the inhibitor of apoptosis protein (IAP) family is expressed during fetal development but becomes undetectable in normal adult tissues. Survivin and its splicing variant survivin-2B is in various types of tumor tissues as well as tumor cell lines, having been identified by immunohistochemistry in a substantial fraction of breast, colon, squamous cell cancers, melanoma, lung and gastric cancers. HLA restricted peptide epitopes have been identified. Full length survivin could be used to induce surviving-specific T cell responses amongst mouse and human T cells *in vitro* [58]. Idenoue, et al.[59] reported on the identification of an HLA-A24-restricted antigenic peptide, survivin-2B80-88 (AYACNTSTL), recognized by CD8+ CTL. HLA-A24/survivin-2B80-88 tetramer analysis revealed that there existed an increased number of CTL precursors in peripheral blood mononuclear cells (PBMC) of HLA-A24+ cancer patients, and *in vitro* stimulation of PBMCs from six breast cancer patients with survivin-2B80–88 peptide could lead to increases of the CTL precursor frequency. Furthermore, CTLs specific for this peptide were successfully induced from PBMCs in all 7 (100%) patients with breast cancers, 6 of 7 (83%) patients with colorectal cancers, and 4 of 7 (57%) patients with gastric cancers. HLA-A2-restricted peptide epitopes have been identified as well [60]. Clinical trials immunizing patients against survivin have demonstrated induction of surviving-specific T cells without obvious autoimmunity [61, 62]. These data support the use of survivin as a "universal" tumor antigen. An interesting advantage for both telomerase and survivin is that antigen loss variants might no longer have survival capacity due to loss of survivin or telomerase.

MUC1 mucins are highly glycosylated, cell surface-expressed type I glycoproteins expressed by many normal cells, but is also widely expressed, in an aberrantly glycosylated form, across many epithelial (breast, ovarian) and hematologic malignancies (myeloma, AML, and some lymphomas) [63]. An important feature of MUC-1 is an extracellular domain with a variable number of tandem repeats of 20 amino acids [64]. These tandem repeats can be recognized directly by CD8+ T cells without the need for MHC presentation, but also may be presented within MHC class I molecules as well [64–66]. One 9-mer peptide, M1.1, is derived from the tandem repeat region of the MUC1 protein; another, M1.2, is localized within the signal sequence of MUC1 [65, 67]. These peptides can be recognized by CTLs. The availability of epitopes and the overexpression of MUC1 in many malignancies have made MUC1 a broadly applicable target for cancer vaccination strategies [68]. For example, Wierecky, et al.[69] vaccinated patients with advanced cancer using dendritic cells pulsed with MUC1 derived peptides. Of 20 patients with metastatic renal cell carcinoma, 6 patients showed regression of metastases with 3 objective responses. In patients responding to treatment, T cell responses for antigens not used for treatment occurred suggesting that antigen spreading *in vivo* might be a possible mechanism of mediating antitumor effects.

UNIQUE TUMOR-SPECIFIC ANTIGENS

Unique tumor antigens are those found exclusively in tumors and in many situations are mutated proteins or fusion molecules associated with malignant transformation and/or progression. Most of these mutations are likely to be unique to a patient and not broadly applicable, but some are mutations that occur in many patients' tumors. For example, many colon, pancreatic, and lung cancers harbor point mutations in the *ras* gene at codon 12, where the normal Gly residue is substituted with either a Val, Asp or Cys residue. This mutated region has been the focus of cancer vaccines because A theoretically the antigens are foreign to the immune system. particularly interesting scenario is that of hereditary nonpolyposis colon cancer caused by defects in mismatch repair genes that lead to the microsatellite instability (MSI+) phenotype. Multiple genes are affected and their products are proteins with novel mutations. For example, Saeterdal, et al.[70] described a peptide SLVRLSSCVP-VALMSAMTTSSSQ, representing a common frameshift mutation in TGF betaRII, that was recognized by T cells from patients with MSI+ colon cancers. This group [71] also described an HLA-A2-restricted, CD8+ T cell epitope (RLSSCVPVA), resulting from a common frameshift mutation in TGF betaRII. A CTL clone generated against this peptide was able to kill an HLA-A2+ colon cancer cell line with mutated TGF betaRII.

Fusions molecules created by translocations of chromosomes are very interesting potential tumor-specific antigens. While some of these fusion molecules truly give rise to a unique epitope spanning the fusion region (e.g. FVEHDDESPGL an HLA-A2-restricted peptide derived from the BCR-abl fusion in CML [72] others may be found exclusively in one of the partners to the translocation, but because the aberrant molecules over-expressed, the peptide epitope is also overexpressed. A number of HLA class II-restricted epitopes have been described as well [72, 73].

CONCLUSION

The identification of defined tumor antigens has raised a number of important questions. The first is whether, in fact, defined or undefined antigens would be preferred in cancer immunotherapy strategies. It is possible that the actual tumor rejection antigen might differ for each patient and might even be a molecule without previously defined epitopes. Therefore, using all the "antigens" derived from a patient's tumor would be appealing. Unfortunately, it is difficult to monitor these responses. The second question is whether to use one or multiple antigens in a vaccine. As described above, not all antigens will induce specific immune responses and thus using a vaccine with several antigens increases the likelihood of inducing a potent immune response. It might also prevent development of antigen loss escape mutants. Use of multiple epitopes complicates the vaccine and the development of epitope and antigen spreading suggests that immune responses against antigens not part of the vaccine may occur following immune attack on the tumor through cross presentation of antigen from destroyed tumors. Finally, the choice of the type of antigen could be debated. Are widely expressed antigens such as telomerase to be preferred because they could be part of a "universal" vaccine or are antigens unique to a person's tumor (such as mutated antigens) better? While there are no answers to these questions yet, they must be addressed each time a clinical trial of a new platform for inducing immune responses is to be tested.

REFERENCES

1. P. van der Bruggen, C. Traversari, P. Chomez, C. Lurquin, E. De Plaen, B. Van den Eynde, et al. A gene encoding an antigen recognized by cytolytic T lymphocytes on a human melanoma, *Science* 254, 1643–7(1991).
2. L. Novellino, C. Castelli, G. Parmiani, A listing of human tumor antigens recognized by T cells: March 2004 update. *Cancer Immunol. Immunother.* 54(3), 187–207 (2005).
3. M. Probst-Kepper, V. Stroobant, R. Kridel, B. Gaugler, C. Landry, F. Brasseur, J.P. Cosyns, B. Weynand, T. Boon, B.J. Van Den Eynde, An alternative open reading frame of the human macrophage colony-stimulating factor gene is independently translated and codes for an antigenic peptide of 14 amino acids recognized by tumor-infiltrating CD8 T lymphocytes, *J. Exp. Med.* 193, 1189 (2001).
4. Y. Hirohashi, T. Torigoe, A. Maeda, Y. Nabeta, K. Kamiguchi, T. Sato, J. Yoda, H. Ikeda, K. Hirata, N. Yamanaka, N. Sato, An HLA-A24-restricted cytotoxic T lymphocyte epitope of a tumor-associated protein, survivin. *Clin. Cancer Res.* 8, 1731 (2002).
5. K. Hanada, J.W. Yewdell, J.C. Yang, Immune recognition of a human renal cancer antigen through post-translational protein splicing, *Nature* 427, 252 (2004).
6. B.J. Van Den Eynde, B. Gaugler, M. Probst-Kepper, L. Michaux, O. Devuyst, F. Lorge, P. Weynants, T. Boon, A new antigen recognized by cytolytic T lymphocytes on a human kidney tumor results from reverse strand transcription, *J. Exp. Med.* 190, 1793–800 (1999).
7. D. Valmori, U. Gileadi, C. Servis, P.R. Dunbar, J.C. Cerottini, P. Romero, et al. Modulation of proteasomal activity required for the generation of a cytotoxic T lymphocyte-defined peptide derived from the tumor antigen MAGE-3. *J. Exp. Med.* 189, 895–906 (1999).
8. P. van der Bruggen, C. Traversari, P. Chomez, C. Lurquin, E. De Plaen, B. Van den Eynde, et al. A gene encoding an antigen recognized by cytolytic T lymphocytes on a human melanoma, *Science* 254, 1643–7 (1991).
9. C. Traversari, P. van der Bruggen, I.F. Luescher, C. Lurquin, P. Chomez, A. Van Pel, E. De Plaen, A. Amar-Costesec, T. Boon, A nonapeptide encoded by human gene MAGE-1 is recognized on HLA-A1 by cytolytic T lymphocytes directed against tumor antigen MZ2-E, *J. Exp. Med.* 176, 1453–7(1992).
10. T. Itoh, W.J. Storkus, E. Gorelik, M.T. Lotze, Partial purification of murine tumor-associated peptide epitopes common to histologically distinct tumors, melanoma and sarcoma, that are presented by H-2Kb molecules and recognized by CD8+ tumor-infiltrating lymphocytes, *J. Immunol.* 153(3),1202–15 (1994).
11. H. Rammensee, J. Bachmann, N.P. Emmerich, O.A. Bachor, S. Stevanovic, SYFPEITHI: database for MHC ligands and peptide motifs, *Immunogenetics* 50, 213–9 (1999).
12. E. Keogh, J. Fikes, S. Southwood, E. Celis, R. Chesnut, A. Sette, Identification of new epitopes from four different tumor-associated antigens: recognition of naturally processed epitopes correlates with HLA-A*0201-binding affinity, *J. Immunol.* 167, 787–796 (2001).
13. M.R. Parkhurst, M.L. Salgaller, S. Southwood, P.F. Robbins, A. Sette, S.A. Rosenberg et al. Improved induction of melanoma-reactive CTL with peptides from the melanoma antigen gp100 modified at HLA-A*0201-binding residues, *J. Immunol.* 157, 2539–2548 (1996).
14. B. Fisk, C. Savary, J.M. Hudson, C.A. O'Brian , J.L. Murray, J.T. Wharton et al. Changes in an HER-2 peptide upregulating HLA-A2 expression affect both conformational epitopes and CTL recognition: implications for optimization of antigen presentation and tumor-specific CTL induction, *J. Immunother.* 18, 197–209 (1996).

15. M.W. Schreurs, E.W. Kueter, K.B. Scholten, D. Kramer, C.J. Meijer, E. Hooijberg, Identification of a potential human telomerase reverse transcriptase-derived, HLA-A1-restricted cytotoxic T-lymphocyte epitope, *Cancer Immunol. Immunother.* (2005).
16. J.E. Slansky, F.M. Rattis, L.F. Boyd, T. Fahmy, E.M. Jaffee, J.P. Schneck et al. Enhanced antigen-specific antitumor immunity with altered peptide ligands that stabilize the MHC-peptide-TCR complex, *Immunity* 13, 529–538 (2000).
17. S. Zaremba, E. Barzaga, M.Z. Zhu, N. Soares, K.Y. Tsang, J. Schlom, Identification of an enhancer agonist cytotoxic T lymphocyte peptide from human carcinoembryonic antigen, *Cancer Res.* 57, 4570–4577 (1997).
18. L. Fong, Y. Hou, A. Rivas, C. Benike, A. Yuen, G.A. Fisher et al. Altered peptide ligand vaccination with Flt3 ligand expanded dendritic cells for tumor immunotherapy, *Proc Natl Acad Sci USA* 98, 8809–8814 (2001).
19. M. Alsheimer, T. Drewes, W. Schutz, R. Benavente, The cancer/testis antigen CAGE-1 is a component of the acrosome of spermatids and spermatozoa, *Eur. J. Cell. Biol.* 84, 445–52 (2005).
20. G. Cronwright, K. Le Blanc, C. Gotherstrom, P. Darcy, M. Ehnman, B. Brodin, Cancer/testis antigen expression in human mesenchymal stem cells: down-regulation of SSX impairs cell migration and matrix metalloproteinase 2 expression, *Cancer. Res.* 65, 2207–15 (2005).
21. C. De Smet, C. Lurquin, B. Lethe, V. Martelange, T. Boon, DNA methylation is the primary silencing mechanism for a set of germ line- and tumor-specific genes with a CpG-rich promoter, *Mol. Cell. Biol.* 19, 7327 (1999).
22. J.H. Lim, S.P. Kim, E. Gabrielson, Y.B. Park, J.W. Park, T.K. Kwon, Activation of human cancer/testis antigen gene, XAGE-1, in tumor cells is correlated with CpG island hypomethylation, *Int. J. Cancer* (2005).
23. L. Sigalotti, E. Fratta, S. Coral, S. Tanzarella, R. Danielli, F. Colizzi, E. Fonsatti, C. Traversari, M. Altomonte, M. Maio, Intratumor heterogeneity of cancer/testis antigens expression in human cutaneous melanoma is methylation-regulated and functionally reverted by 5-aza-2'-deoxycytidine, *Cancer Res.* 64 (24), 9167–71 (2004).
24. M.J. Scanlan, A.J. Simpson, L.J. Old, The cancer/testis genes: review, standardization, and commentary, *Cancer Immun.* 4, 1 (2004).
25. K. Mashino, N. Sadanaga, F. Tanaka, H. Yamaguchi, H. Nagashima, H. Inoue, K. Sugimachi, M. Mori, Expression of multiple cancer-testis antigen genes in gastrointestinal and breast carcinomas, *Br. J. Cancer* 85, 713–20 (2001).
26. A.A. Jungbluth, S. Ely, M. Diliberto, R. Niesvizky, B. Williamson, D. Frosina, Y.T. Chen, N. Bhardwaj, S. Chen-Kiang, L.J. Old, H.J. Cho, The Cancer-Testis antigens CT7 (MAGE-C1) and MAGE-A3/6 are commonly expressed in multiple myeloma and correlate with plasma cell proliferation, *Blood* (2005).
27. G. Melloni, A.J. Ferreri, V. Russo, L. Gattinoni, G. Arrigoni, G.L. Ceresoli, P. Zannini, C. Traversari, Prognostic significance of cancer-testis gene expression in resected non-small cell lung cancer patients, *Oncol. Rep.* 12, 145–51 (2004).
28. M. Li, Y.H. Yuan, Y. Han, Y.X. Liu, L. Yan, Y. Wang, J. Gu, Expression profile of cancer-testis genes in 121 human colorectal cancer tissue and adjacent normal tissue, *Clin. Cancer Res.* 11, 1809–14 (2005).
29. M. Mandic, C. Almunia, S. Vicel, D. Gillet, B. Janjic, K. Coval, BB. Maillere, J.M. Kirkwood, H.M. Zarour, The alternative open reading frame of LAGE-1 gives rise to multiple promiscuous HLA-DR-restricted epitopes recognized by T-helper 1-type tumor-reactive CD4+ T Cells, *Cancer Res.* 63, 6506–15 (2003).
30. J. Ries, S. Schultze-Mosgau, F. Neukam, E. Diebel, J. Wiltfang, Investigation of the expression of melanoma antigen-encoding genes (MAGE-A1 to -A6) in oral squamous cell carcinomas to determine potential targets for gene-based cancer immunotherapy, *Int. J. Oncol.* 26, 817–24 (2005).
31. N.H. Segal, N.E. Blachere, J.A. Guevara-Patino, H.F. Gallardo, H.Y. Shiu, A. Viale, C.R. Antonescu, J.D. Wolchok, A.N. Houghton, Identification of cancer-testis genes expressed by melanoma and soft tissue sarcoma using bioinformatics, *Cancer Immun.* 5, 2 (2005).

32. T. Utsunomiya, H. Inoue, F. Tanaka, H. Yamaguchi, M. Ohta, M. Okamoto, K. Mimori, M. Mori, Expression of cancer-testis antigen (CTA) genes in intrahepatic cholangiocarcinoma, *Ann. Surg. Oncol.* 11, 934–40 (2004).
33. L. Zhao, D.C. Mou, X.S. Leng, J.R. Peng, W.X. Wang, L. Huang, S. Li, J.Y. Zhu, Expression of cancer-testis antigens in hepatocellular carcinoma, *World J. Gastroenterol.* 10, 2034–8 (2004).
34. M. Li, Y.H. Yuan, Y. Han, Y.X. Liu, L. Yan, Y. Wang, J. Gu, Expression profile of cancer-testis genes in 121 human colorectal cancer tissue and adjacent normal tissue, *Clin. Cancer Res.* 11(5), 1809–14 (2005).
35. K.A. Chianese-Bullock, J. Pressley, C. Garbee, S. Hibbitts, C. Murphy, G. Yamshchikov, G.R. Petroni, E.A. Bissonette, P.Y. Neese, W.W. Grosh, P. Merrill, R. Fink, E.M. Woodson, C.J. Wiernasz, J.W. Patterson, C.L. Slingluff Jr., MAGE-A1-, MAGE-A10-, and gp100-derived peptides are immunogenic when combined with granulocyte-macrophage colony-stimulating factor and montanide ISA-51 adjuvant and administered as part of a multipeptide vaccine for melanoma, *J. Immunol.* 17, 3080–6 (2005).
36. J. Xiao, H.S. Chen, Biological functions of melanoma-associated antigens. *World J. Gastroenterol.* 10(13), 1849–53 (2004).
37. M.A. Morse, J. Garst, T. Osada, S. Khan, A. Hobeika, T.M. Clay, N. Valente, R. Shreeniwas, M.A. Sutton, A. Delcayre, D.H. Hsu, J.B. Le Pecq, H.K. Lyerly, A phase I study of dexosome immunotherapy in patients with advanced non-small cell lung cancer, *J. Transl. Med.* 3(1), 9 (2005).
38. D. Atanackovic, N.K. Altorki, E. Stockert, B. Williamson, A.A. Jungbluth, E. Ritter, D. Santiago, C.A. Ferrara, M. Matsuo, A. Selvakumar, B. Dupont, Y.T. Chen, E.W. Hoffman, G. Ritter, L.J. Old, S. Gnjatic, Vaccine-induced CD4+ T cell responses to MAGE-3 protein in lung cancer patients, *J. Immunol.* 172(5), 3289–96 (2004).
39. S. Graff-Dubois, O. Faure, D.A. Gross, P. Alves, A. Scardino, S. Chouaib, F.A. Lemonnier, K. Kosmatopoulos, Generation of CTL recognizing an HLA-A*0201-restricted epitope shared by MAGE-A1, -A2, -A3, -A4, -A6, -A10, and -A12 tumor antigens: implication in a broad-spectrum tumor immunotherapy, *J. Immunol.* 169(1), 575–80 (2002).
40. E. Jager, Y.T. Chen, J.W. Drijfhout, J. Karbach, M. Ringhoffer, D. Jager, et al. Simultaneous humoral and cellular immune response against cancer-testis antigen NY-ESO-1: definition of human histocompatibility leukocyte antigen (HLA)-A2-binding peptide epitopes, *J. Exp. Med.* 187, 265–270 (1998).
41. R.F. Wang, S.L. Johnston, G. Zeng, S.L.Topalian, D.J. Schwartzentruber, S.A. Rosenberg, A breast and melanoma-shared tumor antigen: T cell responses to antigenic peptides translated from different open reading frames, *J. Immunol.* 161, 598–3606 (1998).
42. M. Schirle, W. Keilholz, B. Weber, et al. Identification of tumor-associated MHC class I ligands by a novel T cell-independent approach, *Eur. J. Immunol.* 30, 2216–2225 (2000).
43. N.L. Berinstein, Carcinoembryonic antigen as a target for therapeutic anticancer vaccines: a review, *J. Clin. Oncol.* 20(8), 2197–207 (2002).
44. J.L. Marshall, J.L. Gulley, P.M. Arlen, P.K. Beetham, K.Y. Tsang, R. Slack, J.W. Hodge, S. Doren, D.W. Grosenbach, J. Hwang, E. Fox, L. Odogwu, S. Park, D. Panicali, J. Schlom, Phase I study of sequential vaccinations with fowlpox-CEA(6D)-TRICOM alone and sequentially with vaccinia-CEA(6D)-TRICOM, with and without granulocyte-macrophage colony-stimulating factor, in patients with carcinoembryonic antigen-expressing carcinomas, *J. Clin. Oncol.* 23(4), 720–31 (2005).
45. M.A. Morse, T.M. Clay, A.C. Hobeika, T. Osada, S. Khan, S. Chui, D. Niedzwiecki, D. Panicali, J. Schlom, H.K. Lyerly, Phase I study of immunization with dendritic cells modified with fowlpox encoding carcinoembryonic antigen and costimulatory molecules, *Clin. Cancer Res.* 11(8), 3017–24 (2005).
46. M. Salio, D. Shepherd, P.R. Dunbar, M. Palmowski, K. Murphy, L. Wu, V. Cerundolo, Mature dendritic cells prime functionally superior Melan-A-specific CD8þ lymphocytes as compared with nonprofessional APC, *J. Immunol.* 167, 1188–1197 (2001).

47. F.O. Nestle, S. Alijac, M. Gilliet, Y. Sun, S. Grabbe, R. Dummer, G. Burg, D. Schadendorf, Vaccination of melanoma patients with peptide or tumor lysate-pulsed dendritic cells, *Nat. Med.* 4, 328–332 (1998).
48. P. Romero, N. Gervois, J. Schneider, P. Escobar, D. Valmori, C. Pannetier, A. Steinle, T. W€olfel, D. Lienard, V. Brichard, A. Van Pel, F. Jotereau, J.C. Cerottini, Cytolytic T lymphocyte recognition of the immunodominant HLA-A*0201 restricted Melan-A/MART-1 antigenic peptide in melanoma, *J. Immunol.* 158, 2366–2374 (1997).
49. D. Valmori, J.F. Fonteneau, C. Lizana, N. Gervois, D. Lienard, D. Rimoldi, V. Jongeneel, F. Jotereau, J.C. Cerottini, P. Romero, Enhanced generation of specific tumor-reactive CTL in vitro by selected Melan-A/MART-1 immunodominant peptide analogues, *J. Immunol.* 160, 1750–1758 (1998).
50. G. Guichard, A. Zerbib, F.A. Le Gal, J. Hoebeke, F. Connan, J. Choppin, J.P. Briand, J.G.Guillet, Melanoma peptide MART-1(27–35) analogues with enhanced binding capacity to the human class I histocompatibility molecule HLA-A2 by introduction of a beta-amino acid residue: implications for recognition by tumor-infiltrating lymphocytes, *J. Med. Chem.* 43(20), 3803–8 (2000).
51. Y. Men, I. Miconnet, D. Valmori, D. Rimoldi, J.C. Cerottini, P. Romero, Assessment of immunogenicity of human Melan-A peptide analogues in HLA-A*0201/Kb transgenic mice, *J. Immunol.* 162, 3566–3573 (1999).
52. R. Wong, R. Lau, J. Chang, T. Kuus-Reichel, V. Brichard, C. Bruck, J. Weber, Immune responses to a class II helper peptide epitope in patients with stage III/IV resected melanoma, *Clin. Cancer Res.* 10(15), 5004–13 (2004).
53. P. Hersey, S.W. Menzies, G.M. Halliday, T. Nguyen, M.L. Farrelly, C. DeSilva, M. Lett, Phase I/II study of treatment with dendritic cell vaccines in patients with disseminated melanoma, *Cancer Immunol. Immunother.* 53(2), 125–34 (2004).
54. G.Q. Phan, C.E. Touloukian, J.C. Yang, N.P. Restifo, R.M. Sherry, P. Hwu, S.L. Topalian, D.J. Schwartzentruber, C.A. Seipp, L.J. Freezer, K.E. Morton, S.A. Mavroukakis, D.E. White, S.A. Rosenberg, Immunization of patients with metastatic melanoma using both class I- and class II-restricted peptides from melanoma-associated antigens, *J. Immunother.* 26(4), 349–56 (2003).
55. V. Pullarkat, P.P. Lee, R. Scotland, V. Rubio, S. Groshen, C. Gee, R. Lau, J. Snively, S. Sian, S.L. Woulfe, R.A. Wolfe, J.S.Weber, A phase I trial of SD-9427 (progenipoietin) with a multipeptide vaccine for resected metastatic melanoma, *Clin. Cancer Res.* 9(4), 1301–12 (2003).
56. Z. Su, J. Dannull, B.K. Yang, P. Dahm, D. Coleman, D. Yancey, S. Sichi, D. Niedzwiecki, D. Boczkowski, E. Gilboa, J.Vieweg, Telomerase mRNA-transfected dendritic cells stimulate antigen-specific CD8+ and CD4+ T cell responses in patients with metastatic prostate cancer, *J. Immunol.* 174(6), 3798–807 (2005).
57. M. Zanetti, X. Hernandez, P. Langlade-Demoyen, Telomerase reverse transcriptase as target for anti-tumor T cell responses in humans, *Springer Semin. Immunopathol.* (2005).
58. M. Zeis, S. Siegel, A. Wagner, M. Schmitz, M. Marget, R. Kuhl-Burmeister, I. Adamzik, D. Kabelitz, P. Dreger, N. Schmitz, A.Heiser, Generation of cytotoxic responses in mice and human individuals against hematological malignancies using survivin-RNA-transfected dendritic cells, *J. Immunol.* 170(11), 5391–7 (2003).
59. S. Idenoue, Y. Hirohashi, T. Torigoe, Y. Sato, Y. Tamura, H. Hariu, M. Yamamoto, T. Kurotaki, T. Tsuruma, H. Asanuma, T. Kanaseki, H. Ikeda, K. Kashiwagi, M. Okazaki, K. Sasaki, T. Sato, T. Ohmura, F. Hata, K. Yamaguchi, K. Hirata, N. Sato, A potent immunogenic general cancer vaccine that targets survivin, an inhibitor of apoptosis proteins, *Clin. Cancer Res.* 11(4), 1474–82 (2005).
60. S.M. Schmidt, K. Schag, M.R. Muller, M.M. Weck, S. Appel, L. Kanz, F. Grunebach, P. Brossart, Survivin is a shared tumor-associated antigen expressed in a broad variety of malignancies and recognized by specific cytotoxic T cells, *Blood* 102, 571–576 (2003).
61. K. Otto, M.H. Andersen, A. Eggert, P. Keikavoussi, L.O. Pedersen, J.C. Rath, M. Bock, E.B. Brocker, P.T. Straten, E. Kampgen, J.C. Becker, Lack of toxicity of therapy-induced T cell responses against the universal tumour antigen survivin, *Vaccine* 23(7), 884–9 (2005).
62. T. Tsuruma, F. Hata, T. Torigoe, T. Furuhata, S. Idenoue, T. Kurotaki, M. Yamamoto, A. Yagihashi, T. Ohmura, K. Yamaguchi, T. Katsuramaki, T. Yasoshima, K. Sasaki, Y. Mizushima, H. Minamida,

H. Kimura, M. Akiyama, Y. Hirohashi, H. Asanuma, Y. Tamura, K. Shimozawa, N. Sato, K. Hirata, Phase I clinical study of anti-apoptosis protein, survivin-derived peptide vaccine therapy for patients with advanced or recurrent colorectal cancer, *J. Transl. Med.* 2(1), 19 (2004).
63. S.J. Gendler, A.P.Spicer, Epithelial mucin genes, *Annu. Rev. Physiol.* 57, 607–634 (1995).
64. S. Gendler, J. Taylor-Papadimitriou, T. Duhig, J. Rothbard, J.Burchell, Highly immunogenic region of a human polymorphic epithelial mucin expressed by carcinomas is made up of tandem repeats, *J. Biol. Chem.* 263, 12820–12823 (1988).
65. T. Takahashi, Y. Makiguchi, Y. Hinoda, H. Kakiuchi, N. Nakagawa, K. Imai, A. Yachi, Expression of MUC1 on myeloma cells and induction of HLA-unrestricted CTL against MUC1 from a multiple myeloma patient, *J. Immunol.* 153, 2102–2109 (1994).
66. P. Brossart, K.S. Heinrich, G. Stuhler, L. Behnke, V.L. Reichardt, S. Stevanovic, A. Muhm, H.G. Rammensee, L. Kanz, W. Brugger, Identification of HLA-A2-restricted T-cell epitopes derived from the MUC1 tumor antigen for broadly applicable vaccine therapies, *Blood* 93, 4309–4317 (1999).
67. V. Apostolopoulos, V. Karanikas, J.S. Haurum, I.F. McKenzie, Induction of HLA-A2-restricted CTLs to the mucin 1 human breast cancer antigen, *J. Immunol.* 159, 5211–5218 (1997).
68. O.J. Finn, K.R. Jerome, R.A. Henderson, G. Pecher, N. Domenech, J. Magarian-Blander, S.M. Barratt-Boyes, MUC-1 epithelial tumor mucin-based immunity and cancer vaccines, *Immunol. Rev.* 145, 61–89 (1995).
69. J. Wierecky, M. Mueller, P. Brossart. Dendritic cell-based cancer immunotherapy targeting MUC-1, *Cancer Immunol. Immunother.* 55, 63–7 (2006).
70. I. Saeterdal, J. Bjorheim, K. Lislerud, M.K. Gjertsen, I.K. Bukholm, O.C. Olsen, J.M. Nesland, J.A. Eriksen, M. Moller, A. Lindblom, G. Gaudernack, Frameshift-mutation-derived peptides as tumor-specific antigens in inherited and spontaneous colorectal cancer, *Proc. Natl. Acad. Sci. USA* 98, 13255–60 (2001).
71. I. Saeterdal, M.K. Gjertsen, P. Straten, J.A. Eriksen, G. Gaudernack, A TGF betaRII frameshift-mutation-derived CTL epitope recognised by HLA-A2-restricted CD8+ T cells, *Cancer Immunol. Immunother.* 50, 469–76 (2001).
72. W.M. Wagner, Q. Ouyang, G. Pawelec, The abl/bcr gene product as a novel leukemia-specific antigen: peptides spanning the fusion region of abl/bcr can be recognized by both CD4+ and CD8+ T lymphocytes, *Cancer Immunol. Immunother.* 52, 89 (2003).
73. G.J. ten Bosch, J.H. Kessler, A.M. Joosten, A.A. Bres-Vloemans, A. Geluk, B.C. Godthelp, J. van Bergen, C.J. Melief, O.C. Leeksma, A BCR-ABL oncoprotein p210b2a2 fusion region sequence is recognized by HLA-DR2a restricted cytotoxic T lymphocytes and presented by HLA-DR matched cells transfected with an Ii(b2a2) construct, *Blood* 94, 1038 (1999).

CHAPTER 3

T CELLS AND ANTIGEN RECOGNITION

LEISHA A. EMENS*

Departments of Oncology, The Johns Hopkins University School of Medicine, Sidney Kimmel Comprehensive Cancer Center, Baltimore, MD

INTRODUCTION

The immune response is broadly classified into either the innate, antigen-nonspecific response, or the adaptive, antigen-specific response. Leukocytes of the innate immune system reside in peripheral tissues and circulate through the blood and secondary lymphoid tissues (the spleen and the lymph nodes), serving as immunologic sentinels for detecting general signs of danger. Similarly, B and T lymphocytes traverse the body to mediate the adaptive immune response. These cells express a comprehensive repertoire of antigen-specific receptors (cell surface immunoglobulin receptors for B cells, and cell surface T cell receptors (TCR) for T cells) that can recognize over one million distinct antigens [1]. Whereas the B cell antigen receptor directly binds to antigenic determinants present on soluble proteins, carbohydrates, or nucleic acids, the T cell antigen receptor binds most commonly to short fragments of antigens that have been broken down and loaded onto Major Histocompatibility Complex (MHC) molecules. Thus, B cells can see antigen directly, and respond by differentiating into immunoglobulin-secreting plasma cells. In contrast, T cells see processed antigen in the context of self MHC molecules, thereby providing a basis for self-nonself discrimination [2]. Two major subsets of T cells collaborate to mediate an effective immune response. $CD4^+$ helper T cells are activated after binding peptide antigen presented by MHC Class II molecules,

*Assistant Professor of Oncology, The Johns Hopkins University School of Medicine, Sidney Kimmel Comprehensive Cancer Center at Johns Hopkins, Bunting-Blaustein Cancer Research Building, 1650 Orleans Street, Room 4M90, Baltimore, MD 21231-1000 E-mail: emensle@jhmi.edu

H.L. Kaufman and J.D. Wolchok (eds.), General Principles of Tumor Immunotherapy, 33–53.

and provide cytokine-mediated "help" both to shape the B cell-mediated humoral response, and to maximize the quality and durability of the $CD8^+$ T cell-mediated cytotoxic T lymphocyte (CTL) response [3]. $CD4^+$ T cells can be further divided into T helper type 1 cells, which secrete interleukin-2 (IL-2) and interferon-$\gamma$to promote CTL activity, and T helper type 2 cells, which secrete interleukin-4 (IL-4), interleukin-5 (IL-5), and interleukin-6 (IL-6), and promote humoral and allergic immune responses. Of these two T helper phenotypes, the T helper type 1 phenotype is generally considered to contribute more to antitumor immunity [4]. CTLs are activated after binding antigen presented by MHC Class I molecules, deploying a payload of cytokines and enzymes that can effectively lyse diseased cellular targets. Thus, it is $CD8^+$ effector T cells that are critical for destroying host cells altered by either viral infection or oncogenic transformation.

In order for $CD8^+$ CTL to recognize and destroy diseased cellular targets, they must migrate throughout the body to interact with professional antigen presenting cells (APCs) (DCs, B cells, macrophages, and $\gamma\delta$ T cells) [5,6]. After the priming APC-T cell interaction, $CD8^+$ CTL subsequently engage target cells that have been altered by pathogens or neoplastic transformation. The distinct physical and inflammatory environments in which the priming and effector cross-talk occurs alters the length and character of the cellular interactions [7]. Importantly, these variables impact the ultimate quality and character of the immune response as it is reflected by the size, phenotype (effector, tolerogenic, or memory), and functional status (cytokine secreting, cytotoxic) of the activated T cell repertoire. Due both to their exquisite antigenic specificity and their capacity for a faster, more vigorous secondary response, the use of T cells for the immune-mediated therapy of cancer has attracted great interest. To effectively harness the therapeutic power of T cells, a thorough understanding of the mechanisms regulating how T cells see antigen is required. These mechanisms can be considered at the molecular level (antigen processing and presentation, and accessory signaling pathways for T cell activation), the cellular level (immune priming and target cell destruction), and the environmental level (systemic mechanisms of immune tolerance and the suppressive local tumor microenvironment). Opportunities for therapeutic manipulation exist at each of these levels of T cell control.

SYSTEMIC MECHANISMS OF IMMUNE TOLERANCE

The immune system must be able to respond quickly to foreign antigens, yet remain quiescent toward normal tissues. To achieve this, the available T cell repertoire is shaped by deletional pathways of immune tolerance that occur centrally during the process of thymic education, and peripherally in extrathymic tissues. These processes together create a partially redundant system for physically eliminating a specific self-reactive T cell clone from the T cell repertoire [8]. Tumor cells arise from normal host tissues, and are almost invariably recognized as self. Consequently, components of the antitumor T cell repertoire with the highest affinity for tumor antigens are most frequently eliminated by central thymic deletion. Those that survive thymic education may be deleted in extrathymic tissues by activation-induced cell death (AICD), a scenario that most often occurs in the setting of widely disseminated tumor. These processes are thought to establish a suboptimal antitumor T cell repertoire with a lower recognition efficiency for tumor antigens, and an inadequate functional response upon T cell engagement [9–11]. Multiple groups have recently described persistent, small populations of peripheral T cells with a high recognition efficiency for tumor antigens. These high avidity tumor-specific T cells normally fail to be recruited to the antitumor immune response due to compensatory immunoregulatory mechanisms that keep them suppressed [12–15]. Together, these features of the available T cell repertoire suggest at least three major strategies for inducing effective T cell-mediated antitumor immunity. The first is to disrupt secondary immunosuppressive pathways in order to recruit latent, highly reactive T cells to the antitumor immune response. The second is to augment the tumor antigen recognition efficiency of low avidity T cells by optimizing antigen binding to the TCR and/or MHC molecule. The third is to amplify the net positive signal for T cell activation generated when the T cell recognizes its cognate tumor antigen.

ANTIGEN PROCESSING AND PRESENTATION

T cell activation is initiated at the molecular level by the TCR-mediated recognition of antigenic epitopes bound to MHC molecules. The specificity of most T cell responses is conferred by the αβ TCR [16]; an alternative γδ TCR with limited diversity is present on about 1% to 5% of peripheral T cells, and on the majority of intraepithelial T cells [17]. These TCRs are formed by two transmembrane glycoproteins, each composed of one extracellular variable and constant domain joined by a hinge region to the transmembrane domain. The diversity of the TCR is primarily found in the variable region, which is formed at the DNA level by the juxtaposition of V, D, and J gene segments (β or δchain) or V and J gene segments (α or γ chain). MHC molecules are also highly polymorphic, with multiple alleles of several genes giving rise to the protein products. The final array of molecules expressed by a given individual is referred to as the MHC haplotype. In humans, there are three MHC Class I molecules (HLA-A, -B, and –C) that associate with the co-receptor β_2-microglobulin, and three pairs of MHC Class II α and β polypeptide chains (HLA-DR, -DP, and –DQ); in mice the corresponding molecules are H2-K, H2-D, H2-L, and H2-A, H2-E respectively. The variability inherent in the MHC receptor system is conferred both by the vast number of polymorphic alleles for each gene, and by the ability of distinct alleles from the two chromosomes to associate combinatorially. This MHC diversity impacts antigen recognition by T cells indirectly by controlling peptide binding to the MHC molecule itself, and directly by physical contacts between the TCR and the MHC molecule.

Antigen processing and presentation for subsequent T cell recognition by the αβTCR can occur through two distinct pathways [2]. All nucleated cells, including tumor cells, have the capacity to directly present endogenous antigens in the context of MHC Class I molecules (Figure 1). Intracellular proteins targeted for destruction are first tagged with multiple ubiquitin molecules [18]. Many of these proteins are defective ribosomal products (DRiPS), defective protein products generated by the infidelity in translating genetic information to protein [19]. DRiPS provide one mechanism for the immune system to screen the functional integrity of the host cell. Ubiquitinated protein products then bind to the 26S proteasome, a widely expressed enzyme of the antigen processing pathway that ultimately produces peptides for presentation to $CD8^+$ CTL by MHC Class I molecules. It is composed of a catalytic 20S core complex bound to two 19S gatekeeper complexes designed

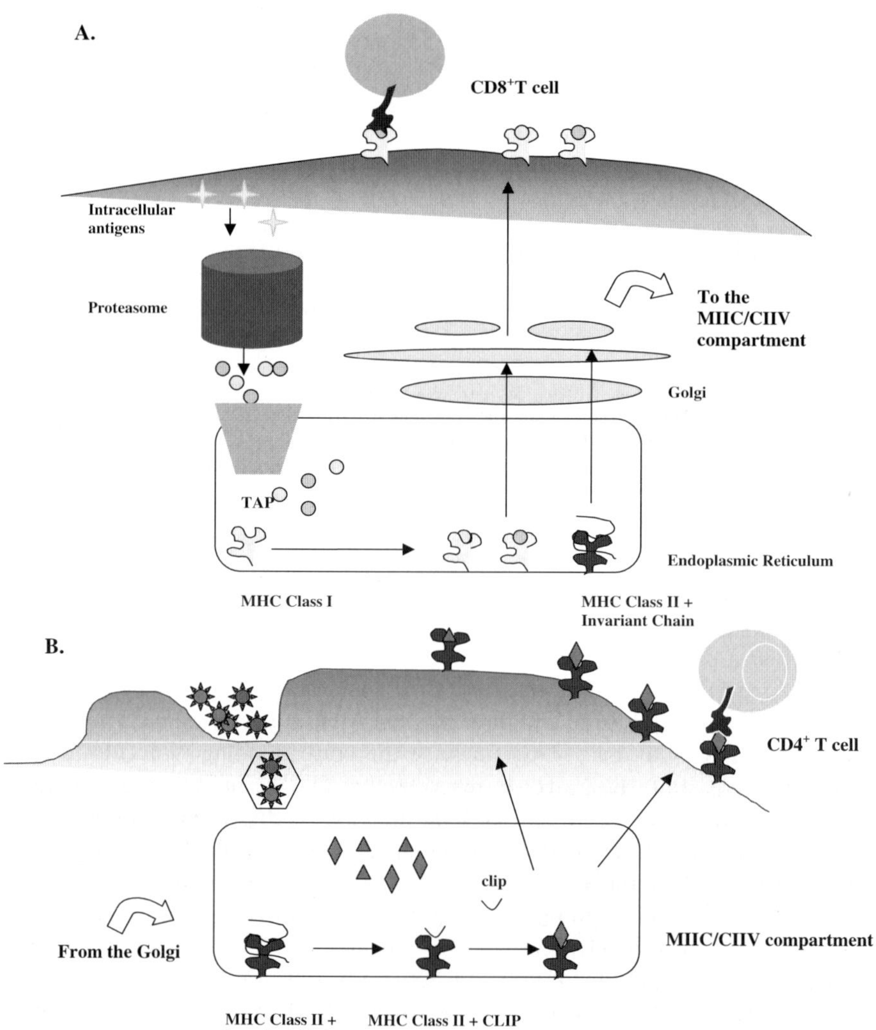

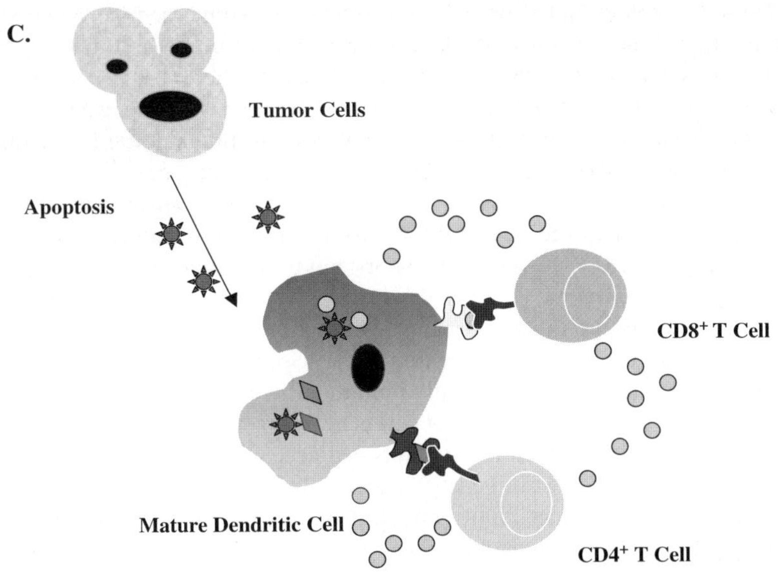

Figure 1. **Direct Priming and Cross Priming of Antigen-Specific T Cell Responses. A.** MHC Class I molecules present peptides from intracellular proteins. These proteins may either be normal cellular proteins, altered self proteins, or the intracellular products of viral or bacterial infection. Intracellular proteins are broken down by the proteasome, and transferred to the endoplasmic reticulum (ER) by the transporter for antigen processing (TAP). They are loaded onto MHC Class I molecules in the ER, and then translocated to the cell surface. **B.** MHC Class II molecules present peptides from proteins of extracellular origin. These proteins enter the cell in endocytic vesicles, and the proteins are broken down in lysosomes. MHC Class II molecules bind to the invariant chain in the ER, which prevents the association of endogenous protein fragments with MHC Class II molecules. The invariant chain is degraded to Class II invariant chain peptide (CLIP), and CLIP is exchanged for the peptide epitope generated by lysosomal cleavage. Peptide-bound MHC Class II molecules are then translocated to the cell surface. **C.** Dendritic cells (DCs) can endocytose antigens from extracellular pathogens and other cells, and display them on MHC Class I molecules by TAP-dependent cross-presentation, and MHC Class II by the classical endocytic route. The use of both of these pathways enables DCs to prime both $CD8^+$ and $CD4^+$ T cells

to feed ubiquitinated protein substrates into the system [18]. One form of the 20S proteasome, c20S, is constitutively expressed by all nucleated cells. A second form, the immunoproteasome (i20S), is expressed under steady state conditions by professional APC, and induced in other nucleated cells upon exposure to IFN-γ, tumor necrosis factor-α (TNF-α) or other inflammatory stimuli [20]. Both proteoasomes are composed of 14 subunits that form four stacked rings containing seven subunits each. The two outer rings are composed of seven α subunits, and the two inner rings are composed of seven β subunits. The catalytic activity of the c20S proteasome is conferred by three β subunits ($\beta 1$, $\beta 2$, and $\beta 5$). These are replaced by the immunosubunits $\beta 1i$ (LMP2, low molecular weight protein 2), $\beta 2i$ (MECL1, multicatalytic endopeptidase complex-like 1), and $\beta 5Ii$ (LMP7) in the i20S immunoproteasome. In nucleated cells, ubiquitinated proteins undergo proteosome-mediated degradation, and these fragments are transported into the endoplasmic reticulum (ER) by the transporter associated with antigen processing (TAP). There, the peptide is loaded onto MHC Class I molecules, and the entire complex is transported to the cell surface for display to the immune system. Notably, peptide binding is essential for stable expression of MHC Class I molecules on the cell surface.

Importantly, immunoproteasomes generate a distinct repertoire of peptide complexes compared to the constitutive proteasomes. This variability contributes to the diversity the $CD8^+$ T cell response by modifying both the T cell repertoire, and by altering the antigenic peptides driving the response [20]. Some self epitopes are not processed by the immunoproteasome, and are consequently not efficiently presented by mature DCs [21]. Also, tumor cells in an inflammatory environment may switch from the constitutive to the immunoproteasome, thereby displaying an epitope that the T cell repertoire cannot detect and respond to well [22]. Conversely, a deficiency in immunoproteasome subunits can decrease the size of the $CD8^+$ CTL repertoire specific for some antigens [23, 24].

Professional APC conduct highly efficient antigen processing and presentation activities that extend well beyond the capabilities of nucleated host cells [6]. Unlike other nucleated cells, they can present antigen bound to *both* MHC Class I and MHC Class II molecules, and can therefore activate *both* $CD8^+$ and $CD4^+$ T cells. For processing through the MHC Class II pathway, extracellular proteins or cell surface proteins are taken up by endocytosis into acidic lysosomes, where they are broken down into peptide fragments of ten to twenty-five amino acids. Endogenous proteins are blocked from binding to MHC Class II molecules by its association with the invariant chain. Subsequently, the invariant chain is degraded to Class II-associated invariant chain peptide (CLIP), and CLIP exchanged for the antigenic lysosomal degradation products. Like MHC Class I molecules, peptide binding is required for the stable expression of MHC Class II molecules on the cell surface.

CROSS-PRESENTATION: AN ALTERNATIVE ROUTE TO MHC CLASS I MEDIATED ANTIGEN PRESENTATION

In addition to processing antigen through the endogenous or classical MHC Class I antigen processing and presentation pathway, DCs and other professional APC can also direct *exogenous* antigen processing through the MHC Class I pathway by a process called cross-presentation [25]. Here, exogenous material from pathogens or diseased host cells are taken up into endosomal vesicles by macropinocytosis, receptor-mediated endocytosis, or phagocytosis. Antigens may be retrotranslocated from the endocytic vesicle to the cytosol to undergo proteosome-mediated proteolysis, followed by loading onto MHC Class I molecules by TAP-mediated transport [26]. The endosome thus may be a self-contained antigen-processing organelle. Alternatively, the lumen of the endosome containing the protein may become contiguous with the lumen of the ER, thereby accessing the classical MHC Class I pathway directly [26]. Regardless, the central concept of cross priming is that protein antigens are transferred from the diseased target to the host professional APC (Figure 1). DCs in particular are highly efficient in capturing exogenous antigens in a variety of physical forms [27]. Notably, processing and presentation of exogenous antigens by DCs may induce (cross prime) or ablate (cross tolerize) $CD8^+$ T cell responses [28]. The ultimate outcome depends both on the maturation state of the presenting DC and on the levels of MHC Class I peptide complexes being presented.

The first demonstration of cross priming involved the injection of homozygous $H2^b$ or $H2^d$ murine spleen cells into heterozygous $H2^{b/d}$recipients [29, 30]. A proportion of recipient $CD8^+$ T cells responded to antigen presented by an H2 Class I allele not present on the homozygous immunizing spleen cells, lysing target cells matched instead to the donor MHC haplotype. Others showed that SV40-transformed tumor cells could induce SV40-specific $CD8^+$ CTLs restricted to the host MHC haplotype [31]. Further supporting cross-priming, CTLs induced by vaccination with a allogeneic granulocyte-macrophage colony-stimulating factor (GM-CSF)-secreting tumor cell line expressing the influenza virus nucleoprotein (NP) recognized NP in the context of host MHC Class I in a TAP-dependent fashion [32,33]. More recently, vaccinated patients with pancreas cancer were found to have mesothelin-specific $CD8^+$ T cells in vaccinated patients restricted to the MHC haplotype of the patient, regardless of the MHC haplotype of the allogeneic immunizing vaccine cells [34]. This is the most robust evidence of *in vivo* cross priming in humans to date.

NAÏVE T CELL STIMULATION BY DENDRITIC CELLS

Peripheral DCs sample and present self and nonself antigens constitutively as they circulate throughout the body [28]. At baseline, they are immature, and process and present antigens inefficiently. In this way they help to maintain peripheral immune tolerance. Upon maturation, specialized components of the immunoproteasome are induced, the trafficking of peptide-loaded MHC molecules within the DC increases, and the cell surface molecules that initiate T cell activation and provide co- and counter-stimulatory signals are upregulated both quanitatively and qualitatively. Additional changes in the expression of chemokines and adhesion molecules facilitates the migration of DCs to regional draining lymph nodes, where they are uniquely licensed to initiate the adaptive immune response by activating naïve T cells.

In the draining lymph node, naïve T cells engage with mature DCs via the TCR:peptide-MHC (TCR:pMHC) interaction. These weak interactions likely help to maintain the peripheral T cell pool by providing subtle activation signals that promote survival, but remain below the threshold required for frank T cell activation and clonal expansion. During inflammation, multiple mature DCs present a discrete antigen repertoire, allowing migrating T cells to scan the surface of many DCs. This way, the T cells receive serial signals that accumulate and ultimately overcome the signaling threshold for activation. These short term interactions result in initial calcium fluxes, which then promote stable T cell-APC interactions to provide sustained signaling and a platform for fine-tuning and consolidating the T cell activation signal.

The TCR:pMHC binding interaction is of relatively low affinity (1 to 50 uM) [16]. The initial weak interaction is compensated for by the confined space between the DC and the T cell, the polyvalent nature of the primary TCR:pMHC interaction itself, and the associated adhesion and co-stimulatory molecules localized at the cell-cell interface [35, 36]. At the time of first cellular engagement, the TCR undergoes conformational changes within its pMHC binding site [36]. This binding site is composed of three complementarity determining region (CDR) loops. The majority of the structural change occurs within the CDR3 loop, which has the most sequence diversity and is the primary determinant of fine antigenic specificity [37–39]. Since the pMHC complex itself changes conformation infrequently, the TCR:pMHC interaction occurs through an induced fit binding process whereby the TCR accommodates the pMHC complex. Alanine scanning mutagenesis studies of the pMHC:TCR interaction have revealed that MHC contact points initiate engagement with the TCR, but that peptide contacts are critical for establishing the final stable binding state [40].

Thus, T cells circulating throughout the body scan their environment for complementary pMHC expressed by mature DCs. To increase the efficiency of this process, endogenous pMHC complexes are brought into the microenvironment at the cell-cell interface of the DC and the T cell in a TCR-dependent fashion [35]. T cell activation is initiated when the TCR encounters a complementary pMHC complex, inducing a tight fit by conformational change to engage peptide contact points, and trigger the signaling cascade for T cell activation [36]. Thus, the peptide antigen present in the MHC protein binding groove plays a central role in directing the intensity of the ensuing immune response. This has significant implications for antitumor immunity and immunotherapy. Mutated self proteins typically represent very subtle alterations of self that the immune system is likely to tolerate. However, mutations introduced into self peptides can increase peptide binding in the MHC Class I or Class II molecules by altering the amino acid residues that anchor the peptide to the MHC binding site [44–49]. This enhanced binding is also reflected as increased TCR affinity for MHC molecules, and increases the density of self peptide at the DC-T cell interface [38]. These enhanced interactions increase the level of TCR-mediated signaling to the threshold required for activating naïve T cells. Notably, T cells primed by an altered peptide ligand may then be activated by the nonmutated wild-type peptide, leading to T cell-dependent rejection of tumors expressing the wild-type peptide [45]. The use of altered peptide ligands (heteroclitic peptide antigens) to raise the T cell recognition efficiency by enhancing MHC Class I or TCR binding is one major strategy under investigation to optimize peptide-based immunization for tumor immunotherapy [44].

THE PRIMING (STABLE) IMMUNOLOGICAL SYNAPSE

The efficiency of the antigen recognition process is enhanced both by the adhesive interactions provided by the co-receptors CD4 and CD8, and by their recruitment of the *lck* signaling kinase to the activation nidus [47]. This compact area of cell-cell contact is a highly specialized area known as the immunologic synapse [35]

(Figure 2). This has been defined as "any stable, flattened interface between a lymphocyte or natural killer (NK) cell and a cell that they are in the process of recognizing" [35]. The development of the immunological synapse occurs in five steps:[1] formation by cellular scanning, contact, and adhesive arrest, [2] early assembly and signaling, [3] maturation and receptor segregation,[4] TCR internalization, and [5] synapse dissolution. Scanning T cells recognize specific cognate pMHC complexes via the TCR, simultaneously undergoing adhesive arrest by the calcium-mediated stop signal generated by the TCR:pMHC interaction and engagement of intercellular adhesion molecule 1 (ICAM1) on the APC with leukocyte function associated-antigen 1 (LFA1) on the surface of the T cell [48]. Importantly, although T cells can detect just one pMHC complex, they require engagement with ten or more pMHC ligands to initiate formation of a stable immunological synapse and sustained calcium signaling [35]. In the absence of CD4, twenty-five to thirty pMHC ligands are required for optimal T cell activation, highlighting the importance of accessory adhesion molecules under conditions of low antigen density [35]. CD4 and CD8 co-receptors move into the vicinity of the engaged TCR, promoting more avid adhesion and delivering the signaling molecule LCK [47]. These changes result in the recruitment of additional signaling molecules, including the CD3ζ chain, ζ-chain-associated protein kinase of 70kDa (ZAP70), and phosphatidylinositol 3-kinase (PI3K). The linker for the activation of T cells (LAT) is also recruited to the complex, serving as a lynchpin for accumulating additional downstream effector molecules [35]. PI3K activity increases local level of membrane-bound phosphatidylinositol-3,4,5-triphosphate (IP_3), which results in the translocation of cytoskeletal proteins and additional protein kinases to the region. The TCR, CD4 or CD8 coreceptors, and other receptors that transduce costimulatory signals (CD28 and CTLA-4 for example) coalesce at one end of the cell along with specialized membrane structure termed lipid rafts, resulting in a polarization of the T cell toward the professional APC [35]. Additionally, the microtubule organizing center (MTOC) translocates to an area immediately adjacent to the cell-cell contact site.

Within five to thirty minutes of continuous signaling, the mature immunological synapse has formed at the cell-cell interface [35]. At this phase, the diverse components of the immunological synapse have undergone molecular segregation into distinct zones denoted by supramolecular activation complexes (SMACs). The central area of the synapse, the cSMAC, is enriched for TCR, associated CD3 complexes, and the signaling molecule protein kinase Cθ(PKCθ). Additional molecules that can be found in the cSMAC are CD28, CTLA4, CD2, CD4, CD45, the IFNγ receptor, and the IL-4 receptor. Immediately surrounding this area is a peripheral ring of adhesion and cytoskeletal molecules enriched for LFA1 and talin; this region is the pSMAC. Larger molecules such as CD43 and CD45 are found even more peripherally in the distal SMAC (dSMAC). The recruitment of a second wave of accessory molecules for T cell activation is dependent on both TCR:pMHC interaction (signal 1), and CD28:B7 or LFA1:ICAM1 interaction (signal 2). After about ten hours of sustained signaling, the TCR is internalized from the cSMAC to cytoplasmic vesicles. While this provides a mechanism for reducing signal intensity,

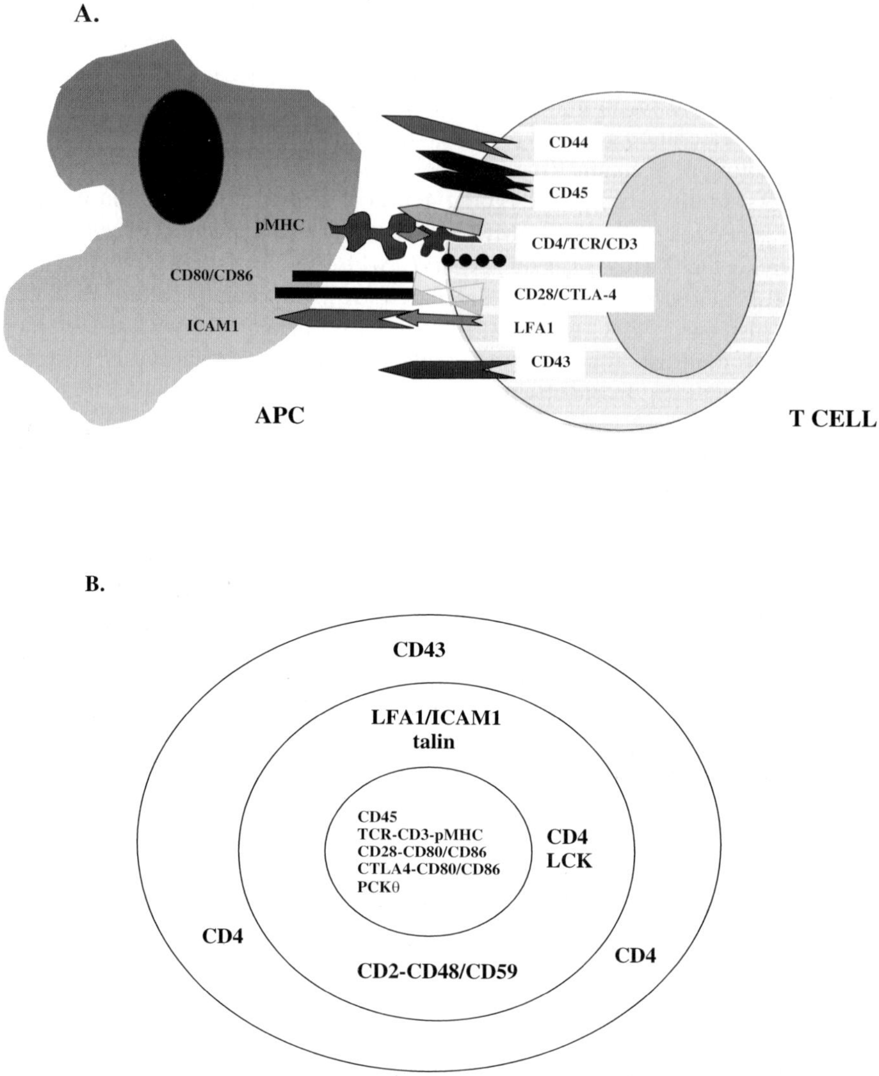

Figure 2. **The Immunological Synapse. A.** The immunological synapse is a complex, highly organized structure that concentrates signaling and adhesion molecules critical for T cell activation within the focal point of contact between the dendritic cell (DC) and the T cell (for the priming synapse), or the target cell and the T cell (for the secretory/effector synapse). **B.** The critical molecules are located centrally in the central supramolecular activation complex (cSMAC), with accessory molecules located in the surrounding zones of the peripheral SMAC (pSMAC) and the distal SMAC (dSMAC)

newly synthesized TCR are recruited back into the synapse, restoring the fully mature synapse within twenty-four hours [49]. To complement TCR downregulation as a means of initiating resolution of the synapse, the negative costimulatory molecule CTLA-4 is progressively recruited into the synapse [50]. Within this specialized space, it competes with CD28 for binding to CD80 and CD86. It also inhibits TCR signaling by recruiting the SRC homology 2 (SH2)-domain-containing tyrosine phosphatase 2 (SHP2) to dephosphorylate activated components of the TCR partner CD3 [51]. Clearly, the immunologic synapse is a dynamic structure, and evolves during the course of T cell activation. This creates a mechanism for the bidirectional cross-talk from the APC to the T cell and back again.

THE EFFECTOR (SECRETORY) IMMUNOLOGIC SYNAPSE

A specialized variant of the stable immunological synapse of immune priming is the secretory (effector) immunologic synapse. The secretory synapse is formed upon engagement of CTLs, T helper cells, and NK cells with their target cells. These activated effector cells contain granules that harbor soluble cytokines, perforins, and/or granzymes. The secretory synapse forms in a manner analogous to the development of the priming synapse. However, with translocation of the MTOC to the area just beneath the cSMAC, secretory granules are railroaded along the cytoskeleton through a specialized area of the cSMAC free of TCR [52]. This configuration allows CTLs to deliver a lethal hit to the target cell by releasing granzymes, perforins, proteoglycans, and lysosomal proteins in a highly directed fashion. It also allows T helper cells to deliver trophic cytokines (IL-2, IL-4, IL-5, IFN-γ) in a focal manner to the area of immediate contact with B cells. In contrast to the priming synapse, which requires ten pMHC ligands and ten to twenty four hours of continuous signaling [49], the initiation of lysis by $CD8^+$ T cells requires the recognition of a minimum of three pMHC ligands, and only three to five minutes of cell-cell contact [35]. Notably, CTL can form synapses with many target cells simultaneously [53], with the T cell MTOC oscillating between target cell sites [54].

CO-STIMULATION AND COUNTER-STIMULATION: THE IMMUNOLOGIC RHEOSTAT

The essential second signal for T cell activation is provided by the interaction of accessory signaling molecules for T cell activation present on the T cell surface with their corresponding ligands present on professional APC. This second signal can be provided by any number of molecules within the B7 or tumor necrosis factor receptor (TNFR) protein families, and ultimately results from the summation of a variety of positive and negative signals transduced by these family members [55]. This system provides a versatile approach for fine-tuning the antigen-specific T cell response, and determines not only the magnitude of the activation signal, but also the character, quality, and duration of the primary T cell response. It also determines the size and phenotype of the memory T cell pool established, and thus the capacity of the immune system to respond to future antigen exposure.

The B7 Family. The B7 family of molecules is a system of receptor-ligand pairs composed of one molecule that transmits a positive signal, and a counter-regulatory molecule that transduces a complementary negative signal [56,57]. This paradigm for the control of T cell activation was established by the identification and characterization of the first set of molecules in the family. B7-1 (CD80) and B7-2 (CD86) interact with CD28 to promote T cell activation, and B7-1/B7-2 interact with the counter-regulatory molecule CTLA-4 to dampen it by feedback inhibition. Highlighting their importance in T cell activation, these molecules modulate the strength of T cell activation in two ways. First, CTLA-4 preferentially attenuates strong signals for T cell activation delivered by the bound TCR in order to limit T cell expansion [50]. Second, CTLA-4 delivers negative signals concomitant with the positive signals transmitted by the bound TCR, thereby raising the threshold for T cell activation [50]. Lending even further flexibility to the signaling system, CD28 and CTLA-4 are preferentially recruited to the immunologic synapse by B7-2 and B7-1 respectively [58]. This preferred partnering tunes the immune response at the molecular and cellular level, where the activating potential of the APC is determined by its relative expression of B7-1 and B7-2.

Newer members of the B7 family can regulate primary immune responses not only at the time of immune priming, but also during the effector phase [59]. Thus, they are expressed by both lymphoid and nonlymphoid tissues. Inducible costimulator (ICOS) is expressed by activated T cells and resting memory T cells, and transmits a positive signal upon engagement with its ligand ICOSL (GL-50, B7RP-1, B7-h, B7H-2). The ICOSL is expressed constitutively by professional APC, and is induced in nonlymphoid tissues under inflammatory conditions. Consistent with its expression pattern, ICOS/ICOSL interactions occur distal to CD28 costimulation. ICOS signaling promotes the T helper type 2 immune response, augmenting interleukin-10 (IL-10) production and $CD4^+$ T cell effector function. It further promotes T cell-dependent humoral immunity by activating the CD40/CD40 ligand (CD40L) pathway [60]. Notably, expression of the ICOSL within the tumor microenvironment facilitates tumor rejection [61]. Thus, the primary role of the ICOS pathway is to support T cell function. However, emerging evidence suggests that it may also exert a negative influence on T cell activation [59]. ICOS-related counter-regulatory mechanisms remain to be elucidated.

B7-H3 is expressed primarily in nonlymphoid tissues. It binds to an unknown ligand expressed by activated T cells to increase T cell proliferation and IFN-γ secretion [62]. Expression of B7-H3 in tumor cells increases their immunogenicity. In a plasmacytoma system, ectopic expression of B7-H3 leads to a vigorous tumor-specific CTL response, resulting in tumor rejection [63]. In an EL-4 lymphoma system, the ectopic expression of B7-H3 by gene transfer induced NK- and $CD8^+$ T cell-dependent tumor regression up to 50% of the time [64]. Despite its ability to promote antitumor immunity, B7-H3 can down regulate the T helper type 1 immune response thought to be optimal for tumor rejection [65]. Thus, it may also downregulate tumor immunity depending upon the context in which it is engaged.

The programmed death-1 (PD-1) receptor group includes PD-1 and its ligands B7-H1 (PD-L1) and B7-DC (PD-L2) [59]. PD-1 is induced by T and B cell activation, and is also expressed by myeloid cells. B7-H1 is constitutively expressed on the surface of T cells, macrophages, and DCs. It is also expressed by normal host tissues, and is upregulated by many tumors. In contrast, B7-DC is expressed primarily by professional APC. It is expressed at high levels by mature DCs, and at lower levels by activated macrophages. The engagement of B7-DC provides a bi-directional signal between the DC and the T cell, and its activation synergizes strongly with signaling through B7-1 and B7-2 to augment T cell proliferation and cytokine production [66]. B7-DC signaling promotes the T helper type 1 phenotype (IFN-γ production) over the T helper type 2 phenotype (IL-4 and IL-10 secretion) [67]. This potent co-stimulatory activity is associated with a receptor distinct from PD-1. Interestingly, the ectopic expression of B7-DC in tumor cells provokes $CD8^+$ T cell-mediated tumor rejection by augmenting both immune priming and T cell effector function [68]. Conversely, B7-DC engagement with its counter-regulatory receptor PD-1 blunts T cell activation, particularly when the signal for T cell activation is weak [69]. To achieve this, B7-DC/PD-1 interactions have an antigen-dependent inhibitory influence on signaling through the B7/CD28 pathway [70]. At low antigen concentrations, strong CD28-mediated signaling is globally inhibited. At high antigen concentrations, CD28 signaling is differentially regulated by B7-DC to maintain T cell proliferation but abrogate cytokine production.

An additional B7 family member, B7-H4, inhibits T and B cell activation by binding to its ligand B and T lymphocyte attenuator-4 (BTLA-4) [59]. Under normal conditions, the expression of B7-H4 is stringently controlled at the translational level, with widespread messenger RNA expression in normal host tissues in the absence of concomitant protein expression. B7-H4 protein expression is induced by inflammation, and is a common feature of many tumors. Given their expression pattern, both B7-H1 and B7-H4 are thought to inhibit immune responses within the tumor microenvironment. B7-H1 engagement causes the apoptosis of tumor reactive T cells [71], and signaling through B7-H4 inhibits TCR-activated T cell proliferation, and the maturation and effector function of $CD8^+$CTL [72].

The TNFR family. The TNFR family plays a central role in the initiation and expansion of the effector T cell response, and in determining its durability [73]. Six receptor-ligand pairs augment T cell activation (CD40/CD40L, OX40/OX40L, 41BB/41BBL, CD27/CD70, CD30/CD30L, and herpes viral entry mediator (HVEM)/LIGHT). CD40 is expressed constitutively by highly proliferative cells, including hematopoietic progenitor cells, epithelial cells, endothelial cells, and on all APC; activated leukocytes express CD40L [74]. The CD40/CD40L pathway is essential for T cell-dependent humoral immunity, and activation of this pathway can substitute for T cell help in priming $CD4^+$ and $CD8^+$ T cell responses. OX40, 41BB, and CD30 are induced by T cell activation, and recruited to the immunologic synapse in a second wave after activation of primary co-stimulatory signaling by the

B7/CD28/CTLA-4 pathways. Accordingly, B7/CD28/CTLA-4 signals determine the level of expression and kinetics of recruitment of these downstream signaling molecules to the immunologic synapse. CD27 and HVEM are expressed under steady state conditions, with downregulation of HVEM upon T cell activation and subsequent restoration of constitutive HVEM levels upon return to the resting state. The ligands for these receptors, OX40L, 41BBL, CD70, and CD30L, are induced with the activation of professional APC. Consistent with the expression profile of HVEM, LIGHT is expressed by immature DCs, and is downregulated with DC maturation. Notably, forced expression of LIGHT within the tumor microenvironment provokes a vigorous $CD8^+$ T cell-dependent tumor rejection response [75].

MANIPULATION OF THE T CELL ENCOUNTER WITH ANTIGEN

Overall, co- and counter-stimulatory molecules function in concert to potentiate T cell activation, and ultimately determine the quality and longevity of the T cell response. Importantly, each of these pathways offers an opportunity for the therapeutic manipulation of the molecular context in which a T cell sees antigen in order to maximize antitumor immunity.

αCTLA-4 Monoclonal Antibodies (MAb). MAbs blocking CTLA-4 have already been tested in several clinical trials. Preclinical studies showed that αCTLA-4 MAbs alone can induce the $CD8^+$ T cell-dependent regression of established tumors, even in the absence of vaccination [51]. They further demonstrated that combining αCTLA-4 blockade with GM-CSF-secreting tumor vaccines produced synergistic tumor regression compared to antibody or vaccination alone [76, 77]. Three clinical trials testing a humanized MAb specific for CTLA-4 have been reported [78–80]. One study included nine previously vaccinated patients with metastatic melanoma or ovarian cancer; five had been immunized with GM-CSF-secreting autologous tumor cells, and four with gp100- or MART-1-specific peptide vaccines for melanoma [78]. Of these patients, three melanoma patients previously vaccinated with GM-CSF-secreting autologous tumor cells developed immune cell infiltrates with extensive tumor necrosis as demonstrated by tumor biopsies, and two ovarian cancer patients had stable or declining levels of the tumor marker CA-125. Two studies tested αCTLA-4 in combination with active peptide vaccination for metastatic melanoma [79, 80]. Both reported clinically significant autoimmune toxicity that appeared to track with clinical benefit as measured by objective tumor regression [79] or freedom from disease relapse [80].

αB7-DC MAb. A naturally occurring IgM antibody specific for B7-DC can augment the antigen processing function of DC, increase cytokine production, and promote their survival [81, 82]. This MAb increases the efficacy of naïve T cell activation by DC, and promotes the induction of a $CD4^+$ and $CD8^+$ T cell-dependent immune response that can reject established B16 melanomas. The development of therapeutics targeting B7-DC is an area of active study.

α B7-H1, αB7-H4, and αICOS MAb. Myeloid DC in the blood, draining lymph nodes, and tumor nodules of patients with ovarian cancer express high levels of B7-H1 [83]. Blocking MAb specific for B7-H1 enhanced the ability of these myeloid DC to prime T cell activation. Another study reported the ability of a MAb that blocks B7-H1 signaling to augment the effectiveness of adoptive T cell immunotherapy for squamous cell carcinoma of the head and neck [84]. Also consistent with its ability to regulate effector T cell function, MAb specific for either B7-H1 or its co-receptor PD-1 can facilitate tumor regression mediated by therapeutic MAb specific for 41BB [85]. Neither B7-H4 nor ICOS-directed immunomodulation has been reported.

α 41BB MAb. MAb specific for 41BB as a single intervention can cause the regression of poorly immunogenic tumors [86]. This activity is dependent on $CD4^+$ and $CD8^+$ T cells as well as NK cells. This antibody can potentiate the function of preactivated $CD8^+$ T cells by prolonging their survival [87]. In combination with active vaccination, α41BB MAb synergizes with immunization to break immunologic ignorance, and facilitates the $CD4^+$ T helper cell response, thereby enlisting pre-exisiting and ineffective tumor-specific immune effectors to provoke vigorous tumor rejection [87, 88]. Therapeutics targeting 41BB have not yet been tested in human clinical trials.

α OX40 MAb. OX40-signaling promotes the activation and survival of effector $CD4^+$ T cells in response to antigen-specific immune priming, potentiating humoral immune response and increasing the size of the $CD4^+$ memory T cell pool [89]. Emerging evidence suggests that it promotes the function of OX40-expressing $CD8^+$ effector T cells directly, and helps T cells traffic through the tumor microvasculature into the tumor mass by binding OX40L expressed by endothelial cells. Agonist MAb specific for OX40 can circumvent $CD4^+$ T cell tolerance [90] by inhibiting peripheral deletion [91] and abrogating the negative influence of $CD4^+CD25^+$ T regs [92, 93]. Administering agonist MAb as a single agent to mice with pre-established tumors results in durable T cell-dependent tumor-free survival in models of melanoma, sarcoma, colon cancer, breast cancer, and glioma [89]. $CD4^+$ memory T cells adoptively transferred from these mice can subsequently protect naïve mice from a challenge with homologous tumor. Lending further credence to the concept of manipulating multiple T cell co-stimulatory pathways, the impact of OX40 ligation is markedly potentiated by concomitant 41BB ligation (in the present of IL-12) [94] or GM-CSF exposure [95]. A human OX40-specific MAb has been developed, and will soon enter clinical testing in patients with advanced malignancies.

αCD40 MAb. Although CD40 is not critical for the activation of naïve T cells, it does play a central role in the activation of antigen-specific memory T cell pools [76]. MAb specific for CD40 are especially effective against B cell malignancies that express high cell surface levels of the molecule, the expression of CD40 by epithelial and mesenchymal tumors suggests that it could have activity against those tumor types as well. Potential mechanisms include promoting tumor cell lysis by direct binding, increasing antigen processing and presentation (particularly for malignant B cells) and enhancing tumor-specific CTL activity. When agonist αCD40 MAbs are combined with tumor vaccines, the maturation of endogenous DC is enhanced. This results in the cross-presentation of relevant tumor antigens, thereby providing a pathway to circumvent established tumor-specific immune tolerance [96, 97]. Agonist CD40 MAbs are just entering human clinical trials.

SYSTEMIC AND LOCAL ENVIRONMENTAL CONSTRAINTS ON ACTIVATED ANTITUMOR T CELLS

It is now clear that functional T cells of low or high avidity may be directly suppressed by a variety of immunoregulatory cells [8]. At least three types of regulatory cells help to keep immune responses in check, including immature DCs, myeloid suppressor cells (MSCs), and $CD4^+CD25^+$ regulatory T cells (Tregs). Inflammatory mediators induce DC maturation, recruiting MSCs in tandem to contain the immune response [98]. Naturally occurring and inducible $CD4^+CD25^+$ Tregs comprise 5% to 10% of $CD4^+$ T cells, and also play a key role in shutting immune responses down [99]. *In vivo*, the abrogation of Treg-mediated suppression promotes effective T cell-mediated antitumor immune responses [15, 100–102].

Multiple parameters control the locoregional priming and migration of antitumor T cells to the local tumor mass, where they recognize and respond to tumor antigens expressed by diseased cells. Once there, additional factors specific to the tumor microenvironment itself frequently hamper T cell activity. Physical antigen recognition itself may be suboptimal due to antigen loss variants, MHC molecule loss variants, or tumor cell-specific mutations in critical components of the antigen processing machinery [103]. Additionally, tumor cells themselves produce a number of factors that promote Treg activity (Cyclooxygenase 2 (COX2)/prostaglandin E2 (PGE-2), or MSC (GM-CSF/VEGF) activity, or that inhibit DC activity (IL-10, TGF-β, VEGF). These latter tumor cell-derived cytokines upregulate the STAT-3 pathway, which itself blocks DC maturation [19, 104, 105]. Additionally, tumor cells express IDO, and recruit IDO-expressing APC, all of which promotes the local development of Tregs. Thus the lack of inflammatory stimuli is compounded by active immunosuppressive factors that prevent antitumor T cell activity where it is most needed. In this case, conditioning the tumor microenvironment to provide a more favorable context for T cell activity might be effective. Genetic strategies that re-program the tumor to effectively present tumor antigens are under active investigation. Additionally, the use of modulatory drugs that block the suppressive influences specific to the tumor microenvironment is receiving increasing attention in immunotherapeutic research.

CONCLUSIONS

Great strides in our understanding of how T cells see antigen at the molecular and cellular level have contributed to recent preclinical and clinical progress in T cell-based immunotherapy. Superimposed on the precise interactions of the TCR with the pMHC complex are additional mechanisms that define the antitumor T cell repertoire, and control its activity. Thus, the larger context in which these T cells recognize antigen is as important as the processes by which they directly see it.

Further scientific progress elucidating the mechanisms controlling antitumor T cell activity will provide the foundation for developing effective clinical strategies that harness the power of the antitumor T cell response in the fight against cancer.

REFERENCES

1. Oltz E. Regulation of antigen receptor gene assembly in lymphocytes. Immunol Res 2001; 23:121–133.
2. Germain R. The biochemistry and cell biology of antigen presentation by MHC Class I and Class II molecules. Implications for development of combination vaccines. Ann NY Acad Sci 1995;754:114–125.
3. Pulendran B. Modulating Th1/Th2 responses with microbes, dendritic cells, and pathogen recognition receptors. Immunol Res 2004;29:187–196.
4. Kidd P. Th1/Th2 balance: the hypothesis, its limitations, and implications for health and disease. Alt Med Rev 2003;8:223–246.
5. Brandes M, Williman K, Moser B. Professional antigen presentation function by human $\gamma\delta$ T cells. Science 2005;309:264–268.
6. Trombetta E, Mellman I. Cell biology of antigen processing *in vitro* and *in vivo* . Ann Rev Immunol 2005;23:975–1028.
7. Huang A, Qi H, Germain R. Illuminating the landscape of *in vivo* immunity: insights from dynamic *in situ* imaging of secondary lymphoid tissues. Immunity 2004;21:331–339.
8. Walker L, Abbas A. The enemy within: keeping self-reactive T cells at bay in the periphery. Nat Rev Immunol 2001;21:11–19.
9. Morgan D, Kreuwel H, Fleck S et al. Activation of low avidity CTL specific for a self epitope results in tumor rejection but not autoimmunity. J Immunol 1998;160:643–651.
10. Lui G, Fairchild P, Smith R et al. Low avidity antigen recognition of self antigen by T cells permits escape from central tolerance. Immunity 1995;3:407–415.
11. De Visser K, Cordaro T, Kessels H et al. Low avidity self-specific T cells display a pronounced expansion defect that can be overcome by altered peptide ligands. J Immunol 2001;167: 3818–3828.
12. Lymann M, Nugent C, Marquardt K et al. The fate of low affinity tumor specific $CD8^+$ T cells in tumor-bearing mice. J Immunol 2005;174:2563–2572.
13. Hernandez J, Ko A, Sherman L. CTLA-4 blockade enhances the CTL responses to the p53 self-tumor antigen. J Immunol 2001;166:3908–3914.
14. Gross D-A, Graff-Dubois S, Opolon P et al. High vaccination efficiency of low affinity epitopes in antitumor immunotherapy. J Clin Invest 2004;113:425–433.
15. Ercolini A, Ladle B, Manning E et al. Recruitment of latent pools of high aviditiy $CD8^+$ T cells to the antitumor immune response. J Exp Med 2005; 201: 1591–1602.
16. Davis M, Boniface J, Rieich Z et al. Ligand recognition by $\alpha\beta$ T cell receptors. Ann Rev Immunol 1998;15:523–544.
17. Jameson J, Witherden D, Havran W. T cell effector mechanisms: gamma delta and CD1d-restricted subsets. Curr Opin Immunol 2003;15:349–353.
18. Mani A, Gelmann E. The ubiquitin-proteasome pathway and its role in cancer. J Clin Oncol 2005;23:4776–4789.
19. Yewdell J, Schuburt U, Bennick J. At the crossroads of cell biology and immunology: DRiPs and other sources of peptide ligands for MHC Class I molecules. J Cell Sci 2001;114:845–851.
20. van den Eynde B, Morel S. Differential processing of Class-I-restricted epitopes by the standard proteasome and the immunoproteasome. Curr Opin Immunol 2001;13:147–153.
21. Morel S, Levy F, Burlet-Schiltz O et al. Processing of some antigens by the standard proteasome but not by the immunoproteasome results in poor presentation by dendritic cells. Immunity 2000;12:107–117.

22. Sun Y, Sijts A, Song M et al. Expression of the proteasome activator PA28 rescues the presentation of a cytotoxic T lymphocyte epitope on melanoma cells. Cancer Res 2002;62:2875–2882.
23. Chen W, Norbury C, Cho Y et al. Immunoproteasomes shape immunodominance hierarchies of antiviral $CD8^+$ T cells at the levels of T cell repertoire and presentation of viral antigens. J Exp Med 2001;193:1319–1326.
24. Toes R, Nussbaum A, Degerman S et al. Discrete cleavage motifs of constitutive and immunoproteasomes revealed by quantitative analysis of cleavage products. J Exp Med 2001;194:1–12.
25. Melief C. Regulation of cytotoxic T lymphocyte responses by dendritic cells: peaceful coexistence of cross-priming and direct priming? Eur J Immunol 2003;33:2645–2654.
26. Ackerman A, Cresswell P. Cellular mechanisms governing cross-presentation of exogenous antigens. Nature Immunol 2004;5:678–684.
27. Heath W, Belz G, Behrens G et al. Cross-presentation, dendritic cell subsets, and the generation of immunity to cellular antigens. Immunol Rev 2004;199:9–26.
28. Heath W, Carbone F. Cross-presentation in viral immunity and self-tolerance. Nature Rev Immunol 2001;1:126–134.
29. Bevan M. Minor H antigens introduced on H-2 different stimulating cells cross-react at the cytotoxic T cell level during *in vivo* priming. J Immunol 1976;117:2233–2238.
30. Bevan M. Cross-priming for a secondary cytotoxic response to minor H antigens with H-2 congenic cells which do not cross-react in the cytotoxic assay. J Exp Med 1976;143:1283–1288.
31. Gooding L, Edwards C. H-2 antigen requirements in the *in vitro* induction of SV-40-specific cytotoxic T lymphocytes. J Immunol 1980;123:125801262.
32. Huang A, Golumbek P, Ahmdzadeh M et al. Role of bone marrow-derived cells in presenting MHC class I-restricted tumor antigens. Science 1994;264:961–965.
33. Huang A, Bruce A, Pardoll D et al. *In vivo* cross-priming of MHC class I-restricted antigens requires TAP transporter. Immunity 1996;4:349–355.
34. Thomas A, Santarsiero L, Lutz E et al. Mesothelin-specific $CD8^+$ T cell responses provide evidence of *in vivo* cross-priming by antigen-presenting cells in vaccinated pancreatic cancer patients. J Exp Med 2004;200:297–306.
35. Huppa J, Davis M. T cell antigen recognition and the immunological synapse. Nature Rev Immunol 2003;3:973–983.
36. Krogsgaard M, Davis M. How T cells 'see' antigen. Nature Immunol 2005;6:239–245.
37. Borg N, Ely L, Beddoe T et al. The CDR3 regions of an immunodominant T cell receptor dictate the 'energetic landscape' of peptide-MHC recognition. Nature Immunol 2005;6:171–180.
38. Reiser R, Gregoire C, Darnault C et al. A T cell receptor CDR3beta loop undergoes conformational changes of unprecedented magnitude upon binding to a peptide/MHC Class I complex. Immunity 2002;16:345–354.
39. Reiser R, Darnault C, Gregoire C et al. CDR3 loop flexibility contributes to the degeneracy of T cell recognition. Nature Immunol 2003;4:241–247.
40. Wu L, Tuot D, Lyons D et al. Two-step binding mechanism for T cell receptor recognition of peptide MHC. Nature 2002;418:553–556.
41. Zhao R, Collins E. Enhancing cytotoxic T cell responses with altered peptide ligands. Arch Immunol Ther Exp 2001; 49: 271–277.
42. Bakker A, van der Burg S, Huijbens R et al. Analogues of CTL epitopes with improved MHC Class I binding capacity elicit anti-melanoma CTL recognizing the wild-type epitope. Int J Cancer 1997;70:302–309.
43. Dyall R, Bowne W, Weber L et al. Heteroclitic immunization induces tumor immunity. J Exp Med 1998;188: 1553–1561.
44. Overwijk W, Tsung A, Irvine K et al. pg100/pmel17 is a murine tumor rejection antigen: induction of "self"-reactive, tumoricidal T cells using high affinity, altered peptide ligand. J Exp Med 1998;188:277–286.
45. Valmori D, Fonteneau J, Valitutti S et al. Optimal activation of tumor-reactive T cells by selected antigenic peptide analogues. Int Immunol 1999;11:1971–1980.

46. Slansky J, Rattis R, Boyd L et al. Enhanced antigen-specific immunity with altered peptide ligands that stabilize the MHC-peptide-TCR complex. Immunity 2000;13:529–538.
47. Li Q-J, Dinner A, Qi S et al. CD4 enhances T cell sensitivity to antigen by coordinating Lck accumulation at the immunological synapse. Nature Immunol 2004;5:791–799.
48. Dustin M. Stop and go traffic to tune T cell responses. Immunity 2004;21:305–314.
49. Huppa J, Gleimer M, Sumen C et al. Continuous T cell receptor signaling required for synapse maintenance and full effector potential. Nature Immunol 2003;4(749–755).
50. Egen J, Allison J. Cytotoxic T lymphocyte antigen-4 accumulation in the immunological synapse is regulated by TCR signal strength. Immunity 2002;16:23–35.
51. Egen J, Kuhns M, Allison J. CTLA-4: new insights into its biological function and use in tumor immunotherapy. Nature Immunol 2002;3:611–618.
52. Stinchcombe J, Bossi G, Booth S et al. The immunological synapse of CTL contains a secretory domain and membrane bridges. Immunity 2001;15:751–761.
53. McGavern D, Christen U, Oldstone M. Molecular anatomy of antigen-specific $CD8^+$ T cell engagement and synapse formation *in vivo*. Nature Immunol 2002;3:918–925.
54. Kuhn J, Poenie M. Dynamic polarization of the microtubule cytoskeleton during CTL-mediated killing. Immunity 2002;16:111–121.
55. Pardoll D. Spinning molecular immunology into successful immunotherapy. Nature Rev Immunol 2002;2:227–238.
56. Greenwald R, Freeman G, Sharpe A. The B7 family revisited. Ann Rev Immunol 2005;23: 515–548.
57. McCoy K, Le Gros G. The role of CTLA-4 in the regulation of T cell immune responses. Immunol Cell Biol 1999;77:1–10.
58. Pentcheva-Hoang T, Egen J, Wojnoonski et al. B7–1 and B7–2 selectively recruit CTLA-4 and CD28 to the immunological synapse. Immunity 2004;21:401–413.
59. Khoury S, Sayegh M. The roles of the new negative T cell costimulatory pathways in regulating autoimmunity. Immunity 2004;20:529–538.
60. McAdam A, Greenwald R, Levin M et al. ICOS is critical for CD40-mediated antibody class-switching. Nature 2001;409:102–105.
61. Wallin J, Liang L, Bakardjiev A et al. New regulatory co-receptors: inducible co-stimulator and PD-1. Curr Opin Immunol 2002;14:779–782.
62. Chapoval A, Ni J, Lau J et al. B7-H3: a costimulatory molecule for T cell activation and IFN-γ production. Nature Immunol 2001;2:269–274.
63. Luo L, Chapoval A, Flies D et al. B7-H3 enhances tumor immunity *in vivo* by costimulating rapid clonal expansion of antigen-specific $CD8^+$ cytolytic T cells. J Immunol 2004;173:5445–5450.
64. Sun X, Richards S, Prasad D et al. Mouse B7-H3 induces antitumor immunity. Gene Ther 2003;10:1728–1734.
65. Suh W, Gajewska B, Okada H et al. The B7 family member B7-H3 preferentially down-regulates T helper type 1-mediated immune responses. Nature Immunol 2003;4:899–906.
66. Shin T, Kennedy G, Gorski K et al. Cooperative B7–1/2 (CD80/86) and B7-DC costimulation of $CD4^+$ T cells independent of the PD-1 receptor. J Exp Med 2003;198:31–38.
67. Tseng B, Otsuji M, Gorski K et al. B7-DC, a new dendritic cell molecule with potent costimulatory properties for T cells. J Exp Med 2001;193:839–845.
68. Liu X, Gao J, Wen J et al. B7-DC/PD-L2 promotes tumor immunity by a PD-1-independent mechanism. J Exp Med 2003;197:1721–1730.
69. Freeman G, Long A, Iwai Y et al. Engagement of the PD-1 immunoinhibitory receptor by a novel B7 family member leads to negative regulation of lymphocyte activation. J Exp Med 2000;192:1027–1034.
70. Latchman Y, Wood C, Chernova T et al. PD-L2 is a second ligand for PD-1 and inhibits T cell activation. Nature Immunol 2001;2:261–268.
71. Dong H, Strome S, Salomao D et al. Tumor-associated B7-H1 promotes T-cell apoptosis: a potential mechanism of immune evasion. Nature Med 2002;8:793–800.

72. Sica G, Choi I, Zhu G et al. B7-H4, a molecule of the B7 family, negatively regulates T cell immunity. Immunity 2003;18:849–861.
73. Watts T. TNF/TNFR family members in costimulation of T cell responses. Ann Rev Immunol 2005;23:23–68.
74. Tong A, Stone M. Prospects for CD40-directed experimental therapy of human cancer. Cancer Gene Ther 2002;10:1–13.
75. Yu P, Lee Y, Liu W et al. Priming of naive T cells inside tumors leads to eradication of established tumors. Nature Immunol 2004;5:141–149.
76. Hurwitz A, Yu T, Leach D, et al. CTLA-4 blockade synergizes with tumor-derived granulocyte-macrophage colony-stimulating factor for treatment of an experimental mammary carcinoma. Proc Natl Acad Sci USA 1998;18:10067–10071.
77. van Elsas A, Hurwitz A, Allison J. Combination immunotherapy of B16 melanoma using anti-cytotoxic T lymphocyte-associated antigen-4 (CTLA-4) and granulocyte-macrophage colony-stimulating factor (GM-CSF)-producing vaccines induces rejection of subcutaneous and metastatic tumors accompanied by autoimmune depigmentation. J Exp Med 1999;190:355–366.
78. Hodi F, Mihm M, Soiffer R et al. Biologic activity of cytotoxic T lymphocyte-associated antigen 4 antibody blockade in previously vaccinated metastatic melanoma and ovarian carcinoma patients. Proc Natl Acad Sci USA 2003;100:4712–4717.
79. Phan G, Yang J, Sherry R et al. Cancer regression and autoimmunity induced by cytotoxic T lymphocyte-associated antigen 4 blockade in patients with metastatic melanoma. Proc Natl Acad Sci USA 2003;100:8372–8377.
80. Sanderson K, Scotland R, Lee P et al. Autoimmunity in a phase I trial of a fully human anti-cytotoxic T-lymphocyte antigen-4 monoclonal antibody with multiple melanoma peptides and Montanide ISA 51 for patients with resected stages III and IV melanoma. J Clin Oncol 2005;23:741–750.
81. Radhakrishnan S, Nguyen L, Ciric B et al. Naturally occurring human IgM antibody that binds B7-DC and potentiates T cell stimulation by dendritic cells. J Immunol 2003;170:1830–1838.
82. Radhakrishnan S, Nguyen L, Ciric B et al. Immunotherapeutic potential of B7-DC (PD-L2) cross-linking antibody in conferring antitumor immunity. Cancer Res 2004;64:4965–4972.
83. Curiel T, Wei S, Dong H et al. Blockade of B7-H1 improves myeloid dendritic cell-mediated antitumor immunity. Nature Med 2003;9:562–567.
84. Strome S, Dong H, Tamura H et al. B7-H1 blockade augments adoptive T-cell immunotherapy for squamous cell carcinoma. Cancer Res 2003;63:6501–6501.
85. Hirano F, Kaneko K, Tamura H et al. Blockade of B7-H1 and PD-1 by monoclonal antibodies potentiates cancer therapeutic immunity. Cancer Res 2005;65:1089–1096.
86. Melero I, Shuford W, Newby S et al. Monoclonal antibodies against the 4–1BB T-cell activation molecule eradicate established tumors. Nature Med 1997;3:682–685.
87. May K, Chen L, Zheng P et al. Anti-4–1BB monoclonal antibody enhances rejection of large tumor burden by promoting survival but not clonal expansion of tumor-specific $CD8^+$ T cells. Cancer Res 2002;62:3459–3465.
88. Ito F, Li Q, Shreiner A, Okuyama R et al. Anti-CD137 monoclonal antibody administration augments the antitumor efficacy of dendritic cell-based vaccines. Cancer Res 2004;64:8411–8419.
89. Sugamura K, Ishii N, Weinberg A. Therapeutic targeting of the effector T-cell co-stimulatory molecule OX40. Nature Rev Immunol 2004;4:420–431.
90. Bansal-Pakala P, Jember A, Croft M. Signaling through OX40 (CD134) breaks peripheral T-cell tolerance. Nature Med 2001;7:907–912.
91. Maxwell J, Weinberg A, Prell R et al. Danger and OX40 receptor signaling synergize to enhance memory T cell survival by inhibiting peripheral deletion. J Immunol 2000;164:107–112.
92. Takeda I, Ine S, Killeen N et al. Distinct roles for the OX40-OX40 ligand interaction in regulatory and nonregulatory T cells. J Immunol 2004;172:3580–3589.
93. Valzasina B, Guiducci C, Dislich H et al. Triggering of OX40 (CD134) on $CD4^+CD25^+$ T cells blocks their inhibitory activity: a novel regulatory role for OX40 and its comparison with GITR. Blood 2005;105:2845–2851.

94. Pan P, Zang Y, Weber K et al. OX40 ligation enhances primary and memory cytotoxic T lymphocyte responses in an immunotherapy for hepatic colon metastases. Molecular Ther 2002;6:528–536.
95. Gri G, Gallo E, Di Carlo E et al. OX40 ligand-transduced tumor cell vaccine synergizes with GM-CSF and requires CD40-APC signaling to boost the host T cell antitumor response. J Immunol 2003;170:99–106.
96. Diehl L, den Boer A, van der Voort E et al. The role of CD40 in peripheral T cell tolerance and immunity. J Mol Med 2000;78:363–371.
97. Sotomayor E, Borrello I, Tubb E et al. Conversion of tumor-specific $CD4^+$ T-cell tolerance to T-cell priming through *in vivo* ligation of CD40. Nature Med 1999;5:780–787.
98. Bronte V, Serafini P, Mazzoni A et al. L-arginine metabolism in myeloid cells controls T-lymphocyte functions. Trends Immunol 2003;24:301–305.
99. O'Garra A, Vierira P. Regulatory T cells and mechanisms of immune system control. Nature Med 2004;10:801–805.
100. Onizuka S, Tawara I, Shimizu J et al. Tumor rejection by *in vivo* administration of anti-CD25 (interleukin-2 receptor alpha) monoclonal antibody. Cancer Res 1999;59:3128–3133.
101. Sutmuller R, van Duivenvoorde L, van Elsas A et al. Synergism of cytotoxic T lymphocyte-associated antigen-4 blockade and depletion of $CD25^+$ regulatory T cells in antitumor therapy reveals alternative pathways for suppression of autoreactive cytotoxic T lymphocyte responses. J Exp Med 2001;194:824–832.
102. Antony P, Piccirillo C, Akpinarli A et al. $CD8^+$ T cell immunity against a tumor/self-antigen is augmented by $CD4^+$ T helper cells and hindered by naturally occurring T regulatory cells. J Immunol 2005;174:2591–2601.
103. Ferrone S, Finerty J, Jaffee E et al. How much longer will tumour cells fool the immune system? Immunol Today 2000;21:70–72.
104. Wang T, Niu G, Kortylewski M et al. Regulation of the innate and adaptive immune responses by Stat-3-signaling in tumor cells. Nature Med 2004;10:48–54.
105. Munn D, Mellor A. IDO and tolerance to tumors. Trends Mol Med 2004;10:15–18.

CHAPTER 4

THE ROLE OF NATURAL KILLER T CELLS IN TUMOR IMMUNITY

MADHAV V. DHODAPKAR*

Laboratory of Tumor Immunology and Immunotherapy, The Rockefeller University, New York, NY; and Hematology Service, Memorial Sloan Kettering Cancer Center, New York, NY 10021

Keywords: innate immunity, cancer vaccine,

The immune system has several cellular components that can theoretically be recruited for protection from tumors [1, 2]. CD4+ and CD8+ T cells are the adaptive components of cell-mediated immunity. These cells differentiate upon antigen encounter to produce cytokines and lytic products, clonally expand, and establish memory. Natural killer (NK) and NKT cells have innate functions, already prepared to produce cytokines and lyse cells upon tumor recognition. NK and NKT cells do proliferate upon exposure to cytokines like IL-2, but they are not known to establish memory with either expanded cell numbers or improved function. In contrast to CD4 and CD8+ T cells that recognize peptide ligands in the context of major histocompatibility complex (MHC) I and II products, the NKT cells respond to glycolipid ligands presented in the context of CD1d on antigen presenting cells. Here I will review the recent data that have emphasized the growing importance of NKT cells in resistance against tumors.

WHAT IS A NKT CELL?

At the outset, it is important to clearly define what we mean by the term "NKT cells". NKT cells were first characterized in mice as cells that express both T cell receptor (TCR) and NK1.1, a C-lectin type NK receptor [3]. This definition however

*The Rockefeller University, 1230 York Avenue, #196, New York, NY 10021
E-mail: dhodapm@rockefeller.edu;

H.L. Kaufman and J.D. Wolchok (eds.), General Principles of Tumor Immunotherapy, 55–66.

does not satisfactorily delineate these innate glycolipid reactive lymphocytes. This has led to a revised nomenclature that emphasizes the CD1d restricted nature of these cells, as analyzed by binding to glycolipid loaded CD1d multimers (Figure 1) [4–7]. Most of the current data in this regard is restricted to CD1d tetramers loaded with a synthetic ligand, α-galactosyl ceramide (α-GalCer). Majority of the α-GalCer-CD1d multimer binding cells express an invariant T cell receptor (Vα14 in mice and Vα24 in humans), and are termed as type I NKT cells or invariant NKT (iNKT) cells [8]. Much of the current literature about the biology of NKT cells is restricted to this subset. These cells are also the subject of most of the discussion below, due to their anti-tumor properties. However, it has also become clear that several of the glycolipid reactive CD1d restricted T cells lack invariant TCR (termed type II NKT cells) [9]. Current data on identification of these cells with diverse TCRs is largely restricted to the α-GalCer-CD1d multimer, however it is likely that improved understanding of ligands naturally recognized by human NKT cells will provide greater insight into the spectrum of these cells. Finally, there is a heterogeneous subset of T cells with diverse TCRs that express NK markers, but are not CD1d restricted or glycolipid reactive, and are termed type III NKT cells [10]. These latter cells are diverse in their phenotypic and functional properties and not discussed here.

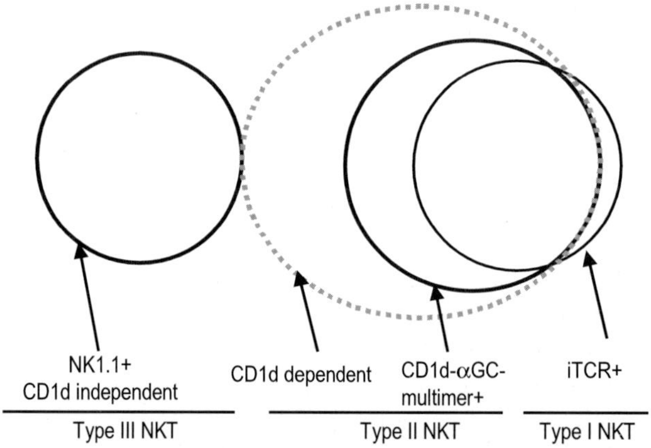

Figure 1. The spectrum of glycolipid reactive/NKT cells. Most of the currently visualized spectrum of glycolipid reactive T cells consists of T cells with invariant T cell receptors (Vα24/Vβ11 in humans; iTCR, termed type I NKT cells); or cells that bind CD1d-α-galactosyl ceramide multimer (CD1d-αGC multimer + cells). A subset of these lacks the invariant TCR and is termed type II NKT cells. The full spectrum of type II NKT cells (dotted line) remains to be elucidated, as the antigenic determinant of these CD1d restricted cells is not yet known. Type III NKT cells consist of T cells with diverse T cell receptors that express NK markers

LIGANDS RECOGNIZED BY INKT CELLS

The recognition of glycolipid ligands by iNKT cells means that these cells recognize ligands generally ignored by conventional T cells. Relatively few examples of ligands recognized by CD1d are known, although the recognition of mycobacterial lipids by other CD1 family molecules is now well recognized [7, 11]. Most of the current data about ligand reactive function for NKT cells is based on a synthetic ligand, α-galactosyl ceramide, which was originally isolated from a marine sponge [12]. α-GalCer is a strong agonist for NKT cells, and when presented by CD1d molecules, elicits strong interferon-γ and IL-4 production by both human and murine NKT cells [13]. Several other glycolipids have been tested for their capacity to stimulate NKT cells, including the ganglioside GD3 [14], glycophosphatidylinositol (GPI) [15], phosphoethanolamine [16], and some forms of β-GalCer [17], which stimulate subsets of these cells. More recently, isoglobotrihexosylceramide 3 (Igb3) [18] and glycolipids derived from the cell wall of a nonpathogenic bacterium, sphingomonas [19–21]; as well as some non-lipidic small molecules [22] were shown to bind murine and human CD1d. However, the nature of ligands recognized by human NKT cells *in vivo*, or the nature of tumor derived ligands for NKT cells remains unclear.

INNATE FUNCTIONS OF iNKT CELLS

A distinct functional property of NKT cells is their "innate effector function", and the ability to produce large amounts of cytokines within 1–2 hours of TCR ligation [6,7]. Individual NKT cells are able to make both Th1 and Th2 type cytokines (Th0 like cytokine pattern), which at face value seems paradoxical, as these cytokines are thought to often oppose biologic functions [23]. However, NKT cells can be skewed at least *in vitro* in either direction, depending on the nature of the activating stimulus, antigen presenting cell, or both. In addition to the prototypic Th1/Th2 cytokines, TCR activated NKT cells produce several other cytokines such as IL-2, tumor necrosis factor, IL-5, IL-13, and GM-CSF. At least in mice, these cells can store preformed mRNA for cytokines, even before activation with exogenous antigens, indicating that these cells are capable of rapidly producing cytokines [24]. The ability of NKT cells to secrete a diverse array of cytokines likely contributes to their immune regulatory function, although they may also have more direct cell contact dependent mechanisms for immune regulation. It is worth noting that the phenotype of NKT cells is at least in part overlapping with the CD4+CD25+ regulatory T cells, as CD4+ NKT cells in humans also express CD25 [6].

Another important feature of NKT cells is their ability to cause rapid activation of several immune cells including NK cells [25,26], DCs [27] and B cells (Figure 2). This has however been largely studied in the context of stimulation with α-GalCer, and may not reflect the situation with more physiologic stimulation *in vivo*. NKT cells can efficiently activate NK cells within hours to secrete interferon-γ and exhibit greater cytolytic activity against NK targets [25,26]. This ability of NKT cells to

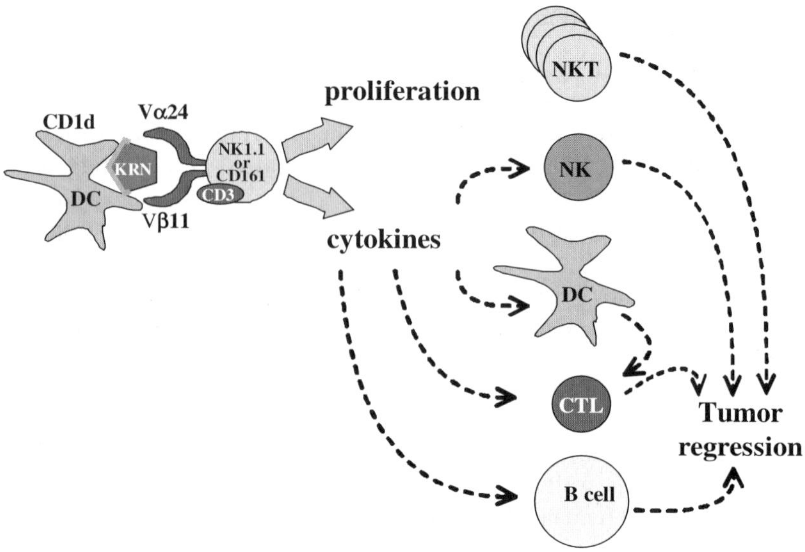

Figure 2. The cascade of immune activation by NKT cells. Activated NKT cells can mediate direct effects on tumor cells, as well as lead to rapid activation of several "downstream" immune cells, such as NK cells, T cells, dendritic cells and B cells

rapidly communicate with other immune cells may be critical to their function. For example, the bulk of systemic interferon-γ release after α-GalCer mediated NKT activation *in vivo* is due to the activity of NK cells [28]. NKT cells can also activate B cells to increase Ig secretion and therefore provide help for the generation of antibody responses [29].

ADJUVANT ROLE OF NKT CELLS IN ADAPTIVE IMMUNITY

Although much of the early work focused on the innate functions of NKT cells, more recent studies have emphasized the impact of NKT cells on the generation of antigen specific T cell responses. α-GalCer mediated activation of NKT cells leads to maturation of dendritic cells *in vivo*, which is associated with enhanced immunostimulatory function [30,31]. NKT mediated DC maturation requires CD40-CD40L interactions [32]. Thus although inflammatory cytokines released by NKT cells can lead to phenotypic changes typically associated with DC maturation, they do not lead to enhanced APC function, a hallmark of the maturation process. The ability of the NKT cells to transmit an "instructional signal" to DCs may be an avenue to link innate and adaptive immunity via DCs. Injection of α-GalCer and resultant NKT activation leads to enhanced T cell immunity to co-administered protein antigen [30,31]. Current studies are trying to extend this approach to other antigens including to whole tumor cells. The NKT-T interaction likely depends on the context in which it occurs, as NKT activation in autoimmune models has been shown to lead to initial activation, but subsequent T cell tolerance in the draining lymph nodes [33]. Further studies are needed to better characterize and exploit the potent ability of NKT cells to modify T cell function *in vivo*.

TISSUE DISTRIBUTION AND SUBSETS OF NKT CELLS

Human NKT cells include at least 2 major subsets, CD4+ and double negative (CD4-CD8-), although CD8+ NKT cells have also been described [34, 35]. Subsets of NKT cells in mice are less clear. Both CD4+ and CD4- subsets of NKT cells exist wherever other NKT cells are found, although the relative frequency may differ depending on the specific tissue. In mice, 20–40% of intrahepatic lymphocytes are iNKT cells. Tissue distribution of NKT cells in humans is less well studied, although they are certainly less frequent in human liver (<1%) compared to mice. Functionally, the different subsets of NKT cells differ in terms of their ability to produce cytokines *in vitro* and expression of chemokine receptors. For example, IL-4 production appears to be largely restricted to the CD4+ subset, while the double negative subset can produce interferon-γ. However the functional and biologic significance of these subsets remains to be clarified.

ANTI-TUMOR PROPERTIES OF NKT CELLS

Several studies have demonstrated the potential importance of NKT cells in tumor rejection [7, 7]. NKT cells were found to be necessary for IL-12 mediated anti-tumor immunity in mice [39]. Indeed, the discovery of α-GalCer as an NKT ligand was driven largely based on its ability to promote NKT and CD1d dependent rejection of a broad range of tumors including melanoma, thymoma, carcinoma, and sarcoma [40]. α-GalCer can also mediate protection against chemical or oncogene dependent tumors in mice [41]. The anti-tumor effects of α-GalCer seem to depend on its ability to induce strong production of interferon-γ *in vivo*, while other potentially NKT associated tumoricidal products such as TNF, Fas ligand, TRAIL, and perforin are also involved but may be dispensable [42]. In addition to the effects on tumor and other immune cells, interferon-γ mediated effects of NKT cells likely also involve inhibition of angiogenesis [43]. Consistent with the prime role for interferon-γ production by NKT cells, a C-glycoside analogue of α-GalCer that is more effective at inducing interferon production was also more effective at mediating tumor rejection as well [44]. In addition to cytokine production and direct cytolytic function, NKT activation can lead to activation of other "downstream" effectors. For example, NKT cells can cause rapid activation of NK cells *in vivo*. NKT cells may also enhance anti-tumor immunity by promoting the activation of antigen presenting dendritic cells (DCs) and IL-12 production via CD40 ligand (CD40 L) upregulation [32, 45].

Studies using α-GalCer support the concept that NKT cells can be recruited for protection against tumors *in vivo*. However they do not address whether these cells play a physiologic role in the protection from tumors *in vivo*. This is particularly important as α-GalCer is a synthetic and an exceptionally strong agonist, and physiologic ligands for NKT cells are not yet well characterized. One model where NKT cells are clearly required for tumor rejection is methylcholanthrene induced sarcomas in mice [46]. In this model, sarcomas formed with greater incidence in NKT deficient *Jα18 -/-* mice. Sarcoma cell lines also grew preferentially in NKT deficient mice and could be treated by adoptive transfer of NKT cells from wild type donors [47]. NKT cells were also shown to mediate tumor rejection in a lung metastasis model of sarcoma [48], wherein they were suppressed by regulatory T cells. As in α-GalCer induced effects, these effects are also interferon-γ dependent and involve downstream activation of both NK and CD8+ killer T cells [36].

ENHANCEMENT OF TUMOR GROWTH BY NKT CELLS

Although the data discussed above support a suppressive effect of NKT cells on tumor growth, NKT cells also appear to paradoxically enhance tumor growth in some models [49,50]. For example, experimental 15-12RM fibrosarcoma and 4T1 mammary tumors were rejected in CD1d -/- mice, but grew progressively in wild type mice. Tumor enhancement in the 15-12RM model was IL-13 dependent/IL-4 independent, and appeared to involve TGF-β production by Gr-1+ myeloid cells, that was associated with impaired CTL responses [51]. In contrast, the effects in 4T1 model were IL-13 independent, suggesting that other mechanisms of tumor enhancement exist. CD1d dependent T cells have also been implicated in UV induced inhibition of skin carcinogenesis [52]. It is perhaps notable that the putative NKT cells in these experiments appear to be CD1d restricted, but have not been clearly shown to be invariant TCR+, and thus could be type II NKT cells. Nonetheless, there is clear evidence from autoimmunity models that iNKT cells can lead to suppression of T cell immunity as well [53]. In other words, this immune regulatory cell appears to have the capacity to regulate T cell responses in either direction, both to boost and suppress immunity [5]. One of the major challenges in the field is to understand the rules by which this is regulated.

STUDIES ON NKT CELLS IN HUMAN CANCER

The recognition that NKT cells can mediate tumor rejection *in vivo* and modulate the function of other downstream immune cells has led several investigators to characterize the nature of NKT cells in cancer patients [54]. Several studies have now reported deficiency in NKT numbers and/or function in the blood of cancer patients [55,56]. One notable exception is patients with glioma, suggesting that the loss of circulating NKT function is related to systemic nature of these cancers [57]. Most of the functional data suggests a loss of interferon-γ producing function of these cells. In many instances such as in multiple myeloma and prostate cancer, this appears to correlate with the clinical behavior of tumors, in that the loss of NKT function is observed in patients with more progressive myeloma or hormone refractory advanced prostate cancer. Nonetheless, these defects can be restored *ex vivo* after stimulation with α-GalCer bearing APCs. Expanded NKT cells can then secrete interferon-γ, and even recognize and kill autologous tumors, if appropriately expanded *in vitro* using α-GalCer loaded DCs. One major caveat of most of the existing data on human NKT cells in cancer is that nearly all the data is based on NKT cells in the blood, and very few studies have analyzed iNKT cells in the tumor tissue itself [56, 58]. Human NKT cells were shown to preferentially infiltrate neuroblastomas expressing the chemokine CCL-2, suggesting that chemokines/other molecules secreted by tumors may recruit or modify the presence and function of NKT cells in the tumor bed [58]. In the case of myeloma, the loss of iNKT cell function in the tumor bed correlates with the presence of clinically progressive disease [56]. The mechanism behind the observed loss of NKT effector function in cancer patients is not known, but current data suggest that suppressive factors in the tumor bed or ligands expressed by tumor cells contribute to NKT dysfunction in cancer.

MANIPULATING HUMAN NKT CELLS *IN VIVO*

The availability of α-GalCer as a clinical grade ligand has encouraged studies to use this ligand to manipulate NKT cells *in vivo* [12]. As discussed above, injection of NKT cells *in vivo* in mice leads to NKT activation and a "cytokine storm", which lead to tumor rejection. The initial studies with the injection of this compound in patients with advanced cancer have been sobering and associated with only modest and transient changes in some serum cytokines, along with a decline in circulating NKT cells [59]. Prior studies have shown that monocyte derived DCs are efficient APCs for the stimulation of human NKT cells in culture and *in vivo* in mice [60–62]. This has led to attempts to inject α-GalCer loaded DCs in patients with advanced cancer. Injection of immature DCs led to only modest and transient NKT activation *in vivo* [63]. Recently, we carried out a phase I trial to test the safety and tolerability of α-GalCer loaded mature DCs in patients with advanced cancer[64]. DC injections were well tolerated in all patients, and led to > 100 fold expansion of several subsets of NKT cells *in vivo*. DC mediated NKT activation was sustained, lasting several months. This was a bit surprising, suggesting that the effects of NKT cells may not be restricted to short term "innate" effects, but may be more long lasting. Importantly, NKT activation was associated with an increase in serum levels of IL-12p40 and interferon-γ inducible protein 10, as well as an increase in virus specific memory CD8+ T cells. Therefore, targeting of NKT cells has now begun to enter the arena of human clinical studies.

CHALLENGES FOR TARGETING NKT CELLS IN THE CLINIC

Although the pre-clinical and early clinical studies provide rationale and hope for targeting NKT cells in the clinic, there remain several challenges before these cells can be safely and effectively targeted in the clinic. One of the central challenges is needed to better understand the rules by which NKT cells can boost or suppress immunity *in vivo*. This property of NKT cells, if properly harnessed, could be very useful for a broad range of human diseases, from autoimmunity to tumors. As discussed above, the nature of antigen presenting cell may be a critical determinant of NKT activation *in vivo* [65]. Therefore, integrating DC mediated NKT targeting, with T cell based approaches may help the generation of a broad immune response including both innate and adaptive immune effectors [2,66]. Development of pharmacologic adjuncts to manipulate NKT cell function in patients, as well as the availability of novel ligands to selectively modify NKT cells, will greatly facilitate the translation of these approaches towards therapy of immune mediated diseases in the clinic.

REFERENCES

1. Sogn, J.A. 1998. Tumor immunology: the glass is half full. *Immunity* 9:757–763.
2. Blattman, J.N., and P.D. Greenberg. 2004. Cancer Immunotherapy: A treatment for the masses. *Science* 305:200–205.
3. Bendelac, A., M.N. Rivera, S.H. Park, and J.H. Roark. 1997. Mouse CD1-specific NK1 T cells: development, specificity, and function. *Annu Rev Immunol* 15:535–562.
4. Godfrey, D.I., H.R. MacDonald, M. Kronenberg, M.J. Smyth, and L. Van Kaer. 2004. NKT cells: what's in a name? *Nat Rev Immunol* 4:231–237.
5. Godfrey, D.I., and M. Kronenberg. 2004. Going both ways: Immune regulation via CD1d-dependent NKT cells. *J Clin Invest* 114:1379–1388.
6. Kronenberg, M. 2005. Toward an understanding of NKT cell biology: progress and paradoxes. *Annu Rev Immunol* 23:877–900.
7. Brigl, M., and M.B. Brenner. 2004. CD1: antigen presentation and T cell function. *Annu Rev Immunol* 22:817–890.
8. Dellabona, P., E. Padovan, G. Casorati, M. Brockhaus, and A. Lanzavecchia. 1994. An invariant V alpha 24-J alpha Q/V beta 11 T cell receptor is expressed in all individuals by clonally expanded CD4–8- T cells. *J Exp Med* 180:1171–1176.
9. Gadola, S.D., N. Dulphy, M. Salio, and V. Cerundolo. 2002. Valpha24-JalphaQ-independent, CD1d-restricted recognition of alpha-galactosylceramide by human CD4(+) and CD8alphabeta(+) T lymphocytes. *J Immunol* 168:5514–5520.
10. Slifka, M.K., R.R. Pagarigan, and J.L. Whitton. 2000. NK markers are expressed on a high percentage of virus-specific CD8+ and CD4+ T cells [published erratum appears in J Immunol 2000 Mar 15;164(6):following 3444]. *J Immunol* 164:2009–2015.
11. Gumperz, J.E., C. Roy, A. Makowska, D. Lum, M. Sugita, T. Podrebarac, Y. Koezuka, S.A. Porcelli, S. Cardell, M.B. Brenner, and S.M. Behar. 2000. Murine CD1d-restricted T cell recognition of cellular lipids. *Immunity* 12:211–221.
12. Hayakawa, Y., D.I. Godfrey, and M.J. Smyth. 2004. Alpha-galactosylceramide: potential immunomodulatory activity and future application. *Curr Med Chem* 11:241–252.
13. Sidobre, S., O.V. Naidenko, B.C. Sim, N.R. Gascoigne, K.C. Garcia, and M. Kronenberg. 2002. The V alpha 14 NKT cell TCR exhibits high-affinity binding to a glycolipid/CD1d complex. *J Immunol* 169:1340–1348.

14. Wu, D.Y., N.H. Segal, S. Sidobre, M. Kronenberg, and P.B. Chapman. 2003. Cross-presentation of disialoganglioside GD3 to natural killer T cells. *J Exp Med* 198:173–181.
15. Schofield, L., M.J. McConville, D. Hansen, A.S. Campbell, B. Fraser-Reid, M.J. Grusby, and S.D. Tachado. 1999. CD1d-restricted immunoglobulin G formation to GPI-anchored antigens mediated by NKT cells. *Science* 283:225–229.
16. Rauch, J., J. Gumperz, C. Robinson, M. Skold, C. Roy, D.C. Young, M. Lafleur, D.B. Moody, M.B. Brenner, C.E. Costello, and S.M. Behar. 2003. Structural features of the acyl chain determine self-phospholipid antigen recognition by a CD1d-restricted invariant NKT (iNKT) cell. *J Biol Chem* 278:47508–47515.
17. Ortaldo, J.R., H.A. Young, R.T. Winkler-Pickett, E.W. Bere, Jr., W.J. Murphy, and R.H. Wiltrout. 2004. Dissociation of NKT stimulation, cytokine induction, and NK activation in vivo by the use of distinct TCR-binding ceramides. *J Immunol* 172:943–953.
18. Zhou, D., J. Mattner, C. Cantu, 3rd, N. Schrantz, N. Yin, Y. Gao, Y. Sagiv, K. Hudspeth, Y.P. Wu, T. Yamashita, S. Teneberg, D. Wang, R.L. Proia, S.B. Levery, P.B. Savage, L. Teyton, and A. Bendelac. 2004. Lysosomal glycosphingolipid recognition by NKT cells. *Science* 306:1786–1789.
19. Mattner, J., K.L. Debord, N. Ismail, R.D. Goff, C. Cantu, 3rd, D. Zhou, P. Saint-Mezard, V. Wang, Y. Gao, N. Yin, K. Hoebe, O. Schneewind, D. Walker, B. Beutler, L. Teyton, P.B. Savage, and A. Bendelac. 2005. Exogenous and endogenous glycolipid antigens activate NKT cells during microbial infections. *Nature* 434:525–529.
20. Kinjo, Y., D. Wu, G. Kim, G.W. Xing, M.A. Poles, D.D. Ho, M. Tsuji, K. Kawahara, C.H. Wong, and M. Kronenberg. 2005. Recognition of bacterial glycosphingolipids by natural killer T cells. *Nature* 434:520–525.
21. Wu, D., G.W. Xing, M.A. Poles, A. Horowitz, Y. Kinjo, B. Sullivan, V. Bodmer-Narkevitch, O. Plettenburg, M. Kronenberg, M. Tsuji, D.D. Ho, and C.H. Wong. 2005. Bacterial glycolipids and analogs as antigens for CD1d-restricted NKT cells. *Proc Natl Acad Sci U S A* 102:1351–1356.
22. Moody, D.B., D.C. Young, T.Y. Cheng, J.P. Rosat, C. Roura-Mir, P.B. O'Connor, D.M. Zajonc, A. Walz, M.J. Miller, S.B. Levery, I.A. Wilson, C.E. Costello, and M.B. Brenner. 2004. T cell activation by lipopeptide antigens. *Science* 303:527–531.
23. Matsuda, J.L., L. Gapin, J.L. Baron, S. Sidobre, D.B. Stetson, M. Mohrs, R.M. Locksley, and M. Kronenberg. 2003. Mouse V alpha 14i natural killer T cells are resistant to cytokine polarization in vivo. *Proc Natl Acad Sci U S A* 100:8395–8400.
24. Stetson, D.B., M. Mohrs, R.L. Reinhardt, J.L. Baron, Z.E. Wang, L. Gapin, M. Kronenberg, and R.M. Locksley. 2003. Constitutive cytokine mRNAs mark natural killer (NK) and NK T cells poised for rapid effector function. *J Exp Med* 198:1069–1076.
25. Carnaud, C., D. Lee, O. Donnars, S.H. Park, A. Beavis, Y. Koezuka, and A. Bendelac. 1999. Cutting edge: Cross-talk between cells of the innate immune system: NKT cells rapidly activate NK cells. *J Immunol* 163:4647–4650.
26. Eberl, G., and H.R. MacDonald. 2000. Selective induction of NK cell proliferation and cytotoxicity by activated NKT cells. *Eur J Immunol* 30:985–992.
27. Vincent, M.S., D.S. Leslie, J.E. Gumperz, X. Xiong, E.P. Grant, and M.B. Brenner. 2002. CD1-dependent dendritic cell instruction. *Nat Immunol* 3:1163–1168.
28. Smyth, M.J., N.Y. Crowe, D.G. Pellicci, K. Kyparissoudis, J.M. Kelly, K. Takeda, H. Yagita, and D.I. Godfrey. 2002. Sequential production of interferon-gamma by NK1.1(+) T cells and natural killer cells is essential for the antimetastatic effect of alpha-galactosylceramide. *Blood* 99:1259–1266.
29. Galli, G., S. Nuti, S. Tavarini, L. Galli-Stampino, C. De Lalla, G. Casorati, P. Dellabona, and S. Abrignani. 2003. CD1d-restricted Help To B Cells By Human Invariant Natural Killer T Lymphocytes. *J Exp Med* 197:1051–1057.
30. Hermans, I.F., J.D. Silk, U. Gileadi, M. Salio, B. Mathew, G. Ritter, R. Schmidt, A.L. Harris, L. Old, and V. Cerundolo. 2003. NKT cells enhance CD4+ and CD8+ T cell responses to soluble antigen in vivo through direct interaction with dendritic cells. *J Immunol* 171:5140–5147.

31. Fujii, S., K. Shimizu, C. Smith, L. Bonifaz, and R.M. Steinman. 2003. Activation of natural killer T cells by alpha-galactosylceramide rapidly induces the full maturation of dendritic cells in vivo and thereby acts as an adjuvant for combined CD4 and CD8 T cell immunity to a coadministered protein. *J Exp Med* 198:267–279.
32. Fujii, S., K. Liu, C. Smith, A.J. Bonito, and R.M. Steinman. 2004. The linkage of innate to adaptive immunity via maturing dendritic cells in vivo requires CD40 ligation in addition to antigen presentation and CD80/86 costimulation. *J Exp Med* 199:1607–1618.
33. Chen, Y.G., C.M. Choisy-Rossi, T.M. Holl, H.D. Chapman, G.S. Besra, S.A. Porcelli, D.J. Shaffer, D. Roopenian, S.B. Wilson, and D.V. Serreze. 2005. Activated NKT cells inhibit autoimmune diabetes through tolerogenic recruitment of dendritic cells to pancreatic lymph nodes. *J Immunol* 174:1196–1204.
34. Gumperz, J.E., S. Miyake, T. Yamamura, and M.B. Brenner. 2002. Functionally distinct subsets of CD1d-restricted natural killer T cells revealed by CD1d tetramer staining. *J Exp Med* 195:625–636.
35. Lee, P.T., K. Benlagha, L. Teyton, and A. Bendelac. 2002. Distinct functional lineages of human V(alpha)24 natural killer T cells. *J Exp Med* 195:637–641.
36. Smyth, M.J., N.Y. Crowe, Y. Hayakawa, K. Takeda, H. Yagita, and D.I. Godfrey. 2002. NKT cells - conductors of tumor immunity? *Curr Opin Immunol* 14:165–171.
37. Smyth, M.J., and D.I. Godfrey. 2000. NKT cells and tumor immunity–a double-edged sword. *Nat Immunol* 1:459–460.
38. Wilson, S.B., and T.L. Delovitch. 2003. Janus-like role of regulatory iNKT cells in autoimmune disease and tumour immunity. *Nat Rev Immunol* 3:211–222.
39. Cui, J., T. Shin, T. Kawano, H. Sato, E. Kondo, I. Toura, Y. Kaneko, H. Koseki, M. Kanno, and M. Taniguchi. 1997. Requirement for Va 14 NKT cells by glycosylceramides. *Science* 278: 1623–1626.
40. Kawano, T., T. Nakayama, N. Kamada, Y. Kaneko, M. Harada, N. Ogura, Y. Akutsu, S. Motohashi, T. Iizasa, H. Endo, T. Fujisawa, H. Shinkai, and M. Taniguchi. 1999. Antitumor cytotoxicity mediated by ligand-activated human V alpha24 NKT cells. *Cancer Res* 59:5102–5105.
41. Hayakawa, Y., S. Rovero, G. Forni, and M.J. Smyth. 2003. Alpha-galactosylceramide (KRN7000) suppression of chemical- and oncogene-dependent carcinogenesis. *Proc Natl Acad Sci USA* 100:9464–9469.
42. Hayakawa, Y., K. Takeda, H. Yagita, S. Kakuta, Y. Iwakura, L. Van Kaer, I. Saiki, and K. Okumura. 2001. Critical contribution of IFN-gamma and NK cells, but not perforin-mediated cytotoxicity, to anti-metastatic effect of alpha-galactosylceramide. *Eur J Immunol* 31:1720–1727.
43. Hayakawa, Y., K. Takeda, H. Yagita, M.J. Smyth, L. Van Kaer, K. Okumura, and I. Saiki. 2002. IFN-gamma-mediated inhibition of tumor angiogenesis by natural killer T-cell ligand, alpha-galactosylceramide. *Blood* 100:1728–1733.
44. Schmieg, J., G. Yang, R.W. Franck, and M. Tsuji. 2003. Superior protection against malaria and melanoma metastases by a C-glycoside analogue of the natural killer T cell ligand alpha-Galactosylceramide. *J Exp Med* 198:1631–1641.
45. Kitamura, H., K. Iwakabe, T. Yahata, S. Nishimura, A. Ohta, Y. Ohmi, M. Sato, K. Takeda, K. Okumura, L. Van Kaer, T. Kawano, M. Taniguchi, and T. Nishimura. 1999. The natural killer T (NKT) cell ligand alpha-galactosylceramide demonstrates its immunopotentiating effect by inducing interleukin (IL)-12 production by dendritic cells and IL-12 receptor expression on NKT cells. *J Exp Med* 189:1121–1128.
46. Smyth, M.J., N.Y. Crowe, and D.I. Godfrey. 2001. NK cells and NKT cells collaborate in host protection from methylcholanthrene-induced fibrosarcoma. *Int Immunol* 13:459–463.
47. Crowe, N.Y., M.J. Smyth, and D.I. Godfrey. 2002. A critical role for natural killer T cells in immunosurveillance of methylcholanthrene-induced sarcomas. *J Exp Med* 196:119–127.
48. Nishikawa, H., T. Kato, K. Tanida, A. Hiasa, I. Tawara, H. Ikeda, Y. Ikarashi, H. Wakasugi, M. Kronenberg, T. Nakayama, M. Taniguchi, K. Kuribayashi, L.J. Old, and H. Shiku. 2003. CD4+ CD25+ T cells responding to serologically defined autoantigens suppress antitumor immune responses. *Proc Natl Acad Sci U S A* 100:10902–10906.

49. Terabe, M., S. Matsui, N. Noben-Trauth, H. Chen, C. Watson, D.D. Donaldson, D.P. Carbone, W.E. Paul, and J.A. Berzofsky. 2000. NKT cell-mediated repression of tumor immunosurveillance by IL-13 and the IL-4R-STAT6 pathway. *Nat Immunol* 1:515–520.
50. Ostrand-Rosenberg, S., V.K. Clements, M. Terabe, J.M. Park, J.A. Berzofsky, and S.K. Dissanayake. 2002. Resistance to metastatic disease in STAT6-deficient mice requires hemopoietic and nonhemopoietic cells and is IFN-gamma dependent. *J Immunol* 169:5796–5804.
51. Terabe, M., S. Matsui, J.M. Park, M. Mamura, N. Noben-Trauth, D.D. Donaldson, W. Chen, S.M. Wahl, S. Ledbetter, B. Pratt, J.J. Letterio, W.E. Paul, and J.A. Berzofsky. 2003. Transforming growth factor-beta production and myeloid cells are an effector mechanism through which CD1d-restricted T cells block cytotoxic T lymphocyte-mediated tumor immunosurveillance: abrogation prevents tumor recurrence. *J Exp Med* 198:1741–1752.
52. Moodycliffe, A.M., D. Nghiem, G. Clydesdale, and S.E. Ullrich. 2000. Immune suppression and skin cancer development: regulation by NKT cells. *Nat Immunol* 1:521–525.
53. Sharif, S., G.A. Arreaza, P. Zucker, Q.S. Mi, J. Sondhi, O.V. Naidenko, M. Kronenberg, Y. Koezuka, T.L. Delovitch, J.M. Gombert, M. Leite-De-Moraes, C. Gouarin, R. Zhu, A. Hameg, T. Nakayama, M. Taniguchi, F. Lepault, A. Lehuen, J.F. Bach, and A. Herbelin. 2001. Activation of natural killer T cells by alpha-galactosylceramide treatment prevents the onset and recurrence of autoimmune Type 1 diabetes. *Nat Med* 7:1057–1062.
54. Smyth, M.J., N.Y. Crowe, Y. Hayakawa, K. Takeda, H. Yagita, and D.I. Godfrey. 2002. NKT cells - conductors of tumor immunity? *Curr Opin Immunol* 14:165–171.
55. Tahir, S.M., O. Cheng, A. Shaulov, Y. Koezuka, G.J. Bubley, S.B. Wilson, S.P. Balk, and M.A. Exley. 2001. Loss of IFN-gamma production by invariant NK T cells in advanced cancer. *J Immunol* 167:4046–4050.
56. Dhodapkar, M.V., M.D. Geller, D.H. Chang, K. Shimizu, S. Fujii, K.M. Dhodapkar, and J. Krasovsky. 2003. A reversible defect in natural killer T cell function characterizes the progression of premalignant to malignant multiple myeloma. *J Exp Med* 197:1667–1676.
57. Dhodapkar, K.M., B. Cirignano, F. Chamian, D. Zagzag, D.C. Miller, J.L. Finlay, and R.M. Steinman. 2004. Invariant natural killer T cells are preserved in patients with glioma and exhibit antitumor lytic activity following dendritic cell-mediated expansion. *Int J Cancer* 109:893–899.
58. Metelitsa, L.S., O.V. Naidenko, A. Kant, H.W. Wu, M.J. Loza, B. Perussia, M. Kronenberg, and R.C. Seeger. 2001. Human NKT cells mediate antitumor cytotoxicity directly by recognizing target cell CD1d with bound ligand or indirectly by producing IL-2 to activate NK cells. *J Immunol* 167:3114–3122.
59. Giaccone, G., C.J. Punt, Y. Ando, R. Ruijter, N. Nishi, M. Peters, B.M. von Blomberg, R.J. Scheper, H.J. van der Vliet, A.J. van den Eertwegh, M. Roelvink, J. Beijnen, H. Zwierzina, and H.M. Pinedo. 2002. A phase I study of the natural killer T-cell ligand alpha-galactosylceramide (KRN7000) in patients with solid tumors. *Clin Cancer Res* 8:3702–3709.
60. Fujii, S., K. Shimizu, R.M. Steinman, and M.V. Dhodapkar. 2003. Detection and activation of human Valpha24+ natural killer T cells using alpha-galactosyl ceramide-pulsed dendritic cells. *J Immunol Methods* 272:147–159.
61. van der Vliet, H.J., J.W. Molling, N. Nishi, A.J. Masterson, W. Kolgen, S.A. Porcelli, A.J. van den Eertwegh, B.M. von Blomberg, H.M. Pinedo, G. Giaccone, and R.J. Scheper. 2003. Polarization of Valpha24+ Vbeta11+ natural killer T cells of healthy volunteers and cancer patients using alpha-galactosylceramide-loaded and environmentally instructed dendritic cells. *Cancer Res* 63:4101–4106.
62. Fujii, S., K. Shimizu, M. Kronenberg, and R.M. Steinman. 2002. Prolonged IFN-gamma-producing NKT response induced with alpha-galactosylceramide-loaded DCs. *Nat Immunol* 3:867–874.
63. Nieda, M., M. Okai, A. Tazbirkova, H. Lin, A. Yamaura, K. Ide, R. Abraham, T. Juji, D.J. Macfarlane, and A.J. Nicol. 2004. Therapeutic activation of Valpha24+Vbeta11+ NKT cells in human subjects results in highly coordinated secondary activation of acquired and innate immunity. *Blood* 103:383–389.

64. Chang, D.H., K. Osman, J. Connolly, A. Kukreja, J. Krasovsky, M. Pack, A. Hutchinson, M. Geller, N. Liu, R. Annable, J. Shay, K. Kirchhoff, N. Nishi, Y. Ando, K. Hayashi, H. Hassoun, R.M. Steinman, and M.V. Dhodapkar. 2005. Sustained expansion of NKT cells and antigen-specific T cells after injection of {alpha}-galactosyl-ceramide loaded mature dendritic cells in cancer patients. *J Exp Med* 201:1503–1517.
65. Fujii, S.I., K. Shimuzu, M. Kronenberg, and R.M. Steinman. 2002. Prolonged interferon-g producing NKT responses induced with a-galactosyl ceramide loaded dendritic cells. *Nature Immunol* 3:867–874.
66. Steinman, R.M., and M. Dhodapkar. 2001. Active immunization against cancer with dendritic cells: the near future. *Int J Cancer* 94:459–473.

CHAPTER 5

IMMUNOMODULATORY MOLECULES OF THE IMMUNE SYSTEM

YVONNE M. SAENGER, ROBERT R. JENQ, AND MIGUEL-ANGEL PERALES*

Memorial Sloan-Kettering Cancer Center
And Weill Medical School and Graduate School of Cornell University 1275 York Avenue New York, NY 10021 USA

INTRODUCTION

Cancer poses a difficult problem for immunotherapy because it arises from the host's own tissues. Many of the target antigens are tissue-specific molecules shared by cancer cells and normal cells. Thus, these are weak antigens that do not typically elicit immunity [1]. In addition, tumor cells have a number of features that make their recognition and destruction by the immune system difficult. These include the loss of expression of antigens that elicit immune responses [2], and the lack of expression of major histocompatibility (MHC) Class II and downregulation of MHC Class I expression, which can lead to non-recognition of tumors by both $CD4^+$ and $CD8^+$ T cells. There is typically no expression of co-stimulatory molecules, leading to inadequate activation of T cells (ignorance) and anergy [3]. Finally, tumors may evade immune recognition through more active mechanisms such as secretion of immunosuppressive cytokines [4]. Despite these obstacles, several strategies for developing effective tumor immunity have been developed. Crucial to these approaches is the discovery and understanding of the immunomodulatory molecules, particularly the co-stimulatory pathways and cytokines that are critical to the generation of an effective immune response to tumors. In this chapter, we review strategies to enhance tumor immunity through the targeting of

*E-mail: peralesm@mskcc.org

H.L. Kaufman and J.D. Wolchok (eds.), General Principles of Tumor Immunotherapy, 67–121.

these immunomodulatory molecules. Given the scope of the subject and ongoing research in this important field, we will focus on the some of the molecules that have been defined in more depth and refer readers to the literature for recent developments.

CO-STIMULATORY MOLECULES

Co-stimulatory molecules are highly active immunomodulatory proteins that play a critical role in the development and maintenance of an immune response. The concept of co-stimulation was first proposed by Bretscher and Cohn three decades ago [5], as it had become apparent that a single on/off switch was insufficient to explain the complexities of lymphocyte activation. Additional studies in the 1970s of allogeneic T cell responses in bone marrow transplantation models demonstrated that only specialized antigen presenting cells (APCs) are capable of inducing a T-cell response [6]. This led to the formulation of a two-signal hypothesis for the activation of naïve T cells. Signal one is the interaction between an antigen bound to an MHC molecule and the T cell receptor (TCR), and signal two results from the interaction of a co-stimulatory molecule and its ligand [7]. In the absence of a second signal, T cell clones can become anergic when the TCR is stimulated [8]. Thus the groundwork was laid for a model whereby specialized APCs, carriers of a co-stimulatory second signal, are able to activate T cell responses following ligation of the TCR. In contrast, somatic tissues, which do not express the second signal, may induce T cell unresponsiveness [8,9].

This model explains peripheral tolerance to self-antigens and has key implications for cancer immunology because tumors rarely express co-stimulatory molecules, thereby lacking this critical "second signal" to activate T cells [10]. This has lead to efforts to artificially insert this "second signal" in tumor cells and render them immunogenic. A number of strategies have been investigated, and early clinical trials have yielded some encouraging results.

More recently, the two-signal hypothesis is being revisited following the recognition that many co-stimulatory molecules can be blocked by co-inhibitory molecules [11] that are expressed by blood vessels [12] as well as by tumor cells [13]. Our current understanding is that interacting immunomodulatory molecules expressed on a wide array of tissues may exert both stimulatory and inhibitory functions depending on the immunologic context [14].

From a structural point of view, cell-surface immunomodulatory molecules can be grouped into two large families of receptors and ligands: the B7/CD28 immunoglobulin family and the Tumor Necrosis Factor (TNF)-related family. Some receptors and ligands have multiple partners. Table 1 lists the most well-described cell-surface immunomodulatory molecules. A number of these co-stimulatory and co-inhibitory molecules have been evaluated in pre-clinical animal models or in clinical trials of cancer immunotherapy.

Table 1. Costimulatory Molecules

Name	Potential Therapeutic Applications	Human Trials[a]	Mouse Studies[a]
CD28/B7 family			
CD28/B7	Tumor cells expressing B7 can be used as vaccines by enhancing T-cell responses.	Yes	Yes
CTLA-4	Anti-CTLA antibodies induce anti-tumor immunity.	Yes	Yes
ICOS/B7h	Transfection of tumors with B7h may allow co-stimulation of ICOS expressing T cells.	No	Yes
PD-1/B7H1 (PDL1)/B7DC (PDL2)	Blocking antibody against PDL1 may prevent tumors from inducing apoptosis in T cells, and may also inhibit myeloid suppressor cells.	No	Yes
TNF family			
CD27/CD70	Tumors transfected with CD70 are rejected, possibly by CD27 expressing NK cells.	No	Yes
OX40/OX40L	Agonist antibodies against OX40, and tumor transfection with OX40L, may co-stimulate memory $CD4^+$ T cells and lead to rejection of tumors	No	Yes
4-1BB/4-1BBL	Agonist antibodies against 4-1BB, and tumor transfection with 4-1BBL, may activate anti-tumor CD8+ T cells	No	Yes
HVEM/LIGHT	LIGHT may directly bind HVEM on tumor cells and induce apoptosis. It can also prime T cells against tumors.	No	Yes
CD40/CD40L	Transfection of tumors with CD40L activates anti-tumor T cells, and ligation of CD40 directly induces apoptosis in solid tumors and some hematologic malignancies.	Yes	Yes
GITR/GITRL	Agonist antibody directed at GITR can stimulate anti-tumor T cells and may impair regulatory T cell function.	No	Yes

[a] Studies are referenced in the text.

CD28/CTLA-4/B7-1/B7-2 Family

Biology

The CD28/CTLA-4/B7-1/B7-2 family represents the classic co-stimulatory axis, and it is in the context of this system that the first experiments were performed showing that effective co-stimulation could cure cancer in mice [15, 16]. B7-1 (CD80), cloned in 1981 [17], as well as the subsequently cloned B7-2 (CD86) [18–20], are expressed on activated APCs and bind to CD28 on T cells, providing the necessary co-stimulation for naïve T-cell activation, inducing IL-2 production, cell division, and the inhibition of activation induced cell death (AICD) [8, 21, 22]. A homologue to CD28, Cytotoxic T lymphocyte-associated antigen 4 (CTLA-4, CD152) [23], binds both B7-1 and B7-2 molecules [24] and, in contrast to CD28, inhibits T-cell proliferation [25]. B7 molecules therefore have two ligands, CD28 and CTLA-4, with opposing effects on T cells.

CTLA-4 was first cloned in 1987 [23], but it took several years until its inhibitory function was more clearly understood [26]. Ligation of CTLA-4 in isolation may cause apoptosis of T cells [27], whereas CTLA-4 ligation in conjunction with signaling via the TCR and CD28 inhibits T-cell activation [25,28]. Accordingly, CTLA-4 -/- mice develop a fatal lymphoproliferative disorder [29–31].

The differential expression, in time and space, of CD28 and CTLA-4 at the cell surface have implications for their respective roles in the generation of immune responses. CD28 is uniformly distributed throughout the membrane but aggregates rapidly to the immunologic synapse with T-cell activation. Conversely, CTLA-4 is present in intracellular vesicles and is mobilized to the cell surface later [32]. Mobilization of CTLA-4 is tightly regulated by B7.1 expression on the APC, and by the strength of TCR stimulation [33]. As a result, the role of CTLA-4 may be to attenuate the T cell response, limiting the activity of high affinity T-cell clones [33].

CTLA-4 has been implicated in multiple aspects of immune regulation. It may cause T-cell anergy [34], modulate memory T-cell responses [35], shape the diversity of a polyclonal T-cell response [36], and raise levels of inhibitory cytokines TGFβ [37] and IL-10 [38]. CTLA-4 may also "back-signal" via B7 to down-regulate dendritic cell activation markers [39]. Intriguingly, there is now emerging evidence that CTLA-4 is expressed on tumor cell lines and that ligation of CTLA-4 may cause apoptosis, potentially an additional mechanism for the tumoricidal effects of anti-CTLA-4 antibodies [13].

In addition, CTLA-4 may play a role in regulatory T-cell (Treg) function [40–42]. CTLA-4 is expressed on Tregs and on cutaneous T cell lymphoma, which may arise from Tregs [43]. Tregs have been noted to accumulate in patients with cancer [44], and there is evidence that they increase with advancing disease [45] and are associated with an unfavorable prognosis [46, 47].

Applications for tumor immunotherapy

The CD28/B7/CTLA-4 co-stimulatory axis has been an area of active investigation as a target for cancer immunotherapy [11]. Initial research focused on the transfection of tumors with B7 molecules [10]. More recently, attention has turned to antibody blockade of the CTLA-4 inhibitory molecule [48]. Anti-CTLA-4 antibodies have the advantage of ease of administration, and have shown promising initial results in clinical trials (see below). Clinical and pre-clinical data using both approaches are summarized in the following sections as well as in tables 2–4.

Lessons learned from B7

As mentioned above, the first successful application of cell-surface immunomodulatory molecules to tumor immunology was the transfection of poorly immunogenic melanoma cell lines with B7.1 [15,16]. In these initial experiments, tumors grew but then regressed in a $CD8^+$ T-cell-dependent process. Furthermore, treated animals became immune to further tumor challenge, demonstrating the induction of immunologic memory. In some tumor models, inoculation with B7-expressing tumor cells caused regression of small pre-existing B7-negative tumors [16, 49, 50]. Larger tumors (greater than 2-3mm), however, were generally not affected [51]. Similar results were seen with B7.2-expressing tumors [52]. This work was then extended to other tumor models including lymphoma [50] and prostate cancer [53]. Irradiation of the B7-expressing tumor cells severely decreased their immunogenicity [54], suggesting that surface molecules were directly contacting and activating T cells, and that B7-transfected tumor cells were functioning as APCs [55].

Lessons learned from B7 models have broad implications for the role of co-stimulation in tumor immunotherapy. First, co-stimulatory molecules are insufficient to trigger an immune response alone. In fact, the intrinsic immunogenicity of the tumor is of critical importance [54]. Some murine tumors are so poorly immunogenic that B7 transfection is insufficient to induce a curative immune response, likely due in part to inadequate expression of MHC complexes or adhesion molecules involved in the formation of the immunologic synapse. In certain models, this could be overcome by additional transfection with genes encoding interferon gamma (IFNγ) [56], other co-stimulatory molecules [57], or more immunogenic epitopes [49]. Second, co-stimulation has been shown in mouse models to broaden the immune response, allowing recognition of otherwise silent sub-dominant epitopes [58]. This may lead to increased recognition of common tumor antigens and explain why vaccination with one B7-expressing tumor sometimes yields protection against other tumors of different tissue origin [50]. The final issue is the role of T-cell subsets in effective tumor responses. In some models, tumor immunity is mediated by $CD8^+$ T cells and does not require $CD4^+$ T cells [59]. However, in other models, tumor immunity is clearly CD4-dependent [49]. These differences may be antigen-dependent [60]. Of note, requirements for other cell types including $\gamma\delta$T cells [61] and NK cells [62] have also been observed.

The results of clinical trials in humans of B7-containing vaccines are summarized in table 2. To date, most of these studies have demonstrated increased immune

Table 2. Targeting B7 in human clinical trials[a]

Vaccine	Tumor	N	Clinical Response	Immune Response[b]		Reference
				T cell	B cell	
Whole cell Vaccine						
Autologous tumors transfected with B7-1 and high dose IL-2	Kidney	13	CR=2, SD=2	6/13	ND	[63]
Allogeneic NSCLC transfected with B7-1 and HLA-A1 or A2	Lung	14	CR=1, SD=4	13/14	12/14	[64]
Allogeneic HLA-matched breast CA transfected with B7-1 and GM-CSF or BCG	Breast	30	SD=4	4/9	17/24	[65, 66]
Recombinant viruses						
Canarypoxvirus expressing CEA and B7.1	Adenocarcinoma	18	SD=3	4/12	10/18	[67]
Canarypoxvirus expressing CEA and B7.1	Adenocarcinoma	39	SD=8	12/15	2/31	[68]
Fowlpox expressing B7-1, ICAM-1 And LFA-3	Adenocarcinoma	58	CR=1, SD=23	10/13	6/33	[69]
Vaccinia virus expressing B7.1	Melanoma	12	PR=2[c], SD=4	4/6	12/12	[70]

[a] CR: complete response, PR: partial response, SD: stable disease, ND: not determined.

[b] Not all patients were evaluated

[c] one of 2 patients with a PR was a long-term survivor

responses, but only limited clinical benefit [63–70]. One of the challenges of using tumor cells transfected with B7 molecules is the requirement for injection of live tumor cells, which may present an obstacle in the clinical setting. One potential approach to overcome this problem is the use of viral vectors expressing B7 [71]. Viral vectors expressing B7.1 in addition to tumor antigens or additional co-stimulatory molecules have also been investigated in clinical trials [67–70]. In a recently reported study, a viral vaccine targeting CEA combined the B7 gene with genes for adhesion molecules ICAM-1 and LFA-3 (TRICOM, Therion Biologics, Inc, Cambridge, MA) and demonstrated increased CEA-specific T cells [69]. Another approach using viral vectors expressing B7.1 has been the direct transfection of tumors. In a study by Kauffman *et al.*[70], intralesional administration of a vaccinia virus expressing B7.1 in patients with melanoma resulted in elevated expression of CD8, IFNγ, and IL-10 in stable or regressing lesions by gene array, compared to growing lesions. This suggested that $CD8^+$ T cells may mediate tumor regression in this system. Further studies should help better define the role for transfection with B7 molecules in clinical practice.

Lessons learned from CTLA-4

The potential for anti-CTLA-4 antibodies in cancer treatment was first demonstrated in James Allison's laboratory in 1996 using murine colon carcinoma and fibrosarcoma [72]. In these models, tumor rejection was observed even when treatment was started one week after tumor injection, when tumors were readily palpable. Anti-CTLA-4 antibodies have also been shown to be effective in murine models of prostate cancer [73], breast cancer [74], and melanoma [75,76], but not in some models of very poorly immunogenic tumors [74,75] (Table 3). Anti-CTLA-4 antibodies have also been combined effectively with tumor-specific therapies, including immunotherapy (vaccines) [74–78] or conventional therapies (surgery, chemotherapy) in mouse models [32,79–81]. Although the exact mechanisms by which CTLA-4 blockade enhances anti-tumor immunity are not fully defined, evidence in mouse models and human studies suggests that the effects are not due to regulatory T cell–mediated suppression but instead to enhanced proliferation of effector T cells through down-regulation of CTLA-4-mediated inhibition [82,83].

A number of phase I/II clinical trials using two different anti-CTLA-4 antibodies (MDX-010, Medarex Inc, Princeton, NJ; and CP-675,206, Pfizer Inc, Groton, CT) have been published to date (Table 4). In the first trial, 7 melanoma patients and 2 ovarian cancer patients, all previous recipients of tumor vaccines, received a single dose of 3mg/kg of antibody (MDX-010) [84]. Patients developed inflammatory reactions within tumors noted clinically and by pathology, and Ca-125 levels declined or stabilized in the two ovarian cancer patients. Side-effects consisted mainly of skin rashes. In a second trial, patients with metastatic melanoma were treated with anti-CTLA-4 (MDX-010) at 3mg/kg every 3 weeks in conjunction with peptide vaccination for melanocyte antigens [85]. Of fourteen patients, two had a complete response and one had a partial response. Six patients had grade

Table 3. Treatment with anti-CTLA-4 antibodies in mouse models

Approach	Tumor	Results (tumor rejection)	Immune Response[a]		Reference
			T cell	B cell	
Antibody alone					
	Prostate	42%	ND	ND	[73]
	Colon, Fibrosarcoma	100%	ND	ND	[72]
Antibody combined with vaccine					
GM-CSF secreting vaccine	Melanoma	80%	ND	ND	[75]
GM-CSF secreting vaccine	Melanoma	80%	$CD8^+$ clones isolated	None	[76]
GM-CSF secreting vaccine	Breast	100%	ND	ND	[74]
GM-CSF secreting vaccine	Prostate	85% vs. 15% (control)	ND	ND	[77]
DNA Vaccine	Prostate, Melanoma	60%	Enhanced $CD8^+$ T-cell responses	ND	[78]
Antibody combined with conventional therapy					
Surgery	Prostate	66%	ND	ND	[79]
Chemotherapy	Plasmocytoma	70% vs 40% (chemotherapy alone)	Tumor-specific T cells	ND	[80]
Radiation therapy	Breast	Prolonged survival	ND	ND	[81]

[a] ND: not determined.

Table 4. Anti-CTLA-4 antibodies in human clinical trials

Therapy	Tumor	N	Clinical Response[a]	Grade 3/4 Autoimmunity	Immune Response	Reference
Published Data						
MDX-010	Melanoma [7] and Ovary [2]	9	Decline/Stabilization in Ca-125	None	Extensive tumor necrosis with immune infiltrates in 5/6 melanoma patients biopsied	[84]
MDX-010 + gp100 peptide vaccine	Melanoma	14	CR=1, PR=2	Dermatitis [3], enterocolitis [1], colitis [1], hypophysistis [1], hepatitis [1]	Not reported	[85][b]
MDX-010 + gp100 peptide vaccine	Melanoma	56	CR=2, PR=5	Colitis [7], dermatitis [4], hepatitis [1], enterocolitis [1],Uveitis [1], Hypophysitis [1]	T cell responses in 18/23 evaluated patients.	[86][b]
MDX-010 + gp100, MART-1, and tyrosinase peptide vaccines	Melanoma	19	7/19 without POD at 28 months.	Diarrhea [3], cramping [1], melena [1]	T cell responses in 15/17 (ELISPOT) and 11/16 (Tetramer).	[88]
MDX-010 + high-dose IL-2	Melanoma	36	CR=3, PR=5	Enterocolitis [4], arthritis [1], uveitis [1]	HLA-DR,CD45-RO, CD25 expression increased	[89]
CP-675,206	Melanoma, Renal cell, Colon	39	CR=2, PR=3	Diarrhea [3], dermatitis [1]	Enhanced tetanus skin responses, increased tetramer staining.	[90]
Unpublished Data						
MDX-010 (arm A) vs. MDX-010 + dacarbazine (arm B)	Melanoma	72	Arm A: PR=2, SD=4ArmB: CR=2, PR=4, SD=4	2 deaths from liver toxicity and PE, colitis [3] requiring colectomy in 1 patient, rash [1], mental status change [1], fever [1], uveitis[1]	Not tested.	Fischkoff et al., ASCO 2005

MDX-010	Prostate	14	2 PSA responses	Pruritis [1]	No increased T cell activation	Davis et al., ASCO 2002
MDX-010 + GM-CSF	Prostate	8	Not Reported	TIA [1]	None.	Fong et al, ASCO 2005
MDX-010	Renal Cell	21	PR=6	Enteritis [9], hypophysitis [2], meningitis [1]	Not reported.	Yang et al., ASCO 2005
CP-675,206	Melanoma	14	CR=1 (another patient NED after WBXRT)	Diarrhea [3]	T cell infiltrates in regressed lesions	Ribas et al, ASCO 2005
CP-675,206	Melanoma	25	PR=5/18 evaluable	Diarrhea, dermatitis (Toxicities not graded.)	Decreased Tregs and IL-10, increased IL-2 in responders.	Reuben et al., ASCO 2005

[a] CR: complete response, PR: partial response, SD: stable disease.
[b] The second report includes 14 patients initially reported in prior publication.

III/IV toxicity including dermatitis, colitis, hypophysitis, and hepatitis. This study was recently updated with additional information on a total of 56 patients [86]. Two patients had ongoing complete responses and 5 patients had a partial response for an overall response rate of 13%. Fourteen patients had grade 3 toxicity, and these patients appeared to have a higher response rate (36%). A majority of patients tested developed immunity to the vaccinating peptide, but there did not appear to be a correlation between immunologic and clinical responses, as noted in prior studies [87]. In another study, nineteen patients with high-risk resected stage III and IV melanoma received anti-CTLA-4 antibody (MDX-010) in conjunction with peptides from gp100, MART-1, and tyrosinase [88]. Immune responses to the wild-type $gp100_{209-217}$ and $MART\text{-}1_{27-35}$ peptides were detected in 6 of 17 and 3 of 17 patients, respectively. No responses to tyrosinase were observed. Reversible dose-related autoimmune adverse events, predominantly skin and GI toxicities, were observed and appeared to correlate with a lower risk of relapse. The Surgical Branch at the NCI has also combined anti-CTLA-4 (MDX-010) with IL-2 in a study of 36 patients with advanced melanoma [89]. The objective response rate of 22% (3 complete responses and 5 partial responses) was consistent with an additive rather than synergistic effect between the two therapies.

A second anti-CTLA-4 antibody (CP-675,206) has been studied in 39 patients with advanced solid malignancies (melanoma, n = 34; renal cell, n = 4; colon, n = 1), resulting in 2 complete responses and 2 partial responses 29 of the patients with melanoma who had measurable disease [90]. Autoimmunity was also observed in this study and included diarrhea, dermatitis, vitiligo, panhypopituitarism and hyperthyroidism. These observations are similar to those reported in studies of other anti-CTLA-4 antibodies [85, 86, 89, 91].

Preliminary results have also been presented from a number of clinical studies of CTLA-4 blockade (using MDX-010) in patients with metastatic renal cancer, prostate cancer and melanoma (in combination with dacarbazine). Additional clinical trials of anti-CTLA-4 antibodies are currently ongoing, including a phase III study of MDX-0101 in patients with advanced melanoma.

These trials demonstrate exciting potential for anti-CTLA-4 antibodies in the clinic, and further studies are currently ongoing. However, as predicted, because CTLA-4 plays an important role in controlling T-cell responses, blocking its activity with antibodies may potentially lead to autoimmunity.

Other members of the CD28/CTLA-4/B7-1/B7-2 family

B7h/Inducible co-stimulator (ICOS) Inducible co-stimulator (ICOS) is a new member of the CD28/B7 family that is expressed on activated T cells [92]. A few limited studies have been carried out in murine cancer models suggesting that ligation of ICOS by B7h can potentiate tumor immunity. B7h transfection was shown to enhance tumor rejection in murine models of fibrosarcoma and plasmacytoma [93–95] and ligation of ICOS with its ligand conjugated to an Fc domain mediates regression of immunogenic tumors in mice [96].

PD-1/PD-L1 (B7-H1), PD-L2 (B7-DC)

Biology

Programmed Death-1 (PD-1), which is expressed by activated T cells, is thought to be primarily an inhibitory modulator, in part because PD-1-deficient mice suffer from autoimmunity [97]. A growing body of evidence has emerged in murine models suggesting that expression of PD-L1 may protect tumors from the immune system. PD-L1 on tumors causes apoptosis in tumor-reactive T cells [98]. A myeloma cell line expressing PD-L1 fails to grow in PD-1 knock-out mice [99]. PD-L1 blocking antibodies cured mice of squamous cell carcinoma in one model [100], and restored responsiveness to immunologic therapy with a 4-1BB (CD137) agonist in another [101]. PD-1 -/- T cells have been shown to have enhanced anti-tumor capabilities [102]. PD-L1 may also play an important role in the function of "suppressor" myeloid cells, as it was recently shown that tumor-associated dendritic cells express high levels of PD-L1, and that culturing dendritic cells in the presence of blocking antibody enhanced the development of T-cell responses against ovarian cancer [103]. One mechanism whereby PD-L1 mediates immune suppression may be through Interleukin-10 (IL-10) production [104]. In contrast, however, the other PD-1 ligand, PD-L2, stimulated immunity in mice to the poorly immunogenic B16 melanoma [105].

Consistent with the role of this pathway in tumor immune evasion, many human cancers have been found to express PD-L1 including tumors of the breast, cervix, lung, ovary, colon, as well as melanoma, glioblastoma and primary T cell lymphomas [98, 106, 107]. Furthermore, expression of PD-L1 may be associated with a poor prognosis in esophageal cancer [108], and renal cell cancer [109]. Similarly, PD-L2 is highly expressed in Hodgkin lymphoma cell lines and may also serve as a prognostic marker [110]. Trials using blocking antibodies against PD-L1 are currently being planned.

TNF Family Members

Tumor necrosis factor receptor (TNFR) family members play a role in maintaining T-cell responses after initial activation. They can signal via a death domain (DD) or a TNF receptor-associated factor (TRAF) protein (Reviewed in [111]). TRAF proteins costimulate T cells through signaling pathways associated with cellular activation, differentiation, and survival. Several of these molecules are being evaluated in the context of cancer immunotherapy.

CD27/CD70

Biology

CD27 is transiently up-regulated on T cells upon activation and is also expressed on NK cells and B cells [112]. Its ligand, CD70, is expressed on mature dendritic cells and activated lymphocytes [113–115]. Loss of CD27 expression on $CD8^+$ T cells is associated with a transition from central-memory to effector-memory phenotype [116]. CD27 -/- mice show impaired memory T cell function as well as decreased accumulation in peripheral tissues during viral infection [117]. Mice with constitutive CD27 expression display the opposite phenotype, accumulating increased T cell populations [118]. Interestingly, these mice develop a paucity of B cells and eventually succumb to a lethal T-cell immunodeficiency, perhaps due to an excessive shift in the T-cell population towards a terminally differentiated, non-reproducing memory phenotype [119].

Applications for tumor immunotherapy

There is significant evidence to support a role for CD27 co-stimulation in tumor rejection. CD70 transgenic mice display enhanced clearance of tumors [120]; transfection of tumor cells with CD70 produces similar results to those observed with B7-transfected tumors [121–123] and ligation of CD27 enhances anti-tumor responses [120]. Intriguingly, rejection of CD70-transfected tumors may be mediated by NK cells expressing CD27 [124].

OX40/OX40L

Biology

OX40 (CD134) expression is restricted to activated T-cells, predominately $CD4^+$ T-cells [125]. Its partner, OX40L, is found on a wide variety of immune cells including activated B cells, T cells, dendritic cells, and vascular epithelial cells [126–128]. Ligation of OX40 on T-cells favors survival, expansion and cytokine production [129]. Studies in knock-out animals show that OX40 is critical for CD4, but not CD8 responses [130]. OX40 is also important for the development and homeostasis of Tregs [131]. Significantly, in the context of immunotherapy, OX40 ligation may reverse T-cell anergy [132] and render silent epitopes immunogenic [133].

Applications for tumor immunotherapy

In mouse models, various strategies to augment OX40 signaling in anti-tumor T cells have shown promise. OX40 ligation increased tumor-free survival and cured some mice in animal models of melanoma, sarcoma, colon cancer, breast cancer or glioma [134–138]. Responses were seen even in poorly immunogenic tumors [134, 138]. In addition, treatment was effective in animal models of metastatic disease [135,137]. Following treatment, mice developed strong anti-tumor T-cell responses, in particular memory $CD4^+$ T-cells, which protected them from further challenge with the same tumor [134]. Vaccines with cells transfected with OX40L and GM-CSF have yielded cures in murine colon cancer models [139]. OX40 ligation has also shown synergy with a combination of 4-1BB ligation and Interleukin 12 (IL-12) [137]. The cumulative evidence from murine studies suggests that ligation of OX40, combined with other immunotherapies, is a promising avenue for research in the treatment of human cancers.

4-1BB/4-1BBL

Biology

4-1BB (CD137) is present on activated T cells [140], as well as NK cells [141], and dendritic cells [142]. 4-1BBL meanwhile can be found on activated APCs [143]. 4-1BB ligation stimulates $CD8^+$ T cells in particular [144], and promotes their differentiation into effectors [145]. Signaling through 4-1BB has been shown to reverse anergy induced by soluble antigens [146], as well as rescue $CD28^{-/-}$ $CD8^+$ T cells [147], which tend to accumulate in elderly persons [148], during chronic inflammation [149], and in cancer [150]. On the other hand, 4-1BB ligation can suppress $CD4^+$ T cells and B cells [151], perhaps due to chronic IFNγ stimulation [111]. In this regard, an agonist anti-4-1BB antibody has been shown to reverse autoimmunity in mice [152].

Applications for tumor immunotherapy

Dramatic responses have been achieved in mice using anti-4-1BB antibodies, with eradication of established tumors (reviewed in [153]). Ligation of 4-1BB by mechanisms including systemically administered antibodies [154–156], as well as therapeutic vaccination with 4-1-BBL expressing tumor cells [156,157] have been shown to result in tumor rejection. Tumor cells transfected with single-chain Fv fragments specific for 4-1BB are also effective [158]. $CD8^+$ T cells are thought to be the primary effectors in these models, but tumor rejection has also been shown in some models to be dependent on both $CD4^+$ T cells and NK cells [159], or on myeloid cells [160]. Significantly, however, ligation of 4-1BB is only effective when CD28 is present and once an immune reaction is already ongoing [161], consistent with *in vitro* models showing a role for 4-1BB later in the immune response [162]. As a result, 4-1BB ligation has therefore been used in combination with CD28 stimulation, with the goal of targeting these two pathways simultaneously [163, 164]. 4-1BB ligation may also be useful in strategies for adoptive immunotherapy because it allows for a greater expansion of $CD8^+$ T cells than CD28 alone [165].

HVEM-LIGHT

Biology

Herpes Virus Entry Mediator (HVEM), initially isolated as the receptor for herpes virus [166], binds at least three receptors: LIGHT, Ltα3 and BTLA [167–169]. LIGHT, in turn, binds two receptors in addition to HVEM: LTβR and CdR3/TR6 [170]. HVEM is expressed on resting T cells, monocytes, and immature dendritic cells, while LIGHT can be found on activated T cells, monocytes and NK cells as well as on immature dendritic cells [170]. LIGHT signaling causes proliferation of T cells stimulated with CD3 or CD3/CD28 [171–173], and it can induce DC maturation [174]. Over-expression of LIGHT causes autoimmunity with increased T cell populations and inflammation of mucosal tissues [175]. Conversely, LIGHT deficiency causes CD8$^+$ T-cell dysfunction [176]. BTLA (B- and T-lymphocyte attenuator) is expressed on activated T cells, B cells and dendritic cells, and its signals can suppress T-cell responses [177, 178].

Applications for tumor immunotherapy

LIGHT is thought to exert its anti-tumor effects through apoptosis induction, as well as through immune activation [179]. LIGHT can kill tumors expressing HVEM via a death-domain pathway [180]. Meanwhile, transfection of tumors with LIGHT causes T-cell-dependent tumor rejection [173, 181]. A very intriguing study showed that tumors transfected with LIGHT induce changes in the tumor stromal cells facilitating the entry of T cells into the tumor [181].

CD40/CD40L

Biology

CD40 is expressed on antigen presenting cells, while CD40L is found on activated T cells. CD40 plays a critical role in humoral immune responses and enables APCs to activate T cells. The CD40/CD40L pathway has been implicated in a wide array of disease pathogenesis, including lupus and arherosclerosis, but the clinical application of anti-CD40L antibodies has been limited to date by thrombotic complications due to CD40 expression on activated platelets [182–184].

CD40 is also present on multiple cancers including hematologic malignancies and solid tumors. In hematologic cancers, signaling via CD40 may mediate growth [185] or regression [186], whereas CD40 signaling is purely tumoricidal in solid tumors [187, 188]. These effects persist in SCID mice, and are therefore likely due to signaling via the TNF death domain [187, 188]. However, there is ample evidence to show that immune modulation also occurs. For example, blockade of the CD40/CD40L pathway mitigates the protective effect of a GM-CSF secreting melanoma vaccine [191].

Applications for tumor immunotherapy

Tumor vaccines expressing CD40L have shown efficacy in cancer models [192–197]. Ligation of CD40 with CD40L or anti-CD40 antibodies has also shown synergy with GM-CSF [198], IFNγ [192], IL-2 [199], and CTLA-4 blockade [200]. A phase I clinical trial in plasma cell leukemia that combined the adoptive transfer of T cells stimulated with CD40-activated tumor cells, a vaccine of CD40-activated tumor cells, and IL-2 has been tested in one patient and yielded a decline in circulating tumor [201]. In addition, a humanized IgG1 anti-human CD40 (SGN-40, Seattle Genetics, Inc., Bothell, WA) has been shown to have activity in pre-clinical models of multiple myeloma and non-hodgkin lymphoma and is currently in a phase I clinical trial in patients with multiple myeloma [202, 203].

Glucocorticoid-induced tumor necrosis factor receptor family-related gene (GITR)

Glucocorticoid-induced TNFR family-related gene (GITR, or TNFRSF18) is a type I transmembrane protein with significant homology to other TNFR family members, including OX40, 4-1BB, and CD27 [204, 205]. GITR is expressed at low levels on resting $CD4^+$ and $CD8^+$ T-cells, and is upregulated on these cells following TCR-mediated activation. Ligation of GITR during activation enhances both $CD4^+$ and $CD8^+$ T-cell proliferation and effector functions, particularly in the setting of suboptimal TCR stimulation [206–210]. In addition, GITR is expressed constitutively at high levels on Tregs, which has lead to its evaluation as a potential target for strategies designed to inhibit suppression. Signaling through GITR, either using agonist anti-GITR antibodies or GITR ligand, has been shown to abrogate the suppressive effects of Tregs *in vitro* and *in vivo*, leading to enhancement of both auto-reactive and allo-reactive T cell responses and exacerbation of disease in autoimmune and graft-versus-host disease models [206, 211–215]. Whether these effects are due primarily to a loss of suppressive activity by Tregs or to an increased resistance to suppression by effector T cells, or both, is currently a subject of debate, but the net effect of GITR signaling is the potential for enhanced ability of effector T cells to recognize and respond to self. As a result, this pathway may also be a useful target in the development of tumor immunotherapy.

CYTOKINES

Cytokines and chemokines are important molecules that form a link between innate and adaptive immunity. They affect immune responses at several levels by modulating the proliferation, differentiation, function and trafficking of immune cells. A number of studies in pre-clinical animal models and in clinical trials have examined the potential for therapeutic use of cytokines in treating cancer. Several cytokines have been approved for use in patients with cancer, including interferon-alpha [216], interleukin-2 (IL-2) [217], and hematopoietic growth factors such as granulocyte colony stimulating factor (G-CSF) [218] and granulocyte-macrophage colony stimulating factor (GM-CSF) [219]. Interferon and Interleukin-2 are discussed in other chapters in this textbook (Chapters 18 and 19). In this section, we will review two broad categories of cytokines, those that enhance immune responses and those that may suppress anti-tumor immunity. For the evolving field of chemokines and their potential role in tumor immunotherapy, the reader is referred to recent reviews on the subject [220–222].

Activating Cytokines

A number of cytokines are currently under investigation based on their ability to enhance immune responses to tumor antigens. In particular, interest has focused on cytokines that affect T-cell responses indirectly through APC activation and chemotaxis (GM-CSF), or directly by increasing T-cell activation (IL-2, IL-12,

IL-15, IL-18) or inducing or maintaining T-cell memory (IL-7, IL-15). In addition, a number of cytokines have been shown to enhance tumor antigen presentation or have direct effects on tumor cells (IFNα, IFNγ and TNF). Many of these cytokines have been given in combination with tumor vaccines, which are detailed in several chapters in Part 2.

Tumor Necrosis Factor (TNF)

Biology

TNF was originally identified for its ability to cause hemorrhagic necrosis of sarcomas [223] and was the first cytokine studied for the treatment of cancer (Reviewed in [224]). TNF is a homotrimer, synthesized as a membrane-bound propeptide, and released after cleavage by TNF-converting enzyme [225]. There are two distinct TNF receptors. TNF-R1 is expressed on all cell types [226], while TNF-R2 is only found on immune and endothelial cells [227]. An important mechanism of TNF regulation is the release of TNF receptors from the cell surface that then circulate in soluble form, binding and inhibiting the activity of TNF [225].

Applications for tumor immunotherapy

TNF has direct antiproliferative and cytotoxic effects on cells, with some selectivity for tumor cells [228]. It also reduces tumor blood flow and causes tumor vascular damage [229, 230]. Finally, TNF may also modulate the immune response by stimulating macrophage and NK cell activity [231, 232].

The clinical use of TNF has been limited by dose-dependent hypotension and capillary leak that can lead to a sepsis-like syndrome. As a result, TNF is currently given only through locoregional drug-delivery systems in order to limit systemic effects. Current applications include isolated limb perfusion for the treatment of sarcomas [233] and in-transit metastatic melanoma [234, 235], as well as isolated hepatic perfusion for unresectable liver tumors [236]. In most cases, TNF is administered with standard cytotoxic agents. Although non-randomized studies have reported higher response rates with the addition of TNF to chemotherapy agents in the locoregional setting [237–239], randomized studies are currently ongoing. Intralesional TNF for treatment of Kaposi's sarcoma was evaluated in a randomized blinded study, and although responses were observed in the injected lesions, there was dose-limiting systemic toxicity due to TNF administration [240].

Several additional approaches to deliver TNF locally are currently under clinical investigation. Injection of adenovirus modified to express TNF is being studied in gastrointestinal malignancies with the goal of increasing responsiveness to chemotherapy and radiation. Preliminary human studies show that the injections are well-tolerated [241], and prospective controlled trials are ongoing. A tumor vasculature-targeted TNF compound has also been developed [242] and is currently undergoing phase I testing in an EORTC trial.

Granulocyte-Macrophage Colony Stimulating Factor (GM-CSF)

Biology

GM-CSF is produced by monocytes/ macrophages and activated T cells [219]. The ability of GM-CSF to act as a growth factor to stimulate and recruit dendritic cells may explain its adjuvant role. In a mouse model study, Dranoff *et al.* [243] found that vaccination with syngeneic mouse melanoma cells secreting GM-CSF stimulated more potent and long-lasting anti-tumor immunity than vaccines that produced other cytokines. Similar results were observed in other tumor models, including lung, colon, renal cell, prostate, lymphoma and leukemia [244–248].

Applications for tumor immunotherapy

GM-CSF (Sargramostin, Berlex, Inc, Montville, NJ) has been given in soluble form in patients with melanoma. In 51 patients with Stage III and IV melanoma treated with adjuvant GM-CSF for up to a year, there was an increased disease-free survival compared to historical controls [249]. A multi-center four-arm phase III trial of GM-CSF given in the adjuvant setting with or without a peptide vaccine (compared to vaccine alone or placebo) is currently ongoing. GM-CSF has also been used extensively in the *in vitro* generation of dendritic cells for vaccines [250, 251] (See Chapter 17).

In most clinical trials, GM-CSF has been used as an immune adjuvant. Various strategies to use GM-CSF in this setting have been explored, including systemic and topical application of soluble GM-CSF, fusion of GM-CSF to other proteins, transfection of tumor cells with GM-CSF, and injection of GM-CSF DNA.

Recombinant GM-CSF has been given as an adjuvant for peptide, protein and viral vaccines (reviewed in [252]). It has been shown to be an effective adjuvant for peptide vaccines in a number of studies in patients with melanoma [253–257] or breast and ovarian cancers [258]. Recombinant GM-CSF has also been given with canarypox viruses expressing tumor antigens [259, 260]. An alternative approach in which the tumor antigen is fused to GM-CSF has demonstrated that GM-CSF can enhance the immunogenicity of the antigen in the fusion protein [261–263].

Several gene-therapy approaches in which the gene for GM-CSF is used instead of recombinant GM-CSF are also under investigation. These include transfection of tumor cells, plasmid DNA and recombinant viruses. Based on the use in mouse models of whole tumor cell vaccines expressing GM-CSF, initial clinical studies using autologous vaccines expressing GM-CSF have demonstrated the feasibility and safety of the approach. In addition, inflammatory responses were observed at the sites of injection, as well as sites of metastatic lesions [264–270]. In the majority of clinical trials using autologous cells, expansion of primary tumor cell cultures for each patient has been a limiting factor. To alleviate the issues of tumor cell recovery and expansion, some investigators have used allogeneic tumor cell lines expressing GM-CSF [271] or a human cell line producing large quantities of human

GM-CSF as universal bystander cells to be mixed with unmodified autologous tumor cells in the formulation of a vaccine [272]. Although clinical responses have been reported in a number of trials investigating cellular vaccines expressing GM-CSF, interpretation of the results is difficult because of relatively small numbers of patients.

The efficacy of recombinant vaccinia viruses expressing murine GM-CSF (rvv-mGM-CSF) has been evaluated in mouse pre-clinical models and shown the adjuvant effects of GM-CSF-based vaccines [273, 274]. Further clinical trials will be needed to elucidate the role of GM-CSF with recombinant viruses.

Finally, our group has previously shown that administration of mouse GM-CSF DNA by particle bombardment into skin induces a significant increase in dendritic cells at the inoculation site and in draining lymph nodes [275, 276]. GM-CSF DNA expression increases T-cell responses following peptide immunization and antibody responses following xenogeneic DNA immunization (see Chapter 15). It also provides increased tumor protection in mice immunized with a melanoma antigen [275,277]. Similarly, other groups have shown that GM-CSF DNA enhances protection of DNA immunization in models of malaria [278] or Dengue fever [279]. We are currently conducting a pilot clinical trial at MSKCC in which patients with advanced melanoma are being given human GM-CSF DNA as an adjuvant for a polypeptide melanoma vaccine.

Interleukin 7 (IL-7)

Biology

IL-7 is a 25 kD glycoprotein produced by stromal cells in the thymus and bone marrow [280], keratinocytes [281], intestinal epithelium [282], and dendritic cells [283]. The IL-7 receptor consists of a specific α chain (CD127) and the common γ chain (CD132), which is also found in the receptors for IL-2, IL-4, IL-9, IL-15 and IL-21 [284–288]. IL-7 and IL-7Rα knockout mice have no $\gamma\delta$ T cells and a 100-fold reduction in thymic cellularity, although a small number of $\alpha\beta$ T cells can develop apparently normally [289, 290]. Patients with mutations in the IL-7Rα or common γ chain develop severe combined immunodeficiency syndrome with a prominent T-cell deficiency.

IL-7 has a variety of effects on lymphocyte development and survival, and is a key regulator of peripheral T-cell homeostasis [291]. It is required at various stages of T-cell development, including the development and survival of memory T cells, and homeostatic proliferation of T cells in peripheral lymphopenia [292, 293]. Administration of IL-7 has several stimulatory effects on T-cell development, including increased thymopoiesis [294–296]). Preclinical studies in mouse hematopoietic stem cell transplant (HSCT) models have demonstrated that post-transplant IL-7 administration can enhance T-cell reconstitution in recipients of a syngeneic or allogeneic HSCT through increased thymopoiesis, increased homeostatic T-cell proliferation and decreased peripheral T-cell apoptosis [295, 297–300].

Applications for tumor immunotherapy

Studies in non-human primates have shown that IL-7 administration has more profound effects on peripheral T cell proliferation than on thymopoiesis and is less effective at promoting B cell development than in rodents [301]. The results of these pre-clinical studies have lead to clinical trials of recombinant human IL-7 (CYT 99 007, Cytheris, Inc, Rockville, MD) in patients with AIDS, tumor-associated immune deficiency and post-transplant immune deficiency, which are currently underway at several centers (R. Buffet, personal communication).

Interleukin 12 (IL-12)

Biology

IL-12 is a heterodimeric pro-inflammatory cytokine formed by two subunits, the p35 and p40 subunits [302,303]. The p40 subunit also combines with a p19 subunit to form interleukin 23 (IL-23), another member of the IL-12 family [304]. IL-12 is primarily produced by dendritic cells and monocytes/macrophages and forms a link between the innate and adaptive immune systems [305]. It induces the production of IFNγ, promotes Th1 differentiation [306, 307], enhances the proliferation of pre-activated T cells and NK cells [303, 308, 309] and induces the production of cytokines (including IFNγ, TNF and GM-CSF) by these cells [302, 310, 311].

Applications for tumor immunotherapy

Systemic administration of recombinant IL-12 is effective in treating tumors in several mouse models [312–314] and has also been shown to provide adjuvant effects for tumor vaccines in mouse preclinical models [315–317]. Recombinant human IL-12 (Wyeth, Cambridge, MA) has been investigated in phase I and phase II clinical trials in patients with a number of malignancies including renal cell cancer and melanoma [318–322], cervical cancer [323], non-Hodgkin's lymphoma (NHL) or Hodgkin's disease (HD) [324] with some limited activity. IL-12 has also been used to enhance responses to peptide vaccines in human studies [325, 326]. Finally, the role of IL-12 DNA as a molecular adjuvant has been demonstrated in infectious disease models [327].

Interleukin 15 (IL-15)

Biology

IL-15 is a pleiotropic cytokine that plays an important role in both the innate and adaptive immune system [328–330]. IL-15 is a member of the 4 alpha-helix bundle family of proteins that includes growth hormone, IL-2, IL-3, IL-6, IL-7, G-CSF and GM-CSF [331–333]. The IL-15 receptor is composed of three subunits: an IL-15Rα subunit, aβ chain subunit (CD122), and the common γ chain. The β chain subunit is shared with IL-2 [328, 330, 334]. IL-15Rα has a wide cellular distribution and is expressed on T cells, NK cells, NKT cells, B cells, macrophages, and in thymic and bone marrow stromal cell lines [334, 335]. IL-15 promotes the activation of neutrophils and macrophages, and is critical to dendritic cell function. In addition, IL-15 promotes the development, activation, homing and survival of immune effector cells, particularly NK, natural killer T (NKT) and $CD8^+$ T cells.

Applications for tumor immunotherapy

IL-15 has been studied as a vaccine adjuvant in a number of infectious diseases, including HIV, HSV and hepatitis B [336–343]. Co-administration of IL-15 DNA enhanced $CD8^+$ T-cell responses to HIV DNA vaccines targeting the *envelope* and *gag* proteins in mouse models [336–339]. Similar results were observed in mice immunized with vaccinia expressing HIV gp160 in conjunction with IL-15 [340]. Interestingly, the latter study also demonstrated that mice injected with vaccinia expressing IL-15 had long-term immunity, whereas the $CD8^+$ T cell-mediated immunity induced by IL-2 was short-lived. These results are consistent with those obtained in rhesus macaques that were immunized against tetanus toxoid and influenza and received daily injections of IL-15 or IL-2 [341].

Interleukin 18 (IL-18)

Biology

IL-18 is a monocyte/macrophage-derived cytokine that participates in the induction of IFNγ and other cytokines [344–346]. In addition to being produced by monocytes/macrophages, IL-18 is also secreted by keratinocytes, dendritic cells, Kuppfer cells in the liver, synovial fibroblasts and osteoblasts [346]. It is structurally related to IL-1β [347]. Similar to the IL-1β precursor, the biologically inactive IL-18 precursor (pro-IL-18) lacks a signal peptide and requires caspase-1 (also known as IL-1β-converting enzyme, or ICE) for cleavage and release of the mature molecule from the intracellular compartment [347–349]. Only mature IL-18 is bioactive, whereas pro-IL-18 is biologically inactive [350]. The importance of the presence of both IL-12 and IL-18 for optimal induction of IFNγ has been demonstrated in IL-18 and ICE knock-out mice [351–353]. In the absence of a costimulus, IL-18 is a weak inducer of IFNγ. However, a synergy for IFNγ production is observed when cells are cultured with IL-18 in the presence of costimuli [354–356]. Different mechanisms may account for this synergy. In particular, IL-12 upregulates the expression of the IL-18 receptor, therefore rendering cells more sensitive to IL-18 [357,358]. In addition, IL-12 and IL-18 regulate the transcriptional activity of the IFNγ promoter at different levels [359], thus providing two distinct signals to the IFNγ-producing cell. IL-12 and IL-18 also regulate each other's production [360, 361].

IL-18 has a number of important biological effects and modulates the activity of T and B cells, NK cells, macrophages, dendritic cells and chondrocytes. In synergy with IL-12 it plays a major role in promoting Th1 responses though the induction of IFNγ.

Applications for tumor immunotherapy

The majority of studies investigating the role of IL-18 in tumor immunotherapy have combined IL-18 with other approaches, in particular with IL-12. Systemic administration of IL-18 enhanced the rejection of IL-12-expressing melanoma in mouse models [362]. Conversely, systemic administration of IL-12 increased tumor rejection induced by intra-tumoral injection of dendritic cells expressing IL-18 [363]. Intra-tumoral gene transfer of IL-12 and IL-18 through electroporation [364], or the use of a tumor cell vaccine expressing both cytokines [365, 366] has been shown to have synergistic effects in mouse models of melanoma and bladder cancer. In addition, the *in vitro* combination of the two cytokines was shown to have synergistic effects on the generation of anti-tumor $CD4^+$ and $CD8^+$ T cells [367]. IL-18 DNA has also been shown to enhance the effects of DNA vaccines targeting gp100 [368] or Fos-related antigen 1, a transcription factor overexpressed by tumor cells [369]. Finally, injection of adenovirus producing IL-18 enhances the effects of cytosine deaminase suicide gene therapy or antibody-targeted superantigen in mouse melanoma models [370, 371]. Phase I studies of recombinant IL-18 (SB-485232, GlaxoSmithKline) are currently ongoing in patients with cancer.

Immunosuppressive Cytokines

In contrast to the above cytokines that are being investigated as therapeutic agents in patients with cancer, certain cytokines have been found to suppress immune responses to tumor antigens. This has lead investigators to develop strategies to block the effects of these cytokines in order to allow effective immunity to proceed.

Transforming Growth Factor-β(TGF-β).

Biology

TGF-β is a potent inhibitor of the immune system, and is one of the proposed mechanisms by which tumor cells evade immune surveillance [4, 372–374]. TGF-β is secreted in a latent inactive form, bound to a protein complex, and is activated by proteases. Three isoforms have been identified, as well as three cell surface receptors.

TGF-β has well-described effects on multiple components of the immune system (Table 5). TGF-β can inhibit T lymphocytes by decreasing their proliferation and stimulation induced by IL-2 [375–378] or IL-12 [379], and suppress the development of Th1 responses [379] and generation and function of cytotoxic T lymphocytes [383, 384]. TGF-β inhibits lymphocyte production of IFNγ, TNF, IL-2, IL-6, IL-4, and IL-5 [385–388]. TGF-β is also thought to be a critical cytokine in the suppressive effects of $CD4^+CD25^+$ regulatory T cells [389]. The inhibitory effects of TGF-β on natural killer cells include decreased proliferation [390], activation [391, 392], cytotoxicity [393, 394] and cytokine production [382]. Similarly, TGF-β decreases the activity and production of lymphokine-activated

Table 5. Effects of TGF-β, IL-10, and IL-13 on Components of the Immune System

Monocytes/macrophages		
TGF-β:	**IL-10:**	**IL-13:**
• inhibits macrophage production in cell cultures [397, 398]. • reduces macrophage activity [399]. • attenuates macrophage responsiveness to cytokine stimulation [399]. • down-regulates macrophage production of cytokines [400, 401].	• down-regulates macrophage production of cytokines [8, 457]. • decreases antigen-presentation by down-regulating co-stimulatory molecules and adhesion molecules [458–460]. • stimulates phagocytic activity [455]. • stimulates macrophage secretion of B cell survival factor in Burkitt's lymphoma [527].	• changes the monocyte phenotype [516]. • inhibits cytotoxic activity [516]. • inhibits cytokine release [516].
T lymphocytes		
TGF-β:	**IL-10:**	**IL-13:**
• blocks ability of IL-2 to stimulate lymphocyte proliferation [375–378]. • blocks stimulatory effects of IL-12 on lymphocytes [379]. • suppresses generation and activity of cytotoxic T lymphocytes [383, 384]. • depresses Th1 responses [380–382]. • down-regulates lymphocyte production of cytokines [385–388]. • central role in development and function of regulatory T cells [389, 528].	• inhibits proliferation of naïve CD4+ T cells [458]. • down-regulates lymphocyte production of cytokines [529]. • along with TGF-β has a central role in development and function of regulatory T cells [528]. • promotes resistance to cytotoxic T cells by reducing MHC class I expression on tumor cells [530].	• may down-regulate $CD8^+$ T cells via TGF-β [519].

(Continued)

Table 5. (Continued)

Monocytes/macrophages		
NK cells		
TGF-β:	**IL-10:**	
• decreases NK cell proliferation [390]. • down-regulates NK cell cytokine production [382] • reduces NK cell activation and cytotoxicity [391–394]. • reduces generation and activity of lymphokine-activated killer cells [385, 395, 396].	• increases NK cell production of cytokines and cytotoxic activity [456]. • up-regulates migration-related genes [531].	
Dendritic cells		
TGF-β:	**IL-10:**	**IL-13:**
• suppresses DC maturation [402]. • may be important in the normal migration of immature DCs [403].	• induces preferential differentiation of monocytes into macrophages rather than DC [461, 462]. • inhibits DC maturation [463]. • down-regulates effective antigen presentation [464].	• stimulates differentiation of monocytes into dendritic cells [532, 533].

killer cells [385,395,396]. TGF-β has also been shown to have an inhibitory effect on monocytes and macrophages [397,400,401]. Finally, although TGF-β suppresses dendritic cell maturation [402], it may play a role in the normal migration of immature dendritic cells [403].

TGF-β is thought to have a complex role in malignancy, capable of both suppressing tumor growth as well as promoting tumor spread by inhibiting immune responses against tumor cells. In addition, it has been shown to enhance tumor invasion, metastasis, and angiogenesis [404, 405]. Whether TGF-β inhibits or promotes malignancy may depend on the stage of the malignant process. Early during the development of a tumor, TGF-β is likely a tumor suppressor, inhibiting cell proliferation by inducing cell cycle arrest [406] as well as possibly augmenting T cell responses through inhibition of IL-6 [407]. Tumor cells likely develop resistance to the anti-proliferative effects of TGF-β by acquiring defects in the TGF-β signaling pathway, including receptor down-regulation [408–410], and mutations in the receptors [411–415] or signaling pathways [409,416–418]. Elevated serum levels of TGF-β have been associated with increased tumor aggressiveness and poorer prognosis [419–422]. Serum levels, however, have not been found to correlate with tumor burden or predict treatment responses in head and neck cancer [423].

Applications for tumor immunotherapy

Several strategies are under investigation to target TGF-β, including the use of antibodies, soluble receptors, TGF-β-associated binding proteins, antisense oligonucleotides and TGF-β-insensitive T cells. Some of these approaches have progressed to clinical trials.

Neutralizing antibodies to TGF-β have had promising results in murine models of melanoma [424], fibrosarcoma [425], and breast cancer [426]. *In vitro* studies suggest that neutralizing antibodies may enhance the efficacy of chemotherapy agents such as cisplatin [427]. Combining antibodies with other modalities of immunotherapy such as IL-2 may have enhanced effects [424,425,428]. Finally, inducing autologous antibodies against TGF-β by using plasmid DNA encoding xenogeneic TGF-β resulted in enhanced efficacy of a plasmid DNA melanoma vaccine in mice [429].

Similarly, preclinical studies using soluble type II TGF-β receptor (TβRII) to bind TGF-β have had promising results in murine models of malignant mesothelioma [430], pancreatic cancer [431,432], melanoma [433], breast cancer [433,434], and thymoma [435].

The use of latency-associated peptide, which binds TGF-β in an inactive form, resulted in decreased tumor size in a murine model of prostate cancer [436]. Decorin, a small TGF-β-binding proteoglycan, also has inhibitory effects on TGF-β. Tumor cells overexpressing decorin have decreased growth in murine models of glioma [437–439] and ovarian cancer [440].

The use of anti-TGF-β antisense oligonucleotides has been shown to be effective in studies in tumors expressing antisense targeting TGF-β1 [441–443], or whole-cell vaccines expressing anti-TGF-β2 antisense were used [444]. In addition, intratumoral administration of antisense targeting TGF-β2 was shown to be beneficial in a murine model of malignant mesothiolioma [445] and antisense TGF-β2 given intrathecally and intraparenchymally for brain tumors has been reported in mice, rabbits, and primates [446].

Adoptive transfer of tumor-reactive TGF-β-insensitive $CD8^+$ T cells has been investigated in murine models of melanoma and prostate cancer. Transplantation of bone marrow expressing a dominant-negative TGF-β type II receptor lead to the generation of mature leukocytes capable of *in vivo* tumor rejection [447]. In another study by the same group, $CD8^+$ T cells infected with a retrovirus containing the dominant-negative TGF-β type II receptor after *in vivo* priming were able to prevent tumor growth in a metastatic prostate cancer model [448]. Transgenic mice with TGF-β-insensitive T cells have also been found to be protected in models of malignant melanoma and thymoma [449].

Clinical trials

To date, the majority of studies targeting TGF-β have been carried out in patients with autoimmune diseases. Despite promising results of a human monoclonal antibody against TGF-β2 (CAT-152, lerdelimumab, Cambridge Antibody Technology, Cambridge, UK) in phase I/II testing in the treatment of scarring due to glaucoma filtration surgery [450], phase III studies were inconclusive and development has been halted. Similarly, a human monoclonal antibody against TGF-β1 (CAT 192, metelimumab, Cambridge Antibody Technology) has not gone beyond phase I testing in patients with scleroderma. A pan-specific human monocolonal antibody against TGF-β (GC-1008) is currently being developed by the same company. Some of these approaches may eventually merit further investigation in patients with cancer. Furthermore, studies with an anti-TGF-β2 antisense oligonucleotide are currently ongoing in patients with high-grade glioma, pancreatic cancer and melanoma [451].

Interleukin 10 (IL-10)

Biology

IL-10 is generally thought to be an immunosuppressive cytokine, although in certain settings it can have stimulatory effects (Table 5). IL-10 is a homodimeric 17-20 kDa glycoprotein, with an alpha-helical tertiary structure [104]. The IL-10 receptor is a member of the IFN receptor family, and has two subunits [104]. The IL-10 receptor-α subunit is primarily expressed on immune cells, with the highest density on monocytes and macrophages, while the β subunit is found ubiquitously [452]. IL-10 is produced be many different components of the immune system, including T cells, B cells, monocytes, dendritic cells, and NK cells [453,454].

IL-10 stimulates macrophage phagocytosis and NK cytotoxicity [455,456], while suppressing inflammatory cytokines [8,457], antigen-presentation [458–464], and T cell responses [458,465]. IL-10 can act as a growth factor for malignant B cells, including myeloma [466] and B cell lymphomas [467, 468]. Finally, animal data suggest that one of the mechanisms of anti-CTLA-4 antibodies may be through a decrease in IL-10 secretion [38]. While the effects of anti-CTLA-4 and anti-IL-10 antibodies were similar, no additive effect was noted when the two were combined.

Tumors have been shown to produce IL-10, including non-small cell lung cancer [469, 470], melanoma [464, 471], glioma [472], leukemia [473], and lymphoma [474, 475]. Furthermore, increased IL-10 production has been observed in tumor-infiltrating lymphocytes from patients with non-small cell lung cancer [476] and peritoneal monocytes from patients with malignant ascites secondary to metastatic ovarian cancer. Elevated IL-10 serum levels represent a poor prognostic factor in NHL [477], CLL [478], Hodgkin's disease [479, 480], cutaneous T-cell lymphoma [481], and some solid tumors [482–486]. Finally, susceptibility to certain malignancies may be predicted by IL-10 promoter polymorphisms [487–489]. These findings suggest that IL-10 may be an important mediator of the ability of tumors to escape immune surveillance. It should be noted, however, that in some instances IL-10 may have a role as a tumor suppressor. Possible mechanisms include inhibiting angiogenesis [490], and preventing tumor metastasis by stimulating NK cell activity [491].

Applications for tumor immunotherapy

Similar to TGF-β, several strategies are being investigated to inhibit IL-10 activity [452, 492]. These include antibodies to IL-10 or its receptor, antisense oligonucleotides, and small interference RNA.

In vitro studies of anti-IL-10 antibodies have shown enhanced monocyte function [493], as well as an increase in sensitivity to chemotherapy in thyroid cancer cells [494], and enhanced sensitivity to rituximab of non-Hodgkin's lymphoma [495,496]. Studies in mouse melanoma models have shown that tumors overexpressing IL-10 were more aggressive, had decreased infiltration by macrophages and that the effects of IL-10 were prevented by treatment with anti-IL-10 antibodies [497]. Similarly, transgenic mice over-expressing IL-10 did poorly when challenged with immunogenic tumors, while anti-IL-10 antibodies restored the anti-tumor response [498]. Regulatory T cells appear to be stimulated by melanoma cells via IL-10, a process which can be blocked by anti-IL-10 antibodies [499]. Anti-IL-10 antibodies were also effective in a murine model of plasmocytoma [38]. In contrast, other studies have shown that anti-IL-10 antibodies could enhance tumor growth in plasmocytoma models, possibly due to a decrease in cytotoxic T cell responses [500]. It is possible that some of these diverging results may be due to the timing of anti-IL-10 antibody administration and this may have bearing on the design of clinical trials.

Another approach under investigation has targeted the IL-10 receptor. The *in vitro* inhibition of T cell proliferation by IL-10-secreting monocytes has been found to be reversible by anti-IL-10 receptor antibodies [501].

Finally, the use of anti-IL-10 antisense and small interference RNA has demonstrated enhanced immune responses through IL-10 blockade. In mouse models of plasmocytoma, whole-cell tumor vaccines were found to be more effective when given with an IL-10 antisense retrovirus [502] or IL-10-specific antisense oligodeoxynucleotides [503]. Similarly, transfection of dendritic cells with small interference RNA resulted in decreased IL-10 expression and augmented Th1 responses [504]. The latter results are consistent with the fact that dendritic cells engineered to be deficient in IL-10 were shown to be potent antigen-presenting cells with a high Th1-activating capacity [505].

Clinical trials

Trials in humans using IL-10 antagonists are in the early stages. One study using a murine anti-IL-10 monoclonal antibody in patients with systemic lupus erythematosus, in which IL-10 contributes to pathogenesis, demonstrated safety and potential benefit [506].

Interleukin 13 (IL-13)

Biology

Interleukin-13 is an important regulatory cytokine that can stimulate immune responses against certain infections and promote anti-tumor activity, while also being involved in the down-regulation of immune surveillance, allowing tumors to escape immune responses (Table 5, recently reviewed in [507, 508]).

The gene for IL-13 is located on chromosome 5q31, close to the gene for IL-4, with which it has roughly 30% homology and shares receptor components [509]. There are two IL-13 receptors. The main IL-13 receptor is composed of two subunits, IL-4Rα and IL-13Rα1 [510–512]. A second receptor, IL-13Rα2, is thought to serve to inactivate IL-13 and down-regulate IL-13 activity [513, 514]. IL-13 is produced by a variety of immune cells, including T cells, B cells, mast cells, basophils, NK cells, and dendritic cells [507]. Like IL-4, IL-13 plays a role in inducing IgE class-switching in B cells [515] and inhibits inflammatory cytokine production [516]. IL-13 is also an important player in resistance to both nematodes and intracellular parasites, and also plays a role in inflammatory lung diseases, tissue modeling, and fibrosis [508].

NKT cells have been implicated as a major source of IL-13. NKT cells from tumor-bearing mice produce more IL-13 compared to cells from control mice [517], and NKT cell-deficient CD1d knockout mice have lower levels of IL-13 production and exhibit high tumor resistance [518]. IL-13 produced by NKT cells has been shown to suppress cytotoxic T-lymphocyte rejection of tumors [518]. IL-13 stimulates $CD11b^{+}GR\text{-}1^{+}$ myeloid cells to produce TGF-β, which then suppresses cytotoxic T-cell activity [519].

Applications for tumor immunotherapy

A variety of tumor types express the IL-13 receptor, including lymphoma, renal cell carcinoma, glioblastoma, head and neck cancer, hepatoma, pancreatic cancer, breast cancer, prostate cancer, and colon cancer [507]. In Hodgkin's lymphoma,

IL-13 acts as an autocrine growth factor for the Reed-Sternberg cells, making it a potential target for therapy [520]. In contrast, IL-13 has been found to inhibit proliferation of a variety of tumor cell lines including breast, renal cell and B-cell lymphoblastic leukemias [508]. Furthermore, tumors engineered to secrete IL-13 or overexpress IL-13Ra2 have been found to be less aggressive [521,522].

The inhibitory effects of IL-13 on tumor immune surveillance have been attributed to its ability to promote a Th2 rather than a Th1 response. Murine knockout models targeting the IL-13 pathway, including Stat6-/- [518,523,524] and IL-4Rα-/- [518] show increased tumor rejection rates. Similar results were obtained when wild-type mice were given an IL-13 inhibitor, soluble IL-13Rα2-Fc [507,518].

Clinical trials

Because many tumor cell types express IL-13 receptors, researchers have tried to exploit this using human IL-13 conjugated to a genetically engineered Pseudomonas exotoxin molecule (IL13-PE38QQR, cintredekin besudotox, NeoPharm Inc, Lake Forest, IL). This compound is currently undergoing phase III testing for adult gliomas and was recently reviewed [525].

CONCLUSION

The past two decades have been marked by a growing understanding of the co-stimulatory pathways and cytokines that are critical to the generation of an effective immune response. Our current understanding is that interacting immunomodulatory molecules expressed on a wide array of tissues may exert both stimulatory and inhibitory functions depending on the immunologic context. In addition, cytokines and chemokines may further influence the development and regulation of immune responses. The discovery of these important pathways has lead to an explosion in the field of therapeutic approaches that may be of benefit to patients with autoimmune diseases or cancer. A number of these molecules are currently being targeted in early stage-clinical trials and some have progressed to phase III studies or are currently in clinical use.

Given the complexity of the generation and regulation of anti-tumor immunity, it is likely that successful therapeutic approaches will ultimately require combining different immunotherapies [526], including vaccines, cytokines and antibodies that enhance immune responses or down-regulate mechanisms of immunosuppression.

REFERENCES

1. Perales MA, Blachere NE, Engelhorn ME et al. Strategies to overcome immune ignorance and tolerance. Semin Cancer Biol 2002; 12: 63–71.
2. Jager E, Ringhoffer M, Karbach J et al. Inverse relationship of melanocyte differentiation antigen expression in melanoma tissues and CD8+ cytotoxic-T-cell responses: evidence for immunoselection of antigen-loss variants in vivo. Int J Cancer 1996; 66: 470–476.
3. Dessureault S, Graham F, Gallinger S. B7–1 gene transfer into human cancer cells by infection with an adenovirus-B7 (Ad-B7) expression vector. Ann Surg Oncol 1996; 3: 317–324.

4. Wojtowicz-Praga S. Reversal of tumor-induced immunosuppression: a new approach to cancer therapy [see comments]. J Immunother 1997; 20: 165–177.
5. Bretscher P, Cohn M. A theory of self-nonself discrimination. Science 1970; 169: 1042–1049.
6. Lafferty KJ, Woolnough J. The origin and mechanism of the allograft reaction. Immunol Rev 1977; 35: 231–262.
7. Baxter AG, Hodgkin PD. Activation rules: the two-signal theories of immune activation. Nat Rev Immunol 2002; 2: 439–446.
8. Jenkins MK, Schwartz RH. Antigen presentation by chemically modified splenocytes induces antigen-specific T cell unresponsiveness in vitro and in vivo. J Exp Med 1987; 165: 302–319.
9. Quill H, Schwartz RH. Stimulation of normal inducer T cell clones with antigen presented by purified Ia molecules in planar lipid membranes: specific induction of a long-lived state of proliferative nonresponsiveness. J Immunol 1987; 138: 3704–3712.
10. Vesosky B, Hurwitz AA. Modulation of costimulation to enhance tumor immunity. Cancer Immunol Immunother 2003; 52: 663–669.
11. Chambers CA, Kuhns MS, Egen JG, Allison JP. CTLA-4-mediated inhibition in regulation of T cell responses: mechanisms and manipulation in tumor immunotherapy. Annu Rev Immunol 2001; 19: 565–594.
12. Chen L. Co-inhibitory molecules of the B7-CD28 family in the control of T-cell immunity. Nat Rev Immunol 2004; 4: 336–347.
13. Contardi E, Palmisano GL, Tazzari PL et al. CTLA-4 is constitutively expressed on tumor cells and can trigger apoptosis upon ligand interaction. Int J Cancer 2005.
14. Taylor PA, Lees CJ, Fournier S et al. B7 expression on T cells down-regulates immune responses through CTLA-4 ligation via R-T interactions. J Immunol 2004; 172: 34–39.
15. Townsend SE, Allison JP. Tumor rejection after direct costimulation of CD8+ T cells by B7-transfected melanoma cells. Science 1993; 259: 368–370.
16. Chen L, Ashe S, Brady WA et al. Costimulation of antitumor immunity by the B7 counterreceptor for the T lymphocyte molecules CD28 and CTLA-4. Cell 1992; 71: 1093–1102.
17. Yokochi T, Holly RD, Clark EA. B lymphoblast antigen (BB-1) expressed on Epstein-Barr virus-activated B cell blasts, B lymphoblastoid cell lines, and Burkitt's lymphomas. J Immunol 1982; 128: 823–827.
18. Azuma M, Ito D, Yagita H et al. B70 antigen is a second ligand for CTLA-4 and CD28. Nature 1993; 366: 76–79.
19. Freeman GJ, Borriello F, Hodes RJ et al. Murine B7–2, an alternative CTLA-4 counter-receptor that costimulates T cell proliferation and interleukin 2 production. J. Exp. Med. 1993; 178: 2185–2192.
20. Freeman GJ, Gribben JG, Boussiotis VA et al. Cloning of B7–2: a CTLA-4 counter-receptor that costimulates human T cell proliferation. Science 1993; 262: 909–911.
21. Martin PJ, Ledbetter JA, Morishita Y et al. A 44 kilodalton cell surface homodimer regulates interleukin 2 production by activated human T lymphocytes. J Immunol 1986; 136: 3282–3287.
22. Boise LH, Minn AJ, Noel PJ et al. CD28 costimulation can promote T cell survival by enhancing the expression of Bcl-XL. Immunity 1995; 3: 87–98.
23. Brunet JF, Denizot F, Luciani MF et al. A new member of the immunoglobulin superfamily–CTLA-4. Nature 1987; 328: 267–270.
24. Linsley PS, Brady W, Urnes M et al. CTLA-4 is a second receptor for the B cell activation antigen B7. J Exp Med 1991; 174: 561–569.
25. Krummel MF, Allison JP. CD28 and CTLA-4 have opposing effects on the response of T cells to stimulation. J Exp Med 1995; 182: 459–465.
26. Thompson CB, Allison JP. The emerging role of CTLA-4 as an immune attenuator. Immunity 1997; 7: 445–450.
27. Scheipers P, Reiser H. Fas-independent death of activated CD4(+) T lymphocytes induced by CTLA-4 crosslinking. Proc Natl Acad Sci U S A 1998; 95: 10083–10088.
28. Walunas TL, Lenschow DJ, Bakker CY et al. CTLA-4 can function as a negative regulator of T cell activation. Immunity 1994; 1: 405–413.

29. Tivol EA, Borriello F, Schweitzer AN et al. Loss of CTLA-4 leads to massive lymphoproliferation and fatal multiorgan tissue destruction, revealing a critical negative regulatory role of CTLA-4. Immunity 1995; 3: 541–547.
30. Waterhouse P, Penninger JM, Timms E et al. Lymphoproliferative disorders with early lethality in mice deficient in Ctla-4. Science 1995; 270: 985–988.
31. Chambers CA, Cado D, Truong T, Allison JP. Thymocyte development is normal in CTLA-4-deficient mice. Proc Natl Acad Sci U S A 1997; 94: 9296–9301.
32. Egen JG, Kuhns MS, Allison JP. CTLA-4: new insights into its biological function and use in tumor immunotherapy. Nat Immunol 2002; 3: 611–618.
33. Pentcheva-Hoang T, Egen JG, Wojnoonski K, Allison JP. B7–1 and B7–2 selectively recruit CTLA-4 and CD28 to the immunological synapse. Immunity 2004; 21: 401–413.
34. Perez VL, Van Parijs L, Biuckians A et al. Induction of peripheral T cell tolerance in vivo requires CTLA-4 engagement. Immunity 1997; 6: 411–417.
35. Metz DP, Farber DL, Taylor T, Bottomly K. Differential role of CTLA-4 in regulation of resting memory versus naive CD4 T cell activation. J Immunol 1998; 161: 5855–5861.
36. Kuhns MS, Epshteyn V, Sobel RA, Allison JP. Cytotoxic T lymphocyte antigen-4 (CTLA-4) regulates the size, reactivity, and function of a primed pool of CD4+ T cells. Proc Natl Acad Sci U S A 2000; 97: 12711–12716.
37. Chen W, Jin W, Wahl SM. Engagement of cytotoxic T lymphocyte-associated antigen 4 (CTLA-4) induces transforming growth factor beta (TGF-beta) production by murine CD4(+) T cells. J Exp Med 1998; 188: 1849–1857.
38. Jovasevic VM, Gorelik L, Bluestone JA, Mokyr MB. Importance of IL-10 for CTLA-4-mediated inhibition of tumor-eradicating immunity. J Immunol 2004; 172: 1449–1454.
39. Orabona C, Grohmann U, Belladonna ML et al. CD28 induces immunostimulatory signals in dendritic cells via CD80 and CD86. Nat Immunol 2004; 5: 1134–1142.
40. Read S, Malmstrom V, Powrie F. Cytotoxic T lymphocyte-associated antigen 4 plays an essential role in the function of CD25(+)CD4(+) regulatory cells that control intestinal inflammation. J Exp Med 2000; 192: 295–302.
41. Salomon B, Lenschow DJ, Rhee L et al. B7/CD28 costimulation is essential for the homeostasis of the CD4+CD25+ immunoregulatory T cells that control autoimmune diabetes. Immunity 2000; 12: 431–440.
42. Takahashi T, Tagami T, Yamazaki S et al. Immunologic self-tolerance maintained by CD25(+)CD4(+) regulatory T cells constitutively expressing cytotoxic T lymphocyte-associated antigen 4. J Exp Med 2000; 192: 303–310.
43. Berger CL, Tigelaar R, Cohen J et al. Cutaneous T-cell lymphoma: malignant proliferation of T-regulatory cells. Blood 2005; 105: 1640–1647.
44. Marshall NA, Christie LE, Munro LR et al. Immunosuppressive regulatory T cells are abundant in the reactive lymphocytes of Hodgkin lymphoma. Blood 2004; 103: 1755–1762.
45. Kono K, Kawaida H, Takahashi A et al. CD4(+)CD25(high) regulatory T cells increase with tumor stage in patients with gastric and esophageal cancers. Cancer Immunol Immunother 2005; 1–8.
46. Wolf AM, Wolf D, Steurer M et al. Increase of regulatory T cells in the peripheral blood of cancer patients. Clin Cancer Res 2003; 9: 606–612.
47. Wolf D, Wolf AM, Rumpold H et al. The Expression of the Regulatory T Cell-Specific Forkhead Box Transcription Factor FoxP3 Is Associated with Poor Prognosis in Ovarian Cancer. Clin Cancer Res 2005; 11: 8326–8331.
48. Hurwitz AA, Kwon ED, van Elsas A. Costimulatory wars: the tumor menace. Curr Opin Immunol 2000; 12: 589–596.
49. Li Y, McGowan P, Hellstrom I et al. Costimulation of tumor-reactive CD4+ and CD8+ T lymphocytes by B7, a natural ligand for CD28, can be used to treat established mouse melanoma. J Immunol 1994; 153: 421–428.
50. Townsend SE, Su FW, Atherton JM, Allison JP. Specificity and longevity of antitumor immune responses induced by B7-transfected tumors. Cancer Res 1994; 54: 6477–6483.

51. Baskar S, Glimcher L, Nabavi N et al. Major histocompatibility complex class II+B7–1+ tumor cells are potent vaccines for stimulating tumor rejection in tumor-bearing mice. J Exp Med 1995; 181: 619–629.
52. Yang G, Hellstrom KE, Hellstrom I, Chen L. Antitumor immunity elicited by tumor cells transfected with B7–2, a second ligand for CD28/CTLA-4 costimulatory molecules. J Immunol 1995; 154: 2794–2800.
53. Hull GW, McCurdy MA, Nasu Y et al. Prostate cancer gene therapy: comparison of adenovirus-mediated expression of interleukin 12 with interleukin 12 plus B7–1 for in situ gene therapy and gene-modified, cell-based vaccines. Clin Cancer Res 2000; 6: 4101–4109.
54. Chen L, McGowan P, Ashe S et al. Tumor immunogenicity determines the effect of B7 costimulation on T cell-mediated tumor immunity. J Exp Med 1994; 179: 523–532.
55. Ostrand-Rosenberg S. Tumor immunotherapy: the tumor cell as an antigen-presenting cell. Curr Opin Immunol 1994; 6: 722–727.
56. Hurwitz AA, Townsend SE, Yu TF et al. Enhancement of the anti-tumor immune response using a combination of interferon-gamma and B7 expression in an experimental mammary carcinoma. Int J Cancer 1998; 77: 107–113.
57. Li Y, Hellstrom KE, Newby SA, Chen L. Costimulation by CD48 and B7–1 induces immunity against poorly immunogenic tumors. J Exp Med 1996; 183: 639–644.
58. Johnston JV, Malacko AR, Mizuno MT et al. B7-CD28 costimulation unveils the hierarchy of tumor epitopes recognized by major histocompatibility complex class I-restricted CD8+ cytolytic T lymphocytes. J Exp Med 1996; 183: 791–800.
59. Harding FA, Allison JP. CD28-B7 interactions allow the induction of CD8+ cytotoxic T lymphocytes in the absence of exogenous help. J Exp Med 1993; 177: 1791–1796.
60. Houghton AN, Gold JS, Blachere NE. Immunity against cancer: lessons learned from melanoma. Curr Opin Immunol 2001; 13: 134–140.
61. Li Y, Newby SA, Johnston JV et al. Protective immunity induced by B7/CD28-costimulated gamma delta T cells to the EL-4 lymphoma in allogenic athymic mice. J Immunol 1995; 155: 5705–5710.
62. Wu TC, Huang AY, Jaffee EM et al. A reassessment of the role of B7–1 expression in tumor rejection. J Exp Med 1995; 182: 1415–1421.
63. Antonia SJ, Seigne J, Diaz J et al. Phase I trial of a B7–1 (CD80) gene modified autologous tumor cell vaccine in combination with systemic interleukin-2 in patients with metastatic renal cell carcinoma. J Urol 2002; 167: 1995–2000.
64. Raez LE, Cassileth PA, Schlesselman JJ et al. Induction of CD8 T-cell-Ifn-gamma response and positive clinical outcome after immunization with gene-modified allogeneic tumor cells in advanced non-small-cell lung carcinoma. Cancer Gene Ther 2003; 10: 850–858.
65. Dols A, Smith JW, 2nd, Meijer SL et al. Vaccination of women with metastatic breast cancer, using a costimulatory gene (CD80)-modified, HLA-A2-matched, allogeneic, breast cancer cell line: clinical and immunological results. Hum Gene Ther 2003; 14: 1117–1123.
66. Dols A, Meijer SL, Hu HM et al. Identification of tumor-specific antibodies in patients with breast cancer vaccinated with gene-modified allogeneic tumor cells. J Immunother 2003; 26: 163–170.
67. Horig H, Lee DS, Conkright W et al. Phase I clinical trial of a recombinant canarypoxvirus (ALVAC) vaccine expressing human carcinoembryonic antigen and the B7.1 co-stimulatory molecule. Cancer Immunol Immunother 2000; 49: 504–514.
68. von Mehren M, Arlen P, Tsang KY et al. Pilot study of a dual gene recombinant avipox vaccine containing both carcinoembryonic antigen (CEA) and B7.1 transgenes in patients with recurrent CEA-expressing adenocarcinomas. Clin Cancer Res 2000; 6: 2219–2228.
69. Marshall JL, Gulley JL, Arlen PM et al. Phase I study of sequential vaccinations with fowlpox-CEA(6D)-TRICOM alone and sequentially with vaccinia-CEA(6D)-TRICOM, with and without granulocyte-macrophage colony-stimulating factor, in patients with carcinoembryonic antigen-expressing carcinomas. J Clin Oncol 2005; 23: 720–731.
70. Kaufman HL, Deraffele G, Mitcham J et al. Targeting the local tumor microenvironment with vaccinia virus expressing B7.1 for the treatment of melanoma. J Clin Invest 2005; 115: 1903–1912.

71. Hodge JW, McLaughlin JP, Abrams SI et al. Admixture of a recombinant vaccinia virus containing the gene for the costimulatory molecule B7 and a recombinant vaccinia virus containing a tumor-associated antigen gene results in enhanced specific T-cell responses and antitumor immunity. Cancer Res 1995; 55: 3598–3603.
72. Leach DR, Krummel MF, Allison JP. Enhancement of antitumor immunity by CTLA-4 blockade. Science 1996; 271: 1734–1736.
73. Kwon ED, Hurwitz AA, Foster BA et al. Manipulation of T cell costimulatory and inhibitory signals for immunotherapy of prostate cancer. Proc Natl Acad Sci U S A 1997; 94: 8099–8103.
74. Hurwitz AA, Yu TF, Leach DR, Allison JP. CTLA-4 blockade synergizes with tumor-derived granulocyte-macrophage colony-stimulating factor for treatment of an experimental mammary carcinoma. Proc Natl Acad Sci U S A 1998; 95: 10067–10071.
75. van Elsas A, Hurwitz AA, Allison JP. Combination immunotherapy of B16 melanoma using anti-cytotoxic T lymphocyte-associated antigen 4 (CTLA-4) and granulocyte/macrophage colony-stimulating factor (GM-CSF)-producing vaccines induces rejection of subcutaneous and metastatic tumors accompanied by autoimmune depigmentation. J Exp Med 1999; 190: 355–366.
76. van Elsas A, Sutmuller RP, Hurwitz AA et al. Elucidating the autoimmune and antitumor effector mechanisms of a treatment based on cytotoxic T lymphocyte antigen-4 blockade in combination with a B16 melanoma vaccine: comparison of prophylaxis and therapy. J Exp Med 2001; 194: 481–489.
77. Hurwitz AA, Foster BA, Kwon ED et al. Combination immunotherapy of primary prostate cancer in a transgenic mouse model using CTLA-4 blockade. Cancer Res 2000; 60: 2444–2448.
78. Gregor PD, Wolchok JD, Ferrone CR et al. CTLA-4 blockade in combination with xenogeneic DNA vaccines enhances T-cell responses, tumor immunity and autoimmunity to self antigens in animal and cellular model systems. Vaccine 2004; 22: 1700–1708.
79. Kwon ED, Foster BA, Hurwitz AA et al. Elimination of residual metastatic prostate cancer after surgery and adjunctive cytotoxic T lymphocyte-associated antigen 4 (CTLA-4) blockade immunotherapy. Proc Natl Acad Sci U S A 1999; 96: 15074–15079.
80. Mokyr MB, Kalinichenko T, Gorelik L, Bluestone JA. Realization of the therapeutic potential of CTLA-4 blockade in low-dose chemotherapy-treated tumor-bearing mice. Cancer Res 1998; 58: 5301–5304.
81. Demaria S, Kawashima N, Yang AM et al. Immune-mediated inhibition of metastases after treatment with local radiation and CTLA-4 blockade in a mouse model of breast cancer. Clin Cancer Res 2005; 11: 728–734.
82. Pure E, Allison JP, Schreiber RD. Breaking down the barriers to cancer immunotherapy. Nat Immunol 2005; 6: 1207–1210.
83. Maker AV, Attia P, Rosenberg SA. Analysis of the cellular mechanism of antitumor responses and autoimmunity in patients treated with ctla-4 blockade. J Immunol 2005; 175: 7746–7754.
84. Hodi FS, Mihm MC, Soiffer RJ et al. Biologic activity of cytotoxic T lymphocyte-associated antigen 4 antibody blockade in previously vaccinated metastatic melanoma and ovarian carcinoma patients. Proc Natl Acad Sci U S A 2003; 100: 4712–4717.
85. Phan GQ, Yang JC, Sherry RM et al. Cancer regression and autoimmunity induced by cytotoxic T lymphocyte-associated antigen 4 blockade in patients with metastatic melanoma. Proc Natl Acad Sci U S A 2003; 100: 8372–8377.
86. Attia P, Phan GQ, Maker AV et al. Autoimmunity correlates with tumor regression in patients with metastatic melanoma treated with anti-cytotoxic T-lymphocyte antigen-4. J Clin Oncol 2005; 23: 6043–6053.
87. Perales MA, Chapman PB. Immunizing against partially defined antigen mixtures, gangliosides, or peptides to induce antibody, T cell, and clinical responses. Cancer Chemother Biol Response Modif 2005; 22: 749–760.
88. Sanderson K, Scotland R, Lee P et al. Autoimmunity in a phase I trial of a fully human anti-cytotoxic T-lymphocyte antigen-4 monoclonal antibody with multiple melanoma peptides and Montanide ISA 51 for patients with resected stages III and IV melanoma. J Clin Oncol 2005; 23: 741–750.

89. Maker AV, Phan GQ, Attia P et al. Tumor Regression and Autoimmunity in Patients Treated With Cytotoxic T Lymphocyte-Associated Antigen 4 Blockade and Interleukin 2: A Phase I/II Study. Ann Surg Oncol 2005; 12: 1005–1016.
90. Ribas A, Camacho LH, Lopez-Berestein G et al. Antitumor Activity in Melanoma and Anti-Self Responses in a Phase I Trial With the Anti-Cytotoxic T Lymphocyte-Associated Antigen 4 Monoclonal Antibody CP-675,206. J Clin Oncol 2005.
91. Blansfield JA, Beck KE, Tran K et al. Cytotoxic T-lymphocyte-associated antigen-4 blockage can induce autoimmune hypophysitis in patients with metastatic melanoma and renal cancer. J Immunother 2005; 28: 593–598.
92. Hutloff A, Dittrich AM, Beier KC et al. ICOS is an inducible T-cell co-stimulator structurally and functionally related to CD28. Nature 1999; 397: 263–266.
93. Liu X, Bai XF, Wen J et al. B7H costimulates clonal expansion of, and cognate destruction of tumor cells by, CD8(+) T lymphocytes in vivo. J Exp Med 2001; 194: 1339–1348.
94. Wallin JJ, Liang L, Bakardjiev A, Sha WC. Enhancement of CD8+ T cell responses by ICOS/B7h costimulation. J Immunol 2001; 167: 132–139.
95. Zuberek K, Ling V, Wu P et al. Comparable in vivo efficacy of CD28/B7, ICOS/GL50, and ICOS/GL50B costimulatory pathways in murine tumor models: IFNgamma-dependent enhancement of CTL priming, effector functions, and tumor specific memory CTL. Cell Immunol 2003; 225: 53–63.
96. Ara G, Baher A, Storm N et al. Potent activity of soluble B7RP-1-Fc in therapy of murine tumors in syngeneic hosts. Int J Cancer 2003; 103: 501–507.
97. Nishimura H, Nose M, Hiai H et al. Development of lupus-like autoimmune diseases by disruption of the PD-1 gene encoding an ITIM motif-carrying immunoreceptor. Immunity 1999; 11: 141–151.
98. Dong H, Strome SE, Salomao DR et al. Tumor-associated B7-H1 promotes T-cell apoptosis: a potential mechanism of immune evasion. Nat Med 2002; 8: 793–800.
99. Iwai Y, Ishida M, Tanaka Y et al. Involvement of PD-L1 on tumor cells in the escape from host immune system and tumor immunotherapy by PD-L1 blockade. Proc Natl Acad Sci U S A 2002; 99: 12293–12297.
100. Strome SE, Dong H, Tamura H et al. B7-H1 blockade augments adoptive T-cell immunotherapy for squamous cell carcinoma. Cancer Res 2003; 63: 6501–6505.
101. Hirano F, Kaneko K, Tamura H et al. Blockade of B7-H1 and PD-1 by monoclonal antibodies potentiates cancer therapeutic immunity. Cancer Res 2005; 65: 1089–1096.
102. Blank C, Brown I, Peterson AC et al. PD-L1/B7H-1 inhibits the effector phase of tumor rejection by T cell receptor (TCR) transgenic CD8+ T cells. Cancer Res 2004; 64: 1140–1145.
103. Curiel TJ, Wei S, Dong H et al. Blockade of B7-H1 improves myeloid dendritic cell-mediated antitumor immunity. Nat Med 2003; 9: 562–567.
104. Moore KW, de Waal Malefyt R, Coffman RL, O'Garra A. Interleukin-10 and the interleukin-10 receptor. Annu Rev Immunol 2001; 19: 683–765.
105. Radhakrishnan S, Nguyen LT, Ciric B et al. Immunotherapeutic potential of B7-DC (PD-L2) cross-linking antibody in conferring antitumor immunity. Cancer Res 2004; 64: 4965–4972.
106. Brown JA, Dorfman DM, Ma FR et al. Blockade of programmed death-1 ligands on dendritic cells enhances T cell activation and cytokine production. J Immunol 2003; 170: 1257–1266.
107. Wintterle S, Schreiner B, Mitsdoerffer M et al. Expression of the B7-related molecule B7-H1 by glioma cells: a potential mechanism of immune paralysis. Cancer Res 2003; 63: 7462–7467.
108. Ohigashi Y, Sho M, Yamada Y et al. Clinical significance of programmed death-1 ligand-1 and programmed death-1 ligand-2 expression in human esophageal cancer. Clin Cancer Res 2005; 11: 2947–2953.
109. Thompson RH, Gillett MD, Cheville JC et al. Costimulatory B7-H1 in renal cell carcinoma patients: Indicator of tumor aggressiveness and potential therapeutic target. Proc Natl Acad Sci U S A 2004; 101: 17174–17179.
110. Rosenwald A, Wright G, Leroy K et al. Molecular diagnosis of primary mediastinal B cell lymphoma identifies a clinically favorable subgroup of diffuse large B cell lymphoma related to Hodgkin lymphoma. J Exp Med 2003; 198: 851–862.

111. Watts TH. TNF/TNFR family members in costimulation of T cell responses. Annu Rev Immunol 2005; 23: 23–68.
112. van Lier RA, Borst J, Vroom TM et al. Tissue distribution and biochemical and functional properties of Tp55 (CD27), a novel T cell differentiation antigen. J Immunol 1987; 139: 1589–1596.
113. Bowman MR, Crimmins MA, Yetz-Aldape J et al. The cloning of CD70 and its identification as the ligand for CD27. J Immunol 1994; 152: 1756–1761.
114. Lens SM, de Jong R, Hooibrink B et al. Phenotype and function of human B cells expressing CD70 (CD27 ligand). Eur J Immunol 1996; 26: 2964–2971.
115. Oshima H, Nakano H, Nohara C et al. Characterization of murine CD70 by molecular cloning and mAb. Int Immunol 1998; 10: 517–526.
116. Wherry EJ, Teichgraber V, Becker TC et al. Lineage relationship and protective immunity of memory CD8 T cell subsets. Nat Immunol 2003; 4: 225–234.
117. Hendriks J, Gravestein LA, Tesselaar K et al. CD27 is required for generation and long-term maintenance of T cell immunity. Nat Immunol 2000; 1: 433–440.
118. Arens R, Tesselaar K, Baars PA et al. Constitutive CD27/CD70 interaction induces expansion of effector-type T cells and results in IFNgamma-mediated B cell depletion. Immunity 2001; 15: 801–812.
119. Tesselaar K, Arens R, van Schijndel GM et al. Lethal T cell immunodeficiency induced by chronic costimulation via CD27-CD70 interactions. Nat Immunol 2003; 4: 49–54.
120. Arens R, Schepers K, Nolte MA et al. Tumor rejection induced by CD70-mediated quantitative and qualitative effects on effector CD8+ T cell formation. J Exp Med 2004; 199: 1595–1605.
121. Couderc B, Zitvogel L, Douin-Echinard V et al. Enhancement of antitumor immunity by expression of CD70 (CD27 ligand) or CD154 (CD40 ligand) costimulatory molecules in tumor cells. Cancer Gene Ther 1998; 5: 163–175.
122. Nieland JD, Graus YF, Dortmans YE et al. CD40 and CD70 co-stimulate a potent in vivo antitumor T cell response. J Immunother 1998; 21: 225–236.
123. Lorenz MG, Kantor JA, Schlom J, Hodge JW. Anti-tumor immunity elicited by a recombinant vaccinia virus expressing CD70 (CD27L). Hum Gene Ther 1999; 10: 1095–1103.
124. Kelly JM, Darcy PK, Markby JL et al. Induction of tumor-specific T cell memory by NK cell-mediated tumor rejection. Nat Immunol 2002; 3: 83–90.
125. Gramaglia I, Weinberg AD, Lemon M, Croft M. Ox-40 ligand: a potent costimulatory molecule for sustaining primary CD4 T cell responses. J Immunol 1998; 161: 6510–6517.
126. Miura S, Ohtani K, Numata N et al. Molecular cloning and characterization of a novel glycoprotein, gp34, that is specifically induced by the human T-cell leukemia virus type I transactivator p40tax. Mol Cell Biol 1991; 11: 1313–1325.
127. Stuber E, Neurath M, Calderhead D et al. Cross-linking of OX40 ligand, a member of the TNF/NGF cytokine family, induces proliferation and differentiation in murine splenic B cells. Immunity 1995; 2: 507–521.
128. Chen AI, McAdam AJ, Buhlmann JE et al. Ox40-ligand has a critical costimulatory role in dendritic cell:T cell interactions. Immunity 1999; 11: 689–698.
129. Weinberg AD, Wegmann KW, Funatake C, Whitham RH. Blocking OX-40/OX-40 ligand interaction in vitro and in vivo leads to decreased T cell function and amelioration of experimental allergic encephalomyelitis. J Immunol 1999; 162: 1818–1826.
130. Blazar BR, Sharpe AH, Chen AI et al. Ligation of OX40 (CD134) regulates graft-versus-host disease (GVHD) and graft rejection in allogeneic bone marrow transplant recipients. Blood 2003; 101: 3741–3748.
131. Takeda I, Ine S, Killeen N et al. Distinct roles for the OX40-OX40 ligand interaction in regulatory and nonregulatory T cells. J Immunol 2004; 172: 3580–3589.
132. Bansal-Pakala P, Jember AG, Croft M. Signaling through OX40 (CD134) breaks peripheral T-cell tolerance. Nat Med 2001; 7: 907–912.
133. Gerloni M, Xiong S, Mukerjee S et al. Functional cooperation between T helper cell determinants. Proc Natl Acad Sci U S A 2000; 97: 13269–13274.

134. Weinberg AD, Rivera MM, Prell R et al. Engagement of the OX-40 receptor in vivo enhances antitumor immunity. J Immunol 2000; 164: 2160–2169.
135. Kjaergaard J, Tanaka J, Kim JA et al. Therapeutic efficacy of OX-40 receptor antibody depends on tumor immunogenicity and anatomic site of tumor growth. Cancer Res 2000; 60: 5514–5521.
136. Kjaergaard J, Peng L, Cohen PA et al. Augmentation versus inhibition: effects of conjunctional OX-40 receptor monoclonal antibody and IL-2 treatment on adoptive immunotherapy of advanced tumor. J Immunol 2001; 167: 6669–6677.
137. Pan PY, Zang Y, Weber K et al. OX40 ligation enhances primary and memory cytotoxic T lymphocyte responses in an immunotherapy for hepatic colon metastases. Mol Ther 2002; 6: 528–536.
138. Morris A, Vetto JT, Ramstad T et al. Induction of anti-mammary cancer immunity by engaging the OX-40 receptor in vivo. Breast Cancer Res Treat 2001; 67: 71–80.
139. Gri G, Gallo E, Di Carlo E et al. OX40 ligand-transduced tumor cell vaccine synergizes with GM-CSF and requires CD40-Apc signaling to boost the host T cell antitumor response. J Immunol 2003; 170: 99–106.
140. Kwon BS, Weissman SM. cDNA sequences of two inducible T-cell genes. Proc Natl Acad Sci U S A 1989; 86: 1963–1967.
141. Wilcox RA, Tamada K, Strome SE, Chen L. Signaling through NK cell-associated CD137 promotes both helper function for CD8+ cytolytic T cells and responsiveness to IL-2 but not cytolytic activity. J Immunol 2002; 169: 4230–4236.
142. Wilcox RA, Chapoval AI, Gorski KS et al. Cutting edge: Expression of functional CD137 receptor by dendritic cells. J Immunol 2002; 168: 4262–4267.
143. Goodwin RG, Din WS, Davis-Smith T et al. Molecular cloning of a ligand for the inducible T cell gene 4–1BB: a member of an emerging family of cytokines with homology to tumor necrosis factor. Eur J Immunol 1993; 23: 2631–2641.
144. Takahashi C, Mittler RS, Vella AT. Cutting edge: 4–1BB is a bona fide CD8 T cell survival signal. J Immunol 1999; 162: 5037–5040.
145. Bukczynski J, Wen T, Ellefsen K et al. Costimulatory ligand 4–1BBL (CD137L) as an efficient adjuvant for human antiviral cytotoxic T cell responses. Proc Natl Acad Sci U S A 2004; 101: 1291–1296.
146. Wilcox RA, Tamada K, Flies DB et al. Ligation of CD137 receptor prevents and reverses established anergy of CD8+ cytolytic T lymphocytes in vivo. Blood 2004; 103: 177–184.
147. Bukczynski J, Wen T, Watts TH. Costimulation of human CD28- T cells by 4–1BB ligand. Eur J Immunol 2003; 33: 446–454.
148. Azuma M, Phillips JH, Lanier LL. CD28- T lymphocytes. Antigenic and functional properties. J Immunol 1993; 150: 1147–1159.
149. Schmidt D, Goronzy JJ, Weyand CM. CD4+ CD7- CD28- T cells are expanded in rheumatoid arthritis and are characterized by autoreactivity. J Clin Invest 1996; 97: 2027–2037.
150. Sze DM, Giesajtis G, Brown RD et al. Clonal cytotoxic T cells are expanded in myeloma and reside in the CD8(+)CD57(+)CD28(-) compartment. Blood 2001; 98: 2817–2827.
151. Myers L, Takahashi C, Mittler RS et al. Effector CD8 T cells possess suppressor function after 4–1BB and Toll-like receptor triggering. Proc Natl Acad Sci U S A 2003; 100: 5348–5353.
152. Sun Y, Lin X, Chen HM et al. Administration of agonistic anti-4–1BB monoclonal antibody leads to the amelioration of experimental autoimmune encephalomyelitis. J Immunol 2002; 168: 1457–1465.
153. Hellstrom KE, Hellstrom I. Therapeutic vaccination with tumor cells that engage CD137. J Mol Med 2003; 81: 71–86.
154. Melero I, Shuford WW, Newby SA et al. Monoclonal antibodies against the 4–1BB T-cell activation molecule eradicate established tumors. Nat Med 1997; 3: 682–685.
155. Diehl L, van Mierlo GJ, den Boer AT et al. In vivo triggering through 4–1BB enables Th-independent priming of CTL in the presence of an intact CD28 costimulatory pathway. J Immunol 2002; 168: 3755–3762.

156. Taraban VY, Rowley TF, O'Brien L et al. Expression and costimulatory effects of the TNF receptor superfamily members CD134 (OX40) and CD137 (4–1BB), and their role in the generation of anti-tumor immune responses. Eur J Immunol 2002; 32: 3617–3627.
157. Martinet O, Ermekova V, Qiao JQ et al. Immunomodulatory gene therapy with interleukin 12 and 4–1BB ligand: long- term remission of liver metastases in a mouse model. J Natl Cancer Inst 2000; 92: 931–936.
158. Ye Z, Hellstrom I, Hayden-Ledbetter M et al. Gene therapy for cancer using single-chain Fv fragments specific for 4–1BB. Nat Med 2002; 8: 343–348.
159. Melero I, Johnston JV, Shufford WW et al. NK1.1 cells express 4–1BB (CDw137) costimulatory molecule and are required for tumor immunity elicited by anti-4–1BB monoclonal antibodies. Cell Immunol 1998; 190: 167–172.
160. Pan PY, Gu P, Li Q et al. Regulation of dendritic cell function by NK cells: mechanisms underlying the synergism in the combination therapy of IL-12 and 4–1BB activation. J Immunol 2004; 172: 4779–4789.
161. Wilcox RA, Flies DB, Zhu G et al. Provision of antigen and CD137 signaling breaks immunological ignorance, promoting regression of poorly immunogenic tumors. J Clin Invest 2002; 109: 651–659.
162. Bertram EM, Lau P, Watts TH. Temporal segregation of 4–1BB versus CD28-mediated costimulation: 4–1BB ligand influences T cell numbers late in the primary response and regulates the size of the T cell memory response following influenza infection. J Immunol 2002; 168: 3777–3785.
163. Melero I, Bach N, Hellstrom KE et al. Amplification of tumor immunity by gene transfer of the co-stimulatory 4–1BB ligand: synergy with the CD28 co-stimulatory pathway. Eur J Immunol 1998; 28: 1116–1121.
164. Guinn BA, DeBenedette MA, Watts TH, Berinstein NL. 4–1BBL cooperates with B7–1 and B7–2 in converting a B cell lymphoma cell line into a long-lasting antitumor vaccine. J Immunol 1999; 162: 5003–5010.
165. Shuford WW, Klussman K, Tritchler DD et al. 4–1BB costimulatory signals preferentially induce CD8+ T cell proliferation and lead to the amplification in vivo of cytotoxic T cell responses. J Exp Med 1997; 186: 47–55.
166. Montgomery RI, Warner MS, Lum BJ, Spear PG. Herpes simplex virus-1 entry into cells mediated by a novel member of the TNF/NGF receptor family. Cell 1996; 87: 427–436.
167. Mauri DN, Ebner R, Montgomery RI et al. LIGHT, a new member of the TNF superfamily, and lymphotoxin alpha are ligands for herpesvirus entry mediator. Immunity 1998; 8: 21–30.
168. Sedy JR, Gavrieli M, Potter KG et al. B and T lymphocyte attenuator regulates T cell activation through interaction with herpesvirus entry mediator. Nat Immunol 2005; 6: 90–98.
169. Gonzalez LC, Loyet KM, Calemine-Fenaux J et al. A coreceptor interaction between the CD28 and TNF receptor family members B and T lymphocyte attenuator and herpesvirus entry mediator. Proc Natl Acad Sci U S A 2005; 102: 1116–1121.
170. Granger SW, Rickert S. LIGHT-HVEM signaling and the regulation of T cell-mediated immunity. Cytokine Growth Factor Rev 2003; 14: 289–296.
171. Harrop JA, McDonnell PC, Brigham-Burke M et al. Herpesvirus entry mediator ligand (HVEM-L), a novel ligand for HVEM/TR2, stimulates proliferation of T cells and inhibits HT29 cell growth. J Biol Chem 1998; 273: 27548–27556.
172. Tamada K, Shimozaki K, Chapoval AI et al. LIGHT, a TNF-like molecule, costimulates T cell proliferation and is required for dendritic cell-mediated allogeneic T cell response. J Immunol 2000; 164: 4105–4110.
173. Tamada K, Shimozaki K, Chapoval AI et al. Modulation of T-cell-mediated immunity in tumor and graft-versus-host disease models through the LIGHT co-stimulatory pathway. Nat Med 2000; 6: 283–289.
174. Morel Y, Truneh A, Sweet RW et al. The TNF superfamily members LIGHT and CD154 (CD40 ligand) costimulate induction of dendritic cell maturation and elicit specific CTL activity. J Immunol 2001; 167: 2479–2486.
175. Shaikh RB, Santee S, Granger SW et al. Constitutive expression of LIGHT on T cells leads to lymphocyte activation, inflammation, and tissue destruction. J Immunol 2001; 167: 6330–6337.

176. Scheu S, Alferink J, Potzel T et al. Targeted disruption of LIGHT causes defects in costimulatory T cell activation and reveals cooperation with lymphotoxin beta in mesenteric lymph node genesis. J Exp Med 2002; 195: 1613–1624.
177. Watanabe N, Gavrieli M, Sedy JR et al. BTLA is a lymphocyte inhibitory receptor with similarities to CTLA-4 and PD-1. Nat Immunol 2003; 4: 670–679.
178. Han P, Goularte OD, Rufner K et al. An inhibitory Ig superfamily protein expressed by lymphocytes and APCs is also an early marker of thymocyte positive selection. J Immunol 2004; 172: 5931–5939.
179. Zhai Y, Guo R, Hsu TL et al. LIGHT, a novel ligand for lymphotoxin beta receptor and TR2/HVEM induces apoptosis and suppresses in vivo tumor formation via gene transfer. J Clin Invest 1998; 102: 1142–1151.
180. Rooney IA, Butrovich KD, Glass AA et al. The lymphotoxin-beta receptor is necessary and sufficient for LIGHT-mediated apoptosis of tumor cells. J Biol Chem 2000; 275: 14307–14315.
181. Yu P, Lee Y, Liu W et al. Priming of naive T cells inside tumors leads to eradication of established tumors. Nat Immunol 2004; 5: 141–149.
182. Grewal IS, Flavell RA. CD40 and CD154 in cell-mediated immunity. Annu Rev Immunol 1998; 16: 111–135.
183. Boumpas DT, Furie R, Manzi S et al. A short course of BG9588 (anti-CD40 ligand antibody) improves serologic activity and decreases hematuria in patients with proliferative lupus glomerulonephritis. Arthritis Rheum 2003; 48: 719–727.
184. Sidiropoulos PI, Boumpas DT. Lessons learned from anti-CD40L treatment in systemic lupus erythematosus patients. Lupus 2004; 13: 391–397.
185. Kluin-Nelemans HC, Beverstock GC, Mollevanger P et al. Proliferation and cytogenetic analysis of hairy cell leukemia upon stimulation via the CD40 antigen. Blood 1994; 84: 3134–3141.
186. Funakoshi S, Longo DL, Beckwith M et al. Inhibition of human B-cell lymphoma growth by CD40 stimulation. Blood 1994; 83: 2787–2794.
187. Ghamande S, Hylander BL, Oflazoglu E et al. Recombinant CD40 ligand therapy has significant antitumor effects on CD40-positive ovarian tumor xenografts grown in SCID mice and demonstrates an augmented effect with cisplatin. Cancer Res 2001; 61: 7556–7562.
188. Hirano A, Longo DL, Taub DD et al. Inhibition of human breast carcinoma growth by a soluble recombinant human CD40 ligand. Blood 1999; 93: 2999–3007.
189. Posner MR, Cavacini LA, Upton MP et al. Surface membrane-expressed CD40 is present on tumor cells from squamous cell cancer of the head and neck in vitro and in vivo and regulates cell growth in tumor cell lines. Clin Cancer Res 1999; 5: 2261–2270.
190. Yamada M, Shiroko T, Kawaguchi Y et al. CD40-CD40 ligand (CD154) engagement is required but not sufficient for modulating MHC class I, ICAM-1 and Fas expression and proliferation of human non-small cell lung tumors. Int J Cancer 2001; 92: 589–599.
191. Mackey MF, Gunn JR, Ting PP et al. Protective immunity induced by tumor vaccines requires interaction between CD40 and its ligand, CD154. Cancer Res 1997; 57: 2569–2574.
192. Noguchi M, Imaizumi K, Kawabe T et al. Induction of antitumor immunity by transduction of CD40 ligand gene and interferon-gamma gene into lung cancer. Cancer Gene Ther 2001; 8: 421–429.
193. Grangeon C, Cormary C, Douin-Echinard V et al. In vivo induction of antitumor immunity and protection against tumor growth by injection of CD154-expressing tumor cells. Cancer Gene Ther 2002; 9: 282–288.
194. Grossmann ME, Brown MP, Brenner MK. Antitumor responses induced by transgenic expression of CD40 ligand. Hum Gene Ther 1997; 8: 1935–1943.
195. Liu Y, Zhang X, Zhang W et al. Adenovirus-mediated CD40 ligand gene-engineered dendritic cells elicit enhanced CD8(+) cytotoxic T-cell activation and antitumor immunity. Cancer Gene Ther 2002; 9: 202–208.
196. Sun Y, Peng D, Lecanda J et al. In vivo gene transfer of CD40 ligand into colon cancer cells induces local production of cytokines and chemokines, tumor eradication and protective antitumor immunity. Gene Ther 2000; 7: 1467–1476.

197. Xiang R, Primus FJ, Ruehlmann JM et al. A dual-function DNA vaccine encoding carcinoembryonic antigen and CD40 ligand trimer induces T cell-mediated protective immunity against colon cancer in carcinoembryonic antigen-transgenic mice. J Immunol 2001; 167: 4560–4565.
198. Chiodoni C, Paglia P, Stoppacciaro A et al. Dendritic cells infiltrating tumors cotransduced with granulocyte/macrophage colony-stimulating factor (GM-CSF) and CD40 ligand genes take up and present endogenous tumor-associated antigens, and prime naive mice for a cytotoxic T lymphocyte response. J Exp Med 1999; 190: 125–133.
199. Peter I, Nawrath M, Kamarashev J et al. Immunotherapy for murine K1735 melanoma: combinatorial use of recombinant adenovirus expressing CD40L and other immunomodulators. Cancer Gene Ther 2002; 9: 597–605.
200. Ito D, Ogasawara K, Iwabuchi K et al. Induction of CTL responses by simultaneous administration of liposomal peptide vaccine with anti-CD40 and anti-CTLA-4 mAb. J Immunol 2000; 164: 1230–1235.
201. Schultze JL, Anderson KC, Gilleece MH et al. A pilot study of combined immunotherapy with autologous adoptive tumour-specific T-cell transfer, vaccination with CD40-activated malignant B cells and interleukin 2. Br J Haematol 2001; 113: 455–460.
202. Hayashi T, Treon SP, Hideshima T et al. Recombinant humanized anti-CD40 monoclonal antibody triggers autologous antibody-dependent cell-mediated cytotoxicity against multiple myeloma cells. Br J Haematol 2003; 121: 592–596.
203. Law CL, Gordon KA, Collier J et al. Preclinical antilymphoma activity of a humanized anti-CD40 monoclonal antibody, SGN-40. Cancer Res 2005; 65: 8331–8338.
204. Nocentini G, Giunchi L, Ronchetti S et al. A new member of the tumor necrosis factor/nerve growth factor receptor family inhibits T cell receptor-induced apoptosis. Proc Natl Acad Sci U S A 1997; 94: 6216–6221.
205. Gurney AL, Marsters SA, Huang RM et al. Identification of a new member of the tumor necrosis factor family and its receptor, a human ortholog of mouse GITR. Curr Biol 1999; 9: 215–218.
206. Kohm AP, Williams JS, Miller SD. Cutting edge: ligation of the glucocorticoid-induced TNF receptor enhances autoreactive CD4+ T cell activation and experimental autoimmune encephalomyelitis. J Immunol 2004; 172: 4686–4690.
207. Kanamaru F, Youngnak P, Hashiguchi M et al. Costimulation via glucocorticoid-induced TNF receptor in both conventional and CD25+ regulatory CD4+ T cells. J Immunol 2004; 172: 7306–7314.
208. Ronchetti S, Zollo O, Bruscoli S et al. GITR, a member of the TNF receptor superfamily, is costimulatory to mouse T lymphocyte subpopulations. Eur J Immunol 2004; 34: 613–622.
209. Tone M, Tone Y, Adams E et al. Mouse glucocorticoid-induced tumor necrosis factor receptor ligand is costimulatory for T cells. Proc Natl Acad Sci U S A 2003; 100: 15059–15064.
210. Stephens GL, McHugh RS, Whitters MJ et al. Engagement of glucocorticoid-induced TNFR family-related receptor on effector T cells by its ligand mediates resistance to suppression by CD4+CD25+ T cells. J Immunol 2004; 173: 5008–5020.
211. Shimizu J, Yamazaki S, Takahashi T et al. Stimulation of CD25(+)CD4(+) regulatory T cells through GITR breaks immunological self-tolerance. Nat Immunol 2002; 3: 135–142.
212. McHugh RS, Whitters MJ, Piccirillo CA et al. CD4(+)CD25(+) immunoregulatory T cells: gene expression analysis reveals a functional role for the glucocorticoid-induced TNF receptor. Immunity 2002; 16: 311–323.
213. Muriglan SJ, Ramirez-Montagut T, Alpdogan O et al. GITR activation induces an opposite effect on alloreactive CD4(+) and CD8(+) T cells in graft-versus-host disease. J Exp Med 2004; 200: 149–157.
214. Suri A, Shimizu J, Katz JD et al. Regulation of autoimmune diabetes by non-islet-specific T cells – a role for the glucocorticoid-induced TNF receptor. Eur J Immunol 2004; 34: 447–454.
215. Valzasina B, Guiducci C, Dislich H et al. Triggering of OX40 (CD134) on CD4(+)CD25+ T cells blocks their inhibitory activity: a novel regulatory role for OX40 and its comparison with GITR. Blood 2005; 105: 2845–2851.

216. Kirkwood J. Cancer immunotherapy: the interferon-alpha experience. Semin Oncol 2002; 29: 18–26.
217. Atkins MB. Interleukin-2: clinical applications. Semin Oncol 2002; 29: 12–17.
218. Welte K, Gabrilove J, Bronchud MH et al. Filgrastim (r-metHuG-CSF): the first 10 years. Blood 1996; 88: 1907–1929.
219. Armitage JO. Emerging applications of recombinant human granulocyte-macrophage colony-stimulating factor. Blood 1998; 92: 4491–4508.
220. Coscia M, Biragyn A. Cancer immunotherapy with chemoattractant peptides. Semin Cancer Biol 2004; 14: 209–218.
221. Zlotnik A. Chemokines in neoplastic progression. Semin Cancer Biol 2004; 14: 181–185.
222. Conti I, Rollins BJ. CCL2 (monocyte chemoattractant protein-1) and cancer. Semin Cancer Biol 2004; 14: 149–154.
223. Carswell EA, Old LJ, Kassel RL et al. An endotoxin-induced serum factor that causes necrosis of tumors. Proc Natl Acad Sci U S A 1975; 72: 3666–3670.
224. Mocellin S, Rossi CR, Pilati P, Nitti D. Tumor necrosis factor, cancer and anticancer therapy. Cytokine Growth Factor Rev 2005; 16: 35–53.
225. Bemelmans MH, van Tits LJ, Buurman WA. Tumor necrosis factor: function, release and clearance. Crit Rev Immunol 1996; 16: 1–11.
226. Aggarwal BB. Signalling pathways of the TNF superfamily: a double-edged sword. Nat Rev Immunol 2003; 3: 745–756.
227. Chen G, Goeddel DV. TNF-R1 signaling: a beautiful pathway. Science 2002; 296: 1634–1635.
228. Herrmann F, Bambach T, Bonifer R et al. The suppressive effects of recombinant human tumor necrosis factor-alpha on normal and malignant myelopoiesis: synergism with interferon-gamma. Int J Cell Cloning 1988; 6: 241–261.
229. MacPherson GG, North RJ. Endotoxin-mediated necrosis and regression of established tumours in the mouse. A correlative study of quantitative changes in blood flow and ultrastructural morphology. Cancer Immunol Immunother 1986; 21: 209–216.
230. Palladino MA, Jr., Shalaby MR, Kramer SM et al. Characterization of the antitumor activities of human tumor necrosis factor-alpha and the comparison with other cytokines: induction of tumor-specific immunity. J Immunol 1987; 138: 4023–4032.
231. Vujanovic NL. Role of TNF family ligands in antitumor activity of natural killer cells. Int Rev Immunol 2001; 20: 415–437.
232. Mocellin S, Provenzano M, Lise M et al. Increased TIA-1 gene expression in the tumor microenvironment after locoregional administration of tumor necrosis factor-alpha to patients with soft tissue limb sarcoma. Int J Cancer 2003; 107: 317–322.
233. Grunhagen DJ, Brunstein F, ten Hagen TL et al. TNF-based isolated limb perfusion: a decade of experience with antivascular therapy in the management of locally advanced extremity soft tissue sarcomas. Cancer Treat Res 2004; 120: 65–79.
234. Grunhagen DJ, Brunstein F, Graveland WJ et al. One hundred consecutive isolated limb perfusions with TNF-alpha and melphalan in melanoma patients with multiple in-transit metastases. Ann Surg 2004; 240: 939–947; discussion 947–938.
235. Di Filippo F, Cavaliere F, Garinei R et al. TNFa-based isolated hyperthermic limb perfusion (HILP) in the treatment of limb recurrent melanoma: update 16 years after its first clinical application. J Chemother 2004; 16 Suppl 5: 62–65.
236. Grover A, Alexander HR, Jr. The past decade of experience with isolated hepatic perfusion. Oncologist 2004; 9: 653–664.
237. Lejeune FJ. Clinical use of TNF revisited: improving penetration of anti-cancer agents by increasing vascular permeability. J Clin Invest 2002; 110: 433–435.
238. Rossi CR, Foletto M, Pilati P et al. Isolated limb perfusion in locally advanced cutaneous melanoma. Semin Oncol 2002; 29: 400–409.
239. Rossi CR, Mocellin S, Pilati P et al. TNFalpha-based isolated perfusion for limb-threatening soft tissue sarcomas: state of the art and future trends. J Immunother 2003; 26: 291–300.

240. Kahn JO, Kaplan LD, Volberding PA et al. Intralesional recombinant tumor necrosis factor-alpha for AIDS-associated Kaposi's sarcoma: a randomized, double-blind trial. J Acquir Immune Defic Syndr 1989; 2: 217–223.
241. Senzer N, Mani S, Rosemurgy A et al. TNFerade biologic, an adenovector with a radiation-inducible promoter, carrying the human tumor necrosis factor alpha gene: a phase I study in patients with solid tumors. J Clin Oncol 2004; 22: 592–601.
242. Curnis F, Sacchi A, Borgna L et al. Enhancement of tumor necrosis factor alpha antitumor immunotherapeutic properties by targeted delivery to aminopeptidase N (CD13). Nat Biotechnol 2000; 18: 1185–1190.
243. Dranoff G, Jaffee E, Lazenby A et al. Vaccination with irradiated tumor cells engineered to secrete murine granulocyte-macrophage colony-stimulating factor stimulates potent, specific, and long-lasting anti-tumor immunity. Proceedings of the National Academy of Sciences of the United States of America 1993; 90: 3539–3543.
244. Kielian T, Nagai E, Ikubo A et al. Granulocyte/macrophage-colony-stimulating factor released by adenovirally transduced CT26 cells leads to the local expression of macrophage inflammatory protein 1alpha and accumulation of dendritic cells at vaccination sites in vivo. Cancer Immunol Immunother 1999; 48: 123–131.
245. Shinohara H, Yano S, Bucana CD, Fidler IJ. Induction of chemokine secretion and enhancement of contact-dependent macrophage cytotoxicity by engineered expression of granulocyte-macrophage colony-stimulating factor in human colon cancer cells. J Immunol 2000; 164: 2728–2737.
246. Sanda MG, Ayyagari SR, Jaffee EM et al. Demonstration of a rational strategy for human prostate cancer gene therapy. Journal of Urology 1994; 151: 622–628.
247. Dunussi-Joannopoulos K, Dranoff G, Weinstein HJ et al. Gene immunotherapy in murine acute myeloid leukemia: granulocyte-macrophage colony-stimulating factor tumor cell vaccines elicit more potent antitumor immunity compared with B7 family and other cytokine vaccines. Blood 1998; 91: 222–230.
248. Levitsky HI, Montgomery J, Ahmadzadeh M et al. Immunization with granulocyte-macrophage colony-stimulating factor-transduced, but not B7-1-transduced, lymphoma cells primes idiotype-specific T cells and generates potent systemic antitumor immunity. J Immunol 1996; 156: 3858–3865.
249. Spitler LE, Grossbard ML, Ernstoff MS et al. Adjuvant therapy of stage III and IV malignant melanoma using granulocyte-macrophage colony-stimulating factor. J Clin Oncol 2000; 18: 1614–1621.
250. Chang DH, Dhodapkar MV. Dendritic cells and immunotherapy for cancer. Int J Hematol 2003; 77: 439–443.
251. Buchler T, Michalek J, Kovarova L et al. Dendritic cell-based immunotherapy for the treatment of hematological malignancies. Hematology 2003; 8: 97–104.
252. Chang DZ, Lomazow W, Joy Somberg C et al. Granulocyte-macrophage colony stimulating factor: an adjuvant for cancer vaccines. Hematology 2004; 9: 207–215.
253. Schaed SG, Klimek VM, Panageas KS et al. T-cell responses against tyrosinase 368–376(370D) peptide in HLA(*)A0201(+) melanoma patients: randomized trial comparing incomplete Freund's adjuvant, granulocyte macrophage colony-stimulating factor, and QS-21 as immunological adjuvants. Clin Cancer Res 2002; 8: 967–972.
254. Jager E, Ringhoffer M, Dienes HP et al. Granulocyte-macrophage-colony-stimulating factor enhances immune responses to melanoma-associated peptides in vivo. Int J Cancer 1996; 67: 54–62.
255. Scheibenbogen C, Schmittel A, Keilholz U et al. Phase 2 trial of vaccination with tyrosinase peptides and granulocyte-macrophage colony-stimulating factor in patients with metastatic melanoma. J Immunother 2000; 23: 275–281.
256. Scheibenbogen C, Schadendorf D, Bechrakis NE et al. Effects of granulocyte-macrophage colony-stimulating factor and foreign helper protein as immunologic adjuvants on the T-cell response to vaccination with tyrosinase peptides. Int J Cancer 2003; 104: 188–194.

257. Weber J, Sondak VK, Scotland R et al. Granulocyte-macrophage-colony-stimulating factor added to a multipeptide vaccine for resected Stage II melanoma. Cancer 2003; 97: 186–200.
258. Disis ML, Grabstein KH, Sleath PR, Cheever MA. Generation of immunity to the HER-2/neu oncogenic protein in patients with breast and ovarian cancer using a peptide-based vaccine. Clin Cancer Res 1999; 5: 1289–1297.
259. von Mehren M, Arlen P, Gulley J et al. The influence of granulocyte macrophage colony-stimulating factor and prior chemotherapy on the immunological response to a vaccine (ALVAC-CEA B7.1) in patients with metastatic carcinoma. Clin Cancer Res 2001; 7: 1181–1191.
260. Ullenhag GJ, Frodin JE, Mosolits S et al. Immunization of colorectal carcinoma patients with a recombinant canarypox virus expressing the tumor antigen Ep-CAM/KSA (ALVAC-KSA) and granulocyte macrophage colony- stimulating factor induced a tumor-specific cellular immune response. Clin Cancer Res 2003; 9: 2447–2456.
261. Kwak LW, Young HA, Pennington RW, Weeks SD. Vaccination with syngeneic, lymphoma-derived immunoglobulin idiotype combined with granulocyte/macrophage colony-stimulating factor primes mice for a protective T-cell response. Proc Natl Acad Sci U S A 1996; 93: 10972–10977.
262. Timmerman JM, Levy R. Linkage of foreign carrier protein to a self-tumor antigen enhances the immunogenicity of a pulsed dendritic cell vaccine. J Immunol 2000; 164: 4797–4803.
263. Pasquini S, Peralta S, Missiaglia E et al. Prime-boost vaccines encoding an intracellular idiotype/GM-CSF fusion protein induce protective cell-mediated immunity in murine pre-B cell leukemia. Gene Ther 2002; 9: 503–510.
264. Ellem KA, O'Rourke MG, Johnson GR et al. A case report: immune responses and clinical course of the first human use of granulocyte/macrophage-colony-stimulating-factor-transduced autologous melanoma cells for immunotherapy. Cancer Immunol Immunother 1997; 44: 10–20.
265. Dranoff G, Soiffer R, Lynch T et al. A phase I study of vaccination with autologous, irradiated melanoma cells engineered to secrete human granulocyte-macrophage colony stimulating factor. Hum Gene Ther 1997; 8: 111–123.
266. Soiffer R, Lynch T, Mihm M et al. Vaccination with irradiated autologous melanoma cells engineered to secrete human granulocyte-macrophage colony-stimulating factor generates potent antitumor immunity in patients with metastatic melanoma. Proc Natl Acad Sci U S A 1998; 95: 13141–13146.
267. Chang AE, Li Q, Bishop DK et al. Immunogenetic therapy of human melanoma utilizing autologous tumor cells transduced to secrete granulocyte-macrophage colony-stimulating factor. Hum Gene Ther 2000; 11: 839–850.
268. Soiffer R, Hodi FS, Haluska F et al. Vaccination with irradiated, autologous melanoma cells engineered to secrete granulocyte-macrophage colony-stimulating factor by adenoviral-mediated gene transfer augments antitumor immunity in patients with metastatic melanoma. J Clin Oncol 2003; 21: 3343–3350.
269. Simons JW. Bioactivity of human GM-CSF gene therapy in metastatic renal cell carcinoma and prostate cancer. Hinyokika Kiyo 1997; 43: 821–822.
270. Simons JW, Mikhak B, Chang JF et al. Induction of immunity to prostate cancer antigens: results of a clinical trial of vaccination with irradiated autologous prostate tumor cells engineered to secrete granulocyte-macrophage colony-stimulating factor using ex vivo gene transfer. Cancer Res 1999; 59: 5160–5168.
271. Jaffee EM, Dranoff G, Cohen LK et al. High efficiency gene transfer into primary human tumor explants without cell selection. Cancer Research 1993; 53: 2221–2226.
272. Borrello I, Sotomayor EM, Cooke S, Levitsky HI. A universal granulocyte-macrophage colony-stimulating factor-producing bystander cell line for use in the formulation of autologous tumor cell-based vaccines. Hum Gene Ther 1999; 10: 1983–1991.
273. Qin H, Chatterjee SK. Cancer gene therapy using tumor cells infected with recombinant vaccinia virus expressing GM-CSF. Hum Gene Ther 1996; 7: 1853–1860.
274. Kass E, Parker J, Schlom J, Greiner JW. Comparative studies of the effects of recombinant GM-CSF and GM-CSF administered via a poxvirus to enhance the concentration of antigen- presenting cells in regional lymph nodes. Cytokine 2000; 12: 960–971.

275. Bowne WB, Wolchok JD, Hawkins WG et al. Injection of DNA encoding granulocyte-macrophage colony-stimulating factor recruits dendritic cells for immune adjuvant effects. Cytokines Cell Mol Ther 1999; 5: 217–225.
276. Perales MA, Fantuzzi G, Goldberg SM et al. GM-CSF DNA induces specific patterns of cytokines and chemokines in the skin: implications for DNA vaccines. Cytokines Cell Mol Ther 2002; 7: 125–133.
277. Bowne WB, Srinivasan R, Wolchok JD et al. Coupling and uncoupling of tumor immunity and autoimmunity. J Exp Med 1999; 190: 1717–1722.
278. Weiss WR, Ishii KJ, Hedstrom RC et al. A plasmid encoding murine granulocyte-macrophage colony-stimulating factor increases protection conferred by a malaria DNA vaccine. J Immunol 1998; 161: 2325–2332.
279. Raviprakash K, Ewing D, Simmons M et al. Needle-free Biojector injection of a dengue virus type 1 DNA vaccine with human immunostimulatory sequences and the GM-CSF gene increases immunogenicity and protection from virus challenge in Aotus monkeys. Virology 2003; 315: 345–352.
280. Sakata T, Iwagami S, Tsuruta Y et al. Constitutive expression of interleukin-7 mRNA and production of IL-7 by a cloned murine thymic stromal cell line. J. Leukoc. Biol. 1990; 48: 205–212.
281. Heufler C, Topar G, Grasseger A et al. Interleukin 7 is produced by murine and human keratinocytes. J. Exp. Med. 1993; 178: 1109–1114.
282. Madrigal-Estebas L, McManus R, Byrne B et al. Human small intestinal epithelial cells secrete interleukin-7 and differentially express two different interleukin-7 mRNA Transcripts: implications for extrathymic T-cell differentiation. Hum. Immunol. 1997; 58: 83–90.
283. Fry TJ, Mackall CL. Interleukin-7: from bench to clinic. Blood 2002; 99: 3892–3904.
284. Noguchi M, Nakamura Y, Russell SM et al. Interleukin-2 receptor gamma chain: a functional component of the interleukin-7 receptor [see comments]. Science 1993; 262: 1877–1880.
285. Goodwin RG, Friend D, Ziegler SF et al. Cloning of the human and murine interleukin-7 receptors: demonstration of a soluble form and homology to a new receptor superfamily. Cell 1990; 60: 941–951.
286. He YW, Malek TR. The structure and function of gamma c-dependent cytokines and receptors: regulation of T lymphocyte development and homeostasis. Crit Rev Immunol 1998; 18: 503–524.
287. Uribe L, Weinberg KI. X-linked SCID and other defects of cytokine pathways. Semin Hematol 1998; 35: 299–309.
288. Asao H, Okuyama C, Kumaki S et al. Cutting edge: the common gamma-chain is an indispensable subunit of the IL-21 receptor complex. J Immunol 2001; 167: 1–5.
289. von Freeden-Jeffry U, Vieira P, Lucian LA et al. Lymphopenia in interleukin (IL)-7 gene-deleted mice identifies IL-7 as a nonredundant cytokine. J Exp Med 1995; 181: 1519–1526.
290. Peschon JJ, Morrissey PJ, Grabstein KH et al. Early lymphocyte expansion is severely impaired in interleukin 7 receptor-deficient mice. J Exp Med 1994; 180: 1955–1960.
291. Alpdogan O, van den Brink MR. IL-7 and IL-15: therapeutic cytokines for immunodeficiency. Trends Immunol 2005; 26: 56–64.
292. Schluns KS, Kieper WC, Jameson SC, Lefrancois L. Interleukin-7 mediates the homeostasis of naive and memory CD8 T cells in vivo. Nat Immunol 2000; 1: 426–432.
293. Kaech SM, Tan JT, Wherry EJ et al. Selective expression of the interleukin 7 receptor identifies effector CD8 T cells that give rise to long-lived memory cells. Nat Immunol 2003; 4: 1191–1198.
294. Sempowski GD, Gooding ME, Liao HX et al. T cell receptor excision circle assessment of thymopoiesis in aging mice. Mol Immunol 2002; 38: 841–848.
295. Bolotin E, Smogorzewska M, Smith S et al. Enhancement of thymopoiesis after bone marrow transplant by *in vivo* interleukin-7. Blood 1996; 88: 1887–1894.
296. Okamoto Y, Douek DC, McFarland RD, Koup RA. Effects of exogenous interleukin-7 on human thymus function. Blood 2002; 99: 2851–2858.
297. Alpdogan O, Muriglan SJ, Eng JM et al. IL-7 enhances peripheral T cell reconstitution after allogeneic hematopoietic stem cell transplantation. J Clin Invest 2003; 112: 1095–1107.

298. Abdul-Hai A, Or R, Slavin S et al. Stimulation of immune reconstitution by interleukin-7 after syngeneic bone marrow transplantation in mice. Exp Hematol 1996; 24: 1416–1422.
299. Alpdogan O, Schmaltz C, Muriglan SJ et al. Administration of interleukin-7 after allogeneic bone marrow transplantation improves immune reconstitution without aggravating graft-versus-host disease. Blood 2001; 98: 2256–2265.
300. Mackall CL, Fry TJ, Bare C et al. IL-7 increases both thymic-dependent and thymic-independent T-cell regeneration after bone marrow transplantation. Blood 2001; 97: 1491–1497.
301. Storek J, Gillespy T, 3rd, Lu H et al. Interleukin-7 improves CD4 T-cell reconstitution after autologous CD34 cell transplantation in monkeys. Blood 2003; 101: 4209–4218.
302. Kobayashi M, Fitz L, Ryan M et al. Identification and purification of natural killer cell stimulatory factor (NKSF), a cytokine with multiple biologic effects on human lymphocytes. J Exp Med 1989; 170: 827–845.
303. Stern AS, Podlaski FJ, Hulmes JD et al. Purification to homogeneity and partial characterization of cytotoxic lymphocyte maturation factor from human B-lymphoblastoid cells. Proc Natl Acad Sci U S A 1990; 87: 6808–6812.
304. Oppmann B, Lesley R, Blom B et al. Novel p19 protein engages IL-12p40 to form a cytokine, IL-23, with biological activities similar as well as distinct from IL-12. Immunity 2000; 13: 715–725.
305. Trinchieri G. Interleukin-12 and the regulation of innate resistance and adaptive immunity. Nat Rev Immunol 2003; 3: 133–146.
306. Manetti R, Parronchi P, Giudizi MG et al. Natural killer cell stimulatory factor (interleukin 12 [IL-12]) induces T helper type 1 (Th1)-specific immune responses and inhibits the development of IL-4-producing Th cells. J Exp Med 1993; 177: 1199–1204.
307. Manetti R, Gerosa F, Giudizi MG et al. Interleukin 12 induces stable priming for interferon gamma (IFN-gamma) production during differentiation of human T helper (Th) cells and transient IFN-gamma production in established Th2 cell clones. J Exp Med 1994; 179: 1273–1283.
308. Perussia B, Chan SH, D'Andrea A et al. Natural killer (NK) cell stimulatory factor or IL-12 has differential effects on the proliferation of TCR-alpha beta+, TCR-gamma delta+ T lymphocytes, and NK cells. J Immunol 1992; 149: 3495–3502.
309. Bertagnolli MM, Lin BY, Young D, Herrmann SH. IL-12 augments antigen-dependent proliferation of activated T lymphocytes. J Immunol 1992; 149: 3778–3783.
310. Gately MK, Desai BB, Wolitzky AG et al. Regulation of human lymphocyte proliferation by a heterodimeric cytokine, IL-12 (cytotoxic lymphocyte maturation factor). J Immunol 1991; 147: 874–882.
311. Murphy EE, Terres G, Macatonia SE et al. B7 and interleukin 12 cooperate for proliferation and interferon gamma production by mouse T helper clones that are unresponsive to B7 costimulation. J Exp Med 1994; 180: 223–231.
312. Noguchi Y, Jungbluth A, Richards EC, Old LJ. Effect of interleukin 12 on tumor induction by 3-methylcholanthrene. Proc Natl Acad Sci U S A 1996; 93: 11798–11801.
313. Brunda MJ, Luistro L, Warrier RR et al. Antitumor and antimetastatic activity of interleukin 12 against murine tumors. J Exp Med 1993; 178: 1223–1230.
314. Cavallo F, Signorelli P, Giovarelli M et al. Antitumor efficacy of adenocarcinoma cells engineered to produce interleukin 12 (IL-12) or other cytokines compared with exogenous IL-12. J Natl Cancer Inst 1997; 89: 1049–1058.
315. Noguchi Y, Richards EC, Chen YT, Old LJ. Influence of interleukin 12 on p53 peptide vaccination against established Meth A sarcoma. Proc Natl Acad Sci U S A 1995; 92: 2219–2223.
316. Irvine KR, Rao JB, Rosenberg SA, Restifo NP. Cytokine enhancement of DNA immunization leads to effective treatment of established pulmonary metastases. J Immunol 1996; 156: 238–245.
317. Nanni P, Nicoletti G, De Giovanni C et al. Combined allogeneic tumor cell vaccination and systemic interleukin 12 prevents mammary carcinogenesis in HER-2/neu transgenic mice. J Exp Med 2001; 194: 1195–1205.
318. Atkins MB, Robertson MJ, Gordon M et al. Phase I evaluation of intravenous recombinant human interleukin 12 in patients with advanced malignancies. Clin Cancer Res 1997; 3: 409–417.

319. Portielje JE, Kruit WH, Schuler M et al. Phase I study of subcutaneously administered recombinant human interleukin 12 in patients with advanced renal cell cancer. Clin Cancer Res 1999; 5: 3983–3989.
320. Gollob JA, Mier JW, Veenstra K et al. Phase I trial of twice-weekly intravenous interleukin 12 in patients with metastatic renal cell cancer or malignant melanoma: ability to maintain IFN-gamma induction is associated with clinical response. Clin Cancer Res 2000; 6: 1678–1692.
321. Gollob JA, Veenstra KG, Parker RA et al. Phase I trial of concurrent twice-weekly recombinant human interleukin-12 plus low-dose IL-2 in patients with melanoma or renal cell carcinoma. J Clin Oncol 2003; 21: 2564–2573.
322. Alatrash G, Hutson TE, Molto L et al. Clinical and immunologic effects of subcutaneously administered interleukin-12 and interferon alfa-2b: phase I trial of patients with metastatic renal cell carcinoma or malignant melanoma. J Clin Oncol 2004; 22: 2891–2900.
323. Wadler S, Levy D, Frederickson HL et al. A phase II trial of interleukin-12 in patients with advanced cervical cancer: clinical and immunologic correlates. Eastern Cooperative Oncology Group study E1E96. Gynecol Oncol 2004; 92: 957–964.
324. Younes A, Pro B, Robertson MJ et al. Phase II clinical trial of interleukin-12 in patients with relapsed and refractory non-Hodgkin's lymphoma and Hodgkin's disease. Clin Cancer Res 2004; 10: 5432–5438.
325. Lee KH, Wang E, Nielsen MB et al. Increased vaccine-specific T cell frequency after peptide-based vaccination correlates with increased susceptibility to in vitro stimulation but does not lead to tumor regression. J Immunol 1999; 163: 6292–6300.
326. Lee P, Wang F, Kuniyoshi J et al. Effects of interleukin-12 on the immune response to a multi-peptide vaccine for resected metastatic melanoma. J Clin Oncol 2001; 19: 3836–3847.
327. Boyer JD, Cohen AD, Ugen KE et al. Therapeutic immunization of HIV-infected chimpanzees using HIV-1 plasmid antigens and interleukin-12 expressing plasmids. Aids 2000; 14: 1515–1522.
328. Grabstein KH, Eisenman J, Shanebeck K et al. Cloning of a T cell growth factor that interacts with the beta chain of the interleukin-2 receptor. Science 1994; 264: 965–968.
329. Burton JD, Bamford RN, Peters C et al. A lymphokine, provisionally designated interleukin T and produced by a human adult T-cell leukemia line, stimulates T-cell proliferation and the induction of lymphokine-activated killer cells. Proc Natl Acad Sci U S A 1994; 91: 4935–4939.
330. Bamford RN, Grant AJ, Burton JD et al. The interleukin (IL) 2 receptor beta chain is shared by IL-2 and a cytokine, provisionally designated IL-T, that stimulates T-cell proliferation and the induction of lymphokine-activated killer cells. Proc Natl Acad Sci U S A 1994; 91: 4940–4944.
331. Waldmann T, Tagaya Y, Bamford R. Interleukin-2, interleukin-15, and their receptors. Int Rev Immunol 1998; 16: 205–226.
332. Bazan JF. Structural design and molecular evolution of a cytokine receptor superfamily. Proc Natl Acad Sci U S A 1990; 87: 6934–6938.
333. Bazan JF. Haemopoietic receptors and helical cytokines. Immunol Today 1990; 11: 350–354.
334. Carson WE, Giri JG, Lindemann MJ et al. Interleukin (IL) 15 is a novel cytokine that activates human natural killer cells via components of the IL-2 receptor. J Exp Med 1994; 180: 1395–1403.
335. Anderson DM, Kumaki S, Ahdieh M et al. Functional characterization of the human interleukin-15 receptor alpha chain and close linkage of IL15RA and IL2RA genes. J Biol Chem 1995; 270: 29862–29869.
336. Kim JJ, Trivedi NN, Nottingham LK et al. Modulation of amplitude and direction of in vivo immune responses by co-administration of cytokine gene expression cassettes with DNA immunogens. Eur J Immunol 1998; 28: 1089–1103.
337. Xin KQ, Hamajima K, Sasaki S et al. IL-15 expression plasmid enhances cell-mediated immunity induced by an HIV-1 DNA vaccine. Vaccine 1999; 17: 858–866.
338. Moore AC, Kong WP, Chakrabarti BK, Nabel GJ. Effects of antigen and genetic adjuvants on immune responses to human immunodeficiency virus DNA vaccines in mice. J Virol 2002; 76: 243–250.
339. McKee HJ, T'Sao P Y, Vera M et al. Durable cytotoxic immune responses against gp120 elicited by recombinant SV40 vectors encoding HIV-1 gp120 +/- IL-15. Genet Vaccines Ther 2004; 2: 10.

340. Oh S, Berzofsky JA, Burke DS et al. Coadministration of HIV vaccine vectors with vaccinia viruses expressing IL-15 but not IL-2 induces long-lasting cellular immunity. Proc Natl Acad Sci U S A 2003; 100: 3392–3397.
341. Villinger F, Miller R, Mori K et al. IL-15 is superior to IL-2 in the generation of long-lived antigen specific memory CD4 and CD8 T cells in rhesus macaques. Vaccine 2004; 22: 3510–3521.
342. Cui FD, Asada H, Jin ML et al. Cytokine genetic adjuvant facilitates prophylactic intravascular DNA vaccine against acute and latent herpes simplex virus infection in mice. Gene Ther 2004.
343. Kwissa M, Kroger A, Hauser H et al. Cytokine-facilitated priming of CD8+ T cell responses by DNA vaccination. J Mol Med 2003; 81: 91–101.
344. Dinarello CA. Interleukin-18. Methods 1999; 19: 121–132.
345. Akira S. The role of IL-18 in innate immunity. Curr Opin Immunol 2000; 12: 59–63.
346. McInnes IB, Gracie JA, Leung BP et al. Interleukin 18: a pleiotropic participant in chronic inflammation. Immunol Today 2000; 21: 312–315.
347. Bazan JF, Timans JC, Kastelein RA. A newly defined interleukin-1? Nature 1996; 379: 591.
348. Gu Y, Kuida K, Tsutsui H et al. Activation of interferon-gamma inducing factor mediated by interleukin-1beta converting enzyme. Science 1997; 275: 206–209.
349. Ghayur T, Banerjee S, Hugunin M et al. Caspase-1 processes IFN-gamma-inducing factor and regulates LPS-induced IFN-gamma production. Nature 1997; 386: 619–623.
350. Puren AJ, Razeghi P, Fantuzzi G, Dinarello CA. Interleukin-18 enhances lipopolysaccharide-induced interferon-gamma production in human whole blood cultures. J Infect Dis 1998; 178: 1830–1834.
351. Takeda K, Tsutsui H, Yoshimoto T et al. Defective NK cell activity and Th1 response in IL-18-deficient mice. Immunity 1998; 8: 383–390.
352. Hyodo Y, Matsui K, Hayashi N et al. IL-18 up-regulates perforin-mediated NK activity without increasing perforin messenger RNA expression by binding to constitutively expressed IL-18 receptor. J Immunol 1999; 162: 1662–1668.
353. Fantuzzi G, Puren AJ, Harding MW et al. Interleukin-18 regulation of interferon gamma production and cell proliferation as shown in interleukin-1beta-converting enzyme (caspase-1)-deficient mice. Blood 1998; 91: 2118–2125.
354. Okamura H, Tsutsi H, Komatsu T et al. Cloning of a new cytokine that induces IFN-gamma production by T cells. Nature 1995; 378: 88–91.
355. Ushio S, Namba M, Okura T et al. Cloning of the cDNA for human IFN-gamma-inducing factor, expression in Escherichia coli, and studies on the biologic activities of the protein. J Immunol 1996; 156: 4274–4279.
356. Robinson D, Shibuya K, Mui A et al. IGIF does not drive Th1 development but synergizes with IL-12 for interferon-gamma production and activates IRAK and NFkappaB. Immunity 1997; 7: 571–581.
357. Yoshimoto T, Takeda K, Tanaka T et al. IL-12 up-regulates IL-18 receptor expression on T cells, Th1 cells, and B cells: synergism with IL-18 for IFN-gamma production. J Immunol 1998; 161: 3400–3407.
358. Ahn HJ, Maruo S, Tomura M et al. A mechanism underlying synergy between IL-12 and IFN-gamma-inducing factor in enhanced production of IFN-gamma. J Immunol 1997; 159: 2125–2131.
359. Barbulescu K, Becker C, Schlaak JF et al. IL-12 and IL-18 differentially regulate the transcriptional activity of the human IFN-gamma promoter in primary CD4+ T lymphocytes. J Immunol 1998; 160: 3642–3647.
360. Bohn E, Sing A, Zumbihl R et al. IL-18 (IFN-gamma-inducing factor) regulates early cytokine production in, and promotes resolution of, bacterial infection in mice. J Immunol 1998; 160: 299–307.
361. Lauw FN, Dekkers PE, te Velde AA et al. Interleukin-12 induces sustained activation of multiple host inflammatory mediator systems in chimpanzees. J Infect Dis 1999; 179: 646–652.
362. Nagai H, Hara I, Horikawa T et al. Antitumor effects on mouse melanoma elicited by local secretion of interleukin-12 and their enhancement by treatment with interleukin-18. Cancer Invest 2000; 18: 206–213.

363. Yamanaka R, Tsuchiya N, Yajima N et al. Induction of an antitumor immunological response by an intratumoral injection of dendritic cells pulsed with genetically engineered Semliki Forest virus to produce interleukin-18 combined with the systemic administration of interleukin-12. J Neurosurg 2003; 99: 746–753.
364. Kishida T, Asada H, Satoh E et al. In vivo electroporation-mediated transfer of interleukin-12 and interleukin-18 genes induces significant antitumor effects against melanoma in mice. Gene Ther 2001; 8: 1234–1240.
365. Asada H, Kishida T, Hirai H et al. Significant antitumor effects obtained by autologous tumor cell vaccine engineered to secrete interleukin (IL)-12 and IL-18 by means of the EBV/lipoplex. Mol Ther 2002; 5: 609–616.
366. Hikosaka S, Hara I, Miyake H et al. Antitumor effect of simultaneous transfer of interleukin-12 and interleukin-18 genes and its mechanism in a mouse bladder cancer model. Int J Urol 2004; 11: 647–652.
367. Li Q, Carr AL, Donald EJ et al. Synergistic effects of IL-12 and IL-18 in skewing tumor-reactive T-cell responses towards a type 1 pattern. Cancer Res 2005; 65: 1063–1070.
368. Yamanaka R, Xanthopoulos KG. Induction of antigen-specific immune responses against malignant brain tumors by intramuscular injection of sindbis DNA encoding gp100 and IL-18. DNA Cell Biol 2005; 24: 317–324.
369. Luo Y, Zhou H, Mizutani M et al. A DNA vaccine targeting Fos-related antigen 1 enhanced by IL-18 induces long-lived T-cell memory against tumor recurrence. Cancer Res 2005; 65: 3419–3427.
370. Ju DW, Yang Y, Tao Q et al. Interleukin-18 gene transfer increases antitumor effects of suicide gene therapy through efficient induction of antitumor immunity. Gene Ther 2000; 7: 1672–1679.
371. Wang Q, Yu H, Ju DW et al. Intratumoral IL-18 gene transfer improves therapeutic efficacy of antibody-targeted superantigen in established murine melanoma. Gene Ther 2001; 8: 542–550.
372. Kirkbride KC, Blobe GC. Inhibiting the TGF-beta signalling pathway as a means of cancer immunotherapy. Expert Opin Biol Ther 2003; 3: 251–261.
373. Iyer S, Wang ZG, Akhtari M et al. Targeting TGFbeta Signaling for Cancer Therapy. Cancer Biol Ther 2005; 4.
374. Elliott RL, Blobe GC. Role of transforming growth factor Beta in human cancer. J Clin Oncol 2005; 23: 2078–2093.
375. Kehrl JH, Wakefield LM, Roberts AB et al. Production of transforming growth factor beta by human T lymphocytes and its potential role in the regulation of T cell growth. J Exp Med 1986; 163: 1037–1050.
376. Inge TH, McCoy KM, Susskind BM et al. Immunomodulatory effects of transforming growth factor-beta on T lymphocytes. Induction of CD8 expression in the CTLL-2 cell line and in normal thymocytes. J Immunol 1992; 148: 3847–3856.
377. Ebert EC. Inhibitory effects of transforming growth factor-beta (TGF-beta) on certain functions of intraepithelial lymphocytes. Clin Exp Immunol 1999; 115: 415–420.
378. Ahuja SS, Paliogianni F, Yamada H et al. Effect of transforming growth factor-beta on early and late activation events in human T cells. J Immunol 1993; 150: 3109–3118.
379. Pardoux C, Asselin-Paturel C, Chehimi J et al. Functional interaction between TGF-beta and IL-12 in human primary allogeneic cytotoxicity and proliferative response. J Immunol 1997; 158: 136–143.
380. Ludviksson BR, Seegers D, Resnick AS, Strober W. The effect of TGF-beta1 on immune responses of naive versus memory CD4+ Th1/Th2 T cells. Eur J Immunol 2000; 30: 2101–2111.
381. Lin JT, Martin SL, Xia L, Gorham JD. TGF-beta 1 uses distinct mechanisms to inhibit IFN-gamma expression in CD4+ T cells at priming and at recall: differential involvement of Stat4 and T-bet. J Immunol 2005; 174: 5950–5958.
382. Laouar Y, Sutterwala FS, Gorelik L, Flavell RA. Transforming growth factor-beta controls T helper type 1 cell development through regulation of natural killer cell interferon-gamma. Nat Immunol 2005; 6: 600–607.

383. Mule JJ, Schwarz SL, Roberts AB et al. Transforming growth factor-beta inhibits the in vitro generation of lymphokine-activated killer cells and cytotoxic T cells. Cancer Immunol Immunother 1988; 26: 95–100.
384. Smyth MJ, Strobl SL, Young HA et al. Regulation of lymphokine-activated killer activity and pore-forming protein gene expression in human peripheral blood CD8+ T lymphocytes. Inhibition by transforming growth factor-beta. J Immunol 1991; 146: 3289–3297.
385. Espevik T, Figari IS, Ranges GE, Palladino MA, Jr. Transforming growth factor-beta 1 (TGF-beta 1) and recombinant human tumor necrosis factor-alpha reciprocally regulate the generation of lymphokine-activated killer cell activity. Comparison between natural porcine platelet-derived TGF-beta 1 and TGF-beta 2, and recombinant human TGF-beta 1. J Immunol 1988; 140: 2312–2316.
386. Espevik T, Waage A, Faxvaag A, Shalaby MR. Regulation of interleukin-2 and interleukin-6 production from T-cells: involvement of interleukin-1 beta and transforming growth factor-beta. Cell Immunol 1990; 126: 47–56.
387. Fargeas C, Wu CY, Nakajima T et al. Differential effect of transforming growth factor beta on the synthesis of Th1- and Th2-like lymphokines by human T lymphocytes. Eur J Immunol 1992; 22: 2173–2176.
388. Ahmadzadeh M, Rosenberg SA. TGF-beta 1 attenuates the acquisition and expression of effector function by tumor antigen-specific human memory CD8 T cells. J Immunol 2005; 174: 5215–5223.
389. Nakamura K, Kitani A, Fuss I et al. TGF-beta 1 plays an important role in the mechanism of CD4+CD25+ regulatory T cell activity in both humans and mice. J Immunol 2004; 172: 834–842.
390. Su HC, Leite-Morris KA, Braun L, Biron CA. A role for transforming growth factor-beta 1 in regulating natural killer cell and T lymphocyte proliferative responses during acute infection with lymphocytic choriomeningitis virus. J Immunol 1991; 147: 2717–2727.
391. Lee JC, Lee KM, Kim DW, Heo DS. Elevated TGF-beta1 secretion and down-modulation of NKG2D underlies impaired NK cytotoxicity in cancer patients. J Immunol 2004; 172: 7335–7340.
392. Malygin AM, Meri S, Timonen T. Regulation of natural killer cell activity by transforming growth factor-beta and prostaglandin E2. Scand J Immunol 1993; 37: 71–76.
393. Bellone G, Aste-Amezaga M, Trinchieri G, Rodeck U. Regulation of NK cell functions by TGF-beta 1. J Immunol 1995; 155: 1066–1073.
394. Rook AH, Kehrl JH, Wakefield LM et al. Effects of transforming growth factor beta on the functions of natural killer cells: depressed cytolytic activity and blunting of interferon responsiveness. J Immunol 1986; 136: 3916–3920.
395. Kuppner MC, Hamou MF, Bodmer S et al. The glioblastoma-derived T-cell suppressor factor/transforming growth factor beta 2 inhibits the generation of lymphokine-activated killer (LAK) cells. Int J Cancer 1988; 42: 562–567.
396. Brooks B, Chapman K, Lawry J et al. Suppression of lymphokine-activated killer (LAK) cell induction mediated by interleukin-4 and transforming growth factor-beta 1: effect of addition of exogenous tumour necrosis factor-alpha and interferon-gamma, and measurement of their endogenous production. Clin Exp Immunol 1990; 82: 583–589.
397. Strassmann G, Cole MD, Newman W. Regulation of colony-stimulating factor 1-dependent macrophage precursor proliferation by type beta transforming growth factor. J Immunol 1988; 140: 2645–2651.
398. Sato Y, Kobori S, Sakai M et al. Lipoprotein(a) induces cell growth in rat peritoneal macrophages through inhibition of transforming growth factor-beta activation. Atherosclerosis 1996; 125: 15–26.
399. Pinson DM, LeClaire RD, Lorsbach RB et al. Regulation by transforming growth factor-beta 1 of expression and function of the receptor for IFN-gamma on mouse macrophages. J Immunol 1992; 149: 2028–2034.
400. Jun CD, Choi BM, Kim SU et al. Down-regulation of transforming growth factor-beta gene expression by antisense oligodeoxynucleotides increases recombinant interferon-gamma-induced nitric oxide synthesis in murine peritoneal macrophages. Immunology 1995; 85: 114–119.

401. Imai K, Takeshita A, Hanazawa S. Transforming growth factor-beta inhibits lipopolysaccharide-stimulated expression of inflammatory cytokines in mouse macrophages through downregulation of activation protein 1 and CD14 receptor expression. Infect Immun 2000; 68: 2418–2423.
402. Yamaguchi Y, Tsumura H, Miwa M, Inaba K. Contrasting effects of TGF-beta 1 and TNF-alpha on the development of dendritic cells from progenitors in mouse bone marrow. Stem Cells 1997; 15: 144–153.
403. Sato K, Kawasaki H, Nagayama H et al. TGF-beta 1 reciprocally controls chemotaxis of human peripheral blood monocyte-derived dendritic cells via chemokine receptors. J Immunol 2000; 164: 2285–2295.
404. Maehara Y, Kakeji Y, Kabashima A et al. Role of transforming growth factor-beta 1 in invasion and metastasis in gastric carcinoma. J Clin Oncol 1999; 17: 607–614.
405. Pepper MS. Transforming growth factor-beta: vasculogenesis, angiogenesis, and vessel wall integrity. Cytokine Growth Factor Rev 1997; 8: 21–43.
406. Ravitz MJ, Wenner CE. Cyclin-dependent kinase regulation during G1 phase and cell cycle regulation by TGF-beta. Adv Cancer Res 1997; 71: 165–207.
407. Becker C, Fantini MC, Schramm C et al. TGF-beta suppresses tumor progression in colon cancer by inhibition of IL-6 trans-signaling. Immunity 2004; 21: 491–501.
408. Paterson IC, Matthews JB, Huntley S et al. Decreased expression of TGF-beta cell surface receptors during progression of human oral squamous cell carcinoma. J Pathol 2001; 193: 458–467.
409. West J, Munoz-Antonia T, Johnson JG et al. Transforming growth factor-beta type II receptors and smad proteins in follicular thyroid tumors. Laryngoscope 2000; 110: 1323–1327.
410. Fujiwara K, Ikeda H, Yoshimoto T. Abnormalities in expression of genes, mRNA, and proteins of transforming growth factor-beta receptor type I and type II in human pituitary adenomas. Clin Neuropathol 1998; 17: 19–26.
411. Park K, Kim SJ, Bang YJ et al. Genetic changes in the transforming growth factor beta (TGF-beta) type II receptor gene in human gastric cancer cells: correlation with sensitivity to growth inhibition by TGF-beta. Proc Natl Acad Sci U S A 1994; 91: 8772–8776.
412. Markowitz S, Wang J, Myeroff L et al. Inactivation of the type II TGF-beta receptor in colon cancer cells with microsatellite instability. Science 1995; 268: 1336–1338.
413. Garrigue-Antar L, Munoz-Antonia T, Antonia SJ et al. Missense mutations of the transforming growth factor beta type II receptor in human head and neck squamous carcinoma cells. Cancer Res 1995; 55: 3982–3987.
414. Lucke CD, Philpott A, Metcalfe JC et al. Inhibiting mutations in the transforming growth factor beta type 2 receptor in recurrent human breast cancer. Cancer Res 2001; 61: 482–485.
415. Kim SJ, Im YH, Markowitz SD, Bang YJ. Molecular mechanisms of inactivation of TGF-beta receptors during carcinogenesis. Cytokine Growth Factor Rev 2000; 11: 159–168.
416. Imai Y, Kurokawa M, Izutsu K et al. Mutations of the Smad4 gene in acute myelogeneous leukemia and their functional implications in leukemogenesis. Oncogene 2001; 20: 88–96.
417. Hu W, Wu W, Nash MA et al. Anomalies of the TGF-beta postreceptor signaling pathway in ovarian cancer cell lines. Anticancer Res 2000; 20: 729–733.
418. Villanueva A, Garcia C, Paules AB et al. Disruption of the antiproliferative TGF-beta signaling pathways in human pancreatic cancer cells. Oncogene 1998; 17: 1969–1978.
419. Giannelli G, Fransvea E, Marinosci F et al. Transforming growth factor-beta1 triggers hepatocellular carcinoma invasiveness via alpha3beta1 integrin. Am J Pathol 2002; 161: 183–193.
420. Saito H, Tsujitani S, Oka S et al. An elevated serum level of transforming growth factor-beta 1 (TGF-beta 1) significantly correlated with lymph node metastasis and poor prognosis in patients with gastric carcinoma. Anticancer Res 2000; 20: 4489–4493.
421. Shim KS, Kim KH, Han WS, Park EB. Elevated serum levels of transforming growth factor-beta1 in patients with colorectal carcinoma: its association with tumor progression and its significant decrease after curative surgical resection. Cancer 1999; 85: 554–561.
422. Guzinska-Ustymowicz K, Kemona A. Transforming growth factor beta can be a parameter of aggressiveness of pT1 colorectal cancer. World J Gastroenterol 2005; 11: 1193–1195.

423. Feltl D, Zavadova E, Pala M, Hozak P. The dynamics of plasma transforming growth factor beta 1 (TGF-beta1) level during radiotherapy with or without simultaneous chemotherapy in advanced head and neck cancer. Oral Oncol 2005; 41: 208–213.
424. Wojtowicz-Praga S, Verma UN, Wakefield L et al. Modulation of B16 melanoma growth and metastasis by anti-transforming growth factor beta antibody and interleukin-2. J Immunother Emphasis Tumor Immunol 1996; 19: 169–175.
425. Gridley DS, Sura SS, Uhm JR et al. Effects of anti-transforming growth factor-beta antibody and interleukin-2 in tumor-bearing mice. Cancer Biother 1993; 8: 159–170.
426. Arteaga CL, Hurd SD, Winnier AR et al. Anti-transforming growth factor (TGF)-beta antibodies inhibit breast cancer cell tumorigenicity and increase mouse spleen natural killer cell activity. Implications for a possible role of tumor cell/host TGF-beta interactions in human breast cancer progression. J Clin Invest 1993; 92: 2569–2576.
427. Ohmori T, Yang JL, Price JO, Arteaga CL. Blockade of tumor cell transforming growth factor-betas enhances cell cycle progression and sensitizes human breast carcinoma cells to cytotoxic chemotherapy. Exp Cell Res 1998; 245: 350–359.
428. Mao XW, Kettering JD, Gridley DS. Immunotherapy with low-dose interleukin-2 and anti-transforming growth factor-beta antibody in a murine tumor model. Cancer Biother 1994; 9: 317–327.
429. Jia ZC, Zou LY, Ni B et al. Effective induction of antitumor immunity by immunization with plasmid DNA encoding TRP-2 plus neutralization of TGF-beta. Cancer Immunol Immunother 2005; 54: 446–452.
430. Suzuki E, Kapoor V, Cheung HK et al. Soluble type II transforming growth factor-beta receptor inhibits established murine malignant mesothelioma tumor growth by augmenting host antitumor immunity. Clin Cancer Res 2004; 10: 5907–5918.
431. Rowland-Goldsmith MA, Maruyama H, Kusama T et al. Soluble type II transforming growth factor-beta (TGF-beta) receptor inhibits TGF-beta signaling in COLO-357 pancreatic cancer cells in vitro and attenuates tumor formation. Clin Cancer Res 2001; 7: 2931–2940.
432. Rowland-Goldsmith MA, Maruyama H, Matsuda K et al. Soluble type II transforming growth factor-beta receptor attenuates expression of metastasis-associated genes and suppresses pancreatic cancer cell metastasis. Mol Cancer Ther 2002; 1: 161–167.
433. Yang YA, Dukhanina O, Tang B et al. Lifetime exposure to a soluble TGF-beta antagonist protects mice against metastasis without adverse side effects. J Clin Invest 2002; 109: 1607–1615.
434. Bandyopadhyay A, Zhu Y, Cibull ML et al. A soluble transforming growth factor beta type III receptor suppresses tumorigenicity and metastasis of human breast cancer MDA-MB-231 cells. Cancer Res 1999; 59: 5041–5046.
435. Won J, Kim H, Park EJ et al. Tumorigenicity of mouse thymoma is suppressed by soluble type II transforming growth factor beta receptor therapy. Cancer Res 1999; 59: 1273–1277.
436. Tuxhorn JA, McAlhany SJ, Yang F et al. Inhibition of transforming growth factor-beta activity decreases angiogenesis in a human prostate cancer-reactive stroma xenograft model. Cancer Res 2002; 62: 6021–6025.
437. Biglari A, Bataille D, Naumann U et al. Effects of ectopic decorin in modulating intracranial glioma progression in vivo, in a rat syngeneic model. Cancer Gene Ther 2004; 11: 721–732.
438. Engel S, Isenmann S, Stander M et al. Inhibition of experimental rat glioma growth by decorin gene transfer is associated with decreased microglial infiltration. J Neuroimmunol 1999; 99: 13–18.
439. Stander M, Naumann U, Dumitrescu L et al. Decorin gene transfer-mediated suppression of TGF-beta synthesis abrogates experimental malignant glioma growth in vivo. Gene Ther 1998; 5: 1187–1194.
440. Yamaguchi Y, Mann DM, Ruoslahti E. Negative regulation of transforming growth factor-beta by the proteoglycan decorin. Nature 1990; 346: 281–284.
441. Park JA, Wang E, Kurt RA et al. Expression of an antisense transforming growth factor-beta1 transgene reduces tumorigenicity of EMT6 mammary tumor cells. Cancer Gene Ther 1997; 4: 42–50.

442. Liau LM, Fakhrai H, Black KL. Prolonged survival of rats with intracranial C6 gliomas by treatment with TGF-beta antisense gene. Neurol Res 1998; 20: 742–747.
443. Dorigo O, Shawler DL, Royston I et al. Combination of transforming growth factor beta antisense and interleukin-2 gene therapy in the murine ovarian teratoma model. Gynecol Oncol 1998; 71: 204–210.
444. Maggard M, Meng L, Ke B et al. Antisense TGF-beta2 immunotherapy for hepatocellular carcinoma: treatment in a rat tumor model. Ann Surg Oncol 2001; 8: 32–37.
445. Marzo AL, Fitzpatrick DR, Robinson BW, Scott B. Antisense oligonucleotides specific for transforming growth factor beta2 inhibit the growth of malignant mesothelioma both in vitro and in vivo. Cancer Res 1997; 57: 3200–3207.
446. Schlingensiepen R, Goldbrunner M, Szyrach MN et al. Intracerebral and Intrathecal Infusion of the TGF-beta2-Specific Antisense Phosphorothioate Oligonucleotide AP 12009 in Rabbits and Primates: Toxicology and Safety. Oligonucleotides 2005; 15: 94–104.
447. Shah AH, Tabayoyong WB, Kundu SD et al. Suppression of tumor metastasis by blockade of transforming growth factor beta signaling in bone marrow cells through a retroviral-mediated gene therapy in mice. Cancer Res 2002; 62: 7135–7138.
448. Zhang Q, Yang X, Pins M et al. Adoptive transfer of tumor-reactive transforming growth factor-beta-insensitive CD8+ T cells: eradication of autologous mouse prostate cancer. Cancer Res 2005; 65: 1761–1769.
449. Gorelik L, Flavell RA. Immune-mediated eradication of tumors through the blockade of transforming growth factor-beta signaling in T cells. Nat Med 2001; 7: 1118–1122.
450. Siriwardena D, Khaw PT, King AJ et al. Human antitransforming growth factor beta(2) monoclonal antibody–a new modulator of wound healing in trabeculectomy: a randomized placebo controlled clinical study. Ophthalmology 2002; 109: 427–431.
451. Schlingensiepen KH, Schlingensiepen R, Steinbrecher A et al. Targeted tumor therapy with the TGF-beta2 antisense compound AP 12009. Cytokine Growth Factor Rev 2005.
452. Sabat R, Asadullah K. Interleukin-10 in Cancer Immunity. In Stuhler G, Walden P (eds): Cancer immune therapy: current and future strategies, Edition Weinheim: Wiley-VCH 2002; 155–175.
453. Becker JC, Czerny C, Brocker EB. Maintenance of clonal anergy by endogenously produced IL-10. Int Immunol 1994; 6: 1605–1612.
454. Cooper MA, Fehniger TA, Turner SC et al. Human natural killer cells: a unique innate immunoregulatory role for the CD56(bright) subset. Blood 2001; 97: 3146–3151.
455. Buchwald UK, Geerdes-Fenge HF, Vockler J et al. Interleukin-10: effects on phagocytosis and adhesion molecule expression of granulocytes and monocytes in a comparison with prednisolone. Eur J Med Res 1999; 4: 85–94.
456. Carson WE, Lindemann MJ, Baiocchi R et al. The functional characterization of interleukin-10 receptor expression on human natural killer cells. Blood 1995; 85: 3577–3585.
457. Hart PH, Hunt EK, Bonder CS et al. Regulation of surface and soluble TNF receptor expression on human monocytes and synovial fluid macrophages by IL-4 and IL-10. J Immunol 1996; 157: 3672–3680.
458. de Waal Malefyt R, Yssel H, de Vries JE. Direct effects of IL-10 on subsets of human CD4+ T cell clones and resting T cells. Specific inhibition of IL-2 production and proliferation. J Immunol 1993; 150: 4754–4765.
459. Creery WD, Diaz-Mitoma F, Filion L, Kumar A. Differential modulation of B7–1 and B7–2 isoform expression on human monocytes by cytokines which influence the development of T helper cell phenotype. Eur J Immunol 1996; 26: 1273–1277.
460. Willems F, Marchant A, Delville JP et al. Interleukin-10 inhibits B7 and intercellular adhesion molecule-1 expression on human monocytes. Eur J Immunol 1994; 24: 1007–1009.
461. Buelens C, Verhasselt V, De Groote D et al. Interleukin-10 prevents the generation of dendritic cells from human peripheral blood mononuclear cells cultured with interleukin-4 and granulocyte/macrophage-colony-stimulating factor. Eur J Immunol 1997; 27: 756–762.
462. Allavena P, Piemonti L, Longoni D et al. IL-10 prevents the differentiation of monocytes to dendritic cells but promotes their maturation to macrophages. Eur J Immunol 1998; 28: 359–369.

463. Corinti S, Albanesi C, la Sala A et al. Regulatory activity of autocrine IL-10 on dendritic cell functions. J Immunol 2001; 166: 4312–4318.
464. Gerlini G, Tun-Kyi A, Dudli C et al. Metastatic melanoma secreted IL-10 down-regulates CD1 molecules on dendritic cells in metastatic tumor lesions. Am J Pathol 2004; 165: 1853–1863.
465. Taga K, Mostowski H, Tosato G. Human interleukin-10 can directly inhibit T-cell growth. Blood 1993; 81: 2964–2971.
466. Klein B, Lu ZY, Gu ZJ et al. Interleukin-10 and Gp130 cytokines in human multiple myeloma. Leuk Lymphoma 1999; 34: 63–70.
467. Beatty PR, Krams SM, Martinez OM. Involvement of IL-10 in the autonomous growth of EBV-transformed B cell lines. J Immunol 1997; 158: 4045–4051.
468. Czarneski J, Lin YC, Chong S et al. Studies in NZB IL-10 knockout mice of the requirement of IL-10 for progression of B-cell lymphoma. Leukemia 2004; 18: 597–606.
469. Huang M, Stolina M, Sharma S et al. Non-small cell lung cancer cyclooxygenase-2-dependent regulation of cytokine balance in lymphocytes and macrophages: up-regulation of interleukin 10 and down-regulation of interleukin 12 production. Cancer Res 1998; 58: 1208–1216.
470. Smith DR, Kunkel SL, Burdick MD et al. Production of interleukin-10 by human bronchogenic carcinoma. Am J Pathol 1994; 145: 18–25.
471. Sato T, McCue P, Masuoka K et al. Interleukin 10 production by human melanoma. Clin Cancer Res 1996; 2: 1383–1390.
472. Huettner C, Czub S, Kerkau S et al. Interleukin 10 is expressed in human gliomas in vivo and increases glioma cell proliferation and motility in vitro. Anticancer Res 1997; 17: 3217–3224.
473. Mori N, Prager D. Interleukin-10 gene expression and adult T-cell leukemia. Leuk Lymphoma 1998; 29: 239–248.
474. Bargou RC, Mapara MY, Zugck C et al. Characterization of a novel Hodgkin cell line, HD-MyZ, with myelomonocytic features mimicking Hodgkin's disease in severe combined immunodeficient mice. J Exp Med 1993; 177: 1257–1268.
475. Voorzanger N, Touitou R, Garcia E et al. Interleukin (IL)-10 and IL-6 are produced in vivo by non-Hodgkin's lymphoma cells and act as cooperative growth factors. Cancer Res 1996; 56: 5499–5505.
476. Ortegel JW, Staren ED, Faber LP et al. Cytokine biosynthesis by tumor-infiltrating T lymphocytes from human non-small-cell lung carcinoma. Cancer Immunol Immunother 2000; 48: 627–634.
477. Blay JY, Burdin N, Rousset F et al. Serum interleukin-10 in non-Hodgkin's lymphoma: a prognostic factor. Blood 1993; 82: 2169–2174.
478. Fayad L, Keating MJ, Reuben JM et al. Interleukin-6 and interleukin-10 levels in chronic lymphocytic leukemia: correlation with phenotypic characteristics and outcome. Blood 2001; 97: 256–263.
479. Bohlen H, Kessler M, Sextro M et al. Poor clinical outcome of patients with Hodgkin's disease and elevated interleukin-10 serum levels. Clinical significance of interleukin-10 serum levels for Hodgkin's disease. Ann Hematol 2000; 79: 110–113.
480. Visco C, Vassilakopoulos TP, Kliche KO et al. Elevated serum levels of IL-10 are associated with inferior progression-free survival in patients with Hodgkin's disease treated with radiotherapy. Leuk Lymphoma 2004; 45: 2085–2092.
481. Asadullah K, Docke WD, Haeussler A et al. Progression of mycosis fungoides is associated with increasing cutaneous expression of interleukin-10 mRNA. J Invest Dermatol 1996; 107: 833–837.
482. Neuner A, Schindel M, Wildenberg U et al. Prognostic significance of cytokine modulation in non-small cell lung cancer. Int J Cancer 2002; 101: 287–292.
483. Galizia G, Lieto E, De Vita F et al. Circulating levels of interleukin-10 and interleukin-6 in gastric and colon cancer patients before and after surgery: relationship with radicality and outcome. J Interferon Cytokine Res 2002; 22: 473–482.
484. Nemunaitis J, Fong T, Shabe P et al. Comparison of serum interleukin-10 (IL-10) levels between normal volunteers and patients with advanced melanoma. Cancer Invest 2001; 19: 239–247.
485. Chau GY, Wu CW, Lui WY et al. Serum interleukin-10 but not interleukin-6 is related to clinical outcome in patients with resectable hepatocellular carcinoma. Ann Surg 2000; 231: 552–558.

486. De Vita F, Orditura M, Galizia G et al. Serum interleukin-10 is an independent prognostic factor in advanced solid tumors. Oncol Rep 2000; 7: 357–361.
487. Cunningham LM, Chapman C, Dunstan R et al. Polymorphisms in the interleukin 10 gene promoter are associated with susceptibility to aggressive non-Hodgkin's lymphoma. Leuk Lymphoma 2003; 44: 251–255.
488. Havranek E, Howell WM, Fussell HM et al. An interleukin-10 promoter polymorphism may influence tumor development in renal cell carcinoma. J Urol 2005; 173: 709–712.
489. Langsenlehner U, Krippl P, Renner W et al. Interleukin-10 promoter polymorphism is associated with decreased breast cancer risk. Breast Cancer Res Treat 2005; 90: 113–115.
490. Stearns ME, Kim G, Garcia F, Wang M. Interleukin-10 induced activating transcription factor 3 transcriptional suppression of matrix metalloproteinase-2 gene expression in human prostate CPTX-1532 Cells. Mol Cancer Res 2004; 2: 403–416.
491. Zheng LM, Ojcius DM, Garaud F et al. Interleukin-10 inhibits tumor metastasis through an NK cell-dependent mechanism. J Exp Med 1996; 184: 579–584.
492. Vicari AP, Trinchieri G. Interleukin-10 in viral diseases and cancer: exiting the labyrinth? Immunol Rev 2004; 202: 223–236.
493. Baj-Krzyworzeka M, Baran J, Szatanek R et al. Prevention and reversal of tumor cell-induced monocyte deactivation by cytokines, purified protein derivative (PPD), and anti-IL-10 antibody. Cancer Immun 2004; 4: 8.
494. Stassi G, Todaro M, Zerilli M et al. Thyroid cancer resistance to chemotherapeutic drugs via autocrine production of interleukin-4 and interleukin-10. Cancer Res 2003; 63: 6784–6790.
495. Alas S, Bonavida B. Rituximab inactivates signal transducer and activation of transcription 3 (STAT3) activity in B-non-Hodgkin's lymphoma through inhibition of the interleukin 10 autocrine/paracrine loop and results in down-regulation of Bcl-2 and sensitization to cytotoxic drugs. Cancer Res 2001; 61: 5137–5144.
496. Alas S, Emmanouilides C, Bonavida B. Inhibition of interleukin 10 by rituximab results in down-regulation of bcl-2 and sensitization of B-cell non-Hodgkin's lymphoma to apoptosis. Clin Cancer Res 2001; 7: 709–723.
497. Garcia-Hernandez ML, Hernandez-Pando R, Gariglio P, Berumen J. Interleukin-10 promotes B16-melanoma growth by inhibition of macrophage functions and induction of tumour and vascular cell proliferation. Immunology 2002; 105: 231–243.
498. Hagenbaugh A, Sharma S, Dubinett SM et al. Altered immune responses in interleukin 10 transgenic mice. J Exp Med 1997; 185: 2101–2110.
499. Seo N, Hayakawa S, Takigawa M, Tokura Y. Interleukin-10 expressed at early tumour sites induces subsequent generation of CD4(+) T-regulatory cells and systemic collapse of antitumour immunity. Immunology 2001; 103: 449–457.
500. Specht C, Bexten S, Kolsch E, Pauels HG. Prostaglandins, but not tumor-derived IL-10, shut down concomitant tumor-specific CTL responses during murine plasmacytoma progression. Int J Cancer 2001; 91: 705–712.
501. Loercher AE, Nash MA, Kavanagh JJ et al. Identification of an IL-10-producing HLA-DR-negative monocyte subset in the malignant ascites of patients with ovarian carcinoma that inhibits cytokine protein expression and proliferation of autologous T cells. J Immunol 1999; 163: 6251–6260.
502. Qin Z, Noffz G, Mohaupt M, Blankenstein T. Interleukin-10 prevents dendritic cell accumulation and vaccination with granulocyte-macrophage colony-stimulating factor gene-modified tumor cells. J Immunol 1997; 159: 770–776.
503. Kim BG, Joo HG, Chung IS et al. Inhibition of interleukin-10 (IL-10) production from MOPC 315 tumor cells by IL-10 antisense oligodeoxynucleotides enhances cell-mediated immune responses. Cancer Immunol Immunother 2000; 49: 433–440.
504. Liu G, Ng H, Akasaki Y et al. Small interference RNA modulation of IL-10 in human monocyte-derived dendritic cells enhances the Th1 response. Eur J Immunol 2004; 34: 1680–1687.
505. He Q, Moore TT, Eko FO et al. Molecular basis for the potency of IL-10-deficient dendritic cells as a highly efficient APC system for activating Th1 response. J Immunol 2005; 174: 4860–4869.

506. Llorente L, Richaud-Patin Y, Garcia-Padilla C et al. Clinical and biologic effects of anti-interleukin-10 monoclonal antibody administration in systemic lupus erythematosus. Arthritis Rheum 2000; 43: 1790–1800.
507. Terabe M, Park JM, Berzofsky JA. Role of IL-13 in regulation of anti-tumor immunity and tumor growth. Cancer Immunol Immunother 2004; 53: 79–85.
508. Wynn TA. IL-13 effector functions. Annu Rev Immunol 2003; 21: 425–456.
509. McKenzie AN, Li X, Largaespada DA et al. Structural comparison and chromosomal localization of the human and mouse IL-13 genes. J Immunol 1993; 150: 5436–5444.
510. Obiri NI, Debinski W, Leonard WJ, Puri RK. Receptor for interleukin 13. Interaction with interleukin 4 by a mechanism that does not involve the common gamma chain shared by receptors for interleukins 2, 4, 7, 9, and 15. J Biol Chem 1995; 270: 8797–8804.
511. Aman MJ, Tayebi N, Obiri NI et al. cDNA cloning and characterization of the human interleukin 13 receptor alpha chain. J Biol Chem 1996; 271: 29265–29270.
512. Hilton DJ, Zhang JG, Metcalf D et al. Cloning and characterization of a binding subunit of the interleukin 13 receptor that is also a component of the interleukin 4 receptor. Proc Natl Acad Sci U S A 1996; 93: 497–501.
513. Chiaramonte MG, Mentink-Kane M, Jacobson BA et al. Regulation and function of the interleukin 13 receptor alpha 2 during a T helper cell type 2-dominant immune response. J Exp Med 2003; 197: 687–701.
514. Wood N, Whitters MJ, Jacobson BA et al. Enhanced interleukin (IL)-13 responses in mice lacking IL-13 receptor alpha 2. J Exp Med 2003; 197: 703–709.
515. Punnonen J, Aversa G, Cocks BG et al. Interleukin 13 induces interleukin 4-independent IgG4 and IgE synthesis and CD23 expression by human B cells. Proc Natl Acad Sci U S A 1993; 90: 3730–3734.
516. de Waal Malefyt R, Figdor CG, Huijbens R et al. Effects of IL-13 on phenotype, cytokine production, and cytotoxic function of human monocytes. Comparison with IL-4 and modulation by IFN-gamma or IL-10. J Immunol 1993; 151: 6370–6381.
517. Smyth MJ, Crowe NY, Pellicci DG et al. Sequential production of interferon-gamma by NK1.1(+) T cells and natural killer cells is essential for the antimetastatic effect of alpha-galactosylceramide. Blood 2002; 99: 1259–1266.
518. Terabe M, Matsui S, Noben-Trauth N et al. NKT cell-mediated repression of tumor immunosurveillance by IL-13 and the IL-4R-STAT6 pathway. Nat Immunol 2000; 1: 515–520.
519. Terabe M, Matsui S, Park JM et al. Transforming growth factor-beta production and myeloid cells are an effector mechanism through which CD1d-restricted T cells block cytotoxic T lymphocyte-mediated tumor immunosurveillance: abrogation prevents tumor recurrence. J Exp Med 2003; 198: 1741–1752.
520. Skinnider BF, Kapp U, Mak TW. The role of interleukin 13 in classical Hodgkin lymphoma. Leuk Lymphoma 2002; 43: 1203–1210.
521. Kawakami K, Kawakami M, Snoy PJ et al. In vivo overexpression of IL-13 receptor alpha2 chain inhibits tumorigenicity of human breast and pancreatic tumors in immunodeficient mice. J Exp Med 2001; 194: 1743–1754.
522. Lebel-Binay S, Laguerre B, Quintin-Colonna F et al. Experimental gene therapy of cancer using tumor cells engineered to secrete interleukin-13. Eur J Immunol 1995; 25: 2340–2348.
523. Kacha AK, Fallarino F, Markiewicz MA, Gajewski TF. Cutting edge: spontaneous rejection of poorly immunogenic P1.HTR tumors by Stat6-deficient mice. J Immunol 2000; 165: 6024–6028.
524. Ostrand-Rosenberg S, Clements VK, Terabe M et al. Resistance to metastatic disease in STAT6-deficient mice requires hemopoietic and nonhemopoietic cells and is IFN-gamma dependent. J Immunol 2002; 169: 5796–5804.
525. Rainov NG, Soling A. Technology evaluation: cintredekin besudotox, NeoPharm/Nippon. Curr Opin Mol Ther 2005; 7: 170–181.
526. Hodge JW, Chakraborty M, Kudo-Saito C et al. Multiple costimulatory modalities enhance CTL avidity. J Immunol 2005; 174: 5994–6004.

527. Ogden CA, Pound JD, Batth BK et al. Enhanced apoptotic cell clearance capacity and B cell survival factor production by IL-10-activated macrophages: implications for Burkitt's lymphoma. J Immunol 2005; 174: 3015–3023.
528. Levings MK, Bacchetta R, Schulz U, Roncarolo MG. The role of IL-10 and TGF-beta in the differentiation and effector function of T regulatory cells. Int Arch Allergy Immunol 2002; 129: 263–276.
529. Taga K, Tosato G. IL-10 inhibits human T cell proliferation and IL-2 production. J Immunol 1992; 148: 1143–1148.
530. Matsuda M, Salazar F, Petersson M et al. Interleukin 10 pretreatment protects target cells from tumor- and allo-specific cytotoxic T cells and downregulates HLA class I expression. J Exp Med 1994; 180: 2371–2376.
531. Mocellin S, Panelli M, Wang E et al. IL-10 stimulatory effects on human NK cells explored by gene profile analysis. Genes Immun 2004; 5: 621–630.
532. Piemonti L, Bernasconi S, Luini W et al. IL-13 supports differentiation of dendritic cells from circulating precursors in concert with GM-CSF. Eur Cytokine Netw 1995; 6: 245–252.
533. Lutz MB, Schnare M, Menges M et al. Differential functions of IL-4 receptor types I and II for dendritic cell maturation and IL-12 production and their dependency on GM-CSF. J Immunol 2002; 169: 3574–3580.

CHAPTER 6

HLA CLASS I ANTIGEN ABNORMALITIES IN TUMORS

BARBARA SELIGER[1] AND SOLDANO FERRONE[2]

Institute of Medical Immunology, Martin Luther University, 06112 Halle, Germany and Department of Immunology, Roswell Park Cancer Institute, Buffalo, NY 14263, USA

Abbreviations: APM, antigen processing machinery; β_2-m, β_2-microglobulin; BIP, immunoglobulin binding protein; CTL, cytotoxic T lymphocyte(s); DC, dendritic cell; EC, endothelial cell(s); ER, endoplasmic reticulum; HC, heavy chain; HLA, human leukocyte antigen; HNSCC, head and neck squamous cell carcinoma; HPV, human papilloma virus; IFN, interferon; LMP, low molecular mass polypeptides; mAb, monoclonal antibody(ies), MHC, major histocompatibility complex; MIC, MHC class I-related molecules; sMIC, soluble MIC; NK, natural killer cell(s); SNPs, single nucleotide polymorphisms; TAM, tumor-associated macrophage; TAP, transporter associated with antigen processing; TCR, T cell receptor; TIL, tumor infiltrating lymphocyte(s); TNF, tumor necrosis factor; T_{regs}, regulatory T cell(s)

INTRODUCTION

Compelling evidence indicates that patients with malignant disease may spontaneously mount an immune response against antigens expressed by their own tumors and that this immune response can be induced or enhanced by a variety of immunization strategies. In contrast to the findings in animal model systems [1], tumor antigen (TA)-specific immune responses are in general not paralleled by clinical responses [2]. These disappointing results have stimulated interest in defining the mechanisms by which tumor cells evade recognition and destruction by the host's immune system. Multiple strategies have been found to be utilized by tumor cells to escape immune surveillance. They include abnormalities in the TA-specific immune response, in the ability of immune cells to migrate and infiltrate into tumor lesions, in the expression and/or function of molecules crucial for recognition by immune cells, in the effector functions of immune cells and in the susceptibility of tumor cells to cell death (Figure 1). In this review we focus on the

H.L. Kaufman and J.D. Wolchok (eds.), General Principles of Tumor Immunotherapy, 123–144.

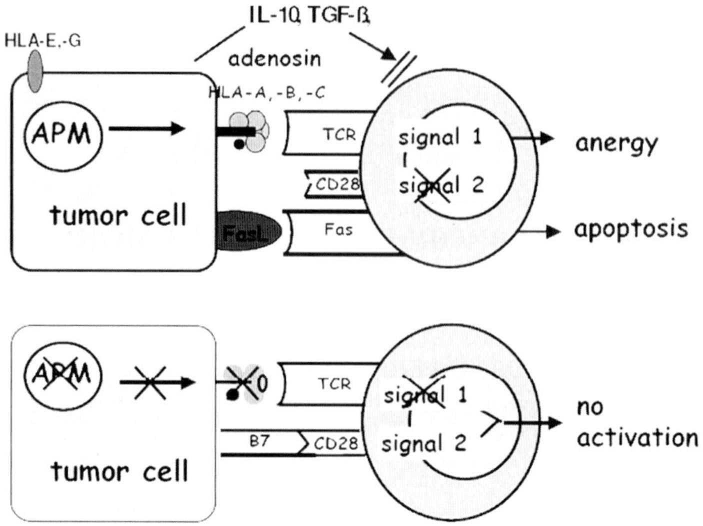

Figure 1. Mechanisms utilized by tumor cells to escape T cell responses

frequency, the molecular mechanisms, functional role and clinical significance of changes in the expression of classical and non-classical HLA class I antigens and MHC class I-related molecules (MIC) by malignant cells.

Characteristics of Classical and Non-classical HLA Class I and MIC Antigens

The superfamily of major histocompatibility complex (MHC) class I antigens can be divided into three subgroups based on their polymorphism, structure, expression and function: (i) the classical HLA class I antigens, (ii) the non-classical HLA class I antigens and (iii) the MHC related antigens MIC (Table 1). The classical HLA class Ia antigens HLA-A, -B and –C are highly polymorphic molecules. This polymorphism represents the structural basis for the presentation of a wide array of peptide antigens to the cellular immune system. HLA class Ia antigens are heterodimers consisting of a 45 kDa glycosylated polymorphic polypeptide, named heavy chain (HC), non-covalently associated with a 12 kDa monomorphic peptide, named β_2-microglobulin (β_2-m). HLA-A, -B, C antigens are loaded with peptides in their groove by the peptide transporter associated with antigen processing (TAP). Their proper assembly with peptides is required for their stable cell surface expression.

Like the classical HLA class Ia antigens, the non-classical HLA class Ib molecules HLA-E, -F, -G, are composed of a polymorphic HC non-covalently associated with β_2-m and are loaded with peptides translocated by TAP [3,4]. However, they differ from classical HLA class Ia antigens in their extent of polymorphism. HLA-E, -F,

Table 1. Characteristics of classical and non-classical HLA class I antigens and the MHC-related antigens MIC

molecule	association with $\beta_2 m$	TAP	presentation of peptides	expression pattern	recognized by NK cells	recognized by T cells
HLA-A, -B, -C	+	+	+	broad	–	+
HLA-E	+	+	+	epithelial tissues	+	+
HLA-F	+	+	+	placenta	?	?
HLA-G	+	+	+	different tissues	++	+
MIC	–	–	–	epithelial cells, stress-induced	+	–

-G antigens are characterized by low levels of allelic polymorphism, which may reflect their respective specialized functions, truncated cytoplasmic/transmembrane domains and/or multiple alternative splicing patterns [5–8]. The MHC class I-related molecules (MICs) are highly glycosylated membrane-anchored MHC class I like molecules that are induced by stress [9–11]. The MIC proteins share some features with classical HLA class I molecules such as chromosomal localization and high polymorphism. At variance with HLA class Ia and Ib molecules they are not associated with β_2-m, do not bind peptides and are therefore not involved in antigen presentation [10].

HLA-A, -B, -C antigens have a broad distribution in normal tissues as they are constitutively expressed on all adult tissues, except erythrocytes, brain cortex, cerebellum, sympathetic ganglia, hypophysis, parathyroid gland, thyroid, exocrine pancreas, hepatocytes, sperms, seminiferous tubules, skeletal muscles and smooth muscles [12]. Their expression can be induced by IFNγ. In comparison, HLA -E, –F, -G antigens exhibit a selective cell surface expression and tissue distribution [13]. HLA-G antigens are transcribed at a basal level without protein expression in several cell types including cytotrophoblasts, epithelial cells and cornea [14–16]. Transcription of HLA-E antigens occurs in most fetal and adult tissues. The analysis of the HLA-E antigen surface expression has been mainly hampered by the lack of HLA-E-specific antibodies with the appropriate characteristics. The expression of HLA-E and HLA-G antigens, like that of HLA-A, -B, -C antigens, can be enhanced by interferon (IFN)-γ. Furthermore, HLA-E HC competes with HLA class Ia HC for β_2-m suggesting that the presence or absence of HLA class Ia HC regulates HLA-E antigen expression [3]. HLA-F protein is intracellularly expressed in a number of tissues including liver, bladder and skin, whereas its cell surface expression is mainly confined to B cells, tonsils, thymus and fetal liver [17]. Like MHC class Ib molecules MIC proteins have a restricted tissue distribution. MICA (MHC class I-related sequence A) is constitutively expressed only by intestinal epithelial cells [18]. However, its expression can be upregulated by heat shock in many cells of epithelial origin [19].

Like classical HLA class Ia antigens, non-classical HLA class Ib antigens as well as MIC antigens have specialized functions with regard to the regulation of immune responses. While HLA-A and -B antigens are recognized by $CD8^+$ cytotoxic T lymphocytes (CTL), HLA-C antigens interact with KIR's on NK cells and HLA-E and -G molecules modulate both CTL and/or NK cell function. Recent studies in mice demonstrate that MHC class Ib antigens can also serve as restricting elements for TA-specific CTL and mediate protective immune responses [20]. HLA-G antigens inhibit NK cell cytotoxicity by binding to the three NK cell inhibitory receptors ILT2, ILT4 and KIR2DL4, whereas HLA-E antigens bind to the NK inhibitory receptors CD94/NKG2A expressed on the cell surface of NK and T cells [21–24]. MICA/-B antigens are ligands of the C-type lectin stimulatory immune receptor NKG2D which is expressed by human NK cells and by both α/β and γ/δ T cells [25–27]. The NKG2D-mediated immune activation can be triggered by its ligands and overcomes the inhibitory signal mediated by MHC class I antigen binding to inhibitory NK cell receptors of NK cells [28, 29]. Thus, cells expressing MIC antigens on the cell surface are susceptible to NK and T cell mediated immunity.

The MHC Class I Antigen Processing and Presentation Pathway

Recognition of tumor cells by HLA class I antigen-restricted, TA-specific CTL is mediated by complexes resulting from the loading of β_2-m-associated HLA class I HC with TA derived peptides. The generation and transport of these complexes to the cell membrane depends on interactions among components of the antigen processing machinery which has been extensively characterized in recent years [30] (Figure 2). Proteasomes generate antigenic peptides from mainly, but not exclusively endogenous proteins. Extracellular proteins are either taken up by phagocytosis or endocytosis and are released from phagosomes or endosomes into the cytosol, where they enter the classical MHC class I antigen processing pathway allowing their presentation by MHC class I antigens [31]. The constitutive proteasome complex is composed of 28 subunits arranged in four stacked seven-membered rings; the outer two rings contain the non-catalytic α-subunits, whereas the inner rings contain the β-subunits. Three of the constitutive β-subunits Delta (Y), MB1 (X) and Zeta (Z) have catalytic activity and are replaced upon exposure to IFNγ by the low molecular mass polypeptides (LMP)2, LMP7 and LMP10. The immuno-proteasome generates a distinct set of antigenic peptides with increased affinity to MHC class I antigens [32]. Thus, the CTL response against cells expressing constitutive and IFN-γ inducible proteasomes may differ. The proteasome mainly trims peptides at the C-terminus, whereas cytosolic or ER-resident aminopeptidases trim peptides at their N-terminus [33, 34]. The heterodimeric transporter-associated with antigen processing (TAP) consisting of an 81 and a 76 kDa subunit, named TAP1 and TAP2, respectively, translocates peptides from the cytosol into the ER., where they are loaded onto β_2-m-associated HLA class I HC. Folding and loading of peptides requires the interplay of various ER-resident chaperones such as calnexin, calreticulin, immunoglobulin-binding protein (BiP), oxidoreductase ERp57 and tapasin. The newly synthesized HLA class I HC is cotranslationally

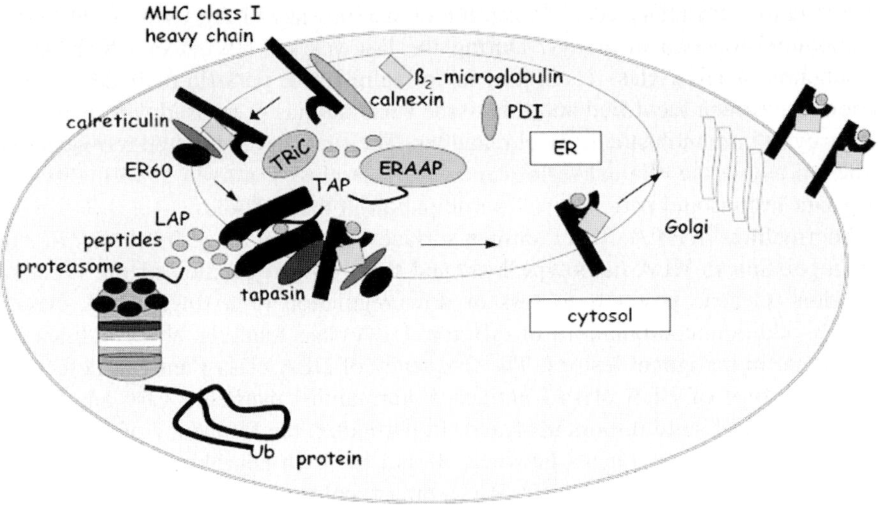

Figure 2. HLA class I antigen processing and presentation pathway

inserted into the ER membrane. Calnexin and BiP transiently interact with the HLA class I HC and promote the folding and assembly with β_2-m. Calnexin is replaced by calreticulin after the heterodimer formation of HC and β_2-m [35]. Together with TAP, ERp57 and tapasin the HC/β_2-m dimer forms the multimeric peptide loading complex. Thus, HLA class I antigen maturation involves interactions with classical chaperones, although most of these proteins have been studied so far only to a limited extent. Upon peptide binding the trimeric HLA class I β_2-m/peptide complex is released and transported via the trans-Golgi to the cell surface. CTL monitor the HLA class I antigens via the T cell receptor (TCR) in combination with the CD8 coreceptor. Cells presenting peptides derived from endogenous abnormal proteins, defective ribosomal products, proteins retrotranslocated to the cytosol from the ER and exogenous, internalized proteins can be recognized and eliminated by $CD8^+$ CTL [30].

Frequency of HLA Class I Antigen Downregulation or Loss in Malignant Tumors

Defects in HLA class I antigen expression have been found in all solid tumors analyzed, although with a different frequency. Flow cytometry and immunohistochemical techniques have been employed to analyze tumor cells isolated from surgically removed malignant lesions and surgically removed tumor sections. The probes utilized include monoclonal antibodies (mAb) recognizing monomorphic, locus- or allele-specific epitopes of HLA class I antigens [36,37]. Most of the mAb which are suitable for immunohistochemical staining recognize antigenic determinants which are not detectable in formalin-fixed, paraffin-embedded tissue sections.

For this reason for many years frozen tumor sections have been used as substrates in immunohistochemical assays. During the last years a few mAb which detect the subunits of HLA class I antigens in formalin-fixed, paraffin-embedded tissue sections have been identified and this tissue substrate has been used with increased frequency in immunohistochemical reactions. Their use has facilitated retrospective studies to assess the clinical significance of HLA class I antigen abnormalities in malignant lesions and pathologists' participation in these studies.

Abnormalities in HLA class I antigen surface expression range from total loss or downregulation to HLA haplotype loss, and from downregulation of the HLA-A, -B and/or -C gene products to loss or downregulation of a single HLA class I allele. In addition, combinations of different HLA class I antigen abnormalities are often found in malignant lesions. The frequency of HLA class I antigen defects as well as the type of HLA class I antigen abnormalities markedly vary among the different types of solid tumors analyzed. In particular, the frequency of HLA class I antigen abnormalities ranges between 50 and 87 % in neuroblastoma, head and neck squamous cell carcinoma (HNSCC), breast, colorectal, prostate, cervical, and ovarian carcinoma lesions, but is markedly lower in melanoma lesions. In addition, HLA class I changes have been only rarely described in hematological malignancies [38–40]. These differences are likely to reflect the extent of tumor cell genetic instability and immunoselective pressure applied to tumor cell populations as well as the time between development of tumors and diagnosis [41–43].

Molecular Mechanisms Underlying HLA Class I Antigen Downregulation or Loss by Malignant Cells

Multiple mechanisms have been shown to underlie HLA class I antigen abnormalities in malignant cells. Their molecular characterization has greatly benefited from the analysis of cell lines with defects in HLA class I antigen expression and/or function. They include structural alterations of the genes involved in HLA class I molecule expression, changes in their methylation pattern and/or dysregulation of HLA class I antigen processing machinery components at the transcriptional and/or posttranscriptional level (Table 2) [44]. Their frequency significantly differs among the tumor types analyzed.

Total HLA class I antigen loss is generally caused by lack of functional β_2-m expression which is required for the transport of HLA class I heavy chain and its

Table 2. Molecular mechanisms underlying HLA class I antigen abnormalities

phenotype	molecular mechanisms
total loss	β_2-m mutation, deletion, rearrangement
total downregulation	downregulation or mutation of APM components
locus- and allele-specific downregulation	mutation in HLA loci/alleles, inhibition of transcription
APM downregulation	methylationtranscriptional/posttranscriptional regulation
single APM component loss	mutations in TAP1 and TAP2

expression on the cell membrane. In the majority of the characterized cell lines and surgically removed tumors lack of functional β_2-m expression is caused by structural abnormalities in one β_2-m gene in combination with loss of the other copy, i.e. loss of heterozygosity. Whether the mutation in one β_2-m gene or the loss of a wild type β_2-m allele occurs first remains to be determined. Whatever the sequence of events, mutations in β_2-m genes range from large to single nucleotide deletions, which in most cases inhibit the translation of mRNA, but do not affect the transcription of β_2-m gene [45]. In spite of the random distribution of mutations in β_2-m a mutation hot spot has been suggested to be located in the CT repeat region in exon 1 within codons 13-15 of the β_2-m gene. It is of interest that this mutation appears to occur preferentially when a strong T cell-mediated selective pressure is applied to tumor cell populations. Thus, this mutation has been found in melanoma cell lines isolated from patients treated with T cell-based immunotherapy [46] and in colon carcinoma lesions displaying a high level microsatellite instability (MSI) phenotype [47, 48]. The high frequency of β_2-m mutations in MSI colon carcinoma lesions suggests that β_2-m is a target gene during MSI-associated carcinogenesis. The latter lesions are characterized by a large number of infiltrating lymphocytes most likely as a result of the cellular immune response triggered by truncated proteins with a carboxy-terminal frameshift peptide expressed by these tumors. Beside melanoma and colon carcinoma cells, β_2-m defects have been described in a lung carcinoma cell line [49]. However they have never been described in other tumor types such HNSCC and renal cell carcinoma (RCC) [45, 50–53].

Total HLA class I antigen downregulation is generally caused by antigen processing machinery (APM) dysfunction which results in defective peptide loading of β_2-m-associated HLA class I HC and instability of β_2-m/HLA class I HC complex on cell surface. The defects which are most frequently responsible for this phenotype are downregulation or loss of one or both TAP subunits and/or tapasin. Due to the potential therapeutic implications of this finding it is noteworthy that these defects can be corrected by cytokines, in particular by IFNγ, in the majority of cases. The frequency and extent of APM component downregulation or loss differ among the tumor types analyzed. In addition to abnormalities in a single APM component multiple combined defects in APM components within a tumor cell population have been found in different tumor types resulting in a coordinated APM component downregulation. A concordant LMP2, LMP7 and LMP10 downregulation has often been found in combination with defects in TAP and/or tapasin expression suggesting that a key regulator mediates these defects [45, 53–55]. It has recently been demonstrated that the promyelocytic leukemia (PML) nuclear bodies might be associated in colorectal tumors with a total MHC class I antigen loss and LMP 7 downregulation [56]. Furthermore, neuroblastoma cells demonstrate impaired LMP2, TAP, HLA class I HC and β_2-m expression in comparison to normal adrenal medulla cells [54]. In melanoma, downregulation of LMPs, TAP, HLA class I and β_2-m as well as calnexin and calreticulin has been described [46, 57]. On the other hand, in RCC cells immunoproteasome subunits and TAP mRNA and protein levels are downregulated, but HLA class I HC and β_2-m expression levels are comparable to those in normal kidney epithelium [53]. Similar results have been obtained in primary ovarian carcinoma lesions [58].

Mutations in the TAP1 and/or TAP2 subunit have been described in a small cell lung carcinoma cell line [49], in MSI colon carcinoma lesions [43], in cervical carcinoma lesions [59] and in a melanoma cell line [57,60]. So far, structural defects in other APM components have not been described in tumors.

Haplotype, locus-specific or allelic losses of HLA-A and –B antigens which result in lack or downregulation of HLA class I antigen surface expression have been identified in different tumor types. Scanty information is only available for HLA-C antigen expression in tumors and the paucity of this information reflects, at least in part, the limited availability of antibodies with the appropriate specificity. The tumors with HLA-A and -B antigen defects include HNSCC, gastric carcinoma, colon carcinoma, cervical carcinoma and melanoma [45, 61, 62]. The molecular mechanisms causing these phenotypes have not been defined in detail. In cervical carcinoma, the HPV E5 protein has been shown to be responsible for HLA-A and –B antigen downregulation without detectable effects on HLA-C and HLA-E antigen expression [63]. The aberrant HLA-A and –B antigen expression has been associated with the integration of high risk human papilloma virus [62]. These data further suggest that a selective E5-mediated downregulation might be responsible for the lack of immune clearance of HPV-infected cells by CTL and NK cells.

Epigenetic modifications are involved in gene silencing and play an important role in tumor development. Thus, one molecular mechanism underlying the differential HLA class I antigen and APM component expression *in vitro* and *in vivo* can be epigenetic repression. Indeed, an aberrant methylation pattern of the HLA class I HC and β_2-m has been described in embryonal tissues and embryonal carcinoma (EC) lesions [64] resulting in reduced or lack of MHC class I surface expression. This could be overcome by IFNγ and 2',5' azacytidine treatment. Furthermore, hypermethylation of the tapasin promoter has recently been detected in melanoma, RCC and colon carcinoma cell lines (Seliger et al. paper in preparation). The frequency of these epigenetic changes appears to be low and comparable to that of β_2-m mutations detected in melanoma and colon carcinoma cell lines.

HLA Class I Antigen Abnormalities and Tumor Microenvironment

The microenvironment can influence the expression of components of the HLA class I pathway due to the cytokines IFNγ and IL-10 that affect the infiltration of tumors with lymphocytes. A major obstacle to the *in vivo* development of TA-specific protective T cell-mediated immune responses is the microenvironment. Therefore adequate tools are needed to tune the best environment. Tumors including breast, RCC, colon, prostate, and ovary carcinoma as well as melanoma often exhibit inflammatory immune cell infiltrates which represent the host's natural defensive activity against the tumor [65–71]. The majority of these tumor infiltrating immune cells are tumor infiltrating lymphocytes (TIL), whereas infiltration with NK cells is relatively limited [72]. HLA class I antigen loss is associated with TIL, but not with NK cell infiltration [72]. A clear association exists between the presence of intratumoral T cells, progression of disease and patients' overall survival. The frequency of T cell infiltration of tumors is heterogeneous indicating an important role for cellular TA-specific immunity. $CD4^+$ and $CD8^+$ intratumoral T cell infiltration has been found to be significantly correlated with MHC class I antigen surface expression, but not with the expression of differentiation antigens, TA and/or MHC class II molecules [71]. Although only described in a few cases, colorectal cancer patients with MHC class I antigen loss develop less metastases than tumors with MHC class I antigen expression suggesting that NK cells might play an important role in the prevention and control of metastatic spread rather than locally in the primary tumor [73].

An impaired T cell function has been observed in many tumors; it could be associated with abnormalities either in HLA class I antigens and/or in T cells [74]. These defects could be mediated by tumor cell-derived immunosuppressive substances or molecules such as TGF-β, vascular endothetial growth factor (VEGF), cellular FLICE inhibitory molecules (cFLIP) and gangliosides [75, 76]. Recent reports suggest a recovery of T cell function during systemic chemotherapy in patients with advanced ovarian carcinoma [77]. T cell function is not permanently suppressed and successful chemotherapy is associated with improved antigen-specific T cell reactivity. These data suggest that the determination of T cell responses during chemotherapy may allow a better timing and optimization of T cell-based immunotherapy [78].

Recently, it has been demonstrated that tumor progression beyond a minimal size is critically dependent on the tumor stroma, which is represented by endothelial cells (EC), fibroblasts, tumor-associated macrophages (TAM) and smooth muscle cells [79]. Inhibition of stromal functions required for tumor growth might reduce the incidence of tumor immune escape [80]. Therefore, tumor stroma represents an important target during T cell-mediated tumor rejection [81]. Indeed, T cells not only recognize TA on tumor cells, but also TAMs, EC and fibroblasts. In this context, it is noteworthy that T cells can indirectly kill antigen loss variants as bystanders because the tumor stroma is eliminated. The elimination of these antigen loss variants coincided with the rapid T cell infiltration of tumors as well as the rapid destruction of the tumor mass [82]. However, they escape bystander killing when stroma cells lack the appropriate HLA class I antigen or when the amount of antigen is too low for effective cross-presentation.

Clinical Significance of HLA Class I Antigen Abnormalities

Although there are conflicting views about the role of immunosurveillance in the control of tumor growth [83,84], several lines of evidence suggest that HLA class I antigen abnormalities have clinical significance. HLA class I antigen defects have a higher frequency in metastases than in primary malignant lesions. Furthermore they are associated with a poor histological differentiation and genetic instability, diminished clinical response to T cell-based immunotherapy and patients' reduced survival [85].

Impaired expression and function of LMP, TAP, tapasin and/or MHC class I antigens may enhance tumorigenicity. Low APM component levels are often associated with the histopathological characteristics of the lesions, metastatic phenotype and/or clinical course of the disease. In some malignancies APM defects are associated with patients' reduced survival [58, 86–92]. It has been convincingly shown that proper APM component expression can limit the malignant potential of tumors [93–95]. Restoration or enhancement of TAP expression in murine and human tumor cells can reconstitute or enhance MHC class I antigen surface expression, antigen presentation and susceptibility to TA-specific CTLs. TAP overexpression significantly delayed tumor growth and increased survival of tumor bearing mice [94, 95]. This result was accompanied by a significant increase of $CD8^+$ and $CD4^+$ T cells as well as $CD11c^+$dendritic cells in malignant lesions. These experimental data have significant implications for the design of T cell-based immunotherapy of malignant diseases [96, 97] since the lack or insufficient presentation of TA via MHC class I molecules results in impaired activation of CTL. Tumors escaping destruction by HLA class I antigen-restricted TA-specific CTLs, can be recognized by NK cells. Although to the best of our knowledge there exists no statistical significance in HLA class I antigen downregulation in non-small cell lung carcinoma, colon carcinoma and uveal melanoma might be associated with a favorable prognosis and improved survival. These results raise the possibility that NK cells may play a major role in the control of these tumor entities [98–101].

Beside deficient expression of APM components due to distinct molecular mechanisms genetic polymorphism of these components has been demonstrated to be associated with some malignancies. Single nucleotide polymorphisms of LMP7 and TAP2 are associated with the risk of the development of HPV-induced esophageal carcinoma [102], whereas polymorphism of TAP1 and TAP2 has been correlated to the risk of cervical cancer. A high frequency of LMP and TAP promoter polymorphism has been detected in RCC, but their role in this disease has not yet been defined [103]. Thus, the biological function of LMP and/or TAP polymorphisms described so far is not clear [104].

Frequency of Non-classical HLA Class Ib Antigen Expression in Tumors

While there is significant amount of information about the involvement of classical MHC class Ia antigens in tumor immunity, little is known about the role of the larger family of non-classical HLA class Ib antigens. HLA-G antigen upregulation correlates with malignant transformation of cells [105]. In a neoplasm like gastric cancer HLA-G antigens are not expressed [61], whereas in other tumor types HLA-G antigens are heterogeneously expressed [106]. A constitutive HLA-G mRNA and

Table 3. Frequency of HLA-G expression in malignant tumors

tumor type	# of analyzed lesions	frequency (%)	
		mRNA	protein
basal cell carcinoma	38	n.d.	90
RCC	36	38	38
lung carcinoma	36	n.d.	33
non-Hodgkin lymphoma	50	n.d.	6
melanoma	79	n.d.	28
bladder carcinoma	42	28	16
glioblastoma	4	n.d.	75
spontaneous B cell lymphoma	10	100	70

n.d. not determined

protein expression has been found in biopsies and/or cell lines of glioma, breast cancer, lung cancer, colorectal carcinoma, RCC, ovary carcinoma, lymphoma, basal cell carcinoma and melanoma [107–115]; (Table 3). Interestingly, HLA-G antigens appear to be most frequently expressed in aggressive tumors [116]. Furthermore, radiotherapy and chemotherapy might cause HLA-G antigen downregulation on tumor cells and/or tumor infiltrating cells. This change is correlated with improved survival [115, 117].

Although HLA-E genes are transcribed in most cell lines, heterogeneous HLA-E antigen surface expression has been detected on 23 % of tumor cell lines of different origin. They include cervical carcinoma, osteosarcoma, leukaemia and melanoma cell lines [118, 119]; (Table 4). In addition, an inverse correlation between classical HLA class I antigen and HLA-E antigen expression has been found [118], most likely because of a competition of their HC for β_2-m. It is noteworthy that HLA-F antigen expression has not yet been analyzed in tumors.

Table 4. HLA-E antigen expression in tumor cell lines

tumor	number of tumor cell lines analyzed	frequencyof HLA-E expression
Burkitt lymphoma	4	0
histiocytic lymphoma	1	1
melanoma	7	3
colon carcinoma	3	0
lung carcinoma	3	0
pancreatic carcinoma	3	1
cervical carcinoma	4	1
leukaemia	3	3
breast carcinoma	2	0
prostate carcinoma	1	0
gastric carcinoma	1	0

Molecular Mechanisms of Non-classical HLA Class Ib Antigen Abnormalities

So far only scanty information is available regarding the molecular mechanisms underlying abnormal HLA class Ib antigen expression in tumors. However, some evidence suggests that different mechanisms regulate HLA class Ib and classical HLA class Ia antigen expression. HLA-G antigen expression is mainly regulated by epigenetic processes. HLA-G gene is silenced by hypermethylation and can be reactivated upon treatment with the demethylating agent 5'aza-2'deoxycytidine. Both HLA-G activation and enhancement of KIR gene expression may occur in the course of treatment with demethylating agents suggesting that epigenetic therapy might in some cases lead to tumor escape [120]. In addition, HLA-G expression can be regulated at the level of mRNA splicing. A rapid switch from cell surface HLA-G1 expression to intracellular HLA-G2 expression has been described in melanoma cells; as a result NK cell-mediated sensitivity of tumor cells is restored. These data suggest that modulation of HLA-G gene at the mRNA splicing level is an efficient way to modulate HLA-G antigen-mediated *in vivo* escape of malignant cells from immune recognition and destruction [121]. Furthermore, HLA-G antigen expression can be upregulated by IFN-β and IFN-γ treatment or by heat shock in melanoma and/or RCC cell lines [110]. However our knowledge of the variables which regulate HLA-G antigen expression in tumor cells is still limited and *in vivo* factors modulating these antigens have to be still defined.

Functional Role of Non-classical HLA Class Ib Antigens in Tumors

HLA-G antigen expression in tumor cells has been hypothesized to play an important role in evasion of tumor cells from CTL and NK cell-mediated lysis. In addition, HLA-G antigen expression can be induced on macrophages and TIL. These TIL also express ILT2 suggesting that the induction of KIR molecules and HLA-G antigens on tumor infiltrating immune cells might represent a novel mechanism of tumor escape [122]. HLA-G antigen bearing tumor cells inhibit immunocompetent cells via their interaction with inhibitory receptors. Furthermore, the immune tolerant properties of HLA-G antigens have been emphasized by their potential role in resistance to interferon-based therapies [123–125]. Lastly soluble HLA-G (sHLA-G) antigens can be shed by tumor cells and induce both apoptosis of CTL and inhibition of NK cell-mediated lysis. It has been suggested that sHLA-G antigens have a negative impact on the clinical course of some malignant diseases such as melanoma [124, 126].

HLA-E antigen upregulation, like that of HLA-G antigens, may allow malignant cells to evade NK cell immune surveillance [127]. However, appropriate HLA class I alleles with leader sequence-derived peptides and HLA-E HC may not be sufficient for HLA-E antigen surface expression on solid tumor cells, a finding which is at variance with the results obtained with cell lines of hematological lineage [119]. Due to the insufficient supply of leader peptides HLA-E antigen surface expression can be also reduced following viral or malignant cell transformation; this abnormality is associated with altered susceptibility to NK cell-mediated lysis [128]. Furthermore, aberrant HLA-E antigen expression might modulate NK cell responses by inhibiting NK cell cytotoxicity due to its interaction with CD94/NKG2A.

Frequency and Clinical Significance of MHC Class I-related Molecules

Low levels of constitutive MIC expression have been found on epithelial cells [25]. MIC can be transcriptionally induced by stress in particular by heat shock on a broad range of human epithelial tumors such as melanoma, breast, lung, colon, hepatocellular and ovarian carcinoma as well as RCC, whereas it is not detected in the corresponding normal tissues [18, 129, 130]. Furthermore, MIC expression can be upregulated in hepatocellular carcinoma cells by retinoic acid treatment [130]. Moreover during tumor cell proliferation and tumor volume increase MICA expression can be downregulated, suggesting a clinical relevance of MIC abnormalities. MICA downregulation may result from release of soluble tumor cell-derived MICA (sMIC;131, 132) Furthermore, a stage-dependent membrane-bound MICA/-B expression was found on low grade uveal melanoma and prostate cancer [133, 134], but is lost during disease progression suggesting the selection of MICA-negative tumor cells during metastases. In contrast, the high expression level of MICA is an indicator of good prognosis in colorectal cancer patients [135].

Role of MIC in Immune Responses

It has been suggested that cell surface expression of MIC may be involved in tumor immune surveillance [136]. MIC-expressing prostate cancer cells are susceptible to NKG2D-mediated NK cell lysis [134]. Thus, MIC can serve as a target for immunotherapy of this disease [137]. However, the MIC/NKG2D-triggered immunity is often impaired in patients with various types of carcinoma [18, 129, 130, 134]. This is due to the shedding of MIC from tumor cells causing NKG2D downregulation on NK cells, tumor infiltrating lymphocytes and peripheral blood T cells [131, 132, 138]. Indeed, a significant increase in serum sMIC levels has been demonstrated in breast, lung, colon and ovarian carcinoma as well as in melanoma [131, 132]. The systemic deficiency associated with sMICA modulates the NKG2D-mediated immune surveillance resulting in severe impairment of the responsiveness of TA-specific effector cells. Therefore it represents a major strategy utilized by tumor cells to evade NK and T cell immune responses [139]. Strategies to counteract surface MIC shedding from tumor cells which then sustain NKG2D-mediated immune response might be useful for enhancing TA immunogenicity. This can be achieved by blocking the metalloproteinases which leads to inhibition of MICA release from tumor cells and its accumulation on the cell surface. In addition, stimulation with cytokines such as IL-2 and IL-15 can also restore sMIC-impaired NKG2D-mediated cytotoxic function in NK cells.

CONCLUSIONS

During the last years the unexpected limited efficacy of immunotherapy has rekindled tumor immunologists' interest in the characterization of abnormalities in the expression and function of classical and non-classical HLA class I antigens as well as MIC antigens on tumor cells of distinct origin. Therefore in a short period of time a tremendous amount of information has been collected on the frequency of HLA class Ia and Ib and MIC antigen abnormalities, their underlying molecular mechanisms, their clinical significance and their impact on immune cell-mediated TA-specific immune responses [36, 45, 114, 140]. It has generally been accepted that $CD8^+$ T cells represent the main effector cells, whereas cytotoxicity mediated by $CD4^+$ T cells is an exception: $CD4^+$ T cells are essential for the activation and survival of CTLs [141]. $CD8^+$ CTLs are mainly responsible for tumor elimination which is dependent on different cytokines such as IFN-γ and tumor necrosis factor (TNF)-γ [142]. However, in uveal melanoma, breast carcinoma and non-small cell lung carcinoma HLA class I antigen downregulation is associated with improved survival, raising the possibility that NK cells may play an important role in the control of some tumor entities [73, 98, 100, 101]. It has been demonstrated that both lack or downregulation of HLA class Ia antigens and upregulation of HLA-G antigens result in escape of tumor cells from lysis by T cells and NK cells. Although the selective upregulation of MICA on tumor cells can activate NK cell-mediated tumor cell lysis, the inhibitory signal generated by HLA-G antigens overcomes the activating signal delivered by MICA. In addition soluble MICA (sMICA) secreted by tumor cells negatively interferes with the cytotoxic function of NK cells. These results suggest that monitoring of HLA-A, -B, -C and HLA-G antigen expression on tumor cells in combination with serum sMICA level in patients with malignant diseases may provide useful information from a prognostic view point. It has to be still taken into account that activation of other immune cells, like TAMs as well as alterations in the activity of T suppressor cells, regulatory T cells (T_{regs}) and DC play an important role in TA-specific immune responses.

These data argue that the pathologist's evaluation of tumors has to include the analysis of the expression of MHC class I antigens and of other molecules crucial for interactions of tumor cells with host's immune system. In addition, characterization of the molecular mechanism(s) underlying the MHC class I antigen abnormalities identified in malignant lesions will contribute to the rational design of approaches to correct these defects. Correlation of these *in vitro* data with the clinical response of patients treated with different types of immunotherapy will determine the clinical significance of this strategy.

ACKNOWLEDGEMENTS

This work was supported by a grant from the Deutsche Forschungsgemeinschaft (DFG; BS) and the Vaillant Stiftung (BS) and by PHS grants RO1 CA67108, RO1 CA 110249 and RO1 CA 113861 awarded by the National Cancer Institute, DHHS. We would like to thank C. Stoerr for excellent secretarial help.

There exist different immune escape strategies of tumors ranging from secretion of immunosuppressive cytokines, fasL expression, lack of costimulatory molecules to abnormalities in the expression of classical and non-classical HLA class I antigens. This results in impaired T cell responses.

REFERENCES

1. Ostrand-Rosenberg S (2004) Animal models of tumor immunity, immunotherapy and cancer vaccines. Curr. Opin. Immunol. 16:143–150
2. Rosenberg SA, Yang JC, Retifo NP (2004) Cancer immunotherapy: moving beyond current vaccines. Nat. Med. 10:909–915
3. Braud V, Jones E Y, McMichel A (1997) The human major histocompatibility complex class Ib molecule HLA-E binds signal sequence-derived peptides with primary anchor residues at positions 2 and 9. Eur. J. Immunol. 27:1164–1169
4. Ulbrecht M, Modrow R, Srivastava R, Pedersen P, Weiss EH (1998) Interaction of HLA-E with peptides and the peptide transporter in vitro: implications for its function in antigen presentation. J. Immunol. 160:4375–4385
5. Ishitani A, Geraghty DE (1992) Alternative splicing of HLA-G transcripts yields proteins with primary structures resembling both class I and class II antigens. Proc. Natl. Acad. Sci. USA 89:3947–3951
6. O' Callaghan CA, Bell JI (1998) Structure and function of the human MHC class Ib molecules HLA-E, HLA-F and HLA-G. Immunol. Rev. 163:129–38
7. Paul P, Cabestre FA, Ibrahim EC, Lefebvre S, Hhalil-Daher I, Vazeux G, Quiles RM, Bermond F, Dausset J, Carosella ED (2000) Identification of HLA-G7 as a new splice variant of the HLA-G mRNA and expression of soluble HLA-G5, -G6, and –G7 transcripts in human transfected cells. Hum. Immunol. 61:1138–1149
8. Kumanovics A, Takada T, Lindahl KF (2003) Genomic organization of the mammalian MHC. Annu. Rev. Immunol. 21:629
9. Bahram S, Spies T (1996) Nucleotide sequence of a human MHC class I MICB cDNA. Immunogenet. 43:230–233
10. Bauer S, Groh V, Wu J, Steinle A, Phillips JH, Lanier LL, Spies T (1999) Activation of NK cells and T cells by NKG2D, a receptor for stress-inducible MICA. Science 285:727–729
11. Bahram S (2000) MIC genes: from genetics to biology. Adv. Immunol. 76:1–60
12. Natali PG, Bigotti A, Nicotra MR, Viora M, Manfredi D, Ferrone S (1984) Distribution of human class I (HLA-A,B,C) histocompatibility antigens in normal and malignant tissues of nonlymphoid origin. Cancer Res. 44:4679–4687
13. Rousseau P, Masternak K, Krawczyk M, Reith W, Dausset J, Carosella ED, Moreau P (2004) In vivo, RFX5 binds differently to the human leukocyte antigen-E, -F, and -G gene promoters and participates in HLA class I protein expression in a cell type-dependent manner. Immunol. 111:53–65
14. Crisa L, McMaster MT, Ishii JK, Fischer SJ, Salomon DR. (1997) Identification of a thymic epithelial cell subset sharing expression of the class Ib HLA-G molecule with fetal trophoblasts. J. Exp. Med. 186:289–298
15. Loke YW, King A, Burrows T, Gardner L, Bowen M, Hiby S, Howlett S, Holmes N, Jacobs D (1997) Evaluation of trophoblast HLA-G antigen with a specific monoclonal antibody. Tissue Antigens 50:135–146
16. Le Discorde M, Moreau P, Sabatier P, Legeais JJ, Carosella ED (2003) Expression of HLA-G in human cornea, an immune-privileged tissue. Hum. Immunol. 64:1039–1044
17.
18. Groh V, Rhinehart R, Secrist H, Bauer S, Grabstein KH, Spies T (1999) Broad tumor-associated expression and recognition by tumor-derived gamma delta T cells of MICA and MICB. Proc. Natl. Acad. Sci. USA 96:6879–6884

19. Groh V, Bahram S, Bauer S, Herman A, Beauchamp M, Spies T (1996) Cell stress-regulated human major histocompatibility complex class I gene expressed in gastrointestinal epithelium. Proc. Natl. Acad. Sci. U S A. 93:12445–12450
20. Chiang EY, Stroynowski I (2004) A non-classical MHC class I molecule restricts CTL-mediated rejection of a syngeneic melanoma tumor. J. Immunol. 173:4394–4401
21. Braud V, Allan DSJ, O'Callaghan CA, Soderstrom K, D'Andrea A, Ogg GS, Lazetic S, Young NT, Bell JI. Phillips JH et al. (1998) HLA-E binds to natural killer cell receptors CD94/NKG2A, B, and C. Nature 391:795–799
22. Lee N, Llano M, Carretero M, Ishitani A, Navarro F, Lopez-Botet M, Geraghty DE (1998) HLA-E is the major ligand for the natural killer inhibitory receptor CD94/NKG2A. Proc. Natl. Acad. Sci. USA 95:5199–5204
23. Khalil-Daher I, Riteau B, Menier C, Sedlik C, Paul P, Dausset J, Carosella ED, Rouas-Freiss N (1999) Role of HLA-G versus HLA-E on NK function: HLA-G is able to inhibit NK cytolysis by itself. J. Reprod. Immunol. 43:175–182
24. Hofmeister V, Weiss EH (2003) HLA-G modulates immune responses by diverse receptor interactions. Semin. Cancer Biol. 13:317–323
25. Groh V, Steinle A, Bauer S, Spies T (1998) Recognition of stress-induced MHC molecules by intestinal epithelial gamma-delta T cells. Science 279:1737–1740
26. Groh V, Rhinehart R, Randolph-Habecker J, Topp MS, Riddell SR, Spies T (2001) Costimulation of CD8 alph/abeta T cells by NKG2D via engagement by MIC induced on virus-infected cells. Nat. Immunol. 2:255–260
27. Cerwenka A, Lanier LL (2003) NKG2D ligands: unconventional MHC class I-like molecules exploited by viruses and cancer, Tissue Antigens 61:335–343
28. Raulet DH (2003) Roles of the NKG2D immunoreceptor and its ligands. Nat. Rev. Immunol. 3:781–790
29. Bahram S, Inoko H, Shiina T, Radosavljevic M (2005) MIC and other NKG2D ligands: from none to too many. Curr. Opin. Immunol.17:505–509
30. Trombetta ES, Mellman I (2005) Cell biology of antigen processing in vitro and in vivo. Ann. Rev. Immunol. 23:975–1028
31. Ackerman A L, Kyritsis C, Tampé R and Cresswell P (2003) Early phagosomes in dendritic cells form a cellular compartment sufficient for cross presentation of exogenous antigens. Proc. Natl. Acad. Si. USA 100:12889–12894
32. Rivett AJ, Hearn AR (2004) Proteasome function in antigen presentation: immunoproteasome complexes, peptide production, and interactions with viral proteins. Curr. Protein Pept. Sci. 5:153–161
33. Saveanu L, Carroll O, Lindo V, Del Val M, Lopez D, Lepelletier Y, Greer F, Schomburg L, Fruci D, Niedermann G, van Endert PM (2002) Concerted peptide trimming by human ERAP1 and ERAP2 aminopeptidase complexes in the endoplasmic reticulum. Nat. Immunol. 6:689–697
34. Serwold T, Gonzalez F, Kim J, Jacob R, Shastri N (2002) ERAAP customizes peptides for MHC class I molecules in the endoplasmic reticulum. Nature 419:480–483
35. Paulsson K, Wang P (2003) Chaperones and folding of MHC class I molecules in the endoplasmic reticulum. Biochim. Biophys. Acta. 1641:1–12
36. Garrido F, Ruiz-Cabello F, Cabrera T, Perez-Villar JJ, Lopez-Botet M, Duggan-Keen M, Stern PL (1997) Implications for immunosurveillance of altered HLA class I phenotypes in human tumours. Immunol. Today 18:89–95
37. Garcia-Lora A, Martinez M, Algarra I, Gaforio JJ, Garrido F (2003) MHC class I-deficient metastatic tumor variants immunoselected by T lymphocytes originate from the coordinated downregulation of APM components. Int. J. Cancer 106:521–527
38. Murray PG, Constandinou CM, Crocker J, Young LS, Ambinder RF (1998) Analysis of major histocompatibility complex class I, TAP expression, and LMP2 epitope sequence in Epstein-Barr virus-positive Hodgkin's disease. Blood 92:2477–83

39. Wetzler M, Baer MR, Stewart SJ, Donohue K, Ford L, Stewart CC, Repasky EA, Ferrone S (2001) HLA class I antigen cell surface expression is preserved on acute myeloid leukemia blasts at diagnosis and at relapse. Leukemia 15:128–133
40. Demant C, Mulder A, Deneys V, Worsham MJ, Maes P, Claas FH, Ferrone S (2004) Down-regulation of HLA-A and HLA-Bw6, but not HLA-Bw4, allospecificities in leukemic cells: an escape mechanism from CTL and NK attack? Blood. 103:3122–30
41. Lehmann F, Marchand M, Hainaut P, Pouillart P, Sastre X, Ikeda H, Boon T, Coulie PG. (1995) Differences in the antigens recognized by cytolytic T cells on two successive metastases of a melanoma patient are consistent with immune selection. Eur. J. Immunol. 25:340–347
42. Restifo NP, Marincola FM, Kawakami Y, Taubenberger J, Yannelli JR, Rosenberg SA. (1996) Loss of functional beta 2-microglobulin in metastatic melanomas from five patients receiving immunotherapy. J Natl Cancer Inst. 88:100–108
43. Kloor M, Becker C, Benner A, Woerner SM, Gebert J, Ferrone S, von Knebel Doeberitz M (2005) Immunoselective pressure and human leukocyte antigen class I antigen machinery defects in microsatellite unstable colorectal cancers. Cancer Research 65:6418–6424
44. Algarra I, Garcia-Lora A. Cabrera T, Ruiz-Cabello F and Garrido F (2004) The selection of tumor variants with altered expression of classical and non-classical MHC class I molecules: implications for tumor immune escape. Cancer Immunol. Immunother. 53:904–910
45. Seliger B, Maeurer MJ, Ferrone S (2000) Antigen-processing machinery breakdown and tumor growth. Immunol. Today. 21:455–64
46. Chang CC, Campoli M, Pestifo NP, Wang X, Ferrone S (2005) Immune selection of hot-spot β_2-microglobulin gene mutations, HLA-A2 allospecificity loss, and antigen-processing machinery component down-regulation in melanoma cells derived from recurrent metastases following immunotherapy. J. Immunol. 174:1462–1474
47. Bicknell DC, Kaklamanis L, Hampson R, Bodmer WF, Karran P (1996) Selection for ß2-microglobulin mutation in mismatch repair defective colorectal carcinomas. Curr. Biol. 6: 1695–1697
48. Cabrera CM, Jimenez P, Cabrera T, Esparza C, Ruiz-Cabello F, Garrido F (2003) Total loss of MHC class I in colorectal tumors can be explained by two molecular pathways: b2-microglobulin inactivation in MSI-positive tumors and LMP7/TAP2 downregulation in MSI-negative tumors. Tissue Antigens 61:211–219
49. Chen HL, Gabrilovich D, Tampe R, Girgis KR, Nadaf S, Carbone DP (1996) A functionally defective allele of TAP1 results in loss of MHC class I antigen presentation in a human lung cancer. Nat. Genet.13:210–213
50. Benitez R, Godelaine D, Lopez-Nevot MA et al. (1998) Mutations of the $ß_2$-microglobulin gene result in a lack of HLA class I molecules on melanoma cells of two patients immunized with MAGE peptides. Tissue Antigens 52:520–529
51. Hicklin DJ, Wang Z, Arienti F, Rivoltini L, Parmiani G, Ferrone S (1998) beta2-microglobulin mutations, HLA class I antigen loss, and tumor progression in melanoma. J. Clin. Invest. 101: 2720–2729
52. Feenstra M, rozemuller E, Duran K, Stuy I, van den Tweel J, Slootweg P, de Weger R, Tilanus M. (1999) Mutation in the beta 2m gene is not a frequent event in head and neck squamous cell carcinomas. Hum Immunol. 60:697–706
53. Atkins D, Ferrone S, Schmahl GE, Storkel S, Seliger B (2004) Down-regulation of HLA class I antigen processing molecules: an immune escape mechanism of renal cell carcinoma. J. Urol. 171:885–889
54. Raffaghello L, Prigione I, Bocca P, Morandi F, Camoriano M, Gambini C, Wang X, Ferrone S, Pistoia V (2005) Multiple defects of the antigen-processing machinery components in human neuroblastoma: immunotherapeutic implications. Oncogene 24:4634–4644
55. Romero JM, Jiménez P, Cabrera T, Cózar JM, Pedrinaci S, Tallada M, Garrido F, Ruiz-Cabello F (2005) Coordinated downregulation of the antigen presentation machinery and HLA class I/$?_2$-microglobulin complex is responsible for HLA-ABC loss in bladder cancer. Int. J. Cancer 113:605–610

56. Cabrera CM, Jimenez P, Concha A, Garrido F, Ruiz-Cabello F (2004) Promyelocytic leukemia (PML) nuclear bodies are disorganized in colorectal tumors with total loss of major histocompatibility complex class I expression and LMP7 downregulation. Tissue Antigens 63:446–452
57. Seliger B, Ritz U, Abele R, Bock M, Tampe R, Sutter G, Drexler I, Huber C, Ferrone S (2001) Immune escape of melanoma: First evidence of structural alterations in two distinct components of the MHC class I antigen processing pathway. Cancer Res. 61:8647–8650
58. Vitale M, Pelusi G, Taroni B, Gobbi G, Micheloni C, Rezzani R, Donato F, Wang X, Ferrone S (2005) HLA class I antigen down-regulation in primari ovary carcinoma lesions: association with disease stage. Clin. Cancer Res. 11:67–72
59. Fowler NL, Frazer IH (2004) Mutations in TAP genes are common in cervical carcinomas. Gynecol. Oncol. 92:914–921
60. Yang T, McNally BA, Ferrone S, Liu Y, Zheng P (2003) A single-nucleotide deletion leads to rapid degradation of TAP-1 mRNA in a melanoma cell line. J. Biol. Chem. 278:15291–15296
61. Dutta N, Majumder D, Gupta A, Mazumber DN, Banerjee S (2005) Analysis of human lymphocyte antigen class I expression in gastric cancer by reverse transcriptase-polymerase chain reaction. Hum. Immunol. 66 :164–169
62. Sheu BC, Chiou SH, Chang WC, Chow SN, Lin HH, Chen RJ, Huang SC, Ho HN, Hsu SM (2005) Integration of high risk human papillomavirus DNA correlates with HLA genotype aberration and reduced HLA class I molecule expression in human cervical carcinoma. Clin. Immunol. 115:295–301
63. Ashrafi GH, Haghshenas MR, Marchetti B, O'Brien PM, Campo MS (2005) E5 protein of human papillomavirus type 16 selectively downregulates surface HLA class I. Int. J. Cancer 113:276–283
64. Seliger B, Dunn T, Schwenzer A, Casper J, Huber C, Schmoll HJ (1997) Analysis of the MHC class I kantigen presentation machinery in human embryonal carcinomas: evidence for deficiencies in TAP, LMP and MHC class I expression and their upregulation by IFN-gamma. Scand J Immunol. 46:625–32
65. Marrogi AJ, Munshi A, Merogi AJ, Ohadike Y, El-Habashi A, Marrogi OL, Freeman SM (1997) Study of tumor infiltrating lymphocytes and transforming growth factor-ß as prognostic factors in breast carcinoma. Int. J. Cancer 74:492–501
66. Naito Y, Saito K, Shiiba K, Ohuchi A, Saigenji K, Nagura H, Ohtani H (1998) $CD8^+$ T cells infiltrated within cancer cell nests as a prognostic factor in human colorectal cancer. Cancer Res. 58:3491–3494
67. Nakano O, Sato M, Naito Y, Suzuki K, Orikasa S, Aizawa M, Suzuki Y, Shintaku I, Nagura H, Ohtani H. (2001) Proliferative activity of intratumoral CD8(+) T-lymphocytes as a prognostic factor in human renal cell carcinoma: clinicopathologic demonstration of antitumor immunity. Cancer Res. 61:5132–5136
68. Schumacher K, Haensch W, Roefzaad C, Schlag PM (2001) Prognostic significance of activated $CD8^+$ T cell infiltrations within esophageal carcinomas. Cancer Res. 61:3932–3936
69. Zhang L, Conejo-Garcia JR, Katsaros D, Gimotty PA, Massobrio M, Regnani G, Makrigiannakis A, Gray H, Schlienger K, Liebman MN, Rubin SC, Coukos G (2003) Intratumoral T cells, recurrence, and survival in epithelial ovarian cancer. N. Engl. J. Med. 348:203–213
70. Prall F, Dührkop T, Weirich V et al (2004) Prognostic role of $CD8^+$ tumor-infiltrating lymphocytes in stage III colorectal cancer with and without microsatellite instability. Hum. Pathol. 35:808–816
71. Al-Batran SE, Rafiyan MR, Atmaca A, Neumann A, Karbach J, Bender A, Weidmann E, Altmannsberger HM, Knuth A and Jager E (2005) Intratumoral T-cell infiltrates and MHC class I expression in patients with stage IV melanoma. Cancer Res. 65:3937–3941
72. Sandel MH, Speetjens FM, Menon AG, Albertsson PA, Basse PH, Hokland M, Nagelkerke JF, Tollenaar RA EM, van de Velde CJH, Kuppen PJK (2005) Natural killer cells infiltrating colorectal cancer and MHC class I expression. Mol. Immunol. 42:541–546
73. Menon AG, Fleuren GJ, Alphenaar EA, Jonges LE., Janssen van Rhijn CM, Ensink NG, Putter H, Tollenaar RA, van de Velde CJ, Kuppen PJ (2002a) A basal membrane-like structure surrounding tumor nodules may prevent intraepithelial leukocyte infiltration in colorectal cancer. Cancer Immunol. Immunother. 52:121–126

74. Scrivener S, Goddard R, Kaminski E, Prentice A (2003) Abnormal T-cell function in B-cell chronic lymphocytic leukaemia. Leuk. Lymphoma 44:383–389
75. Gabrilovich DI, Chen HL, Girgis KR, Cunningham HT, Meny GM, Hadaf S, Kavanaugh D, Carbone DP (1996) Production of vascular endothelial growth factor by human tumors inhibits the functional maturation of dendritic cells. Nat. Med. 2:1096–1103
76. Medema JP, de Jong J, van Hall T, Melief CJ, Offringa R (1999) Immune escape of tumors in vivo by expression of cellular FLICE-inhibitory protein. J. Exp. Med. 190:1033–1038
77.
78. Coleman S, Clayton A, Mason MD, Jasani B, Adams M, Tabi Z (2005) Recovery of CD8$^+$ T-cell function during systemic chemotherapy in advanced ovarian cancer. Cancer Res. 65:7000–7006
79. Liotta LA, Kohn EC (2001) The microenvironment of the tumor-host interface. Nature 411: 375–379
80. Gilboa E (2004) The promise of cancer vaccines. Nat. Rev. Cancer 4:401–411
81. Kammertoens T, Schüler T, Blankenstein T (2005) Immunotherapy: target the stroma to hit the tumor, Trends Mol Med.11:225–31
82. Spiotto MT, Schreiber H. (2005) Rapid destruction of the tumor microenvironment by CTLs recognizing cancer-specific antigens cross-presented by stromal cells. Cancer Immunity 5:8.
83. Qin Z, Blankenstein T (2004) A cancer immunosurveillance controversy. Nat. Immunol. 5:3–4
84. Willimsky G., Blankenstein T (2005) Sporadic immunogenic tumours avoid destruction by inducing T-cell tolerance. Nature 437:141–6
85. Campoli M, Ferrone S, Zea AH, Rodriguez PC, Ochoa AC (2005) Mechanisms of tumor evasion. Cancer Treat. Res. 123:61–88
86. Cromme FV, Airey J, Heemels MT et al. (1994) Loss of transporter protein, encoded by the TAP-1 gene, is highly correlated with loss of HLA expression in cervical carcinomas. J. Exp. Med. 179:335–340
87. Kaklamanis L, Townsend A, Doussis-Anagnostopoulou IA, Mortensen N, Harris AL, Gatter KC (1994) Loss of major histocompatibility complex-encoded transporter associated with antigen presentation (TAP) in colorectal cancer. Am. J. Pathol. 145:505–509
88. Kaklamanis L, Leek R, Koukourakis M, Gatte KC, Harris AL (1995) Loss of transporter in antigen processing 1 transport protein and major histocompatibility complex class I molecules in metastatic versus primary breast cancer. Cancer Res. 55:5191–5194
89. Vitale M, Rezzani R, Rodella L, Zauli G, Grigolato P, Cadei M, Hicklin DJ, Ferrone S (1998) HLA class I antigen and transporter associated with antigen processing (TAP1 and TAP2) down-regulation in high-grade primary breast carcinoma lesions. Cancer Res. 58:737–742
90. Le YS, Kim TE, Kim BK et al (2002) Alterations of HLA class I and class II antigen expressions in borderline, invasive and metastatic ovarian cancers. Exp. Mol. Med. 34:18–26
91. Krishnakumar S, Lakshmi SA, Abhyankar D, Biswa J (2004) Transporter associated protein expression in uveal melanoma. Br. J. Ophthalmol. 88:925–928
92. Meissner M, Reichert TE, Kunkel M, Gooding W, Whiteside TL, Ferrone S, Seliger B (2005) Defects in the human leukocyte antigen class I antigen processing machinery in head and neck squamous cell carcinoma: association with clinical outcome. Clin. Cancer Res. 11:2552–2560
93. Kallfelz M, Jung D, Hilmes C, Knuth A, Jaeger E, Huber C, Seliger B (1999) Induction of immunogenicity of a human renal-cell carcinoma cell line by TAP1-gen transfer. Int. J. Cancer.81: 125–133
94. Qin Z, Harders C, Cao X, Huber C, Blankenstein T, Seliger B (2002) Increased tumorigenicity, but unchanged immunogenicity, of transporter for antigen presentation 1-deficient tumors. Cancer Res. 62:2856–2860
95. Lou Y, Vitalis TZ, Basha G, Cai B, Chen SS, Choi KB, Jeffries AP, Elliott WM, Atkins D, Seliger B, Jefferies WA (2005) Restoration of the expression of transporters associated with antigen processing in lung carcinoma increases tumor-specific immune responses and survival. Cancer Res. 65:7926–7933
96. Parmiani G, Castelli C, Dalerba P, Mortarini R, Rivoltini L, Marincola FM, Anichini A (2002) Cancer immunotherapy with peptide-based vaccines: what have we achieved? Where are we going. J. Natl. Cancer Inst. 94:805–818

97. Agrawal S, Reemtsma K, Bagiella E, Oluwole SF and Braunstein NS (2004) Role of TAP-1 and/or TAP-2 antigen presentation defects in tumorigenicity of mouse melanoma. Cell. Immunol. 228:130–137
98. Jager MJ, Hurks HM, Levitskaya J, Kiessling R (2002) HLA expression in uveal melanoma: there is no rule without some exception. Hum. Immunol. 63:444–451
99. Menon AG, Morreau H, Tollenaar RA, Alphenaar E, Van Puijenbroek M, Putter H, Janssen-Van Rhijn CM, Van De Velde CJ, Fleuren GJ, Kuppen PJ (2002b) Down-regulation of HLA-A expression correlates with a better prognosis in colorectal cancer patients. Lab. Invest. 82: 1725–1733
100. Madjd Z, Spendlove I, Pinder SE, Ellis IO, Durrant LG (2005) Total loss of MHC class I is an independent indicator of good prognosis in breast cancer. Int. J. Cancer 117:248–255
101. Ramnath N, Tan D, Li Q, Hylander BL, Bogner P, Ryes L, Ferrone S (2005) Is downregulation of MHC class I antigen expression in human non-small cell lung carcinoma associated with prolonged survival? Cancer Immunol. Immunother. 27:1–9
102. Cao B, Tian X, Li Y, Jiang P, Ning T, Xing H, Zhao Y, Zhang C, Shi X, Chen D, Shen Y, Ke Y (2005) LMP7/TAP2 gene polymorphisms and HPV infection in esophageal carcinoma patients from a high incidence area in China. Carcinogen. 26:1280–1284
103. Seliger B, Bock M, Ritz U, Huber C (2002) High frequency of a non-functional TAP1/LMP2 promoter polymorphism in human tumors. Int. J. Oncol. 20:349–353 s
104. McCluskey J, Rossjohn J, Purcell AW (2004) TAP genes and immunity. Curr. Opin. Immunol. 16:651–659
105. Ibrahim EC, Aractingi S, Allory Y, Borrini F, Dupuy A, Duvillard P, Carosella ED, Avril MF, Paul P (2004) Analysis of HLA antigen expression in benign and malignant melanocytic lesions reveals that upregulation of HLA-G expression correlates with malignant transformation, high inflammatory infiltration and HLA-A1 genotype. Int. J. Cancer 108:243–250
106. Real LM, Cabrera T, Collado A, Jimenez P, Garcia A, Ruiz-Cabello F, Garrido F (1999) Expression of HLA-G in human tumors is not a frequent event. Int. J. Cancer 81:512–518
107. Fukushima Y, Oshika Y, Nakamura M, Tokunaga T, Hatanaka H, Abe Y, Yamazaki H, Kijima H, Ueyama Y, Tamaoki N (1998) Increased expression of human histocompatibility leucocyte antigen-G in colorectal cancer cells. Int. J. Mol. Med. 2:349–351
108. Paul P, Rouas-Freiss N, Khalil-Daher I, Moreau P, Riteau B, Le Gal FA, Avril MF, Dausset J, Guillet JG, Carosella ED (1998) HLA-G expression in melanoma: a way for tumor cells to escape from immunosurveillance. Proc. Natl. Acad. Sci. USA 95:4510–4515
109. Paul P, Canestre FA, Le Gal FA, Khalil-Daher I, Le Danff C, Schmid M, Mercier S, Avril MF, Dausset J, Guillet JG, Carosella ED (1999) Heterogeneity of HLA-G gene transcription and protein expression in malignant melanoma biopsies. Cancer Res. 59:1954–1960
110. Ibrahim EC, Morange M, Dausset J, Carosella ED, Paul P (2000) Heat shock and arsenite induce expression of the non-classical class I histocompatibility HLA-G gene in tumor cell lines. Cell Stress Chaperones 5:207–218
111. Ibrahim EC, Guerra N, Lacombe MJ, Angevin E, Chouaib S, Carosella ED, Caignard A, Paul P (2001) Tumor up-regulaton of the non-classical class I HLA-G antigen expression in renal carcinoma. Cancer Res. 61: 6838–6845
112. Urosevic M, Kurrer MO, Kamarashev J, Mueller B, Weder W, Burg G, Stahel RA, Dummer R, Trojan A (2001) Human leukocyte antigen G up-regulation in lung cancer associates with high-grade histology human leukocyte antigen class I loss and interleukin-10 production. Am. J. Pathol. 159:817–824
113. Wiendl H, Mitsdoerffer M, Hofmeister V, Wischhusen J, Bornemann A, Meyermann R, Weis EH, Melms A, Weller M (2002) A functional role of HLA-G expression in human gliomas: an alternative strategy of immune escape. J. Immunol. 168:4772–4780
114. Chang CC, Ferrone S (2003) HLA-G in melanoma: can the current controversies be solved? Semin. Cancer Biol. 13:361–369
115. Davidson B, Elstrand MB, McMaster MT, Berner A, Kurman RJ., Risberg B, Trope CG. Shih IM (2005) HLA-G expression in effusions is a possible marker of tumor susceptibility to chemotherapy in ovarian carcinoma. Gynecol. Oncol. 96:42–47

116. Urosevic M, Willers J, Mueller B, Kempf W, Burg G, Dummer R (2002a) HLA-G protein up-regulation in primary cutaneous lymphomas is associated with interleukin-10 expression in large cell T-cell lymphomas and indolent B-cell lymphomas. Blood 99:609–617
117. Urosevic M, Kempf W, Zagrodnik B, Panizzon R, Burg G, Dummer R (2005) HLA-G expression in basal cell carcinomas of the skin recurring after radiotherapy. Clin. Exp. Dermatol. 30:422–425
118. Marin R, Ruiz-Cabello F, Pedrinaci S, Mendez R, Jimenez P, Geraghty DE, Garrido F (2003) Analysis of HLA-E expression in human tumors. Immunogenet. 54:767–775
119. Palmisano GL, Contardi E, Morabito A, Gargaglione V, Ferrara GB, Pistillo MP (2005) HLA-E surface expression is independent of the availability of HLA class I signal sequence-derived peptides in human tumor cell lines. Hum. Immunol. 66:1–12
120. Mouillot G, Marcou C, Rousseau P, Rouas-Freiss N, Carosella ED, Moreau P (2005) HLA-G gene activation in tumor cells involves cis-acting epigenetic changes, Int. J. Cancer 113:928–936
121. Rouas-Freiss N, Bruel S, Menier C, Marcou C, Moreau P, Carosella ED (2005) Switch of HLA-G alternative splicing in a melanoma cell line causes loss of HLA-G1 expression and sensitivity to NK lysis. Int. J. Cancer 117:114–122
122. Urosevic M, Trojan A, Dummer R (2002b) HLA-G and its KIR ligands in cancer-another enigma yet to be solved? J. Pathol. 196:252–253
123. Wagner SN, Rebmann V, Willers CP, Grosse-Wilde H, Goos M (2000) Expression analysis of classic and non classical HLA molecules before interferon alfa-2b treatment of melanoma. Lancet 356:220–221
124. Ugurel S, Rebmann V, Ferrone S, Tilgen W, Grosse-Wilde H, Reinhold U (2001) Soluble human leukocyte antigen-G serum level is elevated in melanoma patient and is further increased by interferon-alpha immunotherapy. Cancer 92:369–376
125. Lefebvre S, Antioin, Uzan S, McMaster M, Dausset J, Carosella ED, Paul P (2002) Specific activation of the non-classical class I histocompatibility HLA-G antigen and expression of the ILT2 inhibitory receptor in human breast cancer. J. Pathol. 196:266–274
126. Rebmann V, Regel J, Stolke D, Grosse-Wilde H. (2003) Secretion of sHLA-G molecules in malignancies. Semin Cancer Biol. 13:371–7
127. Tomasec P, Braud VM, Rickards C, Powell MB, McSharry BP, Gadola S, Cerundolo V, Borysiewicz LK, McMichael AJ, Wilkinson GW (2000) Surface expression of HLA-E, an inhibitor of natural killer cells, enhanced by human cytomegalovirus gpUL40. Science 287:1031
128. Ljunggren HG, Karre K (1985) Host resistance directed selectively against H-2-deficient lymphoma variants: analysis of the mechanism. J. Exp. Med. 162:1745–1759
129. Vetter CS, Groh V, thor Straten P, Spies T, Brocker EB, Becker JC (2002) Expression of stress-induced MHC class I related chain molecules on human melanoma. J. Invest. Dermatol. 118:600–605
130. Jinushi M, Takehara T, Tatsumi T, Kanto T, Groh V, Spies T, Kimura R, Miyagi T, Mochizuki K, Sasaki Y, Hayashi N (2003) Expression and role of MICA and MICB in human hepatocellular carcinomas and their regulation by retinoic acid. Int. J. Cancer. 104:354–361
131. Salih HR, Rammensee HG, Steinle A (2002) Down-regulation of MICA on human tumors by proteolytic shedding. J. Immunol. 169:4098–4102
132. Groh V, Wu J, Yee C, Spies T (2002) Tumour-derived soluble MIC ligands impair expression of NKG2D and T-cell activation. Nature 419:734–738
133. Vetter CS, Lieb W, Bröcker EB, Becker JC (2004) Loss of nonclassical MHC molecules MIC-A/B expression during progression of uveal melanoma. Brit. J. Cancer 91:1495–1499
134. Wu JD, Higgin LM, Steinle A, Cosman D, Haugk K, Plymate SR (2004) Prevalent expression of the immunostimulatory MHC class I chain-related molecule is counteracted by shedding in prostate cancer. J. Clin. Invest. 114:560–568
135. Watson NF, Spendlove I, Madjg Z, McGilvray R, Green AR, Ellis IO, Scholefield JH, Durrant LG (2005) Expression of the stress-related MHC class I chain-related protein MICA is an indicator of good prognosis in colorectal cancer patients. Int. J. Cancer 118:1445–52
136. Cerwenka A, Baron JL, Lanier LL (2001) Ectopic expression of retinoic acid early inducible-1 gene (RAE-1) permits natural killer cell-mediated rejection of a MHC class I-bearing tumor in vivo. Proc. Natl. Acad. Sci. USA 98:11521–11526

137. Germain C, Larbouret C, Cesson V, Donda A, Held W, Mach JP, Pelegrin A, Robert B (2005) MHC class I-related chain A conjugated to antitumor antibodies can sensitize tumor cells to specific lysis by natural killer cells. Clin. Cancer Res. 11:7516–7522
138. Doubrovina ES, Doubrovin MM, Vider E, Sisson RB, O'Reilly RJ, Dupont B, Vyas YM (2003) Evasion from NK cell immunity by MHC class I chain-related molecules expressing colon adenocarcinoma. J. Immunol. 171:6891–6899
139. Wiemann K, Mittrucker HW, Feger U, Welte SA, Yokoyama WM, Spies T, Rammensee HG, Steinle A (2005) Systemic NKG2D down-regulation impairs NK and CD8 T cell responses in vivo. J. Immunol. 175:720–729
140. Rivoltini L, Canese P, Huber V, Iero M, Pilla L, Valenti R, Fais S, Lozupone F, Casati C, Castelli C, Parmiani G (2005) Escape strategies and reasons for failure in the interaction between tumor cells and the immune system: how can we tilt the balance towards immune-mediated cancer control? Expert Opin. Biol. Ther. 5:463–476
141. Mumberg D, Monach PA, Wanderling S, Philip M, Toledano AY, Schreiber RD, Schreiber H (1999) CD4(+) T cells eliminate MHC class II-negative cancer cells in vivo by indirect effects of IFN-gamma. Proc. Natl. Acad. Sci. USA 96:8633–8638
142. Qin Z, Schwartzkopff J, Pradera F, Kammertoens T, Seliger B, Pircher H, Blankenstein T (2003) A critical requirement of interferon gamma-mediated angiostasis for tumor rejection by $CD8^+$ T cells. Cancer Res. 63:4095–4100
143. Chen HL, Gabrilovich D, Virmani A, Ratnani I, Girgis KR, Nadaf-Rahrof S, Fernandez-Vina M, Carbone DP. (1996) Structural and functional analysis of beta2 microglobulin abnormalities in human lung and breast cancer. Int J Cancer. 67:756–63
144. Krishnakumar S, Sundaram A, Abhyankar D, Krishnamurthy V, Shanmugam MP, Gopal L, Sharma T, Biswas J (2004) Major histocompatibility antigens and antigen-processing molecules in retinoblastoma. Cancer 100:1059–1069
145. Lee N, Geraghty DE (2003) HLA-F surface expression on B cell and monocyte cell lines is partially independent from tapasin and completely independent from TAP. J. Immunol. 171:5264–5271
146. York IA, Grant EP, Dahl AM, Rock KL (2005) A mutant cell with a novel defect in MHC class I quality control. J. Immunol. 174:6839–6846

CHAPTER 7

THE LOCAL TUMOR MICROENVIRONMENT

THERESA L. WHITESIDE
University of Pittsburgh Cancer Institute and
Departments of Pathology, Immunology and Otolaryngology
University of Pittsburgh School of Medicine
Hillman Cancer Center, 5117 Centre Avenue, Suite 1.27, Pittsburgh, PA 15213

Keywords: TIL, immune evasion, immune surveillance, tumor escape, inflammation, cancer

INTRODUCTION

Tumors arise as a result of oncogenic transformation, and their progression involves multiple genetic changes, which occur and accumulate in the progeny of the transformed cell over many years [1]. A malignant phenotype established as a result of this series of genetic changes is characterized by uncontrolled growth of transformed cells and their progeny [1]. In parallel, a variety of alterations occur in the surrounding normal tissues, leading to establishment of the tumor microenvironment. These alterations are necessary to accommodate tumor growth and to assure survival of the tumor at the expense of surrounding normal tissue cells. Local tissue response to tumor progression resembles the process of chronic inflammation. Inflammation is a normal component of wound healing or tissue repair. Several years ago, H. Dworak described tumors as wounds that do not heal [2]. Inflammatory reaction is initiated by ischemia, which is followed by the interstitial and cellular edema associated with an appearance in tissue of inflammatory cells, including lymphocytes responsible for mediating an immune reaction and for tissue repair. Finally, a network of blood capillaries and lymphatics necessary for feeding of the repaired tissues is established [3,4]. These phases of inflammatory response progress from an anerobic tissue environment (ischemia) to the development of oxidative metabolism, which uses oxygen to produce energy in the form of ATP [5, 6]. Inflammation is a ubiquitous tissue response common to many normal conditions,

H.L. Kaufman and J.D. Wolchok (eds.), General Principles of Tumor Immunotherapy, 145–167.

including removal of pathogens, embryonic development or tissue re-structuring. It also is a major component of many disease states. Inflammation associated with tumor development is referred to as the "host reaction" to the tumor, and its involvement in shaping the tumor microenvironment has been well recognized.

The tumor appears to be able to attract inflammatory cells early on, and the presence of immune cells in pre-cancerous or benign lesions has been interpreted as an attempt of the host immune system to interfere with tumor development [7–9]. "Immune surveillance" refers to the ability of the host to recognize a danger signal, in this case an incipient tumor, and mount a response designed at its elimination. This implies that the host's immune system can survey, detect and destroy tumor cells, thus preventing tumor progression. However, it appears that tumors progress despite immune surveillance, and thus considerable skepticism has developed about the role of the immune system in the control of tumor growth. Based on the notion that the developing tumor is not a passive target of immune intervention but rather an active participant, the current view is that tumors take advantage of the host response in order to orchestrate their escape. As tumor cells sensitive to immune effector mechanisms are eliminated, others that are resistant to immune intervention expand and replace the sensitive targets. "Immune selection" of resistant tumor cells is one way to assure that only the fittest (i.e., most resistant) tumor cells survive, and to this end, the host immune system is used as a tool for selection, so that it subserves the tumor and not the host. In addition, once selected for resistance, tumor cells also become adept in using a variety of immunosuppressive mechanisms to engineer an escape from the host-mediated anti-tumor effects, a process termed "immune evasion." As a result, the tumor either disables the host immune system or manipulates it to create a local microenvironment favorable to tumor progression. To this end, the host becomes a participant in the establishment and maintenance of the tumor by providing structural and trophic elements required for cancer progression. Lymphocytes, macrophages and dendritic cells (DC) infiltrating the tumor, together with fibroblasts and extracellular matrix forming a scaffold supporting its expansion, contribute to establishing an inflammatory milieu that nourishes the tumor.

The objective of this chapter is to review the role of immune cells in the tumor-host interactions. This topic has been highly controversial in the past, because immune cells accumulating at tumor sites or those present in tumor-involved lymph nodes (LN) may be activated to exercise anti-tumor responses or may be profoundly suppressed by tumor-derived factors [10]. The capabilities of these immune cells to eliminate tumor targets or to serve as a source of growth factors for the tumor are likely to depend on the local milieu established by the tumor.

IMMUNE CELLS IN THE TUMOR MICROENVIRONMENT

Local or locoregional immune responses to malignant cells are mediated by tumor infiltrating lymphocytes (TIL), which accumulate in many human solid tumors and whose role in tumor progression remains controversial; lymphocytes present in tumor-involved LN; and lymphocytes in tumor-draining LN, which may or may not contain tumor cells. It has been well documented in the literature that TIL isolated from various human tumors are functionally compromised as compared to normal circulating or tissue-infiltrating lymphocytes [11]. The same appears to be true of lymphocytes obtained from tumor-involved LN [12]. On the other hand, lymphocytes isolated from tumor-draining lymph nodes have often been found to be able to mediate tumor antigen (TA)-specific responses and even to be enriched in TA-specific effector cells [13]. The impression that emerges from cumulative data is that immune cells in close proximity to tumors, especially large tumors, are more dysfunctional than those located at a distance or in contact with few tumor cells. Lymphocytes in tumor-draining LN interacting with TA may be able to respond, provided tumor-derived inhibitory factors are not present. Circulating lymphocytes in cancer patients may not be functionally impaired, although more recent data indicate that the same functional impairments seen in TIL are found in circulating as well as lymph node lymphocytes of patients with cancer [14]. Together, the available evidence suggests that in the presence of tumors, both local and systemic anti-tumor immunity is compromised in patients with cancer, although the extent of suppression as well as mechanisms engaged may vary. In general, TA-specific as well as non-specific proliferative and cytolytic responses are depressed, delayed-type hypersensitivity responses to recall antigens are weak and those to TA are absent, especially in advanced disease, and the cytokine profile is skewed from Th1 to Th2 [15]. However, this does not mean that patients with cancer are immunodeficient. They do not usually present with frequent, severe or opportunistic infections, and their responses to bacterial and viral antigens remain unimpaired.

Mechanisms responsible for suppression of immune responses of lymphocytes in the tumor environment are numerous, and selected examples are illustrated in Figure 1. Human tumors are known to produce a broad variety of inhibitory factors, including small molecules such as PGE_2 or COX-2, enzymes such as arginase or IDO, immunosuppressive cytokines (IL-10 and/or TGF-β), express immunoinhibitory ligands, release FasL+ microvesicles (MV) and attract regulatory T cells (Treg) to the tumor site [reviewed in 16 and 17].

The cellular composition of infiltrates in human tumors varies, depending on the histologic tumor type and/or tumor stage. In contrast to rodents, human tumors are rarely infiltrated by granulocytes, although eosinophils and basophils tend to be enriched in some head and neck cancers (HNC) and renal cell carcinomas (RCC) [18]. Mononuclear cells are the major component of TIL, although some TIL and all LN-derived cells contain variable proportions of T cells, B cells, dendritic cells (DC) and macrophages. The intensity of cellular infiltrates into tumors and their phenotypic characteristics have been extensively investigated, because of the possible prognostic and survival benefits of these features reported early on for several human tumor types [19]. However, it has been acknowledged that functional properties of infiltrating cells rather than their phenotypic characteristics determine their importance as anti-tumor effector cells.

Tumor-infiltrating T Cells

T cells ($CD3^+TCR^+$) are by far the largest component of mononuclear tumor infiltrates in all human tumors [20], although some tumors may be also highly infiltrated by macrophages [21]. The hypothesis that TIL-T cells represent antitumor-specific cytolytic T cells (CTL) has been promoted; however, early limiting dilution studies performed with TIL-T from various human tumor indicated that the frequency of such CTL was low as compared to peripheral blood T lymphocytes (PBL-T) [22]. Nevertheless, evidence exists that Vβ-restricted clones of T cells are present in some freshly isolated TIL, and that TIL can selectively recognize and kill autologous tumor cells in some cases [23]. Using tetramers and multi-parameter flow cytometry, it has recently been possible to determine the frequency of tumor-peptide-specific (tetramer$^+$) T cells among TIL with greater accuracy in various human tumors [24]. We reported, for example, that TIL obtained from patients with HNC were significantly enriched in wild type (wt) p53 epitope-specific T cells, as compared to autologous peripheral blood mononuclear cells (PBMC) [24]. The frequency of the tetramer$^+$ TIL was highly variable and ranged from 1/800 to 1/5,000 of $CD3^+CD8^+$ TIL, which recognized the wt $p53_{264-272}$ peptide, compared to the mean frequency of 1/6,000 such cells among autologous PBMC [24]. Furthermore, our recent analysis of TcR Vβ restrictions in paired TIL and PBMC of patients with HNC indicated the presence of the same Vβ restrictions in both cell populations. These oligoclonal expansions of T cells were observed in paired TIL and PBMC of all 10 patients with HNC and in 0/10 PBMC samples obtained from normal donors [25]. This type of evidence is also available for melanoma [23, 26], and it indicates that TIL may be enriched in TA-specific T cells.

The phenotypic analysis of T cells in human tumors shows that TIL-T are memory lymphocytes, expressing either CD8 or CD4 markers, although the CD4/CD8 ratio may be highly variable from one tumor to another [11]. Enrichment of TIL in $CD8^+$ T cells has been reported, resulting in a low CD4/CD8 ratio relative to that seen with nonmalignant inflammatory infiltrates, which consist largely of $CD4^+$ T cells [27, 28]. In some studies, high tumor content of $CD8^+$ T cells has been linked to a better prognosis [29, 30], although this is not a consistent finding, as in cervical cancer or RCC, enrichment of TIL in $CD8^+$ T cells seems to be associated with disease progression and a poor prognosis [31, 32]. TIL-T freshly isolated from human tumors generally express an activated phenotype, i.e., are HLA-DR^+CD25^+, which is inconsistent with their functional properties. The TIL-T have significantly depressed proliferative and anti-tumor functions in comparison with normal T cells, as measured in conventional *ex vivo* assays. Further, TIL obtained from advanced or metastatic lesions are more functionally impaired than those from early lesions, suggesting that large or more aggressive tumors are more immunosuppressive. The cytokine profile of TIL-T is also different from that of normal activated T cells, as either no or little type 1 cytokines (IL-2, IFN-γ) were produced by TIL-T and, instead, these cells preferentially secreted down-regulatory cytokines, IL-10 and TGF-β [33]. These functional characteristics of TIL-T do not correlate with the phenotype of activated T lymphocytes [11].

A hypothesis has been advanced that TIL-T may be enriched in $CD4^+CD25^+$ regulatory T cells. Recent reports confirmed the accumulation of regulatory $CD4^+CD25^{bright}$ T cells (Treg) at the tumor site in several human malignancies [24,34,35]. This enrichment in Treg, could provide an explanation for the observed discrepancy between the observed "activation" phenotype of TIL-T and their functional impairments. Treg accumulating in the tumor microenvironment could be responsible for down-regulation of TIL functions [17]. However, until very recently, it was not possible to make a firm distinction between activated $CD4^+$ T cells and Treg due to the lack of specific phenotypic markers for the Treg population.

These cells were identified based on the ability to express message for the FOXp3 gene [36] or functionally, by the ability to suppress activity of other immune cells in *ex vivo* mixing experiments [37]. We have observed a significant increase in the proportion of $CD4^+CD25^+$ T cells in TIL isolated from HNC (a mean of 30% in TIL vs. 11% in autologous PBMC; n = 17) [17]. When the newly available antibodies to FOXp3, a transcription factor expressed in Treg [36], and antibodies to glucocorticoid-induced TNF receptor (GITR) or to CTLA-4 antigen [38,39] were used for staining and flow cytometry of permeabilized TIL obtained from patients with HNC, we observed that nearly all $CD4^+CD25^+$ TIL were positive for these markers. In contrast, only 1–2% of $CD4^+CD25^+$ T cells in PBMC were stained with the antibodies recognizing Treg. These preliminary data indicate that tumors indeed "beckon regulatory T cells" [17]. However, these results have to be confirmed by functional studies demonstrating suppressive capabilities of $CD4^+CD25^+$ T cells isolated from TIL and PBMC of patients with HNC, similar to those recently performed by Curiel and colleagues with TIL obtained from tumor tissues and ascites of patients with ovarian carcinoma [40]. A tentative conclusion that can be drawn from the data available so far is that TIL-T are often, but not always, enriched in CD8+ T cells, some of which may be TA-specific effector cells. Functional paralysis of TIL might, in part, be attributed to suppressive effects mediated by Treg accumulating in the tumor microenvironment. Very recent data suggest that $CD8^+CD28^-$ T cells may also represent a subset of Treg [41]. It is equally likely, however, that other suppressive factors present in the tumor microenvironment (Figure 1) could also contribute to functional defects in TIL-T.

Functional impairments observed with TIL-T could be also explained by sensitivity of these cells to apoptosis. Significant *in situ* apoptosis of TIL-T cells was observed in human solid tumors. In our studies, the numbers of $TUNEL^+CD3^+$ T cells in the tumor was significantly correlated to FasL expression on the tumor cells [14]. As human tumors are known to express a variety of inhibitory ligands (FasL, PDL-1 or 2, TRAIL) and activated T cells express complementary receptors, it is not surprising that TIL-T are especially sensitive to tumor-induced apoptosis. A model of T-cell demise in the tumor microenvironment mediated by FasL expressed on the tumor cell surface is shown in Figure 2. Flow cytometry studies with TIL-T freshly isolated from human tumors confirm that a considerable percentage of these cells

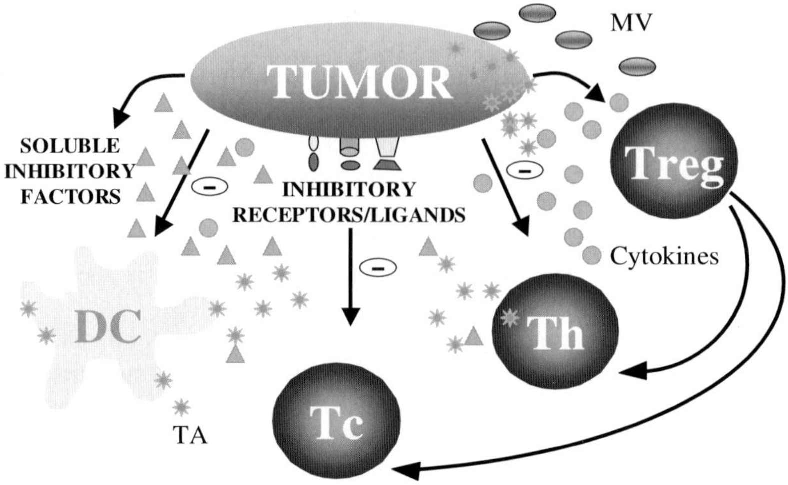

Figure 1. Inhibitory pathways operating in the tumor microenvironment. Immune cells infiltrating human tumors encounter a variety of immunosuppressive factors (e.g., cytokines such as IL-10 or TGF-β; enzymes such as IDO or arginase; gangliosides; small molecules such as PGE_2) or microvesicles (MV) released by the tumor. Regulatory T cells (Treg) accumulate at tumor sites and may down-regulate functions of cytotoxic (Tc) or helper (Th) T cells. Tumors express a variety of inhibitory ligands (e.g., FasL, TRAIL, PDL-1 or -2), and receptors for these ligands are present on activated T cells. Tumor also shed a profusion of tumor antigens, creating an antigen excess in the tumor microenvironment

are in various stages of apoptosis, as indicated by intracellular caspase activation, mitochondrial membrane potential (MMP) changes, or Annexin V binding [42].

In situ studies of signaling molecules in TIL-T also confirm that TIL-T are functionally impaired. Such studies show that expression of the T-cell receptor (TcR)-associated ζ chain as well as that of NF-κB, the transcription factor regulating expression of a number of immune and inflammatory genes, is significantly decreased in TIL-T compared to expression in T cells obtained from the peripheral circulation of normal donors [43,44]. This is particularly evident for TIL evaluated *in situ* or isolated from advanced or metastatic lesions. In a study comprising over 130 cases of human oral squamous cell carcinomas (OSCC), expression of ζ in TIL-T was found to be an independent and highly statistically significant biomarker of prognosis and survival in patients with stage III and IV disease [45]. The patients with tumors infiltrated by T cells with low or absent ζ expression had significantly shorter 5-year survival compared to the patients with tumors infiltrated by T cells with normal ζ expression [45]. Stimulus-dependent activation of NF-κB was found to be impaired in TIL-T cells of patients with RCC. In some patients, the primary defect was the failure of the transactivating complex RelA/NF-κB1 (p50) to accumulate in the nucleus following T-cell activation due to impaired phosphorylation and degradation of the inhibitor IκBα [46,47]. In other patients, NF-κB activation was defective despite normal stimulus-dependent degradation of IκBα [48]. In both situations, this defective state could be induced by exposure of normal

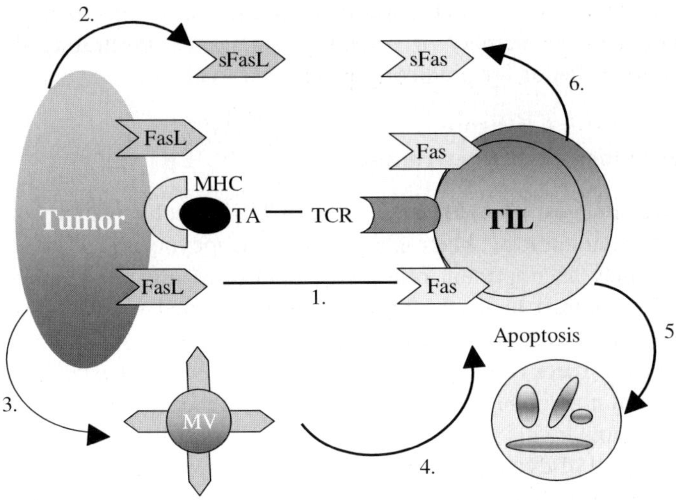

Figure 2. The Fas/FasL pathway and tumor escape from immune surveillance. Tumor cells use this pathway to execute "Fas counter attack." 1. Tumor cells express FasL, while activated T cells (presumably responsive to TA) express Fas, providing an opportunity for a direct interaction between the membrane-anchored receptor and the ligand. 2. Tumor cells enzymatically cleave FasL from the surface membrane and release sFasL. 3. Tumor also releases FasL-containing microvesicles (MV). 4. MV armed with FasL induce Fas-mediated apoptosis of TIL. 5. Apoptosis of TIL is also a result of the direct interactions between TIL and tumor cells. 6. TIL express Fas and can release sFas (as well as sFasL: not shown). sFasL, whether it originates from tumor cells or TIL, does not effectively cross-link its membrane-bound receptor, but it can bind sFas, forming soluble complexes. Tumor cells use the Fas/FasL pathway to induce TIL apoptosis *in situ*

T cells to supernatants of RCC, and the soluble product responsible was identified as an RCC-derived ganglioside [48]. Impaired NF-κB activity may contribute to reduced T-cell function seen in TIL-T present in RCC, since this transcription factor controls expression of a number of genes encoding cytokines, their receptors and other membrane regulatory molecules essential for T-cell activation [49, 50]. It is important to note that defects in function of the ζ chain and activation of NF-κB are observed in TIL-T as well as circulating T cells of patients with cancer [51, 52]. Thus, these signaling defects in T cells are both local and systemic and seem to be related to the tumor burden.

The data obtained from many different laboratories are consistent in demonstrating that the majority of TIL-T obtained from a variety of human solid tumors are functionally incompetent, despite expression of the "activation" phenotype. A reasonable explanation for this finding is that T lymphocytes accumulating in the tumor microenvironment are exposed to a variety of inhibitory signals generated either by the tumor or by activated Treg. It also appears that the degree of tumor-associated inhibition and the loss of functions in TIL-T may relate to tumor aggressiveness, as the most aggressive tumors are characterized by an especially immunoinhibitory microenvironment. However, not all TIL-T are equally immunocompromised and tumors differ in the ability to inhibit T cells, the functional potential of TIL rather than the number or phenotype of T cells infiltrating the tumor may be the important factor for predicting patient survival.

Macrophages in the Tumor Microenevironment

Tumor-associated macrophages (TAM) are $CD45^+CD14^+$ cells which are commonly found in human tumors. Macrophages are phagocytic and antigen-presenting cells, which play an important role in the control of infections and in anti-tumor immunity. In contrast to macrophages found in normal tissues, TAM are re-programmed to inhibit lymphocyte functions through release of inhibitory cytokines, prostaglandins or reactive oxygen species (ROS). It is hypothesized that re-programming of normal macrophages into TAM occurs in the tumor microenvironment as a result of tumor-driven activation [53]. Possibly, macrophages are the main contributors to removal of dying tumor cells, and rapidly proliferating tumors, which are also characterized by high rates of apoptosis, are especially attractive to these scavengers. For example, invasiveness of human tumors, e.g., primary colon carcinomas, is directly related to the number of TAM detected in the tumor [53]. An increased TAM count is an independent predictor of reduced relapse-free survival as well as reduced overall survival in invasive breast cancer [54]. The available data support the active role of TAM in promoting tumor progression, possibly by interfering with anti-tumor functions of TIL. The mechanisms that contribute to TAM-mediated inhibition of immune cells in the tumor milieu are likely to be driven by the tumor. Much attention has been recently devoted to the role of NADPH-dependent ROS, such as superoxide anion or hydrogen peroxide as potential inhibitors of TIL [55,56]. T-cell proliferation and NK-mediated anti-tumor cytotoxicity are profoundly inhibited by macrophage-derived ROS *in vitro* [56]. T and NK cells isolated from human tumors have a decreased expression of CD3ζ and FcγRIII-associated ζ, respectively, and this down-modulation of ζ, a critical signal-transducing molecule associated with TCR, can be induced by ROS produced by TAM [57]. The changes observed in TIL: a loss of normal ζ expression accompanied by a decreased ability to proliferate and subsequent apoptotic cell death, correspond to similar changes induced in T and NK cells co-cultured with activated macrophages [56]. Removal of macrophages from these cultures restores T and NK cell functions [56].

The overall conclusion from these studies of TAM is that tumors acquire the ability to program infiltrating macrophages so that they primarily function as a source of suppressive factors. These immunoinhibitory activities of TAM, whether due to oxidative stress or to release of inhibitory cytokines, such as IL-10, contribute to making the tumor microenvironment a particularly unfriendly milieu for immune cells. In this, TAM appear to reinforce effects mediated by tumor cells, which also produce ROS, PGE_2 and a variety of immunoinhibitory cytokines [16]. In addition to their suppressive activities, TAM were reported to be involved in angiogenesis and progression of breast carcinomas [58].

Dendritic Cells in Human Tumors

Dendritic cells (DC; *Lin*$^-$CD80$^+$CD86$^+$HLA-DR$^+$ cells) are the most potent antigen presenting cells (APC). They are a heterogenous population of highly motile cells that originate from the precursors in the bone marrow and migrate through the blood stream to peripheral non-lymphoid tissues, capturing antigens [59]. They then travel to the lymphoid tissues, where antigen presentation to T cells takes place. DC comprise subpopulations of morphologically and functionally distinct cells, defined by their hematopoietic origin, maturation stage or tissue localization [60]. The two main subpopulations are myeloid-derived DC (DC1) and lymphoid-derived DC (DC2). While in man, this distinction is somewhat blurred, phenotypic and functional differences exist between monocyte-drived CD11c$^+$ DC (MDC) and CD11c$^-$CD123$^+$ (IL-3Rα^{high}) lymphoid-derived DC [54, 60]. The latter subset of DC is much smaller than that of myeloid DC, and most of these cells belong to a relatively rare subset of plasmacytoid DC (pDC), which produce IFN-α in response to viral antigens [54]. Human tumors are frequently infiltrated by MDC but rarely by pDC. The presence of pDC in the tumor is associated with poor prognosis [61]. The DC maturation stage determines their functionality: immature DC are primarily responsible for antigen uptake, while mature CD83$^+$ DC primarily serve as antigen-presenting cells [54].

In tumor-bearing hosts, DC take up, process and cross-present TA to naïve or memory T cells, thus playing a crucial role in the generation of TA-specific effector T cells. DC presentation of TA leads to T cell proliferation, resulting in either immunity or tolerance, depending on the stage of maturation of the presenting DC. In human solid tumors, DC may be present in a substantial number, and they express attributes of immature DC [62]. Because TA-specific immune responses are inefficient in tumor-bearing individuals, it has been suggested that DC, like T cells, are subverted by the tumor [62]. DC infiltrating human tumors as well as DC recovered from the peripheral blood of patients with cancer exhibit phenotypic and functional alterations relative to DC of normal donors [63, 64]. Tumor-associated DC (TADC) lack of expression of CD80 and CD86 (are immature) and have reduced allostimulatory activity [65]. Tumors or tumor-derived factors have been shown to impair DC maturation or induce DC apoptosis [66, 67]. Co-culture of murine or human DC (obtained from isolated CD34$^+$ precursors or plastic-adherent PBMC, respectively) with a variety of tumor cell lines for 4–48 hours resulted in apoptotic death of DC, as verified by morphology, TUNEL assays, Annexin binding, caspase activation and DNA laddering [68, 69]. Tumor cells induced DC apoptosis by direct contact or through release of soluble factors, and TADC isolated from human tumors contained elevated proportions of DC undergoing apoptosis [69]. Tumor-induced apoptosis of DC was inhibited in the presence of IL-12 and IL-15, and these cytokines stimulated expression of Bcl-2 and Bcl-XL in DC [69, 70]. Tumor-derived factors, e.g., gangliosides, inhibited DC generation and their function *in vitro* [70]. This suppressive effect of gangliosides on DC was found to be mediated by tumor-derived VEGF, a known anti-dendropoietic factor [71]. Importantly, cytokines (IL-12, IL-15 and FLT3L) were found to promote DC generation and their functions by exerting a protective anti-apoptotic effect, while tumor-derived factors caused apoptosis in mature DC and inhibited differentiation of hematopoietic precursors into DC. Very recent studies indicate that tumors and tumor supernatants can down-regulate expression of antigen presenting machinery (APM) components in DC, thus interfering with the capacity of these cells to process antigens and present the processed epitopes to T cells [72,73]. Again, tumor-derived gangliosides were identified as the factor responsible for down-modulation of APM components in DC co-incubated with the tumor [73]. These studies underscore the role of the microenvironment in shaping the functional potential of DC and perhaps that of other tumor-infiltrating immune cells.

Despite the above-mentioned functional impairments of TADC, their presence in tumors is associated with improved prognosis [74, 75]. DC infiltrations into tumors have been correlated to significantly prolonged patient survival and reduced incidence of recurrent or metastatic disease in patients with bladder, lung, laryngeal, oral, gastric and nasopharyngeal carcinomas [75–80]. In contrast, patients with lesions reported to be scarcely infiltrated with DC had a relatively poor prognosis [81]. Fewer DC were observed in metastatic than primary tumor lesions [82]. We demonstrated that the number of S-100^{+} DC present in the tumor was by far the strongest independent predictor of overall survival as well as disease-free survival and time to recurrence in 132 patients with OSCC, compared with such well established prognostic factors as disease stage or lymph node involvement [75]. We also observed that the paucity of DC in the tumor was significantly related to the loss of ζ expression in TIL, and these two factors had a highly significant effect on patient overall survival. The poorest survival and the greatest risk was observed in patients with tumors that had small number of DC and little or no ζ expression in TIL ($p = 2.4 \times 10^{-8}$). Our data suggest that both the number of DC and the presence of functionally unimpaired T cells in the tumor microenvironment are important for overall survival of patients with cancer. When DC and T cells present in the tumor are able to interact, TcR-mediated and presumably TA-specific functions of the infiltrated T cells are amplified and sustained. It has been proposed that DC protect T cells from tumor-induced immune suppression, although the mechanism responsible for such protection remains unknown and is being actively investigated.

The correlation between TADC presence in the tumor and patient overall survival or relapse free survival has not been confirmed in other more recent studies, in which immunostaining for MDC and pDC subsets was performed. Thus, in primary breast cancer, a strong association of mature DC with CD3^{+} T cells was observed but did not correlate with prognosis, and it was pDC infiltration that predicted a poor survival in the same series [61]. While this and all other reports based on immunostaining of tumor sections may suffer from a bias related to selection of tissue sections, antibodies used for staining, methods for cell enumeration and patient selection, these data suggest that, similar to T-cell infiltrates, TADC may have considerable biologic significance in cancer.

B Cell Accumulations

Anti-tumor antibodies (Abs) are frequently detected in the circulation of cancer patients. It has been assumed that these Abs are made and secreted by plasma cells situated in the tumor draining lymph nodes, spleen or other lymphoid tissues. Although B lymphocytes ($CD19^+$, $CD20^+$) are uncommon components of human solid tumors, plasma cells have been observed in some carcinomas and, occasionally, represent a substantial infiltrating element [7]. More recent reports indicate that lymphoplasmacytic infiltrates are relatively common in pre-malignant cervical lesions as well as cervical carcinomas [83] and in medullary ductal breast carcinomas [84]. Using antibody phage display, it was possible to show that infiltrating B cells and plasma cells represent an antigen-induced response to human papillomavirus (HPV) infection or transformation in cervical carcinomas [83]. In medullary ductal breast carcinoma, the presence of B and plasma cells is associated with improved prognosis [85]. This finding has generated considerable interest in the role of tumor-infiltrating B cells and their products in tumor progression. The hypothesis was that lymphoplasmacytic infiltrates represented a host humoral response driven by tumor-derived neo-antigens [86–88]. The data based on patterns and levels of TIL-B IgG heavy chain hypermutation suggested that tumor-infiltrating B cells are undergoing antigen-driven proliferation and affinity maturation *in situ*. Abs produced by TIL-B may be TA-specific or may specifically bind an intracellular protein, such as β-actin, translocated to and presented on the cell surface upon tumor cell apoptosis [87]. It has been suggested that Ig variable region analysis could be used for dissection Ab responses in order to select those Abs with high affinity to TA for the purpose of TA isolation [89]. The presence of ectopic germinal centers in breast cancer and perhaps other solid tumors suggests that Ab production can occur in the tumor microenvironment under certain circumstances. The biologic significance or the prognostic importance of this phenomenon is unknown, although it is possible that the ability to make Abs *in situ* might be an important aspect of host defense.

Other Leukocytes in Human Tumors

As indicated above, human tumors are sometimes infiltrated by granulocytes, and nests of eosinophils may be seen in association with tumor cells in various squamous cell carcinomas, for example. By far the most frequent cell in tumors has characteristics of the immature myeloid cell (iMC). The relationship of this cell type to TAM is unclear. The iMC express CD33, a common myeloid marker, but lack markers of mature myeloid or lymphoid cells and HLA-DR [90]. The iMC are equivalent to murine $Gr\text{-}1^+CD11b^+$ cells, which have been shown to inhibit IFN-γ production by $CD8^+$ T cells in response to epitopes presented by MHC class I molecules on the surface of these cells [90]. This inhibition is apparently mediated by ROS produced by iMC, such as H_2O_2, which suppress CD3ζ expression by T cells [91]. Indeed, granulocyte-derived H_2O_2 has been shown to be involved in the inhibition of IFN-γ production and the suppression of CD3ζ expression in circulating T cells of patients with advanced malignancy [92]. In tumors, where the hypoxic environment prevails, H_2O_2-generating iMC might contribute to creating conditions which favor T-cell suppression.

INTERACTIONS BETWEEN THE TUMOR AND INFILTRATING LEUKOCYTES

The presence in tumor and numbers of infiltrating leukocytes are determined by signals in the tumor microenvironment. Their presence in human solid tumors is a consistent feature. It is only reasonable to expect that the type of cellular infiltrates recruited to the tumor is also dependent on the tumor characteristics. Hence, the nature and cellular composition of these infiltrates vary from one tumor type to another or even among individual tumors of the same histologic type. Importantly, the phenotype, numbers and location of infiltrating leukocytes in the tumor (i.e., stroma vs. intraepithelial) have been in many instances correlated to prognosis and patient survival [see, e.g., ref. [93]. However, no unified view on this aspect have emerged to date, and for every report linking the extent of leukocyte infiltration to a better prognosis, a report can be found claiming the opposite. The data available in the literature indicate that the presence of leukocytic infiltrates in the tumor is either good or bad but certainly not neutral. Clearly, an opportunity for a cross-talk between infiltrating cells and the tumor exists in the tumor microenvironment, as illustrated in Figure 3.

In one respect, leukocytic infiltrates can be considered as a component of the inflammatory process representing a "host reaction" to the tumor. This is in spite of the fact that a granulocytic component is not prominent in human tumors. Today, it has become fashionable to establish a connection between inflammation and cancer [94]. This intriguing concept is not without merit. The initial goal of the inflammatory reaction is destruction of the invader, which in this case is the tumor. Consequently, the "immune phase" of tumor-driven inflammation involves an influx of anti-tumor effector cells to the tumor site and their accumulation. The strength of signals initiating an inflammatory response is crucial. While vigorous cellular and antibody responses are generated in tissues during the infection by exogenous pathogens, "danger signals" generated in the tumor microenvironment are weak [95, 96]. The reason for the lack of robust immune responses to the tumor may be that the immune system perceives infections with bacteria or viruses as "danger" and the tumor as "self." Results of recent "antigen discovery" studies indicate that TA are largely self or altered self antigens. Thus, the host immune system responds vigorously to contain the external danger introduced by pathogens and only weakly, if at all, to the tumor. It is also plausible that the attraction of Treg to the tumor is related to an attempt by the host to ill advisedly (in this case) regulate and suppress host response to self. Tolerance to self needs to be overcome before a full-scale immune response to the tumor can develop, and in the presence of progressing tumor, this is unlikely to happen [97]. Interestingly, inflammatory infiltrates in tumors generally contain few, if any, NK cells which mediate innate immunity

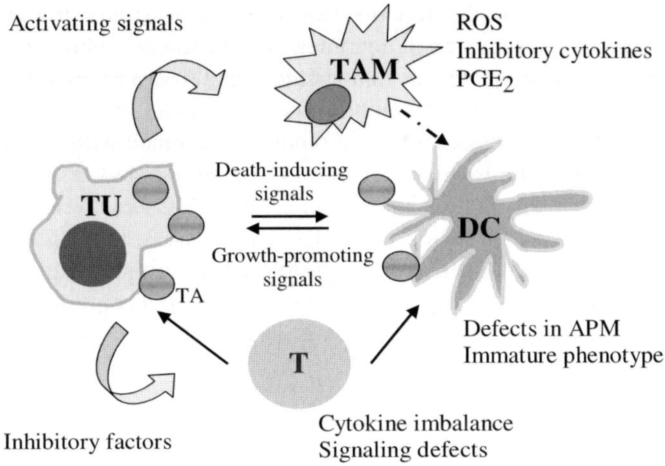

Figure 3. Interactions between immune and tumor cells in the tumor microenvironment. Tumor exerts profound suppressive effects on infiltrating immune cells, including death-inducing signals. At the same time, tumor-associated macrophages (TAM) become activated and induced to secrete ROS and inhibitory cytokines or other inhibitory molecules. DC present in the tumor microenvironment fail to differentiate into APC and express markers associated with the immature phenotype. T lymphocytes are dysfunctional, e.g., have signaling defects, or undergo apoptosis. The cytokine imbalance favors Th2 responses, and the cytokine milieu is altered in favor of cytokines and factors that promote tumor growth. Not shown are stromal cells, which provide a scaffold for tumor growth and are activated, producing pro-inflammatory cytokines

and are rich in perforin- or granzyme-containing granules [98]. NK cells are exquisitely attuned to distinguish self from non-self by virtue of a complex system of inhibitory and activating receptors expressed on their surface [99]. They represent "the first line" of defense against pathogens, and their conspicuous absence from tumor infiltrates or even pre-cancerous lesions [99] suggests that the host's response to the tumor is indeed different in strength and quality from that initiated by exogenous pathogens.

The nature of the tumor microenvironment appears to be quite unique. On the one hand, the tumor creates stress signals, which mobilize the host to initiate an inflammatory cascade. On the other, the tumor microenvironment is characterized by the presence of multiple suppressive factors and by the excess of antigens produced and released from proliferating or dying tumor cells [Figure 1; 100]. Thus, inflammatory cells arrive into this environment to be faced by conflicting signals, which orchestrate the local response. As a result, a somewhat precarious balance is established between the host and the tumor, which clearly favors the tumor, and which has at least two aims: a) to cripple the host immune system so that the tumor can survive, and b) to utilize infiltrating cells and their products for supporting tumor survival. Ample evidence exists to support the existence of both these mechanisms [16].

While tumor escape from the host-mediated surveillance in its various forms has been recently in the limelight [reviewed in 16], those elements of the local inflammatory response that mediate trophic functions and thus support tumor growth have to be recognized as well. Thus, once recruited to the tumor microenvironment, various leukocytes are subjected to non-specific or TA-specific signals and, in response, may produce a variety of soluble products, including cytokines and antibodies. In theory, anti-tumor effects of these products combined with direct cytolytic activity of infiltrating effector cells against tumor targets should result in demise of tumor cells sensitive to immune intervention. In reality, however, the tumor also releases soluble factors, including cytokines, gangliosides, polyamines and other TA which suppress immune cells and at the same time stimulate tumor growth and survival (Figures 1 and 3). The balance between these opposing forces is likely to shift in one direction or another, depending on the nature of the tumor microenvironment.

Inflammation in the Tumor Microenvironment

The tumor microenvironment undergoes continuous alterations in the course of tumor progression, and the nature of inflammatory infiltrates found in the tumor changes as well. Early on, the hypoxic environment prevails. It is created early in the tumor development through activation of hypoxia responsive genes in tumor cells [101]. This microenvironment obviously favors influx of those inflammatory cells that depend on the glycolytic pathway for survival, namely, phagocytic macrophages and granulocytes [102]. These cells can not only survive in the hypoxic environment but actively contribute to it by the hyperproduction of ROS upon their activation, which is supported by apoptosis of rapidly expanding and dying tumor cells requiring phagocytosis. Activating signals delivered to phagocytes lead to massive generation of ROS. In most inflammatory responses, activities of ROS are mediated by the NF-κB pathway, which in turn is regulated by hypoxia and/or re-oxygenation [103]. It has been recently proposed that NF-κB activates signaling pathways in both cancer cells and tumor-associated inflammatory cells, thus promoting malignancy [94]. If progression to malignancy is indeed regulated at the level of NF-κB and a pro-inflammatory mediator TNF-α or other pro-inflammatory cytokines, as some of the animal models of cancer seem to indicate, the missing link between inflammation and cancer may have been identified [104, 105]. These cancer models also underscore the importance of the tumor microenvironment, and its interactions with infiltrating inflammatory cells, in cancer progression. The data suggest that the NF-κB pathway is regulated differently in normal vs. malignant tissues. NF-κB is present as an inactive complex in the cytoplasm of many cells, including inflammatory and tissue cells. During inflammation, activation of NF-κB initiated by, e.g., binding of TNF-α to its receptor (TNFR1) expressed on inflammatory cells in the microenvironment initiates regulated expression of cytokine genes which control cell proliferation and cell death. Tumor cells depend on these cytokines for proliferation, and leukocytes activated in the tumor microenvironment are reprogrammed to continually release these cytokines. Responding to this cytokine cascade, tumor and stromal cells produce a panoply of soluble factors with biologic effects ranging from enhancement of cell proliferation, matrix remodeling, vessel growth, inhibition of cellular differentiation to sustained release of pro-inflammatory mediators. Inhibition of NF-κB activation in tumor cells favors cell death and arrests tumor progression. This model is consistent with observed correlations between the numbers and maturation stages of inflammatory cells in the tumor, levels of cytokines produced and tumor prognosis [106]. The role of TNF-α in driving tumor progression has been emphasized by Balkwill and colleagues [107], and it offers an interesting example of the efficiency of tumors in their ability to usurp normal biologic process of inflammation to promote tumor progression.

In inflammation, the immune phase is followed by the appearance of blood vessels and lymphatics in the repaired tissue. The process of angiogenesis is also a prominent component of the tumor microenvironment [108]. Vascular endothelial growth factor (VEGF) is produced by most tumors and plays a crucial role in the development of tumor vasculature [109]. Increased levels of VEGF in the plasma of patients with cancer were shown to correlate with a poor prognosis [110]. Evidence also identifies VEGF as one of the factors responsible for interfering with DC differentiation in the tumor microenvironment [109]. As TAM play an important role in angiogenesis, it is not surprising that the tumor re-programs the myeloid precursors to express the secretory phenotype and produce VEGF, which serves to promote the vessel development rather than their maturation to DC capable of priming T cells for anti-tumor responses. The appearance of blood vessels in the tumors signals another major change in the tumor microenvironment, namely a switch from the hypoxic to oxidative metabolism. Oxidative phosphorylation with an increase in ATP synthesis is necessary to drive tumor cell proliferation, and it is enabled by angiogenesis promoted by combined activities of tumor-infiltrating leukocytes and tumor cells.

As the successful tumor progression continues, it increasingly assumes the features of chronic inflammation. The nature and composition of the inflammatory infiltrates change in concert with a shift from hypoxic to oxidative metabolism. Fibroblasts continue in the activated mode and cytokine-driven tissue repair phase is extended and subverted to provide for the synthesis of structural elements supporting tumor expansion. The tumor stroma and fibrous septae separating nests of tumor cells provide a scaffold for expanding tumor cells. These cells produce cytokines, MV, TA and other factors, which down-modulate immune responses and favor tumor progression. The tumor never "heals," and the process continues to the detriment of the host. The chronic, persistent nature of the tumor microenvironment is clearly established as a result of the failure of the host's immune system to deal with the "danger signals" generated by the tumor.

The Role of Tumor Cells in Shaping Their Local Environment

The characteristic feature of the tumor microenvironment is that it undergoes alterations in concert with tumor progression. It is for this reason that snapshots of the tumor microenvironment obtained by immunohistology of tumor sections or studies of TIL isolated from tumors at one stage of their progression provide an incomplete picture of cellular interactions *in situ*. Therefore, correlations of the numbers or phenotype of inflammatory cells in the tumor with clinical data or with patient prognosis may not be informative. Indeed, conflicting reports available in the literature regarding the significance of immune cells in the tumor microenvironment reflect the difficulties in interpretation of events that unfold and change in the context of host-tumor interactions. Interestingly, as tumor cells successively modify their microenvironment, they often adopt the phenotypic characteristics of immune cells. They co-opt signaling molecules, chemokines, selectins and their receptors normally expressed by leukocytes to serve for tumor migration, invasion and metastasis. It is likely that soluble factors produced during the immune phase, such as colony-stimulating factor (CSF-1), could contribute to this adoption by tumor cells of a myeloid-like phenotype. The plasticity of tumor cells allows them to express chemokines and chemokine receptors, which usually function as chemoattractants and activating factors in leukocytes. Functions associated with neutrophils, such as the production of extracellular proteases, including matrix metalloproteinases (MMPs) that modify the extracellular matrix and fit it into the tumor scaffolding, are also adopted by tumor cells [111]. The use of a leukocyte-like metabolism by tumor cells, i.e., their ability to metabolize glucose via the glycolytic pathway and to synthesize ROS, is another example of how the properties of leukocytes are co-opted to maintain the hypoxic state in the tumor microenvironment [112]. Masquerading as inflammatory cells, tumor cells acquire the ability to further alter the microenvironment, migrate by responding to signals and pathways normally reserved for the cells of the immune system and establish metastases to organs rich in resident macrophages, where conditions are favorable for proliferation (i.e., lung, liver and bone). Thus, the leukocytes infiltrating the tumor contribute to the maintenance of the cytokine-rich microenvironment, which facilitates adoption of the leukocyte-like phenotype by tumor cells.

Once established, the tumor microenvironment is not a friendly place for infiltrating leukocytes. While they are clearly conscripted by the host to interfere with abnormal tissue growth, once in the tumor, they come in contact with a variety of soluble factors that impede their maturation, inhibit their functions or simply induce their apoptosis [reviewed in 16]. Cytokines are known to be present in tumors and are known to affect maturation, differentiation or functions and survival of immune cells [113]. They include M-CSF, GM-CSF, IL-6, IL-10, TGFβ and other tumor-derived soluble factors [16]. The degree of impairment of immune cells in the tumor microenvironment differs widely in individual tumors. While the inhibitory effects are the strongest in the tumor, they are not confined locally but are systemic, especially in patients with advanced disease [114]. Functional abnormalities and apoptosis of T lymphocytes are seen not only at the tumor site but are common in the circulation of patients with cancer [108]. The mechanisms involved in selective and persistent inhibition of anti-tumor immune responses in patients with cancer are numerous and have been reviewed elsewhere [16].

Tumors grow progressively and metastasize despite prominent leukocyte infiltrations, largely because it evolves strategies for escape from immune intervention [16]. Consequently, the fate of immune cells infiltrating the tumor is to be corrupted by the tumor into helping its progression, to lose their functional attributes or to die. Tumor aggressiveness depends on the efficiency with which this can be accomplished.

CONCLUSIONS

Our perception of *in situ* interactions between infiltrating leukocytes and tumor cells has undergone a considerable revision in recent years, primarily as a result of new insights into molecular immunology in conjunction with newly developed animal models, as discussed above. Current evidence favors the view of the developing tumor as a site of chronic inflammatory reaction that is orchestrated by the tumor. Its success in co-opting functions of leukocytes toward promoting tumor survival depends on a variety of molecular mechanisms, and these are beginning to be elucidated. At least one link between inflammation and cancer has been identified: the NF-κB pathway can either promote survival of cells with the malignant phenotype or sustain the production of pro-inflammatory cytokines by inflammatory cells within the tumor. Thus, the same molecular pathway can be harnessed to mediate opposite effects, depending on the context of signals available in the tumor microenvironment. Dysregulated production of pro-inflammatory cytokines and chemokines, such as exists in the tumor microenvironment, can lead to tissue pathology. The challenge facing oncologists is to understand the complex role of inflammatory infiltrates in the tumor progression and to learn to disrupt the vicious cycle of chronic inflammation. Protection of immune anti-tumor effector cells in the tumor microenvironment and their survival may be the key to designing novel and more effective anti-cancer therapies of the future.

REFERENCES

1. Zhang L, Zhou W, Velculescu VE, Kern SE, Hruban RH, Hamilton SR, Vogelstein B, Kinzler KW (1997) Gene expression profiles in normal and cancer cells. Science 276:1268–72
2. Dworak HF (1986) Tumors: Wounds that do not heal. Similarities between tumor stroma generation and wound healing. N Engl J Med 315:1650–59
3. Aller MA, Arias JL, Nava MP, Arias J (2004) Posttraumatic inflammation is a complex response based on the pathological expression of the nervous, immune and endocrine function systems. Exp Biol Med 229:170–81
4. Ribatti D, Vacca A, Dammacco F (2003) New non-angiogenesis dependent pathways for tumor growth. Eur J Cancer 39:1835–41
5. Balkwill F, Mantovani A (2001) Inflammation and cancer: back to Virehow? Lancet 357 539–45
6. Mareel M, Leroy A (2003) Clinical cellular, and molecular aspects of cancer invasion. Physiol Rev 83:337–76
7. Kornstein MJ, Brooks JS, Elder DE (1983) Immunoperoxidase localization of lymphocyte subsets in the host responses to melanoma and nevi. Cancer Res 43:2749–53

8. Vacarello L, Kanbour A, Kanbour-Shakir A, Whiteside TL (1993) Tumor-infiltrating lymphocytes from ovarian tumors of low malignant potential. Int. J Gynecol Path 12:41–50
9. Von Kleist S, Berling J, Bohle W, Wittekind C (1987) Immunohistochemical analysis of lymphocyte subpopulations infiltrating breast carcinomas and benign lesions. Int J Cancer 40: 18–23
10. Bogenrieder T, Herlyn M (2003) Axis of evil: molecular mechanisms of cancer metastasis. Oncogene 22:6524–36
11. Whiteside TL (1993) Tumor Infiltrating Lymphocytes in Human Malignancies, Medical Intelligence Unit, RG Landes Co, Austin, TX.
12. Letessier E, Sacchi M, Johnson JT, Herberman RB, Whiteside TL (1990) The absence of lymphoid suppressor cells in tumor-involved lymph nodes of patients with head and neck cancer. Cell Immunol 130:446–58
13. Tanaka H, Tanaka J, Kjaergaard J, Shu S (2002) Depletion of CD4+CD25+ regulatory cells augments the generation of specific immune T cells in tumor-draining lymph nodes. J Immunother 25:207–17
14. Reichert TE, Strauss L, Wagner EM, Gooding W, Whiteside TL (2002) Signaling abnormalities and reduced proliferation of circulating and tumor-infiltrating lymphocytes in patients with oral carcinoma. Clin Cancer Res 8:3137–45
15. Fridman WH, Tartour E (1998) Macrophage – and lymphocyte produced Th1 and Th2 cytokines in the tumor microenvironment. Res Immunol 149:651–53
16. Whiteside TL, Campoli M, Ferrone S (2005) Tumor induced immune suppression and immune escape: mechanisms and possible solutions. In: Analyzing T Cell Responses. Nagorsen D, Manincola F (eds), Springer Publishers, pp. 43–82
17. Shevach EM (2004) Fatal attraction: tumors becon regulatory T cells. Nature Med 10:900–01
18. Barnes L (1996) Pathology of the head and neck: general considerations. In: Myers EN, Suen J-Y (eds) Cancer of the head and neck. WB Saunders Co., Philadelphia, PA, pp17–32
19. Chiba T, Ohtani H, Mizoi T, Naito Y, Sato E, Nagura H, Ohuchi A, Ohuchi K, Shiiba K, Kurokawa Y, Satomi S (2004) Intraepithelial CD8+ T-cell-count becomes a prognostic factor after a longer follow-up period in human colorectal carcinoma: possible association with suppression of micrometastasis. Br J Cancer 91:1711–17
20. Mihm MC, Clemente C, Cascinelli N (1996) Tumor infiltrating lymphocytes in lymph node melanoma metastases–a histopathologic prognostic indicator and an expression of local immune response. Lab Invest 74:43–47
21. Lin EY, Nguyen AV, Russell RG, Pollard JW (2001) Colony-stimulating factor 1 promotes progression of mamary tumors to malignancy. J Exp Med 193:727–40
22. Miescher S, Whiteside TL, Moretta L, Von Fliedner V (1987) Clonal and frequency analyses of tumor-infiltrating T lymphocytes from human solid tumors. J Immunol 138:4004–11
23. Weidmann E, Whiteside TL, Giorda R, Herberman RB, Trucco M (1992) The T-cell receptor V beta gene usage in tumor-infiltrating lymphocytes and blood of patients with hepatocellular carcinoma. Cancer Res 52:5913–20
24. Albers AE, Ferris RL, Kim GG, Chikamatsu K, DeLeo AB, Whiteside TL (2005) Immune response to p53 in patients with cancer: enrichment in tetramer+p53 peptide-specific T cells and regulatory T cells at tumor sites. Cancer Immunol Immunother 62:670–79
25. Albers AE, Tsukishiro T, Ferris RL, Whiteside TL, DeLeo AB (2006) T-cell receptor variable gene β-restricted T lymphocytes are sensitive to apoptosis in patients with squamous cell carcinoma of the head and neck. Clin Cancer Res 12:2394–2403
26. Weidmann E, Elder EM, Trucco M, Lotze MT, Whiteside TL (1993) Usage of T-cell receptor V beta chain genes in fresh and cultured tumor-infiltrating lymphocytes from human melanoma. Int J Cancer 54:383–90
27. Whiteside TL (1992) Tumor infiltrating lymphocytes as antitumor effector cells. Biotherapy 5:47–61
28. Whitford P, Mallon EA, George WD, Campbell AM (1990) Flow cytometric analysis of tumour infiltrating lymphocytes in breast cancer. Br J Cancer 62:971–75

29. Baxevanis CN, Dedoussis GV, Papadopoulos NG, Missitzis I, Stathopoulos GP, Papamichail M (1994) Tumor specific cytolysis by tumor infiltrating lymphocytes in breast cancer. Cancer 74:1275–82
30. NaitoY, Saito K, Shiiba K, Ohuchi A, Saigenji K, Nagura H, Ohtani H (1998) CD8+ T cells infiltrated within cancer cell nests as a prognostic factor in human colorectal cancer. Cancer Res 58:3491–94
31. Nakano O, Sato M, Naito Y, Suzuki K, Orikasa S, Aizawa M, Suzuki Y, Shintaku I, Nagura H, Ohtani H (2001) Proliferative activity of intratumoral CD8+ T lymphocytes as a prognostic factor in human renal cell carcinoma: Clinicopathologic demonstration of antitumor immunity. Cancer Res 61:5132–36
32. Sheu BC, Hsu SM, Ho HN, Lin RH, Torng PL, Huang SC (1999) Reversed CD4/CD8 percentages of tumor-infiltrating lymphocytes correlate with disease progression in human cervical cancer. Cancer 86:1537–43
33. Vitolo D, Kanbour A, Johnson JT, Herberman RB, Whiteside TL (1993) In situ hybridization for cytokine gene transcripts in the solid tumor microenvironment. Eur J Cancer 3:371–77
34. Liyanage UK, Moore TT, Joo HG, Tanaka Y, Herrmann V, Doherty G, Drebin JA, Strasberg SM, Eberlein TJ, Goedegebuure PS, Linehan DC (2002) Prevalence of regulatory T cells is increased in peripheral blood and tumor microenvironment of patients with pancreas or breast adenocarcinoma. J Immunol 169:2756–61
35. Woo EY, Chu CS, Goletz TJ, Schlienger K, Yeh H, Coukos G, Rubin SC, Kaiser LR, June CH (2001) Regulatory CD4+ CD25+ T cells in tumors from patients with early-stage non-small cell lung cancer and late stage ovarian cancer. Cancer Res 61:4766–72
36. Ramsdell F (2003) Foxp3 and natural regulatory T cells: key to a cell lineage? Immunity 19:165–68
37. Shevach EM (2000) Regulatory T cells I Autoimmunity. Annu Rev Immunol 18:423–49
38. Lee KM, Chuang E, Griffin M, Khattri R, Hong DK, Zhang W, Straus D, Samelson LE, Thompson CB, Bluestone JA (1998) Molecular basis of T-cell inactivation by CTLA-4. Science 282:2263–66
39. Stephens GL, McHugh RS, Whitters MJ, Young DA, Luxenberg D, Carreno BM, Collins M, Shevach EM (2004) Engagement of glucocorticoid induced TNFR family-related receptor on effector T cells by its ligand mediates resistance to suppression by CD4+CD25+ T cells. J Immunol 173:5008–20
40. Curiel TJ, Coukos G, Zou L, Alvarez X, Cheng P, Mottram P, Evdemon-Hogan M, Conejo-Garcia JR, Zhang L, Burow M, Zhu Y, Wei S, Kryczek I, Daniel B, Gordon A, Myers L, Lackner A, Disis ML, Knutson KL, Chen L, Zou W (2004) Specific recruitment of regulatory T cells in ovarian carcinoma fosters immune privilege and predicts reduced survival. Nature Med 10:942–49
41. Vlad G, Cortesini R, Suciu-Foca N (2005) License to heal: bidirectional interaction of antigen-specific regulatory T cells and tolerogenic APC. J Immunol 174:5907–14
42. Rabinowich H, Reichert EE, Kashii Y, Bell MC, Whiteside TL (1998) Lymphocyte apoptosis induced by Fas ligand-expressing ovarian carcinoma cells: implications for altered expression of TcR in tumor-associated lymphocytes. J Clin Invest 101:2579–88
43. Reichert TE, Rabinowich H, Johnson JT, Whiteside TL (1998) Human immune cells in the tumor microenvironment: mechanisms responsible for signaling and functional defects. J Immunother 21:295–306
44. Li X, Liu J, Park JK, Hamilton TA, Rayman P, Klein E, Edinger M, Tubbs R, Bukowski R, Finke J (1994) T cells from renal cell carcinoma patients exhibit an abnormal pattern of kappa B-specific DNA-binding activity: a preliminary report. Cancer Res 54:5424–29
45. Reichert TE, Day E, Wagner EM, Whiteside TL (1998) Absent of low expression of the ζ chain in T cells at the tumor site correlates with poor survival in patients with oral carcinoma. Cancer Res 58:5344–47
46. Uzzo RG, Rayman P, Kolenko V, Clark PE, Cathcart MK, Bloom T, Novick AC, Bukowski RM, Hamilton T, Finke JH (1999) Renal cell carcinoma-derived gangliosides suppress NFκB activation in T cells. J Clin Invest 104:769–76

47. Ling W, Rayman P, Uzzo R, Clark P, Kim HJ, Tubbs R, Novick A, Bukowski R, Hamilton T, Finke J (1998) Impaired activation of NFκB in T cells from a subset of renal cell carcinoma patients is mediated by inhibition of phosphorylation and degradation of the inhibitor, IκBα. Blood 92:1334–41
48. Uzzo RG, Clark PE, Rayman P, Bloom T, Rybicki L, Novick AC, Bukowski RM, Finke JH (1999) Alterations in NFκB activation in T lymphocytes of patients with renal cell carcinoma. J Nat Cancer Inst 91:718–721
49. Baeuerle PA, Baltimore D (1996) NF-kappa B: ten years after. Cell 87:13–20
50. May MJ, Ghosh S (1998) Signal transduction through NF-κB. Immunol Today 19:80–88
51. Kuss I, Saito T, Johnson JT, Whiteside TL (1999) Clinical significance of decreased ζ chain expression in peripheral blood lymphocytes of patients with head and neck cancer. Clin Cancer Res 5:329–34
52. Whiteside TL (2004) Down-regulation of ζ chain expression in T cells: A biomarker of prognosis in cancer? Cancer Immunol Immunother 53:865–76
53. Al-Sarireh B, Eremin O (2000) Tumour-associated macrophages (TAMS): disordered function, immune suppression and progressive tumour growth. JR Coll Surg Edinb 45:1–16
54. Liu YJ (2001) Dendritic cell subsets and lineages and their functions in innate and adoptive immunity. Cell 106:259–62
55. Hansson M, Asea A, Ericsson U, Hermodsson S, Hellstrand K (1996) Induction of apoptosis in NK cells by monocyte-derived reactive oxygen metabolites. J Immunol 156:42–47
56. Kiessling R, Kono K, Petersson M, Wasserman K (1996) Immunosuppression in human tumor-host interaction: role of cytokines and alterations in signal-transducing molecules. Springer Sem Immunopathol 18:227–42
57. Malmberg KJ, Arulampalam V, Ichihara F, Petersson M, et al (2001) Inhibition of activated/memory (CD45RO(+)) T cells by oxidative stress associated with block of NK-kappaB activation. J Immunol 167:2595–2601
58. Leek RD, Lewis CE, Whitehouse R, Greenall M, Clarke J, Harris AL (1996) Association of macrophage infiltration with angiogenesis and prognosis in invasive breast carcinoma. Cancer Res 56: 4625–29
59. Banchereau J, Briere F, Caux C, Davoust J, et al (2000) Immunobiology of dendritic cells. Annu Rev Immunol 18:767–811
60. Banchereau J, Steinman RM (1998) Dendritic cells and the control of immunity. Nature 392: 245–52
61. Treilleux I, Blay JY, Bendriss-Vermare N, Ray-Coquard K, Bachelot T, Guastalla JP, Bremond A, Goddard S, Pin JJ, Barthelemy-Dubois C, Lebecque S (2004) Dendritic cell infiltration and prognosis of early stage breast cancer. Clin Cancer Res 10:7466–74
62. Gabrilovich D (2004) Mechanisms and functional significance of tumor-induced dendritic cell defects. Nature Med 4:941–52
63. Almand B, Resser JR, Lindman B, Nadaf S, Clark JI, Kwon ED, Carbone DP, Gabrilovich DI (2000) Clinical significance of defective dendritic cell differentiation in cancer. Clin Cancer Res 6:1755–66
64. Hoffmann TK, Dworacki G, Tsukihiro T, Meidenbauer N, Gooding W, Johnson JT, Whiteside TL (2002) Spontaneous apoptosis of circulating T lymphocytes in patients with head and neck cancer and its clinical importance. Clin Cancer Res 8:2553–2562
65. Troy AJ, Summers KL, Davidson PJ, Atkinson CH, Hart DN (1998) Minimal recruitment and activation of dendritic cells in within renal cell carcinoma. Clin Cancer Res 4:585–93
66. Esche C, Shurin GV, Kirkwood JM, Wang GQ, Rabinowich H, Pirtskhalaishvili G, Shurin MR (2001) Tumor necrosis factor-alpha-promoted expression of Bcl-2 and inhibition of mitochondrial cytochrome c release mediated resistance of mature dendritic cells to melanoma-induced apoptosis. Clin Cancer Res 7:974s-79s
67. Gabrilovich DI, Corak J, Ciernik IF, Kavanaugh D, Carbone DP (1997) Decreased antigen presentation by dendritic cells in patients with breast cancer. Clin Cancer Res 3:483–90

68. Esche C, Lokshin A, Shurin GV, Gastman BR, Rabinowich H, Watkins SC, Lotze MT, Shurin MR (1999) Tumor's other immune targets: dendritic cells. J Leukocyte Biol 66:336–44
69. Shurin MR, Esche C, Lokshin A, Lotze MT (1999) Apoptosis in dendritic cells. In: Dendritic Cells: Biology and Clinical Applications, Lotze MT, Thomson AW (eds), Academic Press, New York, pp.673–92
70. Shurin GV, Shurin MR, Bykovskaja S, Shogan J, Lotze MT, Barksdale EM Jr (2001) Neuroblastoma-derived gangliosides inhibit dendritic cell generation and function. Cancer Res 61:363–69
71. Gabrilovich DI, Ishida T, Nadaf S, Ohm JE, Carbone DP (1999) Antibodies to vascular endothelial growth factor enhance the efficacy of cancer immunotherapy by improving endogenous dendritic cell functions. Clin Cancer Res 5:2963–70
72. Whiteside TL, Stanson J, Shurin MR, Ferrone S (2004) Antigen processing machinery (APM) in human dendritic cells: up-regulation by maturation and down-regulation by tumor cells. J Immunol 173:1526–34
73. Tourkova IL, Shurin GV, Chatta GS, Perez L, Finke J, Whiteside TL, Ferrone S, Shurin MR (2005) Restoration by IL-15 of MHC class I antigen processing machinery in human dendritic cells inhibited by tumor-derived gangliosides. J Immunol In Press
74. Becker Y (1993) Dendritic cell activity against primary tumors: an overview. In Vivo 7: 187–91
75. Reichert TE, Scheuer C, Day R, Wagner W, Whiteside TL (2001) The number of intratumoral dendritic cells and ζ-chain expression in T cells as prognostic and survival biomarkers in patients with oral carcinoma. Cancer 91:2136–47
76. Giannini A, Bianchi S, Messerini L, Gallo O, Gallina E, Asprella Libonati G, Olmi P, Zampi G (1991) Prognostic significance of accessory cells and lymphocytes in nasopharygeal carcinoma. Pathol Res Pract 187:496–502
77. Goldman SA, Baker E, Weyant RJ, Clarke MR, Myers JN, Lotze MT (1998) Peritumoral CD1a-positive dendritic cells are associated with improved survival in patients with tongue carcinoma. Arch Otolaryngol Head Neck Surg 124:641–46
78. Furukawa T, Watanabe S, Kodama T, Sato Y, Shimosato Y, Suemasu K (1985) T-zone histiocytes in adenocarcinoma of the lung in relation to postoperative prognosis. Cancer 56:2651–656
79. Lespagnard L, Gancberg D, Rouas G, Leclercq G, de Saint-Aubain Somerhausen N, Di Leo A, Piccart M, Verhest A, Larsimont D (1999) Tumor-infiltrating dendritic cells in adenocarcinomas of the breast: a study of 143 neoplasms with a correlation to usual prognostic factors and to clinical outcome. Int J Cancer 84:309–14
80. Tsujitani S, Furukawa T, Tamada R, Okamura T, Yasumoto K, Sugimachi K (1987) Langerhans cells and prognosis in patients with gastric carcinoma. Cancer 59:501–05
81. Tsujitani S, Kakeji Y, Watanabe A, Kohnoe S, Maehara Y, Sugimachi K (1990) Infiltration of dendritic cells in relation to tumor invasion and lymph node metastasis in human gastric cancer. Cancer 66:2012–16
82. Murphy GF, Radu A, Kaminer M, Berg D (1993) Autologous melanoma vaccine induces inflammatory responses in melanoma metastases: relevance to immunologic regression and immunotherapy. J Invest Dermatol 100:335S-341S
83. O'Brien PM, Tsirimonaki E, Coomber DW, Millan DW, Davis JA, Campo MS (2001) Immunoglobin genes expressed by B-lymphocytes infiltrating cervical carcinomas show evidence of antigen-driven selection. Cancer Immunol Immunother 50:523–32
84. Coronella JA, Telleman P, Kingsbury GA, Truong TD, Hays S, Junghans RP (2001) Evidence for an antigen-driven humoral immune response in medullary ductal breast cancer. Cancer Res 61:7889–99
85. Fisher ER, Kenny JP, Sass R, Dimitrov NV, Siderits RH, Fisher B (1990) Medullary cancer of the breast revisited. Breast Cancer Res Treat 16:215–29
86. Coronella JA, Spier C, Welch M, Trevor KT, Stopeck AT, Villar H, Hersh EM (2002) Antigen-driven oligoclonal expansion of tumor-infiltrating B cells in infiltrating ductal carcinoma of the breast. J Immunol 169:1829–1836

87. Hansen MH, Nielsen HV, Ditzel HJ (2001) The tumor-infiltrating B cell response in medullary breast cancer is oligoclonal and directed against the autoantigen actin exposed on the surface of apoptotic tumor cells. PNAS 98:12659–64
88. Nzula S, Going JJ, Stott DI (2003) Antigen-driven clonal proliferation, somatic hypermutation and selection of B lymphocytes infiltrating human ductal breast carcinomas. Cancer Res 63:3275–80
89. Kotlan B, Simsa P, Foldi J, Fridman WH, Glassy M, McKnight M, Teillaud JL (2003) Immunoglobulin repertoire of B lymphocytes infiltrating breast medullary carcinoma. Hum Antibodies 12:113–21
90. Almand B, Clark JI, Nikitina E, van Beynen J, English NR, Knight SC, Carone DP, Gabrilovich DI (2001) Increased production of immature myeloid cells in cancer patients: a mechanism of immunosuppression in cancer. J Immunol 166:678–89
91. Otsuji M, Kimura Y, Aoe T, Okamoto Y, Saito T (1996) Oxidative stress by tumor-derived macrophagessuppresses the expression of CD3 ζ chain of T-cell receptor complex and antigen-specific cell responses. PNAS 93:13119–24
92. Schmielau J, Finn OJ (2001) Activated granulocytes and granulocyte-derived hydrogen peroxide are the underlying mechanism of suppression of T-cell function in advanced cancer patients. Cancer Res 61:4756–60
93. Phillips SM, Banerjea A, Feakins R, Li SR, Bustin SA, Dorudi S (2004) Tumour-infiltrating lymphocytes in colorectal cancer with microsatellite instability are activated and cytotoxic. Br J Cancer 91:469–75
94. Balkwill F, Coussens LM (2004) Cancer: An inflammatory link. Nature 431:405–06
95. Gallucci S, Matzinger P (2001) Danger signals: SOS to the immune system. Curr Opin Immunol 13:114–19
96. Matzinger P (1998) An innate sense of danger. Semin Immunol 10:399–415
97. Janeway CA, Jr (1992) The immune system evolved to discriminate infectious nonself from noninfectious self. Immunol Today 13:11–16
98. Whiteside TL, Vujanovic NL, Herberman RB (1998) Natural killer cells and tumor therapy. Curr Topics Microbiol Immunol 230:221–44
99. Lanier LL (2003) Natural killer cell receptor signaling. Curr Opin Immunol 15:308–14
100. Whiteside TL, Rabinowich H (1998) The role of Fas/FasL in immunosuppression induced by human tumors. Cancer Immunol Immunother 46:175–184
101. Denko NC, Fontana LA, Hudson KM, Sutphin PD, Raychaudhuri S, Altman R, Giaccia AJ (2003) Investigating hypoxic tumor physiology through gene expression patterns. Oncogene 22:5907–14
102. Sitkovsky MV, Lukashev D, Apasov S, Kojima H, Koshiba M, Caldwell C, Ohta A, Thiel M (2004) Physiological control of immune response and inflammatory tissue damage by hypoxia-inducible factors and adenosine A_{2A} receptors. Annu Rev Immunol 22:21.1–22.26
103. Hanada T, Yoshimura A (2002) Regulation of cytokine signaling and inflammation. Cytokine Growth Factor Rev 13:413–21
104. Greten FR, Eckmann L, Greten TF, Park JM, Li ZW, Egan LJ, Kagnoff MF, Karin M (2004) IKKbeta links inflammation and tumorigenesis in a mouse model of colitis-associated cancer. Cell 118:285–96
105. Pikarsky E, Porat RM, Stein I, Abramovitch R, Amit S, Kasem S, Gutkovich-Pyest E, Urieli-Shoval S, Galun E, Ben-Neriah Y (2004) NF-kappa B functions as a tumor promoter in inflammation-associated cancer. Nature 431:461–66
106. Balkwill F (2004) Cancer and the chemokine network. Nat Rev Cancer 4:540–50
107. Malik STA, Griffin DB, Fiers W, Balkwill FR (1989) Paradoxical effects of tumor necrosis factor in experimental ovarian cancer. Int J Cancer 44:918–25
108. Bamias A, Dimipoulos MA (2003) Angiogenesis in human cancer: implications in cancer therapy. Eur J Intern Med 14:459–69
109. Gabrilovich DI, Chen HL, Girgis KR, Cunningham HT, Meny GM, Nadaf S, Kavanaugh D, Carbone DP (1996) Vascular endothelial growth factor produced by human tumors inhibits the functional maturation of dendritic cells. Nature Med 2:1096–1103
110. Ellis LM, Fidler IJ (1996) Angiogenesis and metastasis. Eur J Cancer 32A:2451–60

111. Engbring JA, Kleinman HK (2003) The basement membrane matrix in malignancy. J Pathol 200:465–70
112. Borregaard N, Herlin T (1982) Energy metabolism of human neutrophils during phagocytosis. J Clin Invest 70:550–57
113. Toi M (2002) Proinflammation in human tumor microenvironment: its status and implication. Med Sci Monit 8:25–26
114. Whiteside TL (2002) Tumor-induced death of immune cells: its mechanisms and consequences. Sem Cancer Biol 12:43–50

PART 2

TUMOR VACCINES

CHAPTER 8

PEPTIDE AND PROTEIN VACCINES FOR CANCER

RAYMOND M. WONG AND JEFFREY S. WEBER

Departments of Molecular Microbiology and Immunology and Medicine, Keck School of Medicine, University of Southern California, Los Angeles, CA

IMMUNE SURVEILLANCE: WHAT IS THE EVIDENCE THAT THE IMMUNE SYSTEM CONTROLS CANCER?

The immune surveillance theory, first proposed by Frank Burnet and Lewis Thomas in the 1950s, hypothesizes that the immune system specifically recognizes and destroys transformed cells [1]. Although debate regarding the relevance of immunity in cancer has persisted over the last half century, the discovery of tumor antigens recognized by T cells provides clear evidence that cellular and serologic immune responses against tumors do exist. Studies in animals have established an important role for both innate and adaptive immunity in tumor rejection and modulation of tumor growth. T cells appear to be critical mediators of adaptive immunity against antigen-expressing tumor cells. Tumor-infiltrating lymphocytes (TILs) isolated from melanoma lesions can recognize autologous and human leukocyte antigen (HLA)-matched tumor cells *in vitro* [2, 3]. Furthermore, T cell reactivity against tumor antigens can often be identified in the peripheral blood of cancer patients and healthy donors. Advances in our understanding of antigen presentation and T cell activation have provided the foundation for rationally-designed immunotherapy strategies that induce anti-tumor immune responses in cancer patients while limiting toxicity. Many of these have shown efficacy in animal models. However, peptide- and protein-based vaccine clinical trials, and clinical trials of adoptive T cell transfer, have thus far been promising but have not demonstrated consistent clinical benefit.

ANTIGEN-PRESENTING CELLS AND T CELL ACTIVATION

Dendritic cells (DCs) are derived from myeloid progenitors within the bone marrow and are involved in initiating immune responses [4]. DCs initially have an immature phenotype characterized by low surface expression of both major histocompatibility

H.L. Kaufman and J.D. Wolchok (eds.), General Principles of Tumor Immunotherapy, 171–192.

complex (MHC) and B7 co-stimulatory molecules [5]. Immature DCs are not potent stimulators of naïve T cells, but are very active in capturing antigens by phagocytosis and macropinocytosis. After persisting at sites of infection for a variable length of time, immature DCs migrate via the lymphatics to the secondary lymphoid tissues where they attain a mature phenotype during interaction with T cells. Mature DCs no longer take up antigen efficiently but express high levels of MHC class I and class II proteins for a prolonged time. They also express high levels of B7, other co-stimulatory and adhesion molecules, and secrete chemokines that specifically attract T cells. These properties help explain their ability to prime naïve T cells and stimulate robust T cell clonal expansion – properties important for generating effective immune responses to tumor antigens.

Specific rejection of tumor tissue requires that transformed cells be distinguished immunologically from their normal counterparts. Peptide fragments presented on the cell surface by MHC molecules provide the basis for specific recognition by T cells. Tumor cells present peptides derived from endogenous and foreign proteins, such as those encoded by viruses. However, tumor cells are not intrinsically immunogenic due to associated immunosuppressive characteristics, such as secretion of cytokines (e.g. TGF-β, IL-10) that down-regulate cellular immunity, antigenic down-modulation, and lack of B7 co-stimulatory molecules and adhesion molecules necessary to interact with and activate naïve T cells. T cell receptor (TCR) signaling in the absence of co-stimulation not only fails to activate naïve T cells, but also leads to anergy (peripheral tolerance). Such self-tolerance can be broken by an intermediary process of immune stimulation initiated by professional APCs such as DCs. DCs presenting "self" peptides and expressing sufficient levels of co-stimulatory molecules can activate self-reactive naïve T cells at the tumor site or distantly in secondary lymphoid organs. Cancer vaccine strategies must exploit this process directly or indirectly in order to break tolerance and generate immune responses against tumor antigens, many of which are "self" antigens as discussed below.

T CELLS RECOGNIZE PEPTIDES DERIVED FROM TUMOR ANTIGENS

The molecular definition of tumor antigens recognized by T cells has provided exciting new possibilities for the development of effective immunotherapy for cancer. In 1991, Boon and colleagues identified the first tumor-associated antigen recognized by T cells [6]. This protein, termed "melanoma-antigen E-1" (MAGE-1), was found in a variety of tumor types as well as normal testis and placental tissue, but no other normal tissue. Other tumor antigens have since been identified using a variety of techniques including (1) "reverse immunology," whereby specific T cells are generated *in vitro* against peptide sequences derived from serologically defined tumor antigens, (2) acid stripping of peptides from tumor cells followed by mass spectroscopy, (3) serological analysis of cDNA expression libraries (SEREX), (4) molecular cloning (5) proteomics, and (6) DNA microarray analysis. To date, over 70 tumor antigens have been identified for a multitude of cancers. Collectively, these studies have demonstrated that true tumor regression antigens exist, and provided additional rationale for their use in treating cancer.

Tumor antigens are broadly classified into two categories: (1) tumor-specific and (2) tumor-associated. They can be thought of as comprising five specific groups (Table 1). Tumor-specific antigens include the E6 and E7 oncoproteins of Human

Table 1. Tumor Antigens Recognized by T Cells

Class	Antigen	Tumor
Viral	HPV E6, E7	Cervical
	EBV LMP1, 2	lymphoma, nasopharyngeal, gastric
	HTLV Env	lymphoma, leukemia
Cancer-Testis	MAGE	melanoma, breast, lung, colon, bladder,head/neck, sarcomas, esophageal, laryngeal, leukemia, thyroid, prostate
	BAGE	melanoma, breast, bladder, head/neck, lung, sarcomas
	RAGE	melanoma, breast, colon, bladder, renal, sarcomas, head/neck
	GAGE	melanoma, breast, lung, esophageal, leukemia, sarcomas, seminoma, head/neck, prostate
	LAGE	lung
	SAGE	lung, sarcomas
	NY-ESO-1	melanoma, breast, lymphoma, bladder, lung, prostate, ovarian, thyroid, head/neck, sarcomas, liver
	SSX	melanoma
Differentiation	Melan A/MART-1	melanoma
	pMel17/gp100	melanoma
	SART-1, 2, 3	lung, esophageal, head/neck, adenocarcinomas, uterine, leukemia, renal, brain
	Tyrosinase	melanoma
	PSA	prostate
	CEA	melanoma, breast, lung, pancreatic, gastric, rectal, colon
	TRP-1, 2	melanoma
	HER-2/Neu	melanoma, breast, ovarian, gastric, pancreatic
Mutations	MUM-1, 2, 3	melanoma
	β-catenin	melanoma
	p14	melanoma
	p16	melanoma
	ras	melanoma
	HLA-A2	renal
	HLA-A11	melanoma
Carbohydrate	MUC-1, 2	breast, colon, ovarian, lymphoma, myeloma, pancreas

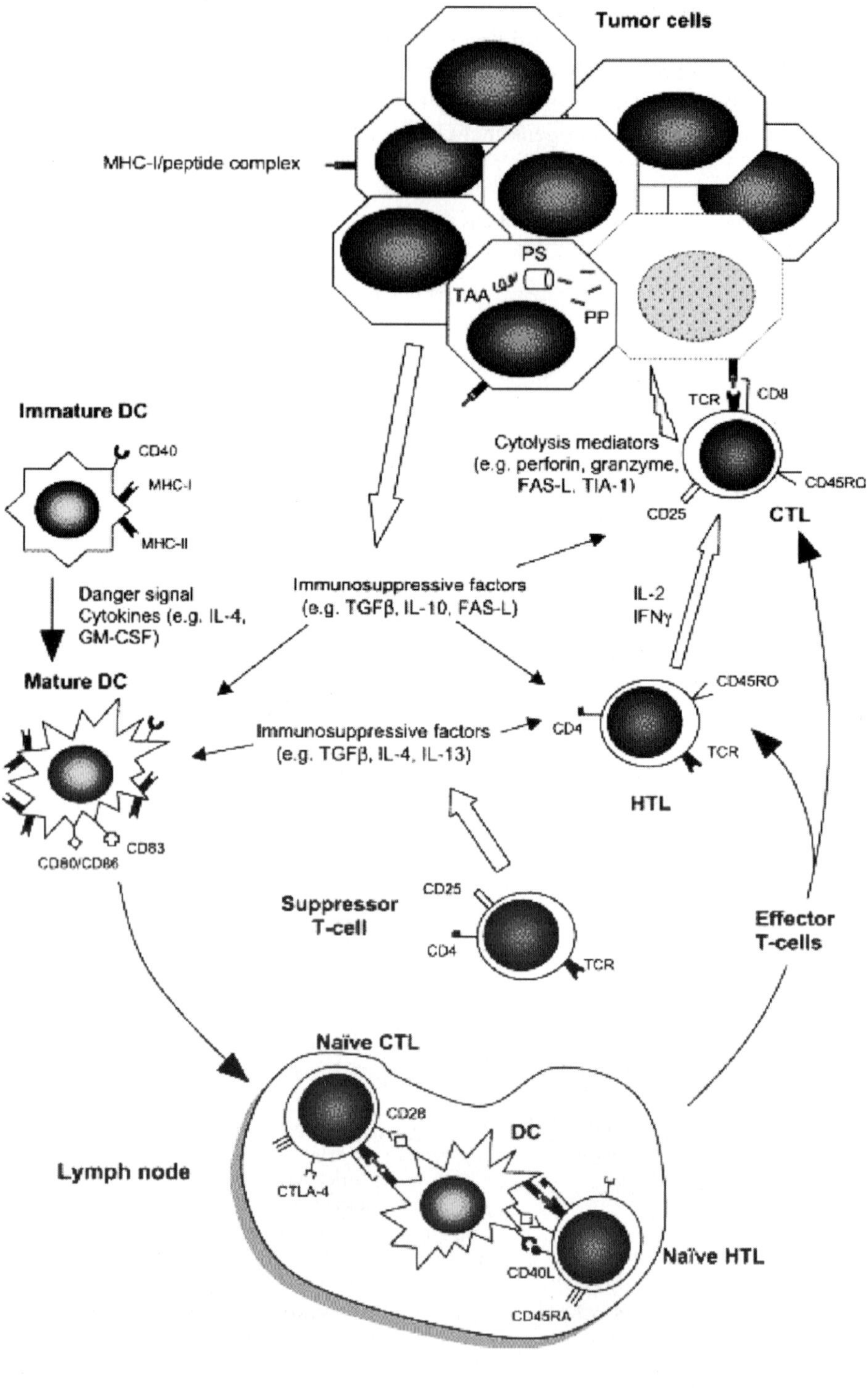
Tumor cells
MHC-I/peptide complex
PS
TAA
PP
Immature DC
CD40
MHC-I
MHC-II
TCR
CD8
Cytolysis mediators
(e.g. perforin, granzyme,
FAS-L, TIA-1)
CD45RO
CD25
CTL
Danger signal
Cytokines (e.g. IL-4,
GM-CSF)
Immunosuppressive factors
(e.g. TGFβ, IL-10, FAS-L)
IL-2
IFNγ
Mature DC
CD45RO
CD4
TCR
Immunosuppressive factors
(e.g. TGFβ, IL-4, IL-13)
HTL
CD80/CD86
CD83
CD25
Suppressor
T-cell
CD4
TCR
Effector
T-cells
Naïve CTL
CD28
DC
Lymph node
CTLA-4
Naïve HTL
CD40L
CD45RA

Papilloma Virus (HPV), a transforming virus associated with human cervical carcinomas [7]. Cells that are transformed by the same virus, such as HPV, express antigens that are distinguished as "non-self" since they are not present in normal tissue. Mutagenic events in tumors can give rise to novel epitopes that are, in turn, also recognized as "non-self" within the context of MHC. For example, TILs from cancer patients have been shown to recognize mutated forms of growth arrest-specific protein 7 (GAS7), glyceraldehyde-3-phosphate dehydrogenase (GAPDH), $p14^{ARF}$, $p16^{INK4A}$, and HLA-A11 [8,9]. Tumors bearing such mutations are antigenically unique, and immune recognition is individually tumor-specific since the likelihood of the same mutation occurring independently in tumors from different patients is low.

Abnormal post-translational modifications of normal cellular proteins can also result in antigenic differences between normal and tumor cells. Mucin 1 (MUC-1), for example, is a transmembrane protein on ductal epithelial cells that is normally heavily glycosylated. Loss of the glycosylation pattern exposes the mucin peptide backbone to T cell recognition, which involves MHC-independent interaction with the αβ TCR in a manner analogous to TCR interaction with bacterial superantigens [10]. MUC-1 can also be a source of peptides presented in association with MHC class I [11].

Most tumor-associated antigens examined thus far result from *de novo* or over-expressed normal cellular proteins. They are present on both transformed and normal tissue, but their appearance on the latter are under conditions (such as lack of MHC expression or low MHC:peptide concentration) that result in tolerance. Cancer-testis antigens (such as the MAGE family, SSX-2, TRP-2, SOX10, and NY-ESO-1) are normally found only in specialized tissues such as the testes and placenta, but are often aberrantly expressed in a variety of different tumor types [12,13]. Differentiation antigens are expressed only during a certain stage of tissue

Figure 1. Scheme of HLA-restricted immune response against cancer. Peptide-loaded mature dendritic cells can prime naïve T cells, which become activated effector cells able to recognize and kill tumor cells expressing the peptide/MHC complex. Tumor cells and regulatory T cells (the latter characterized by the co-expression of CD25 and CD4) can produce immunosuppressive factors that may inhibit both the maturation of dendritic cells, and the activation of T cells. Abbreviations: TAA, tumor associated antigen; PS, proteasome; PP, peptides; DC, dendritic cell; CTL, cytotoxic T lymphocyte; HTL, helper T lymphocyte; IL-2, interleukin-2; IL-4, interleukin-4; IL-10, interleukin-10; IL-13, interleukin-13; IFNγ, interferon-gamma; TGFβ, transforming growth factor-beta; GM-CSF, granulocyte-macrophage colony stimulating factor; TCR, T cell receptor; FAS-L, FAS ligand; TIA-1, cytotoxic granule associated protein; CD40, receptor for CD40L (activation of dendritic cells); CD40L, CD40 ligand; CD83, cell surface antigen expressed by mature dendritic cells; CD80/CD86 (also known as B7.1/B7.2), ligands for CD28 and CTLA-4; CD28, T cell stimulatory receptor (co-stimulatory signal); CTLA-4, T cell inhibitory receptor; CD25, IL-2 receptor; CD45RA and CD45RO, isoforms of CD45 (transmembrane protein tyrosine phosphatase involved in TCR signal transduction) expressed by naïve and effector T cells, respectively. *Reprinted from Biochim Biophys Acta, Volume 1653*(2) *Mocellin S, Rossi CR, Nitti D, Lise M, Marincola FM, Dissecting tumor responsiveness to immunotherapy: the experience of peptide-based melanoma vaccines, Pages 61–71, Copyright 2003, with permission from Elsevier*

development, probably early in embryonic life. Tumors arising from a particular tissue type will often express differentiation antigens characteristic of that tissue. For example, Melan A/MART-1 and pMel17/gp100 are melanosome-related differentiation antigens commonly over-expressed in melanoma cells [14]. These antigens may be uniquely expressed by an individual tumor, although some appear to be shared among tumors of varying origins.

CELLULAR IMMUNOTHERAPY FOR CANCER: T CELL RECOGNITION OF PEPTIDES

Pre-clinical human studies conducted at the National Cancer Institute in the 1980s demonstrated that $CD3^+/CD8^+/CD4^-$ and $CD3^+/CD8^-/CD4^+$ TILs could be isolated from melanoma lesions and expanded *in-vitro* with interleukin(IL)-2 (2). The expanded $CD3^+/CD8^+/CD4^-$ TIL populations lysed autologous and HLA-matched – but not allogeneic – melanoma cells in culture. These findings helped establish the foundation for T cell-based cancer immunotherapy.

In one trial of adoptive T cell transfer in cancer patients, TILs were isolated from melanoma excisional biopsies and rapidly expanded with IL-2, an anti-CD3 antibody, and allogeneic peripheral blood mononuclear feeder cells [15]. Thirty-five patients with metastatic melanoma underwent nonmyeloablative lymphodepleting chemotherapy using cyclophosphamide (60 mg/kg) and fludarabine (25 mg/m^2), followed by intravenous infusion of autologous TILs and high-dose IL-2 (720,000 IU/kg). Partial or complete tumor regression was observed in 18 of the 35 patients. Objective clinical improvements correlated with the *in vivo* persistence of the transferred lymphocyte clonotypes [16].

Biochemical characterizations of TCR and MHC: peptide interactions have furthered our understanding of how T cells are capable of specifically recognizing tumors. $CD8^+$ cytotoxic T lymphocytes (CTLs) recognize short peptides ($\sim$8-12 amino acids), derived from intracellular cytoplasmic proteins, that are presented by MHC class I molecules. Upon activation, CTLs are capable of secreting cytokines and directly killing tumor cells that express sufficient levels of the appropriate MHC class I-restricted peptide epitopes. The anti-tumor cytotoxic function of CTLs is primarily mediated by apoptotic signaling via lytic granule (containing perforin and granzymes) secretion and Fas/Fas Ligand engagement. $CD4^+$ Helper T lymphocytes (HTLs) typically recognize longer peptides (13 amino acids or more) generated in acidified vesicular compartments and subsequently presented within the context of MHC class II. MHC class II molecules are generally loaded with peptides derived from extracellular sources, although it is now evident that they also bind peptides from intracellular-derived proteins. The primary functions of HTLs involve promotion of B cell activation and generation of CTLs. However, a subtype of HTLs reactive to melanoma and lymphomas were shown to have MHC class II-restricted cytotoxic capability against antigen-expressing cells [17–19].

CLINICAL EXPERIENCES WITH PEPTIDE VACCINES: ADJUVANTS, CYTOKINES, AND DENDRITIC CELLS

The largest clinical experience in cancer immunotherapy has been attained with melanoma patients. Melanoma has been considered an immunogenic tumor for a number of reasons: (1) spontaneous regression of the primary lesion is often observed, (2) the clinical prognosis in melanoma is correlated with the lymphocytic infiltrate within the primary lesion, (3) tumor regression can be achieved with immune therapies such as IL-2 and interferon (IFN)-α administration, adoptive transfer of T cells, and vaccine manipulations. Spurred by early findings that $CD8^+$ T cells propagated from patient TIL populations and peripheral blood could lyse melanoma cells *in vitro*, much work has been done to identify MHC class I-restricted peptides capable of inducing anti-tumor CTL responses. With increased focus on the role of HTLs in anti-tumor immunity, identification of immunogenic MHC class II-restricted peptides derived from tumor antigens is progressing rapidly.

Numerous vaccine trials using synthetic peptides derived from some of the tumor antigens listed in Table 1 have been initiated in patients with various types of cancers. Peptides have been administered in aqueous solution or with immune adjuvants including (1) Montanide ISA 51/Incomplete Freund's Adjuvant (2) aluminum hydroxide (3) QS-21 (a natural saponin), and (4) AS02B, which contains QS-21 and monophosphoryl lipid A. In order to maximize T cell generation against tumor antigens, many of which are normal cellular proteins and therefore intrinsically weak immunogens, cancer vaccine regimens often involve repetitive booster immunizations over a period of weeks to months. Induction of T cells against immunizing peptides can be quantified directly from the peripheral blood by MHC:peptide tetramer staining, an assay that utilizes soluble MHC molecules loaded with a peptide of interest. Functional immune responses are often measured *in vitro* by the enzyme-linked immunosorbant assay (ELISA), the enzyme-linked immunospot (ELISpot) assay, cytokine flow cytometry, proliferation assays, and cytotoxicity (lysis) assays.

Spontaneous humoral and CTL immune responses to cancer-testis antigen NY-ESO-1 have been detected in 40–50% of patients with advanced NY-ESO-1-expressing tumors, including melanoma. In one trial, 12 patients with metastatic NY-ESO-1-expressing cancers were vaccinated intradermally with three HLA-A2-binding NY-ESO-1 peptides mixed in a saline solution [20]. Seven patients were NY-ESO-1 serum antibody-negative, and five patients were NY-ESO-1 serum antibody-positive prior to the study. Peptide-specific CTL responses and delayed-type hypersensitivity (DTH) reactivity were generated in 4 of 7 NY-ESO-1 antibody-negative patients. Induction of a specific CTL response to NY-ESO-1 in immunized antibody-negative patients was associated with stabilization of disease and objective regression of individual tumors. Stabilization of disease and regression of individual metastases were observed in 3 of 5 immunized NY-ESO-1 antibody-positive patients, despite the lack of detectable immune responses against the immunizing NY-ESO-1 peptides. This study demonstrated that NY-ESO-1-specific CTLs can be induced by intradermal immunization with NY-ESO-1 peptides.

Exogenous cytokines and other immune stimulants have been included in some cancer vaccine regimens to induce local generation of DCs and/or enhance T cell proliferation. Granulocyte-macrophage colony-stimulating factor (GM-CSF) induces the differentiation of DCs from bone marrow precursors. GM-CSF-transfected cell vaccines can induce specific, long-lasting anti-tumor immunity in mice [21]. In a study comparing adjuvants and differing ways of delivering peptides, melanoma patients were vaccinated with peptides in Montanide ISA 51 + GM-CSF (group 1) or with peptide-loaded DCs (group 2) [22]. In group 1, CTL responses to the immunizing melanoma peptides were observed in 42% of patient peripheral blood lymphocyte (PBL) samples and 80% of patient sentinel immunized nodes (SINs, the node draining a vaccine site). In group 2, they were observed in only 11% and 13%, respectively. The overall immune response was also greater in group 1 ($p < .02$). Furthermore, two objective clinical responses (assessed by measurement of metastatic deposits via computed tomography scan) were observed in group 1, compared to only one in group 2. In a separate study, the same authors combined twelve peptides derived from melanocyte differentiation and cancer-testis antigens in a single mixture and vaccinated patients with resected stage IIB, III, or IV melanoma [23]. Five of the twelve peptides included in this mixture had not previously been evaluated for their *in vivo* immunogenicity. Three of these five peptides (MAGE-A1_{96-104}, MAGE-A$10_{254-262}$, and gp$100_{614-622}$)were immunogenic when administered in Montanide ISA 51 with GM-CSF. T cell IFNγsecretion in response to peptide-loaded target cells was detected in the peripheral blood and in the SIN after three weekly injections. However, immune responses generally diminished quickly over time following the third injection.

Keyhole limpet hemocyanin (KLH), a copper-containing protein found in arthropods and mollusca, is a protein that primes potent HTL responses in humans [24]. The combination of GM-CSF and KLH has been tested to assess if it would enhance CTL responses to a tyrosinase peptide vaccine [25]. Forty-three disease-free, high-risk melanoma patients received six vaccinations with tyrosinase peptides alone, with either GM-CSF or KLH, or with a combination of both adjuvants. The primary end point was the induction of tyrosinase-specific CTLs in the peripheral blood after vaccination. Tyrosinase-specific, IFNγ-secreting CTLs were detected as early as two weeks after the second vaccination in 5 of 9 patients who received the tyrosinase peptides with GM-CSF and KLH, but not in any patient vaccinated without adjuvants or with either adjuvant alone. The combined application of GM-CSF and KLH was associated with early induction of T cell responses and appeared to be an effective adjuvant combination.

Flt3 ligand (FL) is a hematopoietic growth factor shown to increase the number of immature DCs in the blood and other tissues. Subcutaneous injection of FL daily for 14 of every 28 days has been reported to increase immature CD11c^{+} and CD123^{+} peripheral blood DCs in melanoma vaccine patients [26]. Monocytosis, granulocytosis, and thrombocytosis were also observed. Additional topical application of imiquimod, a Toll-like receptor-7 ligand that induces DC maturation, at peptide vaccination sites induced DTH skin reactions to peptide vaccination (influenza, tyrosinase, MART-1, and NY-ESO-1) and enhanced the induction of circulating peptide-specific CTLs, compared to patients not treated with imiquimod. *In vivo* maturation of FL-generated DCs using imiquimod appeared to increase immune responses to tumor antigens after vaccination.

DCs can be cultured *ex vivo* from peripheral blood monocyte precursors using GM-CSF and IL-4. They can be matured using various activating agents including tumor necrosis factor (TNF)-α, IL-1β, IL-6, and prostaglandin-E2. Infusions of peptide-loaded autologous DCs can induce CTL and HTL responses detected in the peripheral blood of patients with various cancer types [27–35]. Despite promising results from early phase clinical trials for a number of different cancers, this strategy is technically complex due to the necessity of obtaining and culturing DC precursors from large leukapheresis specimens.

IL-2 is a lymphoproliferative cytokine that enhances T cell-mediated anti-tumor immunity in mice [36]. TCR stimulation can enhance the responsiveness of T cells to IL-2 by triggering rapid up-regulation of the high-affinity IL-2 receptor. Administration of varying levels of IL-2, either concurrently or on a delayed schedule, with peptide-based melanoma vaccines have been evaluated by a number of investigators. Improved induction of CTLs has generally not been observed with IL-2 administration, and in some cases a surprising reduction in reactivity against immunizing peptides has been observed. In a study assessing the value of low-dose IL-2 as a systemic adjuvant to a peptide vaccine for melanoma, T cell responses to melanoma peptides were observed in 37% of PBLs and 38% of SINs from patients receiving IL-2 with concurrent vaccination [37]. This was compared to 53% of PBLs and 83% of SINs from those receiving IL-2 twenty-eight days after vaccination. The magnitude of T cell responses was higher in the group receiving IL-2 on a delayed schedule. However, clinical benefit (measured by disease-free survival estimates) was noted in the patients receiving IL-2 with concurrent peptide vaccination. This may have been the result of augmented endogenous anti-tumor activity by IL-2, independent of vaccine-induced immunity. The systemic toxicities attributable to IL-2 administration include increased capillary permeability resulting in cardiac depression, pulmonary edema and generalized body edema. However, toxicities associated with low-dose IL-2 regimens have generally been minor, such as low-grade fevers, clinically insignificant hepatic toxicity, mild anemia, and mild thrombocytosis.

IL-12 is involved in the generation of CTLs, natural killer (NK) cells, NK-T cells and the differentiation of $CD4^+$ T helper 1 (Th1) cells [38]. Immunization studies in mice have demonstrated increases in peptide-specific CTL responses with concurrent IL-12 administration, suggesting that the cytokine may be useful for the treatment of a number of diseases including cancer [39, 40]. IL-12 administration with the adjuvants Montanide ISA 51 or aluminum hydroxide in melanoma vaccine patients enhances the induction of CTLs against immunizing peptides, compared to patients receiving only adjuvant and peptides. In one study, patients with high-risk resected melanoma received multiple melanoma peptides in Montanide ISA 51 adjuvant, with or without IL-12 (30 ng/kg) [41]. Transient vaccine-related grade-3, but no grade-4, toxicity was observed and no differences in side effects between the two groups were seen. Eighty-five percent of patients demonstrated an immune response by DTH skin test, ELISA after *in vitro* peptide re-stimulation of PBLs, or MHC:peptide tetramer assays of fresh blood after vaccination. The immune responses in the IL-12 group were greater than without IL-12 ($p < 0.05$). These data suggest that IL-12 may increase the immune response to a peptide vaccine. Further evidence supporting the use of IL-12 as a vaccine adjuvant came in two studies of patients with stage III or IV melanoma expressing MART-1 [42]. IL-12 was administered at doses of 0, 10, 30 and 100 ng/kg, subcutaneously in one study and intravenously in another. The MART-1_{26-35} peptide and the influenza matrix$_{58-66}$ control peptide were administered intradermally on weeks 1, 2, 3, 4 and 9. There was a complete response in a patient with subcutaneous disease, a partial response in a patient with hepatic metastases, and mixed responses in the patients with pulmonary, pleural and nodal disease. Biopsies of accessible tumors showed infiltration with $CD4^+$ and $CD8^+$ lymphocytes capable of lysing MART-1 peptide-loaded targets *in vitro*.

Deoxycytidyl-deoxyguanosin oligodeoxynucleotides (CpG ODNs) trigger signaling through Toll-like receptor 9 expressed on certain DC subsets, resulting in maturation and IL-12 secretion that may enhance the immunogencity of peptide vaccines. The dinucleotide cytosine-guanine occurs at a higher frequency (approximately 1:16 base pairs) in prokaryotic DNA than in eukaryotic DNA (1:50-1:100 base pairs) [43]. Furthermore, eukaryotic DNA is often methylated at CpG residues [44]. These differences appear to account for the immunogenicity of certain prokaryotic DNA sequences containing un-methylated CpG dinucleotides. Studies utilizing CpG ODNs in mice have shown increases in CTL induction and antibody titers against various antigens including those derived from influenza, tetanus, and hepatitis B [45,46]. In a recent study, eight HLA-$A2^+$ melanoma patients received four vaccinations with CpG 7909 mixed with a MART-1 amino-acid altered peptide and Montanide ISA 51 adjuvant [47]. All patients exhibited rapid and strong antigen-specific T cell responses, with the frequency of MART-1-specific T cells reaching over 3% of circulating $CD8^+$ T cells. This was one order of magnitude higher than the frequency seen in eight control patients treated similarly but without the CpG ODN, and several orders of magnitude higher than that seen in previous studies with MART-1 peptide vaccines at the authors' institution. The MART-1-specific T cell populations consisted of effector-memory cells, which in part secreted IFNγ and expressed granzyme B and perforin *ex vivo*.

ALTERED PEPTIDES CAN ENHANCE T CELL INDUCTION

Thymic selection (central tolerance) removes virtually all T cells that have high affinity for self antigens. Furthermore, synthetic peptides derived from tumor-associated antigens generally bind MHC molecules with medium to low affinity [48]. Taken together, these properties may explain the apparent weak *in vivo* immunogenicity of many tumor antigen-derived peptide epitopes selected for use in cancer vaccines. Creation of modified peptide analogs is a strategy to improve immune responses generated by these peptides. There is an established correlation between the MHC class I-binding affinity and immunogenicity of viral antigen-derived peptides [49]. It is therefore plausible that modification of native tumor antigen peptide sequences could be made to increase their affinity for MHC molecules, resulting in increased immunogenicity.

Amino acid substitutions introduced at the MHC class I-binding anchor positions of peptides derived from melanoma-associated antigens MART-1, gp100, and tyrosinase have been achieved. These altered peptides have demonstrated markedly improved *in vitro* immunogenicity in pre-clinical studies, and are also recognized by T cells specific for the native sequence. Altered peptide epitopes have demonstrated usefulness in vaccine strategies. Three melanoma patients were immunized with a MART-1 peptide analog, MART-1_{26-35} (27L), that binds more strongly to HLA-A*0201 and is more immunogenic than the native sequence [50]. This peptide was injected together with a saponin-based adjuvant followed by surgical removal of SINs. *Ex vivo* analysis of SINs revealed differentiated antigen-specific memory $CD8^+$ T cells. *In vitro*, these cells proliferated upon stimulation with the analog peptide, and nearly all (16 of 17) MART-1-specific $CD8^+$ T cell clones generated from these lymph nodes efficiently lysed native melanoma cells *in vitro*. These results demonstrated that the TCR repertoire recruited by the analog peptide is highly specific for the naturally processed MART-1 antigen.

Another amino acid-modified peptide, $gp100_{209-217}$ (210M), and a control peptide, HPV16 $E7_{12-20}$, were mixed in Montanide ISA 51 adjuvant and injected into 30 HLA-$A2^+$ patients with resected melanoma [51]. Patients were randomly assigned to receive vaccinations every two weeks (thirteen vaccinations total) or every three weeks (nine vaccinations total) for six months. An increase of peptide-specific $CD8^+$ T cells in circulating peripheral blood was observed in 28 of 29 examined patients. The median frequency of $CD8^+$ T cells specific for the altered gp100 peptide increased from 0.02% before to 0.34% after vaccination ($p < .0001$), with no significant difference observed between the alternative vaccination schedules. In a subsequent trial from the same group, 35 HLA-$A2^+$ patients with resected melanoma were vaccinated multiple times over six months with the same modified melanoma peptide emulsified in Montanide ISA 51 adjuvant [52]. *Ex vivo* cytokine flow cytometry analysis of post-vaccine PBLs after *in vitro* peptide sensitization showed that, for all of the patients studied, tetramer-positive $CD8^+$ T cells produced IFNγ. Some patients had significant numbers of tetramer-positive, IFNγ-negative $CD8^+$T cells, suggesting that many were functionally anergic. Analysis of cells collected 12–24 months after vaccine therapy demonstrated the durable presence of gp100-specific memory $CD8^+$ T cells with high *in vitro* proliferation potential. These data demonstrate that some melanoma patients can mount a significant antigen-specific $CD8^+$ T cell immune response, with a functionally intact memory component, after receiving a peptide analog vaccine.

CD4^{+} HELPER T CELLS AND ANTI-TUMOR IMMUNITY

The induction of CTLs against immunizing peptides is often achieved in cancer patients, with some patients showing evidence of long-lasting, measurable immunity years after vaccination. In many cases, however, the magnitude of immune responses is low and/or short-lived. Recent studies in mice have provided important insights on the role of HTLs in the generation of memory CTLs. HTL-mediated enhancement of CTL immunity can result from (1) maturation of DCs via CD40 ligation and IFNγ secretion, (2) local secretion of IL-2, and (3) direct cell-to-cell co-stimulation through CD27, CD134, and MHC class II [53]. HTLs may also recruit effector cells of the innate immune system – such as macrophages and eosinophils – into the tumor microenvironment [54]. There is also evidence that HTLs can directly lyse MHC class II-expressing tumors via mechanisms analogous to those used by CTLs, such as perforin/granzyme secretion and Fas/Fas Ligand interaction (17–19). Hence, tumor-specific HTLs can mediate anti-tumor effects through a variety of mechanisms. Induction of tumor antigen-specific HTLs in cancer patients may therefore be a rational mean to generate sustained immunity against tumors.

MHC class II-restricted helper peptide epitopes derived from tumor antigens have been used in some early clinical trials in attempts to boost CTL induction against MHC class I-restricted peptides included in the same vaccine. Despite inconsistent results towards demonstrating enhanced CTL induction by vaccination with T helper peptides, HTL induction against tumor antigens HER-2/neu and MART-1 have been reported in some cancer vaccine patients. In one trial, three resected high-risk metastatic melanoma patients were vaccinated with an HLA-DR4-restricted T helper epitope, MART-1_{51-73} [19]. Immune reactivity to that epitope was detected by HLA-DR4-peptide tetramer staining and ELISpot assay of fresh and *in vitro* re-stimulated CD4^{+} T cells from the patients over the course of a 12-month vaccine regimen. The post-vaccine CD4^{+} T cells exhibited a mixed Th1/ T helper 2 (Th2) phenotype, proliferated in response to the antigen, and promiscuously recognized the peptide epitope bound to different HLA-DRβ alleles. For one HLA-DRβ1*0401^{+} patient, antigen-specific CD4^{+} T cells recognized HLA-matched antigen-expressing melanoma cells, secreted granzyme B, and also lysed antigen-expressing targets in an MHC class II-restricted manner. These data showed that a class II peptide epitope derived from a melanoma-associated antigen was immunogenic *in vivo*.

Currently, there are efforts underway to identify T helper peptide epitopes that contain, within the natural sequence, embedded MHC class I-binding motifs. These peptides have the potential to activate both HTLs and CTLs. A T helper peptide, derived from HER-2/neu, has been reported to induce long-lasting antigen-specific CTLs in patients with HER-2/neu over-expressing cancers [55]. Larger, randomized trials comparing MHC class I vs. MHC class I + II peptide vaccine regimens are needed to further assess the immunological and clinical benefit of HTL induction in cancer patients.

The generation of tumor antigen-specific HTL responses by vaccination, even without concomitant CTL induction, may still provide protective anti-tumor effects. Homing of HTLs to tumor sites may result in a cytokine environment capable of supporting endogenous anti-tumor immune responses. Studies in mice have implicated important roles for both Th1 and Th2 cells in anti-tumor immunity. Th1 cells secrete IFNγ, which activates tumoricidal macrophages that secrete nitric oxide and superoxide [54]. Th1 cells can also modulate antigen expression by local secretion of IFNγ in the tumor bed, which enhances MHC expression in IFN-responsive tumor cells [56]. In studies of melanoma and renal cell carcinoma patients, the presence of tumor antigen-specific Th1 cells in the peripheral blood and TIL populations are associated with spontaneously regressing lesions and remission of disease after therapy [57–59]. Th2 cells may also be important in anti-tumor immune responses through secretion of IL-4 and IL-5, which are critical to the differentiation and recruitment of eosinophils into tumor sites. Eosinophils can mediate tumor destruction by secreting cytotoxic factors, such as major basic protein, and also by modulating macrophage function via secretion of eosinophil peroxidase and macrophage inflammatory protein 1 [54].

BREAKING OF PERIPHERAL TOLERANCE BY CYTOTOXIC T LYMPHOCYTE ANTIGEN-4 (CTLA-4) BLOCKADE

The evolution and function of the immune system has been driven by the absolute need for host defense against pathogenic agents – the "self" vs. "non-self" model. Immunity against cancer represents a paradox in that tumor cells, while expressing specific antigens, often do not fall into the conventional "non-self" category in the same way that microorganisms do. Rather, tumor immunity appears to follow a slightly different model of "self" vs. "altered self." This concept of an "altered self" has important clinical implications for the immunotherapy of some cancers, whereby immune responses are induced against cellular proteins present in both transformed and normal cells.

CTLA-4 is a regulatory molecule expressed on activated T cells and certain subsets of T-regulatory cells. It binds the B7.1 and B7.2 co-stimulatory molecules with higher affinity than the T cell co-stimulatory receptor CD28 [60]. This effectively down-regulates APC-T cell interactions and therefore negatively influences T cell activation. CTLA-4 knock-out mice have a limited lifespan and exhibit profound, uncontrolled lymphoid proliferation and autoimmune phenomena, dying of myocarditis. In animal models, a cell-based vaccine administered with an abrogating antibody against CTLA-4 resulted in cures of established tumors not seen with either component alone [61]. In recent vaccine trials of melanoma patients, a CTLA-4-abrogating antibody (MDX-010) administered with peptide vaccination induced grade III/IV autoimmune manifestations including dermatitis, enterocolitis, hepatitis, and hypophysitis [62, 63]. These observations appeared to correlate with tumor regression in those with metastatic disease, and prolonged time to recurrence in patients with high-risk resected melanoma. It remains to be seen from additional studies if treatment of peptide vaccine patients with a CTLA-4-abrogating antibody correlates with enhanced T cell induction specific for the immunizing peptides. Nonetheless, these results provide evidence for breaking of tolerance to self antigens, and that strategies to augment recognition of "altered self" might be effective for the treatment of cancer.

PROTEIN VACCINES

Random mutations in tumor cells generate unique antigens in each individual, providing a rationale for customized immunotherapy approaches. Srivastava and Amato first proposed that certain heat shock proteins (HSPs) purified from a particular tumor can elicit specific immune responses against that tumor [64, 65]. HSPs are well-conserved, abundant proteins involved in a multitude of cellular processes. Some are induced when a cell is exposed to environmental stress such as temperature fluctuation and oxygen deprivation. Other HSPs are present under normal conditions, many of which are chaperones that aid protein folding and intracellular transport of peptides. Biochemical studies confirmed that low molecular weight peptides are associated with HSP preparations from cells [66, 67]. The peptide-binding pocket of certain HSPs display structural properties similar to that of MHC class I proteins, suggesting that the two have overlapping peptide-binding specificities [68]. Immunological studies have demonstrated that some of the peptides isolated from HSPs of tumor and virus-infected cells are recognized by T cells [69]. The unique repertoire of HSP-associated peptides from tumors includes those resulting from somatic mutations, which create the potential for customized approaches to cellular immunotherapy. Furthermore, autologous HSP preparations circumvent the need to identify individual T cell epitopes and the technical challenges associated with that process. The sheer variety of endogenous HSP-associated peptides may also be effective in maintaining *in vivo* anti-tumor immune responses in the setting of antigen-loss tumor cell variants.

APCs can acquire HSPs through specialized receptors, such as CD91, that mediate their uptake from the extracellular milieu [70]. Once internalized, HSPs traffic to different cellular compartments where chaperoned peptides are released, processed, and assembled onto MHC molecules [71, 72]. In a variety of mouse cancer models, vaccination with certain HSPs (hsp70, hsp90, hsp110, Grp94/gp96, grp170) induces anti-tumor activity via generation of tumor-reactive CTLs and HTLs [73, 74]. In mice with bulky metastatic lesions, slowing of tumor growth is observed and complete tumor regression can be achieved with smaller tumor burdens [75]. HSP treatment in mice after primary tumor resection confers long-lasting immunity against tumor recurrence, with most of the animals achieving a normal lifespan. Recent work has also focused on non-covalent attachment of large protein substrates (e.g. recombinant tumor antigens) to certain HSPs for use in animal vaccination models [76].

Early phase clinical trials using heat shock protein peptide complex 96 (HSPPC96) have been conducted in a number of different cancers including melanoma, pancreatic cancer, gastric cancer, colorectal cancer, renal cell carcinoma, chronic myelogenous leukemia, and non-Hodgkin's lymphoma [77]. Measurable CTL responses against autologous fresh tumor cell preparations and cell lines established from original primary tumors have been achieved in some patients, with immune reactivity correlating with improved clinical outcome and survival time [78–80]. Large, randomized phase III trials using HSPPC96 are currently underway for renal cell carcinoma and metastatic melanoma. Pre-clinical data has also demonstrated that hsp70-associated peptides including those derived from melanoma-associated antigens can activate T cells in an MHC-dependent manner [81, 82].

Recombinant protein vaccines have been reported to induce tumor antigen-specific cellular and humoral immune responses in patients with different cancers. Like HSPs, the use of whole tumor antigen bypasses the need to identify individual peptide epitopes corresponding to different HLA restriction elements, thereby allowing for increased patient inclusion. Pre-clinical studies have demonstrated that MAGE and gp100 recombinant proteins are able to stimulate antigen-reactive T cells *in vitro* [83, 84]. Fusion of MAGE-A3 to immunogens such as the Protein D antigen of *Haemophilus influenzae* has been shown to induce MAGE-A3-specific CTL, HTL, and antibody responses in some metastatic melanoma patients [85].

CONCLUDING REMARKS

Tumor antigen-based peptide and protein vaccines have demonstrated excellent safety profiles characterized primarily by mild, transient side effects such as flu-like symptoms, injection site reactions, and low-grade fevers. Immune responses to tumor antigens have been demonstrated in patients with a variety of different cancers. The accumulated data suggest that peptide and protein vaccines are immunogenic and can generate significant levels of $CD8^+$and $CD4^+$ T cells in the peripheral blood, draining lymph nodes and tumors of cancer patients. Long-lived memory responses can even be seen in some cases. However, these findings have not yet been translated into clinical benefit in randomized clinical trials. Understanding the interaction between tumor cells and the immune system represents a rapidly evolving field. While important advances have been made in understanding the components of effective anti-tumor immune responses, including dendritic cell activation, modulation of tumor antigen expression, control of peripheral tolerance, and the generation of long-lasting T cell memory, that knowledge has not yet been properly applied to cancer vaccine strategies.

The clinical setting for which peptide and protein vaccines are applied is also an important determining factor in the outcomes of cancer immunotherapies. Early trials often focused on treating advanced disease characterized by aggressive and established tumors. With increasing basic knowledge of how tumors induce immunosuppression, it is now evident that the immune system may not effectively induce regression of large tumor burdens. The focus in cancer vaccine studies has therefore shifted towards reduced disease states – including patients with no evidence of disease achieved by appropriate surgery and/or chemotherapy – as more favorable settings to achieve a consistent, positive impact on patient quality of life and survival. Therefore, immunotherapy may be most effective in preventing disease recurrence, as opposed to treating active disease. The ideal vaccine strategy would utilize a potent local or systemic adjuvant, induce both innate and adaptive immunity, incorporate multiple antigenic epitopes, and utilize means of breaking immunological tolerance by provision of some sort of "danger" signal, such as CTLA-4 abrogation.

REFERENCES

1. Burnet FM. The concept of immunological surveillance. Prog Exp Tumor Res. 1970;13:1–27.
2. Topalian SL, Solomon D, Rosenberg SA. Tumor-specific cytolysis by lymphocytes infiltrating human melanomas. J Immunol. 1989 May 15;142(10):3714–25.
3. Lindgren CG, Thompson JA, Higuchi CM, Fefer A. Growth and autologous tumor lysis by tumor-infiltrating lymphocytes from metastatic melanoma expanded in interleukin-2 or interleukin-2 plus interleukin-4. J Immunother. 1993 Nov;14(4):322–8.
4. Banchereau J, Steinman RM. Dendritic cells and the control of immunity. Nature. 1998 Mar 19;392(6673):245–52.
5. Cella M, Sallusto F, Lanzavecchia A. Origin, maturation and antigen presenting function of dendritic cells. Curr Opin Immunol. 1997 Feb;9(1):10–6.
6. van der Bruggen P, Traversari C, Chomez P, Lurquin C, De Plaen E, Van den Eynde B, Knuth A, Boon T. A gene encoding an antigen recognized by cytolytic T lymphocytes on a human melanoma. Science. 1991 Dec 13;254(5038):1643–7.
7. Bosch FX, Manos MM, Munoz N, Sherman M, Jansen AM, Peto J, Schiffman MH, Moreno V, Kurman R, Shah KV. Prevalence of human papillomavirus in cervical cancer: a worldwide perspective. International biological study on cervical cancer (IBSCC) Study Group. J Natl Cancer Inst. 1995 Jun 7;87(11):796–802.
8. Zhou J, Dudley ME, Rosenberg SA, Robbins PF. Persistence of multiple tumor-specific T-cell clones is associated with complete tumor regression in a melanoma patient receiving adoptive cell transfer therapy. J Immunother. 2005 Jan-Feb;28(1):53–62.
9. Huang J, El-Gamil M, Dudley ME, Li YF, Rosenberg SA, Robbins PF. T cells associated with tumor regression recognize frameshifted products of the CDKN2A tumor suppressor gene locus and a mutated HLA class I gene product. J Immunol. 2004 May 15;172(10):6057–64.
10. Barnd DL, Lan MS, Metzgar RS, Finn OJ. Specific, major histocompatibility complex-unrestricted recognition of tumor-associated mucins by human cytotoxic T cells. Proc Natl Acad Sci U S A. 1989 Sep;86(18):7159–63.
11. Apostolopoulos V, Karanikas V, Haurum JS, McKenzie IF. Induction of HLA-A2-restricted CTLs to the mucin 1 human breast cancer antigen. J Immunol. 1997 Dec 1;159(11):5211–8.
12. Chen YT, Gure AO, Tsang S, Stockert E, Jager E, Knuth A, Old LJ. Identification of multiple cancer/testis antigens by allogeneic antibody screening of a melanoma cell line library. Proc Natl Acad Sci U S A. 1998 Jun 9;95(12):6919–23.
13. Khong HT, Wang QJ, Rosenberg SA. Identification of multiple antigens recognized by tumor-infiltrating lymphocytes from a single patient: tumor escape by antigen loss and loss of MHC expression. J Immunother. 2004 May-Jun;27(3):184–90.
14. Kawakami Y, Robbins PF, Rosenberg SA. Human melanoma antigens recognized by T lymphocytes. Keio J Med. 1996 Jun;45(2):100–8.
15. Dudley ME, Wunderlich JR, Yang JC, Sherry RM, Topalian SL, Restifo NP, Royal RE, Kammula U, White DE, Mavroukakis SA, Rogers LJ, Gracia GJ, Jones SA, Mangiameli DP, Pelletier MM, Gea-Banacloche J, Robinson MR, Berman DM, Filie AC, Abati A, Rosenberg SA. Adoptive cell transfer therapy following non-myeloablative but lymphodepleting chemotherapy for the treatment of patients with refractory metastatic melanoma. J Immunother. 2005 May-Jun;28(3):258–67.
16. Huang J, Khong HT, Dudley ME, El-Gamil M, Li YF, Rosenberg SA, Robbins PF. Survival, persistence, and progressive differentiation of adoptively transferred tumor-reactive T cells associated with tumor regression. J Immunother. 2005 May-Jun;28(3):258–67.

17. Zennadi R, Abdel-Wahab Z, Seigler HF, Darrow TL. Generation of melanoma-specific, cytotoxic CD4(+) T helper 2 cells: requirement of both HLA-DR15 and Fas antigens on melanomas for their lysis by Th2 cells. Cell Immunol. 2001 Jun 15;210(2):96–105.
18. Echchakir H, Bagot M, Dorothee G, Martinvalet D, Le Gouvello S, Boumsell L, Chouaib S, Bensussan A, Mami-Chouaib F. Cutaneous T cell lymphoma reactive CD4+ cytotoxic T lymphocyte clones display a Th1 cytokine profile and use a fas-independent pathway for specific tumor cell lysis. J Invest Dermatol. 2000 Jul;115(1):74–80.
19. Wong R, Lau R, Chang J, Kuus-Reichel T, Brichard V, Bruck C, Weber J. Immune responses to a class II helper peptide epitope in patients with stage III/IV resected melanoma. Clin Cancer Res. 2004 Aug 1;10(15):5004–13.
20. Jager E, Gnjatic S, Nagata Y, Stockert E, Jager D, Karbach J, Neumann A, Rieckenberg J, Chen YT, Ritter G, Hoffman E, Arand M, Old LJ, Knuth A. Induction of primary NY-ESO-1 immunity: CD8+ T lymphocyte and antibody responses in peptide-vaccinated patients with NY-ESO-1+ cancers. Proc Natl Acad Sci U S A. 2000 Oct 24;97(22):12198–203.
21. Dranoff G, Jaffee E, Lazenby A, Golumbek P, Levitsky H, Brose K, Jackson V, Hamada H, Pardoll D, Mulligan RC. Vaccination with irradiated tumor cells engineered to secrete murine granulocyte-macrophage colony-stimulating factor stimulates potent, specific, and long-lasting anti-tumor immunity. Proc Natl Acad Sci U S A. 1993 Apr 15;90(8):3539–43.
22. Slingluff CL Jr, Petroni GR, Yamshchikov GV, Barnd DL, Eastham S, Galavotti H, Patterson JW, Deacon DH, Hibbitts S, Teates D, Neese PY, Grosh WW, Chianese-Bullock KA, Woodson EM, Wiernasz CJ, Merrill P, Gibson J, Ross M, Engelhard VH. Clinical and immunologic results of a randomized phase II trial of vaccination using four melanoma peptides either administered in granulocyte-macrophage colony-stimulating factor in adjuvant or pulsed on dendritic cells. J Clin Oncol. 2003 Nov 1;21(21):4016–26
23. Chianese-Bullock KA, Pressley J, Garbee C, Hibbitts S, Murphy C, Yamshchikov G, Petroni GR, Bissonette EA, Neese PY, Grosh WW, Merrill P, Fink R, Woodson EM, Wiernasz CJ, Patterson JW, Slingluff CL Jr. MAGE-A1-, MAGE-A10-, and gp100-derived peptides are immunogenic when combined with granulocyte-macrophage colony-stimulating factor and montanide ISA-51 adjuvant and administered as part of a multipeptide vaccine for melanoma. J Immunol. 2005 Mar 1;174(5):3080–6.
24. DeKruyff RH, Fang Y, Umetsu DT. IL-4 synthesis by in vivo primed keyhole limpet hemocyanin-specific CD4+ T cells. I. Influence of antigen concentration and antigen-presenting cell type. J Immunol. 1992 Dec 1;149(11):3468–76.
25. Scheibenbogen C, Schadendorf D, Bechrakis NE, Nagorsen D, Hofmann U, Servetopoulou F, Letsch A, Philipp A, Foerster MH, Schmittel A, Thiel E, Keilholz U. Effects of granulocyte-macrophage colony-stimulating factor and foreign helper protein as immunologic adjuvants on the T-cell response to vaccination with tyrosinase peptides. Int J Cancer. 2003 Mar 20;104(2):188–94
26. Shackleton M, Davis ID, Hopkins W, Jackson H, Dimopoulos N, Tai T, Chen Q, Parente P, Jefford M, Masterman KA, Caron D, Chen W, Maraskovsky E, Cebon J. The impact of imiquimod, a Toll-like receptor-7 ligand (TLR7L), on the immunogenicity of melanoma peptide vaccination with adjuvant Flt3 ligand. Cancer Immun. 2004 Sep 23;4:9
27. Rieser C, Ramoner R, Holtl L, Rogatsch H, Papesh C, Stenzl A, Bartsch G, Thurnher M. Mature dendritic cells induce T-helper type-1-dominant immune responses in patients with metastatic renal cell carcinoma. Urol Int. 1999;63(3):151–9.
28. Panelli MC, Wunderlich J, Jeffries J, Wang E, Mixon A, Rosenberg SA, Marincola FM. Phase 1 study in patients with metastatic melanoma of immunization with dendritic cells presenting epitopes derived from the melanoma-associated antigens MART-1 and gp100. J Immunother. 2000 Jul-Aug;23(4):487–98.
29. Muderspach L, Wilczynski S, Roman L, Bade L, Felix J, Small LA, Kast WM, Fascio G, Marty V, Weber J. A phase I trial of a human papillomavirus (HPV) peptide vaccine for women with high-grade cervical and vulvar intraepithelial neoplasia who are HPV 16 positive. Clin Cancer Res. 2000 Sep;6(9):3406–16.

30. Lau R, Wang F, Jeffery G, Marty V, Kuniyoshi J, Bade E, Ryback ME, Weber J. Phase I trial of intravenous peptide-pulsed dendritic cells in patients with metastatic melanoma. J Immunother. 2001 Jan-Feb;24(1):66–78.
31. Schuler-Thurner B, Schultz ES, Berger TG, Weinlich G, Ebner S, Woerl P, Bender A, Feuerstein B, Fritsch PO, Romani N, Schuler G. Rapid induction of tumor-specific type 1 T helper cells in metastatic melanoma patients by vaccination with mature, cryopreserved, peptide-loaded monocyte-derived dendritic cells. J Exp Med. 2002 May 20;195(10):1279–88.
32. O'Rourke MG, Johnson M, Lanagan C, See J, Yang J, Bell JR, Slater GJ, Kerr BM, Crowe B, Purdie DM, Elliott SL, Ellem KA, Schmidt CW. Durable complete clinical responses in a phase I/II trial using an autologous melanoma cell/dendritic cell vaccine. Cancer Immunol Immunother. 2003 Jun;52(6):387–95. Epub 2003 Apr 8.
33. Ueda Y, Itoh T, Nukaya I, Kawashima I, Okugawa K, Yano Y, Yamamoto Y, Naitoh K, Shimizu K, Imura K, Fuji N, Fujiwara H, Ochiai T, Itoi H, Sonoyama T, Hagiwara A, Takesako K, Yamagishi H. Dendritic cell-based immunotherapy of cancer with carcinoembryonic antigen-derived, HLA-A24-restricted CTL epitope: Clinical outcomes of 18 patients with metastatic gastrointestinal or lung adenocarcinomas. Int J Oncol. 2004 Apr;24(4):909–17.
34. Yu JS, Liu G, Ying H, Yong WH, Black KL, Wheeler CJ. Vaccination with tumor lysate-pulsed dendritic cells elicits antigen-specific, cytotoxic T-cells in patients with malignant glioma. Cancer Res. 2004 Jul 15;64(14):4973–9.
35. Pandha HS, John RJ, Hutchinson J, James N, Whelan M, Corbishley C, Dalgleish AG. Dendritic cell immunotherapy for urological cancers using cryopreserved allogeneic tumour lysate-pulsed cells: a phase I/II study. BJU Int. 2004 Aug;94(3):412–8.
36. Maas RA, Roest PA, Becker MJ, Weimar IS, Dullens HF, Den Otter W. Effector cells of low-dose IL-2 immunotherapy in tumor bearing mice: tumor cell killing by CD8+ cytotoxic T lymphocytes and macrophages. Immunobiology. 1992 Nov;186(3–4):214–29.
37. Slingluff CL Jr, Petroni GR, Yamshchikov GV, Hibbitts S, Grosh WW, Chianese-Bullock KA, Bissonette EA, Barnd DL, Deacon DH, Patterson JW, Parekh J, Neese PY, Woodson EM, Wiernasz CJ, Merrill P. Immunologic and clinical outcomes of vaccination with a multiepitope melanoma peptide vaccine plus low-dose interleukin-2 administered either concurrently or on a delayed schedule. J Clin Oncol. 2004 Nov 15;22(22):4474–85.
38. Trinchieri G. Interleukin-12 and the regulation of innate resistance and adaptive immunity. Nat Rev Immunol. 2003 Feb;3(2):133–46.
39. Hamajima K, Fukushima J, Bukawa H, Kaneko T, Tsuji T, Asakura Y, Sasaki S, Xin KQ, Okuda K. Strong augment effect of IL-12 expression plasmid on the induction of HIV-specific cytotoxic T lymphocyte activity by a peptide vaccine candidate. Clin Immunol Immunopathol. 1997 May;83(2):179–84.
40. Chattergoon MA, Saulino V, Shames JP, Stein J, Montaner LJ, Weiner DB. Co-immunization with plasmid IL-12 generates a strong T-cell memory response in mice. Vaccine. 2004 Apr16;22(13–14):1744–50.
41. Lee P, Wang F, Kuniyoshi J, Rubio V, Stuges T, Groshen S, Gee C, Lau R, Jeffery G, Margolin K, Marty V, Weber J. Effects of interleukin-12 on the immune response to a multipeptide vaccine for resected metastatic melanoma. J Clin Oncol. 2001 Sep 15;19(18):3836–47.
42. Cebon J, Jager E, Shackleton MJ, Gibbs P, Davis ID, Hopkins W, Gibbs S, Chen Q, Karbach J, Jackson H, MacGregor DP, Sturrock S, Vaughan H, Maraskovsky E, Neumann A, Hoffman E, Sherman ML, Knuth A. Two phase I studies of low dose recombinant human IL-12 with Melan-A and influenza peptides in subjects with advanced malignant melanoma. Cancer Immun. 2003 Jul 16;3:7.
43. Bird AP, Taggart MH, Nicholls RD, Higgs DR. Non-methylated CpG-rich islands at the human alpha-globin locus: implications for evolution of the alpha-globin pseudogene. EMBO J. 1987 Apr;6(4):999–1004.
44. Karl J. Fryxell and Won-Jong Moon. CpG mutation rates in the human genome are highly dependent on local GC content. Mol Biol Evol. 2005 Mar;22(3):650–8. Epub 2004 Nov 10.

45. McCluskie MJ, Davis HL. Oral, intrarectal and intranasal immunizations using CpG and non-CpG oligodeoxynucleotides as adjuvants. Vaccine. 2000 Oct 15;19(4–5):413–22.
46. McCluskie MJ, Weeratna RD, Payette PJ, Davis HL. Parenteral and mucosal prime-boost immunization strategies in mice with hepatitis B surface antigen and CpG DNA. FEMS Immunol Med Microbiol. 2002 Feb 18;32(3):179–85.
47. Speiser DE, Lienard D, Rufer N, Rubio-Godoy V, Rimoldi D, Lejeune F, Krieg AM, Cerottini JC, Romero P. Rapid and strong human CD8+ T cell responses to vaccination with peptide, IFA, and CpG oligodeoxynucleotide 7909. J Clin Invest. 2005 Mar;115(3):739–46.
48. Valmori D, Ayyoub M. Using Modified Antigenic Sequences to Develop Cancer Vaccines: Are We Losing the Focus? PLoS Med. 2004 Nov;1(2):e26. Epub 2004 Nov 30.
49. Sette A, Vitiello A, Reherman B, Fowler P, Nayersina R, Kast WM, Melief CJ, Oseroff C, Yuan L, Ruppert J, et al. The relationship between class I binding affinity and immunogenicity of potential cytotoxic T cell epitopes. J Immunol. 1994 Dec 15;153(12):5586–92.
50. Ayyoub M, Zippelius A, Pittet MJ, Rimoldi D, Valmori D, Cerottini JC, Romero P, Lejeune F, Lienard D, Speiser DE. Activation of human melanoma reactive CD8+ T cells by vaccination with an immunogenic peptide analog derived from Melan-A/melanoma antigen recognized by T cells-1. Clin Cancer Res. 2003 Feb;9(2):669–77.
51. Smith JW 2nd, Walker EB, Fox BA, Haley D, Wisner KP, Doran T, Fisher B, Justice L, Wood W, Vetto J, Maecker H, Dols A, Meijer S, Hu HM, Romero P, Alvord WG, Urba WJ. Adjuvant immunization of HLA-A2-positive melanoma patients with a modified gp100 peptide induces peptide-specific CD8+ T-cell responses. J Clin Oncol. 2003 Apr 15;21(8):1562–73.
52. Walker EB, Haley D, Miller W, Floyd K, Wisner KP, Sanjuan N, Maecker H, Romero P, Hu HM, Alvord WG, Smith JW 2nd, Fox BA, Urba WJ. gp100(209–2M) peptide immunization of human lymphocyte antigen-A2+ stage I-III melanoma patients induces significant increase in antigen-specific effector and long-term memory CD8+ T cells. Clin Cancer Res. 2004 Jan 15;10(2):668–80.
53. Giuntoli RL 2nd, Lu J, Kobayashi H, Kennedy R, Celis E. Direct costimulation of tumor-reactive CTL by helper T cells potentiate their proliferation, survival, and effector function. Clin Cancer Res. 2002 Mar;8(3):922–31.
54. Hung K, Hayashi R, Lafond-Walker A, Lowenstein C, Pardoll D, Levitsky H. The central role of CD4(+) T cells in the antitumor immune response. J Exp Med. 1998 Dec 21;188(12):2357–68.
55. Knutson KL, Schiffman K, Disis ML. Immunization with a HER-2/neu helper peptide vaccine generates HER-2/neu CD8 T-cell immunity in cancer patients. J Clin Invest. 2001 Mar;107(5):553–4.
56. Restifo NP, Esquivel F, Kawakami Y, Yewdell JW, Mule JJ, Rosenberg SA, Bennink JR. Identification of human cancers deficient in antigen processing. J Exp Med. 1993 Feb 1;177(2):265–72.
57. Tatsumi T, Kierstead LS, Ranieri E, Gesualdo L, Schena FP, Finke JH, Bukowski RM, Mueller-Berghaus J, Kirkwood JM, Kwok WW, Storkus WJ. Disease-associated bias in T helper type 1 (Th1)/Th2 CD4(+) T cell responses against MAGE-6 in HLA-DRB10401(+) patients with renal cell carcinoma or melanoma. J Exp Med. 2002 Sep 2;196(5):619–28.
58. Lowes MA, Bishop GA, Crotty K, Barnetson RS, Halliday GM. T helper 1 cytokine mRNA is increased in spontaneously regressing primary melanomas. J Invest Dermatol. 1997 Jun;108(6):914–9.
59. Wittke F, Hoffmann R, Buer J, Dallmann I, Oevermann K, Sel S, Wandert T, Ganser A, Atzpodien J. Interleukin 10 (IL-10): an immunosuppressive factor and independent predictor in patients with metastatic renal cell carcinoma. Br J Cancer. 1999 Mar;79(7–8):1182–4.
60. Chambers CA, Krummel MF, Boitel B, Hurwitz A, Sullivan TJ, Fournier S, Cassell D, Brunner M, Allison JP. The role of CTLA-4 in the regulation and initiation of T-cell responses. Immunol Rev. 1996 Oct;153:27–46.
61. van Elsas A, Hurwitz AA, Allison JP. Combination immunotherapy of B16 melanoma using anti-cytotoxic T lymphocyte-associated antigen 4 (CTLA-4) and granulocyte/macrophage colony-stimulating factor (GM-CSF)-producing vaccines induces rejection of subcutaneous and metastatic tumors accompanied by autoimmune depigmentation. J Exp Med. 1999 Aug 2;190(3):355–66.
62. Phan GQ, Yang JC, Sherry RM, Hwu P, Topalian SL, Schwartzentruber DJ, Restifo NP, Haworth LR, Seipp CA, Freezer LJ, Morton KE, Mavroukakis SA, Duray PH, Steinberg SM,

Allison JP, Davis TA, Rosenberg SA. Cancer regression and autoimmunity induced by cytotoxic T lymphocyte-associated antigen 4 blockade in patients with metastatic melanoma. Proc Natl Acad Sci U S A. 2003 Jul 8;100(14):8372–7. Epub 2003 Jun 25.

63. Sanderson K, Scotland R, Lee P, Liu D, Groshen S, Snively J, Sian S, Nichol G, Davis T, Keler T, Yellin M, Weber J. Autoimmunity in a phase I trial of a fully human anti-cytotoxic T-lymphocyte antigen-4 monoclonal antibody with multiple melanoma peptides and Montanide ISA 51 for patients with resected stages III and IV melanoma. J Clin Oncol. 2005 Feb 1;23(4):741–50.
64. Srivastava PK, Das MR. The serologically unique cell surface antigen of Zajdela ascitic hepatoma is also its tumor-associated transplantation antigen. Int J Cancer. 1984 Mar 15;33(3):417–22.
65. Srivastava PK, DeLeo AB, Old LJ. Tumor rejection antigens of chemically induced sarcomas of inbred mice. Proc Natl Acad Sci U S A. 1986 May;83(10):3407–11.
66. Udono H, Srivastava PK. Heat shock protein 70-associated peptides elicit specific cancer immunity. J Exp Med. 1993 Oct 1;178(4):1391–6.
67. Srivastava PK, Udono H, Blachere NE, Li Z. Heat shock proteins transfer peptides during antigen processing and CTL priming. Immunogenetics. 1994;39(2):93–8.
68. Linderoth NA, Popowicz A, Sastry S. Identification of the peptide-binding site in the heat shock chaperone/tumor rejection antigen gp96 (Grp94). J Biol Chem. 2000 Feb 25;275(8):5472–7.
69. Castelli C, Rivoltini L, Rini F, Belli F, Testori A, Maio M, Mazzaferro V, Coppa J, Srivastava PK, Parmiani G. Heat shock proteins: biological functions and clinical application as personalized vaccines for human cancer. Cancer Immunol Immunother. 2004 Mar;53(3):227–33. Epub 2003 Dec 19.
70. Basu S, Binder RJ, Ramalingam T, Srivastava PK. CD91 is a common receptor for heat shock proteins gp96, hsp90, hsp70, and calreticulin. Immunity. 2001 Mar;14(3):303–13.
71. Suto R, Srivastava PK. A mechanism for the specific immunogenicity of heat shock protein-chaperoned peptides. Science. 1995 Sep 15;269(5230):1585–8.
72. Berwin B, Nicchitta CV. To find the road traveled to tumor immunity: the trafficking itineraries of molecular chaperones in antigen-presenting cells. Traffic. 2001 Oct;2(10):690–7.
73. Udono H, Levey DL, Srivastava PK. Cellular requirements for tumor-specific immunity elicited by heat shock proteins: tumor rejection antigen gp96 primes CD8+ T cells in vivo. Proc Natl Acad Sci U S A. 1994 Apr 12;91(8):3077–81.
74. Tamura Y, Peng P, Liu K, Daou M, Srivastava PK. Immunotherapy of tumors with autologous tumor-derived heat shock protein preparations. Science. 1997 Oct 3;278(5335):117–20.
75. Srivastava PK. Immunotherapy of human cancer: lessons from mice. Nat Immunol. 2000 Nov;1(5):363–6.
76. Wang XY, Manjili MH, Park J, Chen X, Repasky E, Subjeck JR. Development of cancer vaccines using autologous and recombinant high molecular weight stress proteins. Methods. 2004 Jan;32(1):13–20.
77. Lewis JJ. Therapeutic cancer vaccines: using unique antigens. Proc Natl Acad Sci U S A. 2004 Oct 5;101 Suppl 2:14653–6. Epub 2004 Aug 5.
78. Janetzki S, Palla D, Rosenhauer V, Lochs H, Lewis JJ, Srivastava PK. Immunization of cancer patients with autologous cancer-derived heat shock protein gp96 preparations: a pilot study. Int J Cancer. 2000 Oct 15;88(2):232–8.
79. Belli F, Testori A, Rivoltini L, Maio M, Andreola G, Sertoli MR, Gallino G, Piris A, Cattelan A, Lazzari I, Carrabba M, Scita G, Santantonio C, Pilla L, Tragni G, Lombardo C, Arienti F, Marchiano A, Queirolo P, Bertolini F, Cova A, Lamaj E, Ascani L, Camerini R, Corsi M, Cascinelli N, Lewis JJ, Srivastava P, Parmiani G. Vaccination of metastatic melanoma patients with autologous tumor-derived heat shock protein gp96-peptide complexes: clinical and immunologic findings. Clin Oncol. 2002 Oct 15;20(20):4169–80.
80. Mazzaferro V, Coppa J, Carrabba MG, Rivoltini L, Schiavo M, Regalia E, Mariani L, Camerini T, Marchiano A, Andreola S, Camerini R, Corsi M, Lewis JJ, Srivastava PK, Parmiani G. Vaccination with autologous tumor-derived heat-shock protein gp96 after liver resection for metastatic colorectal cancer. Clin Cancer Res. 2003 Aug 15;9(9):3235–45.

81. Castelli C, Ciupitu AM, Rini F, Rivoltini L, Mazzocchi A, Kiessling R, Parmiani G. Human heat shock protein 70 peptide complexes specifically activate anti-melanoma T cells. Cancer Res. 2001 Jan 1;61(1):222–7.
82. Noessner E, Gastpar R, Milani V, Brandl A, Hutzler PJ, Kuppner MC, Roos M, Kremmer E, Asea A, Calderwood SK, Issels RD. Tumor-derived heat shock protein 70 peptide complexes are cross-presented by human dendritic cells. J Immunol. 2002 Nov 15;169(10):5424–32.
83. Manici S, Sturniolo T, Imro MA, Hammer J, Sinigaglia F, Noppen C, Spagnoli G, Mazzi B, Bellone M, Dellabona P, Protti MP. Melanoma cells present a MAGE-3 epitope to CD4(+) cytotoxic T cells in association with histocompatibility leukocyte antigen DR11. J Exp Med. 1999 Mar 1;189(5):871–6.
84. Parkhurst MR, Riley JP, Robbins PF, Rosenberg SA. Induction of CD4+ Th1 lymphocytes that recognize known and novel class II MHC restricted epitopes from the melanoma antigen gp100 by stimulation with recombinant protein. J Immunother. 2004 Mar-Apr;27(2):79–91.
85. Vantomme V, Dantinne C, Amrani N, Permanne P, Gheysen D, Bruck C, Stoter G, Britten CM, Keilholz U, Lamers CH, Marchand M, Delire M, Gueguen M. Immunologic analysis of a phase I/II study of vaccination with MAGE-3 protein combined with the AS02B adjuvant in patients with MAGE-3-positive tumors. J Immunother. 2004 Mar-Apr;27(2):124–35.

ABBREVIATIONS

APC	antigen-presenting cell
ARF	alternative reading frame
CpG ODN	deoxycytidyl-deoxyguanosin oligodeoxynucleotide
CTL	cytotoxic T lymphocyte
CTLA-4	cytotoxic T lymphocyte antigen-4
DC	dendritic cell
DNA	deoxyribonucleic acid
DTH	delayed-type hypersensitivity
FL	Flt3 ligand
ELISA	enzyme-linked immunosorbant assay
ELISPOT	enzyme-linked immunospot assay
GAPDH	glyceraldehyde-3-phosphate dehydrogenase
GAS7	growth arrest-specific gene 7
GM-CSF	granulocyte macrophage colony stimulating factor
HLA	human leukocyte antigen
HTL	helper T lymphocyte
HPV	human papilloma virus
HSP	heat-shock protein
HSPPC96	heath-shock protein peptide complex 96
IFN	interferon gamma
IL	interleukin
IFA	incomplete Freund's Adjuvant
INK	inhibitors of kinase
IU	international unit
KLH	keyhole limpet hemocyanin

kg	kilogram
MAGE	melanoma antigen E
MART-1	melanoma Antigen Recognized by T cells-1
MHC	major histocompatibility complex
MUC-1	mucin-1
ng	nanogram
NK	natural killer
PBMC	peripheral blood mononuclear cells
PBL	peripheral blood lymphocytes
SEREX	serological expression
SIN	sentinel immunized node
TCR	T cell receptor
TGF	transforming growth factor
TNF	tumor necrosis factor
Th	T helper
TIL	tumor-infiltrating lymphocyte
μg	microgram

CHAPTER 9

DNA VACCINES AGAINST CANCER

ADAM D. COHEN AND JEDD D. WOLCHOK*

Department of Medicine, Memorial Sloan-Kettering Cancer Center, Weill Medical College of Cornell University, New York, NY

INTRODUCTION

For over a century, dating back to William Coley's initial experiments with bacterial toxins in cancer patients [1], investigators have been trying to harness the power of the immune system as a means of fighting cancer. The rationale for cancer immunotherapy derives from a number of pre-clinical and clinical observations, including but not limited to: 1) the ability of the immune system to recognize and eliminate tumors of diverse histological types in animal models; 2) the increased incidence of tumor formation in immunodeficient mice; 3) the modest but reproducible response rates seen in melanoma and renal cell carcinoma for cytokine immunostimulants such as interleukin 2 and interferon-alpha; and 4) the identification and isolation of antibodies and tumor-infiltrating lymphocytes from cancer patients which recognize a host of tumor antigens. This rationale has been bolstered further by the success, particularly in patients with hematologic malignancies, of passive immunotherapies such as donor leukocyte infusion following allogeneic stem cell transplantation and monoclonal antibodies such as rituximab. Less successful clinically to date have been attempts at active immunotherapy, despite a number of different immunization strategies designed to induce anti-tumor immunity in recipients (reviewed recently in ref. [2]). DNA vaccination, in which recipients are immunized with bacterially-derived plasmids encoding one or more antigens of interest, represents a relatively novel approach to the active immunotherapy of cancer, and will be reviewed in detail here.

*Department of Medicine Memorial Sloan-Kettering Cancer Center 1275 York Avenue New York, NY 10021 (646) 888-2395, wolchokj@mskcc.org

H.L. Kaufman and J.D. Wolchok (eds.), General Principles of Tumor Immunotherapy, 193–215.

DNA VACCINES: HISTORY, MECHANISM, AND COMPARISON TO OTHER VACCINE STRATEGIES

The first demonstration that plasmid-based immunization could elicit immune responses in animals was reported by Tang and colleagues in 1992. Plasmid DNA encoding human growth hormone or human α1-antitrypsin under the control of a constitutively active promoter was coated onto gold microprojectiles and injected into mouse skin using a "gene gun," and antibodies specific for the encoded proteins were subsequently isolated from the serum of vaccinated recipients [3]. Subsequent studies of DNA vaccines encoding influenza [4, 5], HIV-1 [6], and hepatitis B [7] antigens showed that this approach could generate antibody, CD4 and CD8 T cell responses, as well as protection from pathogenic microbial challenge, and led to its application in a number of infectious disease models. The safety and immunogenicity of DNA vaccines against HIV, malaria, and hepatitis B virus have since been demonstrated in non-human primates, as well as in human clinical trials [8–10].

The mechanism by which DNA vaccines generate immune responses has not been completely elucidated, though two complementary models of immunological priming have been demonstrated in mouse studies, both highlighting the importance of bone-marrow derived antigen-presenting cells (APCs) (Figure 1). The first involves "cross-priming," in which the encoded gene product, having been secreted or released from transfected myocytes or keratinocytes, is taken up by APCs such as dendritic cells which process the antigen and migrate to regional lymph nodes where they can prime naïve T cells [11, 12]. In addition, there is evidence that resident APCs at the site of immunization can be directly transfected by plasmid, leading to endogenous transcription, translation, and antigenic processing of the encoded protein [13, 14].

DNA vaccination offers a number of potential advantages over other vaccination strategies against cancer (Table 1). DNA vaccines are simple and relatively inexpensive to prepare in large quantities, and have a long shelf life compared with traditional protein or peptide vaccines. Because they encode the entire sequence of a tumor antigen, they provide multiple potential epitopes for binding to MHC Class I and Class II molecules as well as to antibodies, and do not require an HLA-restricted patient population, unlike peptide vaccines. Unlike autologous tumor cell or dendritic cell vaccines, they do not require extensive *ex vivo* preparation of patient samples, and unlike live, modified viral vaccines they do not induce potentially neutralizing immunity against immunodominant viral antigens and engender no concerns about virulence in a possibly immunosuppressed patient population. Finally, the bacterial plasmid backbone of a DNA vaccine contains immunostimulatory sequences (ISS) consisting of an unmethylated cytosine-guanine (CpG) dinucleotide flanked by two 5' purines and two 3' pyrimidines (known as a "CpG motif"). These CpG motifs bind to Toll-like receptor 9 (TLR9) on B cells and dendritic cells, promoting B cell activation and leading to NK and T cell activity through activation of dendritic cells and production of interferons and IL-12 [15–17]. These ISS thus provide a natural, inflammatory "danger signal" which bridges both innate and acquired immunity and obviates the need to administer the DNA in a typical vaccine adjuvant.

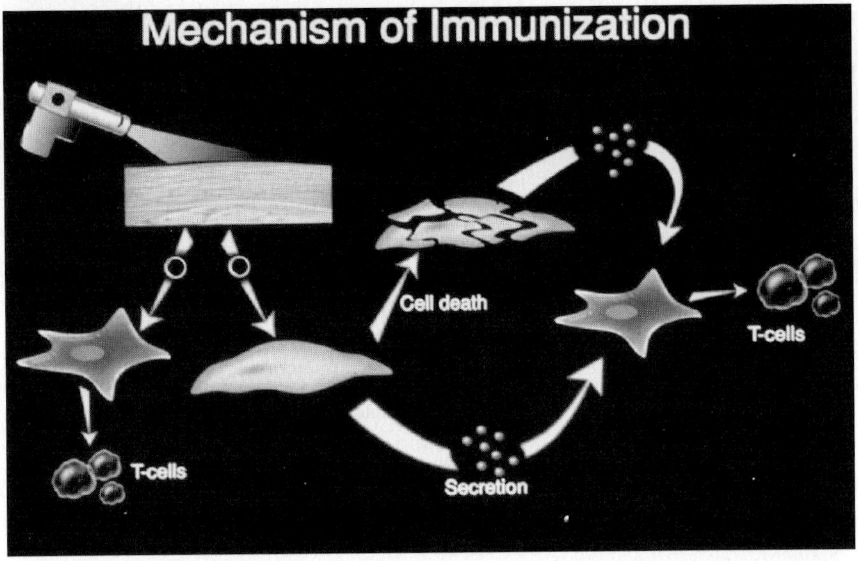

Figure 1. Mechanism of DNA vaccination Antigen-encoding plasmids administered into muscle or skin can be either taken up directly by resident antigen-presenting cells (APCs) (e.g. dendritic cells) or by myocytes/keratinocytes. In the first situation, the encoded protein is translated, processed, and presented as peptide-MHC complexes by the APC to T cells. In the second situation, known as "cross-priming," the encoded antigen is secreted or released by transfected myocytes/keratinocytes, taken up by APC, and subsequently processed and presented to T cells

Source: Reprinted from Cancer Chemotherapy and Biological Response Modifiers: Annual 22, Cohen & Wolchok, "Chapter 35: DNA vaccines for melanoma", p. 762, © 2005, with permission from Elsevier.

DNA vaccines have typically been administered by needle injection or by gene gun, and are most commonly given intramuscularly or intradermally, though mucosal (e.g. oral, intravaginal) and intranodal administrations have been described. Early studies suggested that the site and method of immunization could bias the induced immune response toward a particular T helper cell subtype (i.e. Th1 vs. Th2), with intramuscular and needle-based immunizations leading to Th1 and predominantly cellular immunity, and intradermal and gene gun immunizations leading primarily to Th2 and humoral immunity [18, 19]. The literature on this is inconsistent, however, and we have found that the type of immunity induced depends primarily on the antigen used rather than on the route of immunization [20]. What is clear is that gene gun-based immunization can generate immune responses of similar magnitude to needle injection while using up to 100-fold less DNA, perhaps as a result of greater transfection of resident dendritic cells as the DNA-coated gold particles spread through the epidermis and dermis. However, whether this advantage will translate into greater immune responses clinically has not been tested, and the optimal site and method of DNA immunization therefore remains to be determined.

Table 1. Vaccine strategies for cancer

Type of vaccine	Relative advantages	Relative disadvantages
Autologous tumor cell	Patient-specific, provides multiple tumor antigens	Labor intensive, requires available tumor tissue and extensive ex vivo preparation
Allogeneic tumor cell	"Off the shelf" product, provides multiple tumor antigens	Irrelevant "allo" antigens, difficult to characterize induced immune responses
Peptide	"Off the shelf" product, easy to prepare, easy to quantify immune responses	Limited epitopes, requires HLA restriction, requires adjuvant, minimal antibody responses
Purified protein or carbohydrate	"Off the shelf" product, safety and immunogenicity established in clinical trials, provides multiple epitopes	Purification expensive, requires adjuvant, limited CTL responses
Recombinant viral vector	Stimulates innate immunity, provides multiple epitopes	Safety issues (especially in immunosuppressed), irrelevant viral antigens, neutralizing immunity to vector
Dendritic cell	Potent immunogenicity, can provide multiple epitopes	Labor intensive, requires extensive ex vivo preparation, optimal maturation status unknown
DNA	"Off the shelf" product, easy to prepare and stabilize, provides multiple epitopes, intrinsic immunostimulatory CpG motifs	Little clinical experience to date, optimal delivery method unknown

DNA VACCINES AGAINST CANCER: THE PROBLEM OF "SELF"

A number of tumor antigens (TAs) have been identified in recent years as potential targets for active immunization (Table 2). Some of these TAs, such as viral antigens (e.g. human papillomavirus 16 E6) [21], mutated oncogenes (e.g. CDK4, β-catenin) [22,23], products of translocation events (e.g. bcr-abl) [24], and cancer-testis antigens (e.g. MAGE-A1, NY-ESO-1) [25], represent attractive targets because they contain novel epitopes or were previously sequestered in an immune-privileged site. The most prevalent TAs, however, are true "self" antigens, either widely expressed molecules which are overexpressed on cancer cells (e.g. CEA, MUC1, her2/neu) or differentiation antigens (e.g. gp100, tyrosinase, PSMA) which are expressed only on particular tumors and their normal cell counterparts. Because these TAs are indistinguishable from self, most high-avidity T and B lymphocytes specific for them have already been deleted from the immune repertoire during development, a process known as central tolerance. Furthermore, those self-reactive lymphocytes which manage to escape central tolerance are typically of low avidity and are maintained in an anergic state through the absence of proper co-stimulation and the presence of regulatory T cells, a process known as peripheral

Table 2. Tumor antigens targeted by DNA vaccines

Antigen	Potential applications	References
tyrosinase	melanoma	[39, 64]
gp75/TRP-1	melanoma	[33, 120]
DCT/TRP-2	melanoma	[34, 36]
gp100	melanoma	[35, 37, 38, 40, 63]
melanA/MART-1	melanoma	[65]
CEA	epithelial cancers, including colorectal, lung, breast, head and neck, pancreas, gastric	[42–44, 70]
PSA	prostate carcinoma	[67, 89]
PSMA	prostate, renal cell carcinoma	[66, 129]
her2/neu (erbB2)	epithelial cancers, especially breast, ovarian, pancreas, lung	[49–54]
MUC1	epithelial cancers, especially breast, colorectal, ovarian, pancreas	[61, 62]
Ig idiotype	B-cell NHL, myeloma	[55–57]
TCR idiotype	T cell NHL	[58]
CD20	B-cell NHL	[59]
PML/RARα	APL	[60]
bcr-abl	CML, Ph+ ALL	[135]
HPV E6, E7	cervical carcinoma	[21, 96, 117]
MAGE-1, mage-b	melanoma; myeloma; renal cell, lung, breast, colon, bladder, ovarian carcinomas	[136, 137]
AFP	hepatocellular carcinoma, cholangiocarcinoma, germ cell tumors, ovarian	[138, 139]
WT1	acute leukemias,	[140]
survivin	Most carcinomas; melanoma; neuroblastoma; CLL; NHL	[107]
p53	multiple carcinomas, including gastric, colorectal, pancreas, esophageal, cholangiocarcinoma	[141, 142]
mutant ras	melanoma, pancreas, colorectal, thyroid, lung, cholangiocarcinoma	[143, 144]

Abbreviations: AFP=alpha fetoprotein; APL=acute promyelocytic leukemia; CEA=carcinoembryonic antigen; CLL=chronic lymphocytic leukemia; CML=chronic myelogenous leukemia; DCT=dopachrome tautomerase; HPV=human papillomavirus; Ig=immunoglobulin; MAGE=melanoma antigen; MART-1=melanoma antigen recognized by T cells 1; MUC1=mucin 1; NHL=non-Hodgkins lymphoma; Ph+ ALL=Philadelphia chromosome-positive acute lymphoblastic leukemia; PSA=prostate-specific antigen; PSMA=prostate-specific membrane antigen; TCR=T cell receptor; TRP-1=tyrosinase-related protein 1; TRP-2=tyrosinase-related protein 2; WT1=Wilms tumor 1

tolerance (reviewed in [26]). Overcoming this tolerance is thus one of the central challenges of active immunization against cancer.

DNA Vaccines Against Melanoma Antigens

Among the most extensively-studied TAs are the melanoma differentiation antigens, which are expressed only in melanomas and normal melanocytes, and include tyrosinase, tyrosinase-related protein 1 (TRP-1)/gp75, TRP-2/DCT (dopachrome tautomerase), gp100, and melanA/MART-1. All of these antigens are highly expressed on both melanoma cell lines and primary melanoma patient samples, and have been shown to be recognized by T cells and/or antibodies derived from melanoma patients [27–31]. They therefore are very attractive targets for cancer vaccination strategies. Initial murine studies of active immunization against TRP-1/gp75 demonstrated that immune responses could not be generated by immunizing with an unaltered, syngeneic (i.e. mouse) form of the antigen. However, when mice were immunized with xenogeneic (i.e. human) TRP-1/gp75 protein, which shares 87 % homology with the mouse protein [31], they developed antibodies which recognized both human and mouse TRP-1/gp75 and were protected from an otherwise lethal tumor challenge with the poorly immunogenic, syngeneic B16 melanoma cell line [32]. The human TRP-1/gp75-immunized mice, but not the mouse TRP-1/gp75-immunized mice, also developed autoimmune coat depigmentation, further demonstrating that tolerance to this self melanosomal protein had been broken.

Following this initial study, we [33–35] and others [36–38] demonstrated that DNA vaccines encoding xenogeneic orthologues of these melanoma differentiation antigens were an effective way to break tolerance and induce protective tumor immunity. Immunization of mice with a plasmid encoding human TRP-1/gp75 led to antigen-specific autoantibodies and an 85% decrease in the number of B16 lung metastases compared with unimmunized mice or mice immunized with a mouse TRP-1/gp75 vaccine [33]. Similar protective immunity was seen using DNA vaccines encoding human TRP-2 or gp100, though with these antigens tumor immunity was mediated primarily by CD8+ T cells. Immunization with the human TRP-2 plasmid led to a significant decrease in lung metastases even when started 4 or 10 days after tumor challenge, when metastases were already established, and could also induce protection in an intradermal tumor model [34, 35]. In addition, xenogeneic melanoma DNA vaccines have been studied pre-clinically in an outbred dog population with spontaneously arising melanoma, and have led to documented tumor regressions and prolonged survival compared with historical controls [39]. Thus, xenogeneic DNA immunization can generate both antibody and T cell responses to melanosomal self antigens leading to protective tumor immunity and autoimmunity.

One mechanism by which xenogeneic immunization may break tolerance to self is through key amino acid differences in MHC Class I or Class II epitopes which lead to higher affinity for native MHC molecules than the syngeneic peptide. Such epitopes are known as heteroclitic epitopes, and they represent another strategy by which poorly-recognized self antigens can be altered to become immunogenic. For example, the human form of the MHC class I- restricted $gp100_{25-33}$ epitope, KVPRNQDWL, binds more strongly to the mouse D^b MHC class I molecule than the native mouse peptide, EGSRNQDWL. A DNA vaccine encoding a site-specific mutant of human gp100, in which amino acids 25-27 (KVP) were changed to those seen at positions 25-27 in the mouse (EGS), lost its ability to induce tumor protection. As well, a "minigene" construct encoding just the human $gp100_{25-33}$ epitope was sufficient to induce CTL responses and protect from tumor challenge, while the mouse $gp100_{25-33}$ minigene had no effect [40]. In this system a single heteroclitic epitope is therefore both necessary and sufficient to break tolerance and induce tumor immunity. These results suggest that using site-specific mutagenesis to alter known and potential MHC Class I epitopes in order to enhance binding may be a promising strategy to optimize DNA vaccines against cancer antigens.

DNA Vaccines Against Other Tumor Antigens

Carcinoembryonic antigen (CEA) is a 200-kDa protein expressed in normal fetal and adult gastrointestinal tissue and overexpressed in numerous epithelial malignancies, including colorectal, pancreas, gastric, breast, non-small cell lung, and head and neck carcinomas [41]. Conry et al first showed that DNA vaccination against human CEA could elicit humoral and cellular immune responses and protective immunity against a human CEA-transduced mouse colon cancer cell line [42]. More recent studies have used a more relevant CEA-transgenic mouse model, in which widespread expression of the human CEA protein leads to a state of peripheral tolerance similar to that induced by a self antigen. In this model, a CEA-encoding DNA vaccine could break tolerance and lead to protective immunity against CEA-expressing MC38 colon or Lewis lung carcinomas when the plasmid was administered orally via a bacterial carrier system consisting of an attenuated strain of *Salmonella typhimurium* [43, 44]. The bacterial carrier likely provides natural "danger" signals such as LPS and CpG oligonucleotides, which stimulate innate immunity and provide the inflammatory signals necessary to overcome tolerance, and represents another approach to inducing immunity against self tumor antigens.

Another well-studied antigen used for DNA vaccination is the product of the her-2/neu (erbB-2) oncogene. This 185 kDa member of the epidermal growth factor receptor-tyrosine kinase family is overexpressed in a number of epithelial cancers, including breast, ovarian, lung, and pancreatic cancer, and has been shown to be recognized by naturally-arising antibodies and T cells in cancer patients [45, 46]. The importance of this antigen as a target of immunotherapy has been demonstrated by the success of trastuzumab, a humanized monoclonal antibody specific for the her-2/neu protein, both alone and together with chemotherapy, in improving response rates and survival of women with her-2/neu-overexpressing breast carcinoma [47, 48]. Several investigators have now been able to actively generate immunity against her-2/neu in mice using DNA vaccines encoding human or rat her-2/neu, leading to protection from subsequent challenge with a her-2/neu expressing tumor [49–51]. In addition, her-2/neu DNA vaccination can slow or even reverse the growth of spontaneously arising mammary carcinomas in rat neu transgenic mouse models [52–54]. Protective immunity is mediated by both antibodies and T cells, and can be induced by plasmids encoding truncated her-2/neu proteins lacking the cytoplasmic tyrosine kinase domain, lessening concern about transfecting host cells, even transiently, with a potential oncogene [49–51,53].

These studies and others demonstrate the potential of her-2/neu-targeted active immunotherapy in patients with cancers overexpressing her-2/neu.

While most investigations of DNA immunization to date have focused on antigens expressed by solid tumors such as melanoma or various adenocarcinomas, several DNA vaccines targeting hematologic malignancies are also being developed. The most heavily studied to date are plasmids encoding a unique portion of light and heavy chain variable region sequences derived from the clone-specific immunoglobulin (Ig) expressed by Ig-producing malignancies (i.e. B-cell lymphomas and multiple myeloma). This unique Ig fragment, termed the idiotype (Id), is expressed only by the clonally rearranged neoplastic cell and is a true tumor-specific antigen. It represents a patient-specific antigen as well, as each lymphoma or myeloma patient's neoplastic cells express a unique idiotype. Levy and colleagues first demonstrated that a DNA vaccine encoding a murine B-cell lymphoma idiotype could induce anti-Id antibodies and protection from tumor challenge [55]. Stevenson's group has confirmed and extended these findings in other murine lymphoma and myeloma models using plasmids encoding single chain variable region fragments (scFv) fused to fragment C of tetanus toxin, leading to strong anti-Id antibodies and tumor rejection [56, 57]. This approach can also be used to target T-cell lymphomas, as a DNA vaccine encoding the clonotypic T-cell receptor Vα and Vβ sequences from a murine T-cell lymphoma, again fused to fragment C of tetanus toxin, induced antibody-mediated immunity from in vivo tumor challenge [58]. Finally, Palomba and colleagues have used plasmids encoding all or part of CD20, a surface molecule expressed by the majority of B-cell lymphomas and the target of monoclonal antibody Rituximab, to generate CD20-specific cytotoxic CD8+ T cells and modest tumor protection in the A20 murine B-cell lymphoma model [59].

DNA vaccines encoding a host of additional tumor antigens are currently in various stages of development (Table 2), with potential targets ranging from extremely tumor-specific (e.g. the PML/RARα translocation product in acute promyelocytic leukemia [60]) to extremely broad (e.g. the MUC1 glycoprotein overexpressed in the majority of adenocarcinomas [61, 62]). The extent of this list in Table 2 demonstrates the relative ease of generation of DNA vaccines and their potentially widespread application to cancer therapy.

CLINICAL STUDIES OF DNA VACCINES AGAINST CANCER

Although DNA vaccines have been extensively studied in the pre-clinical setting, there are only scarce data published about DNA vaccine trials in patients with cancer [63–71]. The National Cancer Institute carried out a phase I study of DNA immunization with a plasmid encoding a mutated human gp100 protein in patients with metastatic melanoma [63]. The gene was modified to contain two amino acid substitutions (at positions 210 and 288, respectively) that produced heteroclitic epitopes with increased binding affinity for the HLA-A*0201 class I molecule. The vaccine was administered to 22 HLA-A*0201-positive patients either intramuscularly (n=10) or intradermally (n=12), every month for 4 months. None of the 13 patients evaluable for the induction of T-cell responses after the second vaccination had developed CD8+ responses to the immunodominant $gp100_{209-217}$ or $gp100_{280-288}$ peptides, as measured by an in vitro restimulation assay. Only five patients received all four immunizations, with 3 evaluable, and none showed gp100-specific CD8+ T-cell responses. There was one partial clinical response.

Another phase I trial evaluated the safety and immunogenicity of a DNA vaccine encoding 2 human tyrosinase peptides. The vaccine was administered to 26 patients with stage IV melanoma as a continuous 4-day infusion into an inguinal lymph node, repeated every 2 weeks for 4 treatments. The vaccine was well-tolerated. Although no objective tumor responses were observed, 11 of 24 (46%) evaluable patients had increased peptide-specific T-cell responses, as measured by tetramer assay [64]. A third phase I DNA vaccine trial in melanoma patients, testing escalating doses (100,300, and 1000μg) of a MART-1 plasmid vaccine in 12 patients with resected high-risk melanoma, has recently been reported. The vaccine was injected intramuscularly every 6 weeks for four immunizations, and was well-tolerated. No significant T cell or antibody responses were noted to MART-1 or to a control hepatitis B surface antigen (HBsAg) DNA vaccine that was administered concurrently [65].

A phase I/II study in patients with advanced prostate cancer evaluated the safety of immunization with DNA constructs encoding the extracellular domain of human prostate-specific membrane antigen (PSMA) or PSMA plus the co-stimulatory molecule CD86. Although vaccination with either of these DNA constructs could induce delayed-type hypersensitivity (DTH) responses, the plasmids were less effective than a replication-deficient adenovirus vector expressing PSMA [66]. A separate phase I clinical trial of DNA vaccination with a plasmid expressing prostate-specific antigen (PSA) administered together with the cytokines granulocyte/macrophage-colony stimulating factor (GM-CSF) and IL-2 as vaccine adjuvants was carried out in patients with hormone-refractory prostate cancer. The vaccine was administered to nine patients five times at monthly intervals, and the adjuvants were given concomitantly with the vaccine. The study showed that of the eight evaluable patients, a PSA-specific cellular immune response, measured by IFN-γ production by activated T cells, was detected in 3 patients, and a rise in anti-PSA IgG in two patients treated in the highest dose group (900 μg DNA). One of these patients had a decline in serum PSA levels, though clinical responses were not described [67,68]. Nonetheless, humoral and cellular responses could be induced against PSA in patients vaccinated with PSA DNA and cytokine adjuvants.

A phase I/II clinical trial evaluated safety and immunogenicity of a DNA vaccine encoding a chimeric idiotype protein consisting of the variable heavy and light chains from each patient's tumor linked to a mouse heavy and light chain constant region [69]. Nine of the 12 patients with B-cell lymphoma enrolled in the trial developed anti-mouse immunoglobulin responses, whereas 6 patients (50%) developed modest anti-idiotype humoral or T-cell responses; these responses were usually not solely specific for the patients' own idiotype. DNA vaccination was well-tolerated in all patients evaluated, with mild-moderate injection reactions being the only adverse effect. Finally, in a phase I study for metastatic colon cancer patients, a dual-expression plasmid encoding CEA and hepatitis B surface antigen (HBsAg) induced T-cell proliferative responses to CEA in 4 of 17 patients, but no anti-CEA antibodies or objective clinical responses were reported [70].

Currently, several clinical trials using xenogeneic DNA vaccines are under way at Memorial Sloan-Kettering Cancer Center. We have recently completed accrual of two studies in patients with melanoma who received DNA vaccines encoding the melanosomal differentiation antigens tyrosinase or TRP-1/gp75. Three other studies are under way: one with gp100 DNA for patients with melanoma, one with PSMA DNA for patients with prostate cancer, and one with PSMA DNA for patients with renal cell cancer. These studies should provide important information regarding the immunogenicity of the xenogeneic approach in humans.

While these initial clinical trials have shown DNA vaccines to be safe and well-tolerated in cancer patients, the overall immune and clinical responses generated have been disappointing to date. There are several potential explanations for these observations. First, because most patients in these trials have had advanced metastatic disease and/or have been heavily pre-treated with chemotherapy or immunotherapy, they may not be the optimal population in which to evaluate immune responses to DNA vaccines. More trials testing these vaccines in patients without active disease but at high risk for relapse, as in the MART-1 trial [65], may be necessary to observe evidence of immunity. In addition, it is also possible that the DTH and lymphoproliferation assays commonly used in these initial trials may not have the sensitivity required to detect vaccine-induced immune responses. Newer techniques to measure changes in antigen-specific T cell frequency, including ELISPOT, intracellular cytokine assays, or tetramer assays, may better assess immunogenicity. Third, the optimal schedule, administration site (intramuscular, intradermal or subcutaneous), and administration method (needle and syringe, particle bombardment, or needle-free injection) for DNA vaccines have not been extensively studied in humans, and may markedly influence outcomes. Furthermore, the vaccines' immunogenicity may be dose-dependent, and the doses used to date (100 – 1800 μg) are still 1–2 orders of magnitude lower (on a per-weight basis) than those commonly used in mice.

It is possible, however, that these first-generation DNA vaccines, despite their efficacy in murine tumor models, may simply not be potent enough to induce immune responses in patients with cancer. This may partly be due to differential expression of TLR9, the receptor for immunostimulatory CpG motifs expressed by plasmid vectors, on mouse and human dendritic cell subsets [72, 73], or may reflect the many immunosuppressive and immune-escape mechanisms utilized by tumors in vivo (recently reviewed in [74]). Optimizing the immunogenicity of these vaccines, through many of the strategies described in the next section, may be necessary to generate effective anti-tumor immunity in cancer patients.

MODULATING IMMUNITY TO DNA VACCINES

A well-described feature of DNA vaccination is that the immunization process can be manipulated so that the magnitude of the induced immune response, as well as its bias (e.g. toward cellular vs. humoral immunity, or a Th1 vs. Th2-type response) is altered. This ability to modulate DNA-vaccine induced immunity has been demonstrated using a number of different approaches, including co-immunization with plasmids encoding cytokine or co-stimulatory molecules; fusion of antigens to bacterial or viral products which provide T helper epitopes, alter antigen trafficking, and/or stimulate innate immunity; and blocking inhibitory T cell signaling using monoclonal antibodies, among others (Table 3). Several of these approaches are described briefly below, and in more detail elsewhere in this volume.

Table 3. Modulating immunity to DNA vaccines

Approach	Rationale/Comment	References
Cytokine/chemokine genetic adjuvants		
IL-2	T cell activation and proliferation	[79-81, 84, 85, 88–90]
IL-4	Th2 bias. B cell activation	[84, 90]
IL-12	Th1 bias. Enhances NK and CTL activity.	[80, 84, 87–89, 91]
IL-15	Stimulates effector and memory CD8+ T cells	[80, 88, 93]
IL-18	CD4+ T cell proliferation and IFN-γ production	[80, 89, 91, 94, 95]
GM-CSF	Recruits and activates monocytes and DC's	[83, 84, 86, 88, 92]
IFN-γ	Macrophage activation. Upregulation of MHC complexes	[84, 91]
Flt3L	Expands and matures DC's	[88, 96-99]
MIP-1α	Recruits monocytes and DC's. Synergistic with Flt3L plasmid [97]	[99, 101, 102, 105]
RANTES	Recruits monocytes, T cells	[101, 103, 104]
MCP-1	Recruits monocytes	[101, 103, 105]
SLC/CCL21	CCR7 ligand. Recruits and activates DC's	[80, 106, 107]
Co-stimulatory/adhesion molecule genes		
B7.1/B7.2 (CD80/CD86)	Co-stimulates T cell activation	[92, 109, 110]
CD40 ligand	Activates/matures APCs	[114–116]
ICAM-1 or LFA-3	Facilitate T cell-APC interactions	[145]
Bacterial/viral products	(All enhance innate immunity)	
Tetanus toxoid FrC	Additional T helper epitopes	[56–58]
HSV VP22	Intercellular spread of antigen	[117]
Pseudomonas exotoxin	Alters endosomal trafficking to enhance cross-presentation of antigen	[118, 119]
Alphaviral replicase	Augments antigen expression. Creates dsRNA (TLR3 agonist)	[120]

(*Continued*)

Table 3. (*Continued*)

Approach	Rationale/Comment	References
Klebsiella OmpA	Induces DC maturation and IL-12 production	[146]
Attenuated Salmonella typhimurium	Oral delivery vehicle. Mucosal and systemic immunity	[43, 44, 122, 123]
Mycobacterial HSP70	Enhances MHC Class I presentation of antigen	[147]
Block negative T cell signaling		
Anti-CTLA4 mAb	Blocks B7-CTLA4 interaction.↑ expansion of activated T cells	[129]
Anti-GITR mAb	Inhibits Tregs, co-stimulates activated effector T cells	[133, 134]
Other strategies		
Imiquimod/resiquimod	TLR7 agonist. DC maturation	[148–150]
VEGFR2-, Fra-1-, or PDGF-B-expressing plasmids	Target endothelial cells. Anti-angiogenesis	[151–153]
BCL-xL plasmid	Inhibits apoptosis and prolongs DC survival	[154]
Electroporation	Enhances plasmid delivery/expression	[53, 155]
Low dose cyclophosphamide	Inhibits Tregs or boosts T cell homeostatic proliferation	[153, 156]

Abbreviations: APC=antigen-presenting cell; CTL=cytotoxic T lymphocyte; CTLA4=cytotoxic T lymphocyte antigen 4; DC=dendritic cell; Flt3L=fms-like tyrosine kinase 3 ligand; Fra-1=fos-related antigen 1; FrC=fragment C; GITR=glucocorticoid-induced tumor necrosis factor receptor; GMCSF= granulocyte/monocyte-colony stimulating factor; HSP70=heat shock protein 70; HSV=herpes simplex virus; ICAM-1=intracellular adhesion molecule 1; IFN=interferon; LFA-3=lymphocyte function associated 3; mAb=monoclonal antibody; MHC=major histocompatibility complex; MIP=macrophage inflammatory protein; MCP-1=monocyte chemoattractant protein 1; NK=natural killer; OmpA=outer membrane protein A; PDGF-B=platelet-derived growth factor B; RANTES=regulated upon activation, normal T-cell expressed, and presumably secreted; SLC=secondary lymphoid tissue cytokine; TLR=tolllike receptor; Tregs=CD4+CD25+ regulatory T cells; VEGFR2=vascular endothelial growth factor receptor 2;

Cytokines, Chemokines, and Co-stimulatory Molecules

A multitude of cytokine- and chemokine-expressing plasmids have been tested as "genetic" or "molecular" adjuvants designed to augment DNA-vaccine induced immunity (Table 3) (see references [75–78] for detailed reviews). These are typically administered at the same time or shortly after antigen immunization, and can be effective either as a separate plasmid vector or when co-expressed with antigen in a bi-cistronic vector. The advantages of using the cytokine-encoding gene product rather than recombinant protein include lower cost as well as the ability to generate high concentrations of cytokine at the site of immunization and draining lymph nodes (where the immune response is being primed), with minimal systemic effects.

These local effects can be further enhanced through plasmid vectors which fuse the cytokine to the Fc portion of an IgG immunoglobulin, presumably through greater stability of the protein and longer in vivo half-life [79–81].

Among the best-studied molecular adjuvants are plasmids encoding IL-2, IL-12, or GMCSF. IL-2 constructs have been shown to augment both humoral and cellular immunity, while IL-12 plasmids primarily enhance cytotoxic T cell responses and the generation of memory T cells. GM-CSF constructs are typically given prior to the first vaccination in order to recruit dendritic cells and other APCs to the immunization site [82, 83], leading to greater priming for both antibody and T cell responses. All of these constructs, given in combination with DNA vaccines, have been shown to enhance protection from infectious pathogens or rejection of tumors in both rodent and non-human primate models [75–81, 84–92], and are currently being tested as vaccine adjuvants in clinical trials. Other promising cytokines currently under study in animal models of DNA vaccination include IL-15, which can enhance both effector and memory CD8+ T cell responses [88, 93]; IL-18, which has augmented antigen-specific lymphoproliferative responses and production of the Th1 cytokines IL-2 and IFN-γ [89, 91, 94, 95]; and flt3 (fms-like tyrosine kinase 3) ligand, which expands and matures dendritic cells recruited to the site of immunization, leading to improved priming of both humoral and cellular immunity [88, 96–99].

Chemokines are chemoattractant molecules which function to regulate the trafficking of leukocytes, including monocytes, lymphocytes, dendritic cells, eosinophils, and neutrophils, and are important for the induction of both non-specific inflammatory responses and adaptive immunity [100]. Several animal studies have now shown that plasmids encoding the CCR1/CCR5 agonists MIP (macrophage inflammatory protein)-1α, MIP-1β, and RANTES (regulated upon activation, normal T-cell expressed, and presumably secreted); the CCR2 agonist MCP-1 (monocyte chemoattractant protein-1); and the CCR7 agonist SLC (secondary lymphoid tissue cytokine)/CCL21, among others, have potent adjuvant activity when co-injected with DNA vaccines, due to enhanced recruitment of APCs to the immunization site and increased production of inflammatory cytokines such as IFN-γ [99, 101–107]. In particular, an approach using MIP-1α and flt3L plasmids together to first recruit, and then expand and activate infiltrating dendritic cells synergistically augmented both antibody and T cell responses against an HIV-1 envelope DNA vaccine, demonstrating the potential for combining chemokine and cytokine genetic adjuvants [99]. Interestingly, repeated injections of chemokine-expressing plasmids in a rat autoimmune arthritis model led to neutralizing antibodies against the chemokines and amelioration of autoimmunity [108], suggesting that these constructs may become less effective with repeated administration.

The co-stimulatory molecules CD80 (B7.1) and CD86 (B7.2) are expressed by activated APCs and are critical for the activation of naïve T lymphocytes, via secondary signaling through CD28. Co-delivery of CD80 or CD86 genes during DNA immunization can boost antigen-specific cellular immune responses, presumably by improving the antigen-presenting capability of transfected host cells [92, 109, 110]. CD40 is a co-stimulatory molecule expressed on APCs, including

B cells, macrophages, and dendritic cells, while CD40 ligand (CD40L)/CD154 is expressed by helper CD4+ T cells. Ligation of CD40 sends an activation and maturation stimulus to the APC, allowing it to more effectively activate naïve CD8+ T cells, a process termed "licensing" [111–113], and is one of the primary ways that CD4+ T cells help prime CD8+ T cell responses. DNA immunization with CD40L, either as a separate plasmid or combined with antigen in the same vector, has been shown to enhance both antibody and cytotoxic T lymphocyte responses and improve protection from viral or tumor challenge [114–116].

Bacterial and Viral Products

Another strategy to enhance the immunogenicity of DNA vaccines is to combine the antigen of interest with a component from an infectious organism, either to take advantage of universal T helper epitopes, the functional properties of a particular molecule, the inherent "danger" signals engendered by a microbial product, or some combination of the above. As mentioned previously, fusion of immunoglobulin idiotype genes to fragment C of tetanus toxin, which contains a "promiscuous" MHC Class II binding epitope, induced protective immunity in lymphoma and myeloma mouse models, and is currently undergoing testing in clinical trials [56,57]. Fusion of tumor antigens to the Herpesvirus VP22 tegument protein or the translocation domain of Pseudomonas exotoxin A, which alter inter- or intracellular antigen trafficking, respectively, and enhance MHC Class I presentation, dramatically augmented antigen-specific CD8+ T cell responses and improved protection from tumor challenge [117–119](M Engelhorn, JD Wolchok, and AN Houghton, manuscript in preparation). A DNA vaccine encoding mouse gp75/TRP-1 (mgp75) under control of an alphaviral replicase enzyme was able to break tolerance, induce autoantibodies, and protect mice from challenge with B16 melanoma, while a traditional mgp75-encoding construct was ineffective [120]. Interestingly, this was not due to enhanced antigen expression as predicted, but rather to the production, as a byproduct of replicase-mediated gene expression, of double-stranded RNA (dsRNA), which is a Toll-like receptor 3 (TLR3) agonist and a potent stimulator of innate immunity [121]. Another approach, which delivers DNA vaccines orally using an attenuated Salmonella typhimurium strain as a carrier, has generated strong T cell responses against viral and tumor antigens, and may have promise as a means to induce specific mucosal immunity [43,44,122,123].

Targeting Negative Regulatory Mechanisms

Another strategy to modulate DNA vaccination against cancer is to attempt to block inhibitory responses which result in the suppression of anti-tumor immunity. Two such approaches which have recently been explored in combination with DNA vaccination use monoclonal antibodies to target CTLA-4 (cytotoxic T lymphocyte antigen-4) or GITR (glucocorticoid-induced tumor necrosis factor receptor family-related gene). CTLA-4, a homolog of CD28, binds to CD80 and CD86 and is upregulated on CD4+ and CD8+ cells following TCR-mediation activation. Ligation of CTLA-4 leads to inhibition of T cell activation and therefore controls antigen-specific T cell proliferation and effector activity [124]. CTLA-4 is also constitutively expressed on CD4+CD25+ regulatory T cells (Tregs), though its exact function on these cells remains unclear. Antagonist anti-CTLA-4 antibodies have been shown to enhance T cell responses to whole cell tumor vaccines in murine models [125], and are currently being tested, either alone or in conjunction with peptide vaccination, in cancer patients. Both tumor immunity, manifested as significant clinical responses, and autoimmunity have been observed in early clinical trials to date [126–128]. Gregor et al found that the combination of anti-CTLA-4 antibody with xenogeneic DNA vaccines encoding melanoma or prostate differentiation antigens enhanced antigen-specific CD8+ T cell responses and tumor rejection. Interestingly, this effect was seen only with CTLA-4 blockade during the second or third of three weekly vaccinations. When the antibody was given prior to the initial DNA immunization, no enhancement was observed [129]. This suggests that T cells need to be previously activated for the optimal efficacy of this approach.

GITR is a TNF receptor family member with significant homology to the co-stimulatory molecules OX40, 4-1BB, and CD27. Like CTLA-4, GITR is expressed at low levels on resting CD4+ and CD8+ T cells, is significantly upregulated following T cell activation, and is expressed constitutively at high levels on Tregs [130]. Unlike CTLA-4, however, GITR ligation on activated T cells leads to further co-stimulation and proliferation, while GITR ligation on Tregs abrogates their suppressive activity [131, 132]. Thus, inducing a signal through GITR using an agonist anti-GITR antibody could potentially augment tumor immunotherapy by both co-stimulating tumor-specific effector T cells and inhibiting the immunosuppressive effects of Tregs. Indeed, Sakaguchi and colleagues have demonstrated that an agonist anti-GITR antibody can induce regression of early stage, modestly immunogenic murine tumors, and that this effect is further augmented with combined anti-GITR and anti-CTLA-4 treatment, suggesting the two antibodies may be acting upon distinct cell populations and/or pathways [133]. In addition, we have demonstrated that combining anti-GITR antibody with xenogeneic DNA vaccines encoding the melanoma differentiation antigens gp100 or TRP-2 leads to enhanced primary and recall CD8+ T cell responses and improved rejection of the poorly immunogenic B16 melanoma cell line. Similar to CTLA-4 blockade, GITR ligation was not effective prior to the initial vaccination, but only with subsequent immunizations, again implying a requirement for prior activation of T cells [134]. These initial pre-clinical studies demonstrate the potential for this approach as an adjunct to active immunization against cancer.

CONCLUSIONS

DNA immunization is a relatively novel approach to cancer immunotherapy which has shown significant potency in stimulating both innate and adaptive immunity against a wide variety of tumor antigens. While this promise has yet to be realized in cancer patients, early clinical trials have demonstrated the feasibility and safety of this approach, and a multitude of strategies designed to optimize and augment the immunogenicity of these vaccines (Table 3) have been identified. To move forward in this field, more extensive testing of next-generation vaccines and promising adjuvant strategies must occur in humans, with particular focus on determining the optimal dosing, timing and method of administration in cancer patients, as these parameters may differ significantly from those seen in animal models. Ultimately, combining DNA vaccination with other immunotherapeutic approaches, such as adoptive cellular therapy, other vaccines (e.g. "prime-boosting"), immunomodulatory chemotherapy, or anti-Treg strategies may be the most effective way to develop a comprehensive immune-based treatment regimen for cancer.

REFERENCES

1. Coley WB. The treatment of malignant tumors by repeated inoculations of erysipelas. With a report of ten original cases. Am J Med Sci 1893; 105: 487–511.
2. Rosenberg SA, Yang JC, Restifo NP. Cancer immunotherapy: moving beyond current vaccines. Nat Med 2004; 10: 909–915.
3. Tang DC, DeVit M, Johnston SA. Genetic immunization is a simple method for eliciting an immune response. Nature 1992; 356: 152–154.
4. Ulmer JB, Donnelly JJ, Parker SE et al. Heterologous protection against influenza by injection of DNA encoding a viral protein. Science 1993; 259: 1745–1749.
5. Fynan EF, Webster RG, Fuller DH et al. DNA vaccines: protective immunizations by parenteral, mucosal, and gene-gun inoculations. Proc Natl Acad Sci U S A 1993; 90: 1147811482.
6. Wang B, Ugen KE, Srikantan V et al. Gene inoculation generates immune responses against human immunodeficiency virus type 1. Proc Natl Acad Sci U S A 1993; 90: 4156–4160.
7. Davis HL, Michel ML, Mancini M et al. Direct gene transfer in skeletal muscle: plasmid DNA-based immunization against the hepatitis B virus surface antigen. Vaccine 1994; 12: 15031509.
8. Wang R, Doolan DL, Le TP et al. Induction of antigen-specific cytotoxic T lymphocytes in humans by a malaria DNA vaccine. Science 1998; 282: 476–480.
9. MacGregor RR, Boyer JD, Ugen KE et al. First human trial of a DNA-based vaccine for treatment of human immunodeficiency virus type 1 infection: safety and host response. J Infect Dis 1998; 178: 92–100.
10. Rottinghaus ST, Poland GA, Jacobson RM et al. Hepatitis B DNA vaccine induces protective antibody responses in human non-responders to conventional vaccination. Vaccine 2003; 21: 4604–4608.
11. Casares S, Inaba K, Brumeanu TD et al. Antigen presentation by dendritic cells after immunization with DNA encoding a major histocompatibility complex class II-restricted viral epitope. J Exp Med 1997; 186: 1481–1486.
12. Corr M, von Damm A, Lee DJ, Tighe H. In vivo priming by DNA injection occurs predominantly by antigen transfer. J Immunol 1999; 163: 4721–4727.
13. Porgador A, Irvine KR, Iwasaki A et al. Predominant role for directly transfected dendritic cells in antigen presentation to CD8+ T cells after gene gun immunization. J Exp Med 1998; 188: 1075–1082.
14. 14. Akbari O, Panjwani N, Garcia S et al. DNA vaccination: transfection and activation of dendritic cells as key events for immunity. J Exp Med 1999; 189: 169–178.
15. Krieg AM, Yi AK, Matson S et al. CpG motifs in bacterial DNA trigger direct B-cell activation. Nature 1995; 374: 546–549.
16. Sato Y, Roman M, Tighe H et al. Immunostimulatory DNA sequences necessary for effective intradermal gene immunization. Science 1996; 273: 352–354.
17. Hemmi H, Takeuchi O, Kawai T et al. A Toll-like receptor recognizes bacterial DNA. Nature 2000; 408: 740–745.

18. Feltquate DM, Heaney S, Webster RG, Robinson HL. Different T helper cell types and antibody isotypes generated by saline and gene gun DNA immunization. J Immunol 1997; 158: 2278–2284.
19. Pertmer TM, Roberts TR, Haynes JR. Influenza virus nucleoprotein-specific immunoglobulin G subclass and cytokine responses elicited by DNA vaccination are dependent on the route of vector DNA delivery. J Virol 1996; 70: 6119–6125.
20. Turk MJ, Wolchok JD, Guevara-Patino JA et al. Multiple pathways to tumor immunity and concomitant autoimmunity. Immunol Rev 2002; 188: 122–135.
21. Wlazlo AP, Deng H, Giles-Davis W, Ertl HC. DNA vaccines against the human papillomavirus type 16 E6 or E7 oncoproteins. Cancer Gene Ther 2004; 11: 457–464.
22. Wolfel T, Hauer M, Schneider J et al. A p16INK4a-insensitive CDK4 mutant targeted by cytolytic T lymphocytes in a human melanoma. Science 1995; 269: 1281–1284.
23. Robbins PF, El-Gamil M, Li YF et al. A mutated beta-catenin gene encodes a melanoma-specific antigen recognized by tumor infiltrating lymphocytes. J Exp Med 1996; 183: 1185–1192.
24. Pinilla-Ibarz J, Cathcart K, Korontsvit T et al. Vaccination of patients with chronic myelogenous leukemia with bcr-abl oncogene breakpoint fusion peptides generates specific immune responses. Blood 2000; 95: 1781–1787.
25. Scanlan MJ, Gure AO, Jungbluth AA et al. Cancer/testis antigens: an expanding family of targets for cancer immunotherapy. Immunol Rev 2002; 188: 22–32.
26. O'Garra A, Vieira P. Regulatory T cells and mechanisms of immune system control. Nat Med 2004; 10: 801–805.
27. Brichard V, Van Pel A, Wolfel T et al. The tyrosinase gene codes for an antigen recognized by autologous cytolytic T lymphocytes on HLA-A2 melanomas. J Exp Med 1993; 178: 489–495.
28. Wang RF, Appella E, Kawakami Y et al. Identification of TRP-2 as a human tumor antigen recognized by cytotoxic T lymphocytes. J Exp Med 1996; 184: 2207–2216.
29. Bakker AB, Schreurs MW, de Boer AJ et al. Melanocyte lineage-specific antigen gp100 is recognized by melanoma-derived tumor-infiltrating lymphocytes. J Exp Med 1994; 179: 10051009.
30. Kawakami Y, Eliyahu S, Delgado CH et al. Cloning of the gene coding for a shared human melanoma antigen recognized by autologous T cells infiltrating into tumor. Proc Natl Acad Sci U S A 1994; 91: 3515–3519.
31. Vijayasaradhi S, Bouchard B, Houghton AN. The melanoma antigen gp75 is the human homologue of the mouse b (brown) locus gene product. J Exp Med 1990; 171: 1375–1380.
32. Naftzger C, Takechi Y, Kohda H et al. Immune response to a differentiation antigen induced by altered antigen: a study of tumor rejection and autoimmunity. Proc Natl Acad Sci U S A 1996; 93: 14809–14814.
33. Weber LW, Bowne WB, Wolchok JD et al. Tumor immunity and autoimmunity induced by immunization with homologous DNA. J Clin Invest 1998; 102: 1258–1264.
34. Bowne WB, Srinivasan R, Wolchok JD et al. Coupling and uncoupling of tumor immunity and autoimmunity. J Exp Med 1999; 190: 1717–1722.
35. Hawkins WG, Gold JS, Dyall R et al. Immunization with DNA coding for gp100 results in CD4 T-cell independent antitumor immunity. Surgery 2000; 128: 273–280.
36. Steitz J, Bruck J, Steinbrink K et al. Genetic immunization of mice with human tyrosinase-related protein 2: implications for the immunotherapy of melanoma. Int J Cancer 2000; 86: 89–94.
37. Rakhmilevich AL, Imboden M, Hao Z et al. Effective particle-mediated vaccination against mouse melanoma by coadministration of plasmid DNA encoding Gp100 and granulocyte-macrophage colony-stimulating factor. Clin Cancer Res 2001; 7: 952–961.
38. Schreurs MW, de Boer AJ, Figdor CG, Adema GJ. Genetic vaccination against the melanocyte lineage-specific antigen gp100 induces cytotoxic T lymphocyte-mediated tumor protection. Cancer Res 1998; 58: 2509–2514.
39. Bergman PJ, McKnight J, Novosad A et al. Long-term survival of dogs with advanced malignant melanoma after DNA vaccination with xenogeneic human tyrosinase: a phase I trial. Clin Cancer Res 2003; 9: 1284–1290.

40. Gold JS, Ferrone CR, Guevara-Patino JA et al. A single heteroclitic epitope determines cancer immunity after xenogeneic DNA immunization against a tumor differentiation antigen. J Immunol 2003; 170: 5188–5194.
41. Marshall J. Carcinoembryonic antigen-based vaccines. Semin Oncol 2003; 30: 30–36.
42. Conry RM, LoBuglio AF, Loechel F et al. A carcinoembryonic antigen polynucleotide vaccine has in vivo antitumor activity. Gene Ther 1995; 2: 59–65.
43. Niethammer AG, Primus FJ, Xiang R et al. An oral DNA vaccine against human carcinoembryonic antigen (CEA) prevents growth and dissemination of Lewis lung carcinoma in CEA transgenic mice. Vaccine 2001; 20: 421–429.
44. Zhou H, Luo Y, Mizutani M et al. A novel transgenic mouse model for immunological evaluation of carcinoembryonic antigen-based DNA minigene vaccines. J Clin Invest 2004; 113: 1792–1798.
45. Disis ML, Calenoff E, McLaughlin G et al. Existent T-cell and antibody immunity to HER-2/neu protein in patients with breast cancer. Cancer Res 1994; 54: 16–20.
46. Peoples GE, Goedegebuure PS, Smith R et al. Breast and ovarian cancer-specific cytotoxic T lymphocytes recognize the same HER2/neu-derived peptide. Proc Natl Acad Sci U S A 1995; 92: 432–436.
47. Slamon DJ, Leyland-Jones B, Shak S et al. Use of chemotherapy plus a monoclonal antibody against HER2 for metastatic breast cancer that overexpresses HER2. N Engl J Med 2001; 344: 783–792.
48. Vogel CL, Cobleigh MA, Tripathy D et al. Efficacy and safety of trastuzumab as a single agent in first-line treatment of HER2-overexpressing metastatic breast cancer. J Clin Oncol 2002; 20: 719–726.
49. Chen Y, Hu D, Eling DJ et al. DNA vaccines encoding full-length or truncated Neu induce protective immunity against Neu-expressing mammary tumors. Cancer Res 1998; 58: 1965–1971.
50. Piechocki MP, Pilon SA, Wei WZ. Complementary antitumor immunity induced by plasmid DNA encoding secreted and cytoplasmic human ErbB-2. J Immunol 2001; 167: 33673374.
51. Foy TM, Bannink J, Sutherland RA et al. Vaccination with Her-2/neu DNA or protein subunits protects against growth of a Her-2/neu-expressing murine tumor. Vaccine 2001; 19: 2598–2606.
52. Amici A, Venanzi FM, Concetti A. Genetic immunization against neu/erbB2 transgenic breast cancer. Cancer Immunol Immunother 1998; 47: 183–190.
53. Quaglino E, Iezzi M, Mastini C et al. Electroporated DNA vaccine clears away multifocal mammary carcinomas in her-2/neu transgenic mice. Cancer Res 2004; 64: 2858–2864.
54. Spadaro M, Ambrosino E, Iezzi M et al. Cure of mammary carcinomas in Her-2 transgenic mice through sequential stimulation of innate (neoadjuvant interleukin-12) and adaptive (DNA vaccine electroporation) immunity. Clin Cancer Res 2005; 11: 1941–1952.
55. Syrengelas AD, Chen TT, Levy R. DNA immunization induces protective immunity against B-cell lymphoma. Nat Med 1996; 2: 1038–1041.
56. King CA, Spellerberg MB, Zhu D et al. DNA vaccines with single-chain Fv fused to fragment C of tetanus toxin induce protective immunity against lymphoma and myeloma. Nat Med 1998; 4: 1281–1286.
57. Stevenson FK, Ottensmeier CH, Johnson P et al. DNA vaccines to attack cancer. Proc Natl Acad Sci U S A 2004; 101 Suppl 2: 14646–14652.
58. Thirdborough SM, Radcliffe JN, Friedmann PS, Stevenson FK. Vaccination with DNA encoding a single-chain TCR fusion protein induces anticlonotypic immunity and protects against T-cell lymphoma. Cancer Res 2002; 62: 1757–1760.
59. Palomba ML, Roberts WK, Dao T et al. CD8+ T-cell-dependent immunity following xenogeneic DNA immunization against CD20 in a tumor challenge model of B-cell lymphoma. Clin Cancer Res 2005; 11: 370–379.
60. Padua RA, Larghero J, Robin M et al. PML-RARA-targeted DNA vaccine induces protective immunity in a mouse model of leukemia. Nat Med 2003; 9: 1413–1417.
61. Johnen H, Kulbe H, Pecher G. Long-term tumor growth suppression in mice immunized with naked DNA of the human tumor antigen mucin (MUC1). Cancer Immunol Immunother 2001; 50: 356–360.

62. Kontani K, Taguchi O, Ozaki Y et al. Novel vaccination protocol consisting of injecting MUC1 DNA and nonprimed dendritic cells at the same region greatly enhanced MUC1-specific antitumor immunity in a murine model. Cancer Gene Ther 2002; 9: 330–337.
63. Rosenberg SA, Yang JC, Sherry RM et al. Inability to Immunize Patients with Metastatic Melanoma Using Plasmid DNA Encoding the gp100 Melanoma-Melanocyte Antigen. Hum Gene Ther 2003; 14: 709–714.
64. Tagawa ST, Lee P, Snively J et al. Phase I study of intranodal delivery of a plasmid DNA vaccine for patients with Stage IV melanoma. Cancer 2003; 98: 144–154.
65. Triozzi PL, Aldrich W, Allen KO et al. Phase I study of a plasmid DNA vaccine encoding MART-1 in patients with resected melanoma at risk for relapse. J Immunother 2005; 28: 382–388.
66. Mincheff M, Tchakarov S, Zoubak S et al. Naked DNA and adenoviral immunizations for immunotherapy of prostate cancer: a phase I/II clinical trial. Eur Urol 2000; 38: 208–217.
67. Pavlenko M, Roos AK, Lundqvist A et al. A phase I trial of DNA vaccination with a plasmid expressing prostate-specific antigen in patients with hormone-refractory prostate cancer. Br J Cancer 2004; 91: 688–694.
68. Miller AM, Ozenci V, Kiessling R, Pisa P. Immune monitoring in a phase 1 trial of a PSA DNA vaccine in patients with hormone-refractory prostate cancer. J Immunother 2005; 28: 389–395.
69. Timmerman JM, Singh G, Hermanson G et al. Immunogenicity of a plasmid DNA vaccine encoding chimeric idiotype in patients with B-cell lymphoma. Cancer Res 2002; 62: 5845–5852.
70. Conry RM, Curiel DT, Strong TV et al. Safety and immunogenicity of a DNA vaccine encoding carcinoembryonic antigen and hepatitis B surface antigen in colorectal carcinoma patients. Clin Cancer Res 2002; 8: 2782–2787.
71. Smith CL, Dunbar PR, Mirza F et al. Recombinant modified vaccinia Ankara primes functionally activated CTL specific for a melanoma tumor antigen epitope in melanoma patients with a high risk of disease recurrence. Int J Cancer 2005; 113: 259–266.
72. Kadowaki N, Ho S, Antonenko S et al. Subsets of human dendritic cell precursors express different toll-like receptors and respond to different microbial antigens. J Exp Med 2001; 194: 863–869.
73. Hochrein H, O'Keeffe M, Wagner H. Human and mouse plasmacytoid dendritic cells. Hum Immunol 2002; 63: 1103–1110.
74. Zou W. Immunosuppressive networks in the tumour environment and their therapeutic relevance. Nat Rev Cancer 2005; 5: 263–274.
75. Toka FN, Pack CD, Rouse BT. Molecular adjuvants for mucosal immunity. Immunol Rev 2004; 199: 100–112.
76. Calarota SA, Weiner DB. Enhancement of human immunodeficiency virus type 1-DNA vaccine potency through incorporation of T-helper 1 molecular adjuvants. Immunol Rev 2004; 199: 84–99.
77. Prud'homme GJ. DNA vaccination against tumors. J Gene Med 2005; 7: 3–17.
78. Cohen AD, Boyer JD, Weiner DB. Modulating the immune response to genetic immunization. Faseb J 1998; 12: 1611–1626.
79. Barouch DH, Santra S, Schmitz JE et al. Control of viremia and prevention of clinical AIDS in rhesus monkeys by cytokine-augmented DNA vaccination. Science 2000; 290: 486–492.
80. Ferrone CR, Perales M-A, Somberg CJ et al. Enhancement of CD8 T-cell responses and tumor protection following xenogeneic DNA immunization against a tumor antigen with IL-12/Ig DNA and IL-15/Ig DNA. Submitted for publication.
81. Barouch DH, Truitt DM, Letvin NL. Expression kinetics of the interleukin-2/immunoglobulin (IL-2/Ig) plasmid cytokine adjuvant. Vaccine 2004; 22: 3092–3097.
82. Bowne WB, Wolchok JD, Hawkins WG et al. Injection of DNA encoding granulocyte-macrophage colony-stimulating factor recruits dendritic cells for immune adjuvant effects. Cytokines Cell Mol Ther 1999; 5: 217–225.
83. Perales MA, Fantuzzi G, Goldberg SM et al. GM-CSF DNA induces specific patterns of cytokines and chemokines in the skin: implications for DNA vaccines. Cytokines Cell Mol Ther 2002; 7: 125–133.
84. Chow YH, Chiang BL, Lee YL et al. Development of Th1 and Th2 populations and the nature of immune responses to hepatitis B virus DNA vaccines can be modulated by codelivery of various cytokine genes. J Immunol 1998; 160: 1320–1329.

85. Bertley FM, Kozlowski PA, Wang SW et al. Control of simian/human immunodeficiency virus viremia and disease progression after IL-2-augmented DNA-modified vaccinia virus Ankara nasal vaccination in nonhuman primates. J Immunol 2004; 172: 3745–3757.
86. Weiss WR, Ishii KJ, Hedstrom RC et al. A plasmid encoding murine granulocyte-macrophage colony-stimulating factor increases protection conferred by a malaria DNA vaccine. J Immunol 1998; 161: 2325–2332.
87. Sin JI, Kim JJ, Arnold RL et al. IL-12 gene as a DNA vaccine adjuvant in a herpes mouse model: IL-12 enhances Th1-type CD4+ T cell-mediated protective immunity against herpes simplex virus-2 challenge. J Immunol 1999; 162: 2912–2921.
88. Moore AC, Kong WP, Chakrabarti BK, Nabel GJ. Effects of antigen and genetic adjuvants on immune responses to human immunodeficiency virus DNA vaccines in mice. J Virol 2002; 76: 243–250.
89. Kim JJ, Yang JS, Dang K et al. Engineering enhancement of immune responses to DNA-based vaccines in a prostate cancer model in rhesus macaques through the use of cytokine gene adjuvants. Clin Cancer Res 2001; 7: 882s-889s.
90. Geissler M, Gesien A, Tokushige K, Wands JR. Enhancement of cellular and humoral immune responses to hepatitis C virus core protein using DNA-based vaccines augmented with cytokine-expressing plasmids. J Immunol 1997; 158: 1231–1237.
91. Kim JJ, Nottingham LK, Tsai A et al. Antigen-specific humoral and cellular immune responses can be modulated in rhesus macaques through the use of IFN-gamma, IL-12, or IL-18 gene adjuvants. J Med Primatol 1999; 28: 214–223.
92. Conry RM, Widera G, LoBuglio AF et al. Selected strategies to augment polynucleotide immunization. Gene Ther 1996; 3: 67–74.
93. Kutzler MA, Robinson TM, Chattergoon MA et al. Coimmunization with an optimized IL-15 plasmid results in enhanced function and longevity of CD8 T cells that are partially independent of CD4 T cell help. J Immunol 2005; 175: 112–123.
94. Billaut-Mulot O, Idziorek T, Loyens M et al. Modulation of cellular and humoral immune responses to a multiepitopic HIV-1 DNA vaccine by interleukin-18 DNA immunization/viral protein boost. Vaccine 2001; 19: 2803–2811.
95. Zhu M, Xu X, Liu H et al. Enhancement of DNA vaccine potency against herpes simplex virus 1 by co-administration of an interleukin-18 expression plasmid as a genetic adjuvant. J Med Microbiol 2003; 52: 223–228.
96. Hung CF, Hsu KF, Cheng WF et al. Enhancement of DNA vaccine potency by linkage of antigen gene to a gene encoding the extracellular domain of Fms-like tyrosine kinase 3-ligand. Cancer Res 2001; 61: 1080–1088.
97. Sailaja G, Husain S, Nayak BP, Jabbar AM. Long-term maintenance of gp120-specific immune responses by genetic vaccination with the HIV-1 envelope genes linked to the gene encoding Flt-3 ligand. J Immunol 2003; 170: 2496–2507.
98. Sang H, Pisarev VM, Munger C et al. Regional, but not systemic recruitment/expansion of dendritic cells by a pluronic-formulated Flt3-ligand plasmid with vaccine adjuvant activity. Vaccine 2003; 21: 3019–3029.
99. Sumida SM, McKay PF, Truitt DM et al. Recruitment and expansion of dendritic cells in vivo potentiate the immunogenicity of plasmid DNA vaccines. J Clin Invest 2004; 114: 13341342.
100. Zlotnik A, Yoshie O. Chemokines: a new classification system and their role in immunity. Immunity 2000; 12: 121–127.
101. Kim JJ, Nottingham LK, Sin JI et al. CD8 positive T cells influence antigen-specific immune responses through the expression of chemokines. J Clin Invest 1998;
102. 1112–1124. 102. Lu Y, Xin KQ, Hamajima K et al. Macrophage inflammatory protein-1alpha (MIP1alpha) expression plasmid enhances DNA vaccine-induced immune response against HIV-1. Clin Exp Immunol 1999; 115: 335–341.
103. Pinto AR, Reyes-Sandoval A, Ertl HC. Chemokines and TRANCE as genetic adjuvants for a DNA vaccine to rabies virus. Cell Immunol 2003; 224: 106–113.

104. Sin J, Kim JJ, Pachuk C et al. DNA vaccines encoding interleukin-8 and RANTES enhance antigen-specific Th1-type CD4(+) T-cell-mediated protective immunity against herpes simplex virus type 2 in vivo. J Virol 2000; 74: 11173–11180.
105. Eo SK, Lee S, Chun S, Rouse BT. Modulation of immunity against herpes simplex virus infection via mucosal genetic transfer of plasmid DNA encoding chemokines. J Virol 2001; 75: 569–578.
106. Eo SK, Lee S, Kumaraguru U, Rouse BT. Immunopotentiation of DNA vaccine against herpes simplex virus via co-delivery of plasmid DNA expressing CCR7 ligands. Vaccine 2001; 19: 4685–4693.
107. Xiang R, Mizutani N, Luo Y et al. A DNA vaccine targeting survivin combines apoptosis with suppression of angiogenesis in lung tumor eradication. Cancer Res 2005; 65: 553–561.
108. Youssef S, Maor G, Wildbaum G et al. C-C chemokine-encoding DNA vaccines enhance breakdown of tolerance to their gene products and treat ongoing adjuvant arthritis. J Clin Invest 2000; 106: 361–371.
109. Kim JJ, Bagarazzi ML, Trivedi N et al. Engineering of in vivo immune responses to DNA immunization via codelivery of costimulatory molecule genes. Nat Biotechnol 1997; 15: 641–646.
110. Iwasaki A, Stiernholm BJ, Chan AK et al. Enhanced CTL responses mediated by plasmid DNA immunogens encoding costimulatory molecules and cytokines. J Immunol 1997; 158: 4591–4601.
111. Schoenberger SP, Toes RE, van der Voort EI et al. T-cell help for cytotoxic T lymphocytes is mediated by CD40-CD40L interactions. Nature 1998; 393: 480–483.
112. Bennett SR, Carbone FR, Karamalis F et al. Help for cytotoxic-T-cell responses is mediated by CD40 signalling. Nature 1998; 393: 478–480.
113. Ridge JP, Di Rosa F, Matzinger P. A conditioned dendritic cell can be a temporal bridge between a CD4+ T-helper and a T-killer cell. Nature 1998; 393: 474–478.
114. Mendoza RB, Cantwell MJ, Kipps TJ. Immunostimulatory effects of a plasmid expressing CD40 ligand (CD154) on gene immunization. J Immunol 1997; 159: 5777–5781.
115. Xiang R, Primus FJ, Ruehlmann JM et al. A dual-function DNA vaccine encoding carcinoembryonic antigen and CD40 ligand trimer induces T cell-mediated protective immunity against colon cancer in carcinoembryonic antigen-transgenic mice. J Immunol 2001; 167: 4560–4565.
116. Sin JI, Kim JJ, Zhang D, Weiner DB. Modulation of cellular responses by plasmid CD40L plasmid vectors enhance antigen-specific helper T cell type 1 CD4+ T cell-mediated protective immunity against herpes simplex virus type 2 in vivo. Hum Gene Ther 2001;12: 1091–1102.
117. 117. Hung CF, Cheng WF, Chai CY et al. Improving vaccine potency through intercellular spreading and enhanced MHC class I presentation of antigen. J Immunol 2001; 166: 5733–5740.
118. Hung CF, Cheng WF, Hsu KF et al. Cancer immunotherapy using a DNA vaccine encoding the translocation domain of a bacterial toxin linked to a tumor antigen. Cancer Res 2001; 61: 3698–3703.
119. Rohrbach F, Weth R, Kursar M et al. Targeted delivery of the ErbB2/HER2 tumor antigen to professional APCs results in effective antitumor immunity. J Immunol 2005; 174: 5481–5489.
120. Leitner WW, Hwang LN, deVeer MJ et al. Alphavirus-based DNA vaccine breaks immunological tolerance by activating innate antiviral pathways. Nat Med 2003; 9: 33–39.
121. Alexopoulou L, Holt AC, Medzhitov R, Flavell RA. Recognition of double-stranded RNA and activation of NF-kappaB by Toll-like receptor 3. Nature 2001; 413: 732–738.
122. Xiang R, Lode HN, Chao TH et al. An autologous oral DNA vaccine protects against murine melanoma. Proc Natl Acad Sci U S A 2000; 97: 5492–5497.
123. Woo PC, Wong LP, Zheng BJ, Yuen KY. Unique immunogenicity of hepatitis B virus DNA vaccine presented by live-attenuated Salmonella typhimurium. Vaccine 2001; 19: 29452954.
124. Egen JG, Kuhns MS, Allison JP. CTLA-4: new insights into its biological function and use in tumor immunotherapy. Nat Immunol 2002; 3: 611–618.
125. van Elsas A, Hurwitz AA, Allison JP. Combination immunotherapy of B16 melanoma using anti-cytotoxic T lymphocyte-associated antigen 4 (CTLA-4) and granulocyte/macrophage colony-stimulating factor (GM-CSF)-producing vaccines induces rejection of subcutaneous and metastatic tumors accompanied by autoimmune depigmentation. J Exp Med 1999; 190: 355–366.

126. Phan GQ, Yang JC, Sherry RM et al. Cancer regression and autoimmunity induced by cytotoxic T lymphocyte-associated antigen 4 blockade in patients with metastatic melanoma. Proc Natl Acad Sci U S A 2003; 100: 8372–8377.
127. Hodi FS, Mihm MC, Soiffer RJ et al. Biologic activity of cytotoxic T lymphocyte-associated antigen 4 antibody blockade in previously vaccinated metastatic melanoma and ovarian carcinoma patients. Proc Natl Acad Sci U S A 2003; 100: 4712–4717.
128. Attia P, Phan GQ, Maker AV et al. Autoimmunity Correlates With Tumor Regression in Patients With Metastatic Melanoma Treated With Anti-Cytotoxic T-Lymphocyte Antigen-4. J Clin Oncol 2005.
129. Gregor PD, Wolchok JD, Turaga V et al. Induction of autoantibodies to syngeneic prostate-specific membrane antigen by xenogeneic vaccination. Int J Cancer 2005; 116: 415–421.
130. Nocentini G, Riccardi C. GITR: a multifaceted regulator of immunity belonging to the tumor necrosis factor receptor superfamily. Eur J Immunol 2005; 35: 1016–1022.
131. Shimizu J, Yamazaki S, Takahashi T et al. Stimulation of CD25(+)CD4(+) regulatory T cells through GITR breaks immunological self-tolerance. Nat Immunol 2002; 3: 135–142.
132. McHugh RS, Whitters MJ, Piccirillo CA et al. CD4(+)CD25(+) immunoregulatory T cells: gene expression analysis reveals a functional role for the glucocorticoid-induced TNF receptor. Immunity 2002; 16: 311–323.
133. Ko K, Yamazaki S, Nakamura K et al. Treatment of advanced tumors with agonistic anti-GITR mAb and its effects on tumor-infiltrating Foxp3+CD25+CD4+ regulatory T cells. J Exp Med 2005; 202: 885–891.
134. Cohen AD, Diab A, Perales M-A et al. Agonist anti-GITR antibody enhances DNA vaccine-induced CD8+ T cell responses and tumor immunity against melanoma. Submitted for publication.
135. Sun JY, Krouse RS, Forman SJ et al. Immunogenicity of a p210(BCR-ABL) fusion domain candidate DNA vaccine targeted to dendritic cells by a recombinant adeno-associated virus vector in vitro. Cancer Res 2002; 62: 3175–3183.
136. Park JH, Kim CJ, Lee JH et al. Effective immunotherapy of cancer by DNA vaccination. Mol Cells 1999; 9: 384–391.
137. Sypniewska RK, Hoflack L, Tarango M et al. Prevention of metastases with a Mage-b DNA vaccine in a mouse breast tumor model: potential for breast cancer therapy. Breast Cancer Res Treat 2005; 91: 19–28.
138. Hanke P, Serwe M, Dombrowski F et al. DNA vaccination with AFP-encoding plasmid DNA prevents growth of subcutaneous AFP-expressing tumors and does not interfere with liver regeneration in mice. Cancer Gene Ther 2002; 9: 346–355.
139. Meng WS, Butterfield LH, Ribas A et al. alpha-Fetoprotein-specific tumor immunity induced by plasmid prime-adenovirus boost genetic vaccination. Cancer Res 2001; 61: 8782–8786.
140. Tsuboi A, Oka Y, Ogawa H et al. Cytotoxic T-lymphocyte responses elicited to Wilms'tumor gene WT1 product by DNA vaccination. J Clin Immunol 2000; 20: 195–202.
141. Deng H, Kowalczyk D, O I et al. A modified DNA vaccine to p53 induces protective immunity to challenge with a chemically induced sarcoma cell line. Cell Immunol 2002; 215: 20–31.
142. Tuting T, Gambotto A, Robbins PD et al. Co-delivery of T helper 1-biasing cytokine genes enhances the efficacy of gene gun immunization of mice: studies with the model tumor antigen beta-galactosidase and the BALB/c Meth A p53 tumor-specific antigen. Gene Ther 1999; 6: 629–636.
143. Lindinger P, Mostbock S, Hammerl P et al. Induction of murine ras oncogene peptide-specific T cell responses by immunization with plasmid DNA-based minigene vectors. Vaccine 2003; 21: 4285–4296.
144. Bristol JA, Orsini C, Lindinger P et al. Identification of a ras oncogene peptide that contains both CD4(+) and CD8(+) T cell epitopes in a nested configuration and elicits both T cell subset responses by peptide or DNA immunization. Cell Immunol 2000; 205: 73–83.
145. Kim JJ, Tsai A, Nottingham LK et al. Intracellular adhesion molecule-1 modulates beta-chemokines and directly costimulates T cells in vivo. J Clin Invest 1999; 103: 869–877.

146. Jeannin P, Renno T, Goetsch L et al. OmpA targets dendritic cells, induces their maturation and delivers antigen into the MHC class I presentation pathway. Nat Immunol 2000; 1: 502–509.
147. Chen CH, Wang TL, Hung CF et al. Enhancement of DNA vaccine potency by linkage of antigen gene to an HSP70 gene. Cancer Res 2000; 60: 1035–1042.
148. Otero M, Calarota SA, Felber B et al. Resiquimod is a modest adjuvant for HIV-1 gag-based genetic immunization in a mouse model. Vaccine 2004; 22: 1782–1790.
149. Zuber AK, Brave A, Engstrom G et al. Topical delivery of imiquimod to a mouse model as a novel adjuvant for human immunodeficiency virus (HIV) DNA. Vaccine 2004; 22: 1791–1798.
150. Thomsen LL, Topley P, Daly MG et al. Imiquimod and resiquimod in a mouse model: adjuvants for DNA vaccination by particle-mediated immunotherapeutic delivery. Vaccine 2004; 22: 1799–1809.
151. Niethammer AG, Xiang R, Becker JC et al. A DNA vaccine against VEGF receptor 2 prevents effective angiogenesis and inhibits tumor growth. Nat Med 2002; 8: 1369–1375.
152. Luo Y, Zhou H, Mizutani M et al. Transcription factor Fos-related antigen 1 is an effective target for a breast cancer vaccine. Proc Natl Acad Sci U S A 2003; 100: 8850–8855.
153. Loeffler M, Kruger JA, Reisfeld RA. Immunostimulatory effects of low-dose cyclophosphamide are controlled by inducible nitric oxide synthase. Cancer Res 2005; 65: 5027–5030.
154. Kim TW, Hung CF, Ling M et al. Enhancing DNA vaccine potency by coadministration of DNA encoding antiapoptotic proteins. J Clin Invest 2003; 112: 109–117.
155. Widera G, Austin M, Rabussay D et al. Increased DNA vaccine delivery and immunogenicity by electroporation in vivo. J Immunol 2000; 164: 4635–4640.
156. Hermans IF, Chong TW, Palmowski MJ et al. Synergistic effect of metronomic dosing of cyclophosphamide combined with specific antitumor immunotherapy in a murine melanoma model. Cancer Res 2003; 63: 8408–8413.

CHAPTER 10

RECOMBINANT VIRAL AND BACTERIAL VACCINES

DOUGLAS W. GROSENBACH[1], JARETT FELDMAN[2], JEFFREY SCHLOM[3], AND SCOTT I. ABRAMS[4]

[1]*Laboratory of Tumor Immunology and Biology, CCR, NCI, NIH, 10 Center Drive, Room 8B12 Bethesda, MD 20892-1750 USA*

[2]*Laboratory of Tumor Immunology and Biology, CCR, NCI, NIH, 10 Center Drive, Room 8B12 Bethesda, MD 20892-1750 USA*

[3]*Laboratory of Tumor Immunology and Biology, CCR, NCI, NIH, 10 Center Drive, Room 8B09 Bethesda, MD 20892-1750 USA*

[4]*Laboratory of Tumor Immunology and Biology, CCR, NCI, NIH, 10 Center Drive, Room 5B46 Bethesda, MD 20892-1402 USA*

DEVELOPMENT OF VACCINE-BASED IMMUNOTHERAPY FOR HUMAN CANCER

For many years, oncology has depended on three major clinical options for the treatment of human neoplastic diseases: surgery, radiation or chemotherapy. Recent advances in targeted therapies and the use of monoclonal antibodies have now added to these modalities. In spite of intensive clinical efforts during recent years, treatment of patients with many cancers remains an elusive challenge. This situation has strengthened the need for the design of safer and more effective strategies that better target cancer cells without impacting the integrity of normal cellular compartments.

Active specific immunotherapy is still largely an experimental application for human cancer treatment. The notion that humans can be immunized against their own cancer, and that immunization can evoke a protective or therapeutic anti-neoplastic response rests on resolving several fundamental preclinical and clinical questions: (a) Is the immune response an important factor against neoplastic growth? (b) If so, can the immune response be further "manipulated" to overcome diverse tumor escape mechanisms? and (c) Is cancer vaccination involving recombinant viral or bacterial vectors a viable approach to alter the immune response in favor of cancer cell destruction or prolonged patient survival?

H.L. Kaufman and J.D. Wolchok (eds.), General Principles of Tumor Immunotherapy, 217–250.

In the early 20th century, Ehrlich promoted the idea that the immune system could repress cancer growth. In 1957, Burnet and Thomas formally presented the concept of "cancer immune surveillance" [14], which hypothesized that cells of the immune system continuously surveyed the host for newly arising abnormal cells. Once recognized, the immune system would then destroy these aberrant cells before they became cancerous. Two new lines of experimental observations currently strongly support the conclusion, both in principle and application, that the immune system is crucial for the control of neoplastic development and growth. In comprehensive mouse studies using genetic approaches, Schreiber and colleagues [36,70,160] demonstrated that the loss or impairment of immune function, especially of T cells and IFN-γ production or responsiveness, resulted in a significantly elevated incidence of spontaneous or chemically induced tumor formation. In human studies, Rosenberg and colleagues [31–34] demonstrated that in certain cases tumor-specific immune cells could be isolated from biopsied lesions of patients with metastatic melanoma. After appropriate propagation *ex vivo*, such tumor-infiltrating lymphocytes (TIL) could be returned via adoptive transfer in an autologous manner, which could mediate profound tumor regression in at least some patients, especially under conditions of non-myeloablative chemotherapy. Collectively, in both mouse and human studies, these observations indicate that the immune response does play an important role against the neoplastic process, and if appropriately manipulated could mediate tumor regression.

Another important corollary from these studies is that neoplastic cells are naturally antigenic, but poorly immunogenic. However, the basis of immunogenicity is complex and remains to be fully understood. Despite that, a general consensus is that down-regulation of major histocompatibility complex (MHC) or costimulatory proteins on neoplastic cells underlies a molecular basis of diminished T cell activation or expansion [12,41,136]. Moreover, how such neoplastic clones emerge in the first place represents another layer of complexity. One notion is that an intrinsic adaptive immune response actually facilitates the selection and outgrowth of neoplastic clones expressing those tumorigenic phenotypes [35].

Thus, considerable interest has been committed to the notion that a *de novo* or pre-existing antitumor lymphocyte response may be further intensified by immune-based interventions, which have been classified as: (a) active immunotherapy, also known as therapeutic vaccination [38,41], and (b) passive or adoptive cellular immunotherapy [31,33]. The former classification of immunotherapy will be the subject of this chapter, with particular emphasis on the development and application of recombinant viral and bacterial vectors as cancer vaccines to improve immunogenicity.

CHALLENGES FACING EFFECTIVE CANCER VACCINATION WITH RECOMBINANT LIVE VIRAL OR BACTERIAL VECTORS

A crucial issue in the use of cancer vaccines is how best to overcome potential mechanisms of immune suppression, immune privilege, or central or peripheral tolerance against antigenic, but weakly immunogenic neoplasms. It is noteworthy that based on preclinical studies in transgenic mouse models expressing self-tumor-associated antigens (TAA) [69,130,155,199] and clinical studies [31,105], it appears likely that tumor-specific lymphoid precursors do exist in the periphery, but remain in a relatively unresponsive or "anergized" state.

An additional consideration for the use of active immunotherapy in humans, particularly involving live viral or bacterial-based vectors, reflects the nature of the patient population. The original intention of immunotherapy was to use it in patients with metastatic cancer or disease refractory to conventional treatments. From an ethical standpoint, it was appropriate to enroll such patients in newer experimental therapy protocols because "standard-of-care" treatment was unsuccessful in such patients. From a scientific or practical standpoint, however, such patient populations may be far from optimal to test experimental immunotherapies because disease progression or prior therapies may have already compromised immune function. By its very nature, however, immunotherapy requires a functional immune system.

Another consideration rests with appreciating the sophistication of the host-tumor relationship. By the time cancer is clinically detectable, it likely had already evolved to the point where it can efficiently evade host immune recognition and attack. In fact, as pointed out earlier, studies in mouse models of chemically induced tumor formation support this notion, which has been termed "cancer immunoediting" [35, 160] and reflects a refinement of the original concept of "cancer immunosurveillance" [14]. Thus, although cancer is considered a genetic disease [56, 181], interactions of developing neoplasms with the immune system over many years may serve to influence the immunogenic content of malignant subpopulations that eventually emerge and constitute the clinically detectable mass.

An expanding principle in the field of immunology and immunotherapy is that the dendritic cell (DC) is central to the initiation of the adaptive immune response. But to make the DC functionally useful for this essential role, the DC requires prior activation by elements of the innate immune response. Thus, the DC is thought to be the cellular bridge linking innate and adaptive immunity. However, it has been reported that DC subpopulations from cancer patients may be functionally impaired as a consequence of tumor-derived suppressive factors, such as vascular endothelial growth factor (VEGF), IL-10 or gangliosides [44, 202]. Cancer vaccine strategies aimed to augment the maturation and activation of the DC, therefore, would then likely improve immunogenicity and the production of a more robust T cell response. One way to achieve this outcome is through the use of live viral or bacterial-based vectors, which by their nature generate potent type-1 inflammatory reactions. These reactions, in turn, would antagonize at least to some extent anti-inflammatory elements of the tumorigenic process.

It is now known that microbial products, such as those inherent in certain viruses and bacteria (BCG), also are potent activators of the DC because they contain agonists of toll-like receptors (TLR). TLR are expressed by DC (and other innate immune cell types), and comprise a family of approximately 10–15 receptors that bind to a number of different microbial components, namely lipopolysaccharide

(LPS), RNA species and CpG motifs [72, 129]. Activation of DC via their TLR augments expression of adhesion molecules, chemokine receptors and chemokines, which, in turn, regulate cellular trafficking to sites of inflammation. Thus, the biological consequences of TLR engagement lead to inflammation, characterized by the recruitment of key immune and non-immune effector cells to mediate pathogen destruction. In regard to TLR agonists, CpG motifs constitute the most studied of these sequences [73,84,187]. It is thought, therefore, that some of the immunogenic properties of viral or bacterial constructs can be attributed to the fact that they also contain numerous CpG motifs. In addition, certain cytokines have been shown to enhance the level of DC function *in vitro* and *in vivo*. For example, GM-CSF has been demonstrated to enhance Ag-specific T cell responses, such as proliferative, CTL, delayed-type hypersensitivity reactions or antitumor responses [30,38,77,137,157,186,194]. It should be noted, however, that GM-CSF most likely acts indirectly via recruitment and activation of host DC populations. Increased DC competence correlates with heightened levels of MHC, adhesion, and costimulatory molecules, which serve to improve immune system interactions overall.

At the induction phase, vaccination should elicit a potent tumor-reactive immune response, at both quantitative and qualitative levels. Quantitative factors reflect significant rises in tumor-reactive T lymphocyte precursor frequencies, while qualitative factors reflect improvements in the potency, specificity and sensitivity of those lymphocytes for recognition and destruction of the Ag-bearing target. This is particularly important in light of the possibility that by the time cancer is clinically diagnosed the resulting lesions may have already evaded or have been reshaped by the naturally occurring innate and adaptive immune interactions over many years. At the effector phase of the host-tumor interaction, the vaccine-induced immune cells must be able to achieve a number of sequentially complex steps. The immune cells must be able to migrate to and accumulate at the sites of neoplastic growth. Once they collect at those sites, these immune cells must be able to penetrate lesions at sufficiently high levels so that the *in vivo* "effector/target ratios" favor the immune response over the tumor load, as well as to overcome various cancer-directed countermeasures which serve to disable effector function. Notably, the presence of immune regulatory cell populations, such as NKT cells [169], $CD4^+CD25^+$ Treg cells [26] and myeloid suppressor $CD11b^+Gr\text{-}1^+$ cells [108] have been reported to downregulate T_h1-type and CTL activity. Furthermore, this is further compounded by the production of numerous tumor-derived inhibitory factors, such as TGF-β, VEGF and IL-10, which further abrogate immune reactivity in the host-tumor microenvironment [44, 162, 202].

Finally, in the event a therapeutic T cell response is initiated and executed, the possibility exists for the development of undesirable immune reactions. For example, if vaccines are directed against a given TAA, the induction of immunity toward the tumor may also eventually lead to the induction of immunity to normal tissues also expressing that TAA. This has been the case for immune responses to some melanoma-associated Ag, where vitiligo has been induced, in both experimental [132] and clinical studies [31]. It is noteworthy that, in preclinical vaccine studies, the induction of antitumor immunity in transgenic mice expressing TAA has not led to the induction of autoimmunity in normal tissues expressing those same TAA [69, 130, 155, 199]. So far, in clinical trials using recombinant viral vaccines directed against carcinomas, no autoimmunity has been observed, including those cases in which positive clinical outcomes have been reported [104, 105].

VIRAL VECTORS

The central concept in the construction of a recombinant viral vaccine for cancer therapy resides within its ability to productively activate the immune response. The gene encoding a target Ag, most often a TAA, is recombined into the genome of a live virus. Upon infection, the target Ag is then expressed among other viral gene products, thus exposing the Ag to the immune system for recognition and activation of T lymphocytes. This model further postulates that activated T lymphocytes then migrate from the site of induction, enter the circulation via the lymphatics, infiltrate the tumor site(s) and mediate tumor cell destruction. T cell recognition is governed by the clonotypic T cell receptor, which recognizes antigenic fragments or "epitopes" derived from endogenous proteins displayed on the tumor cell surface generally in the context of MHC class I molecules.

This mechanism for the introduction of Ag to the immune system is attractive for several reasons: (a) viruses infect many cell types including professional APC leading to both direct and indirect presentation of Ag to the immune system; (b) viral infection tends to send the appropriate "danger signals" concurrently resulting in the activation of the innate immune response which creates an inflammatory milieu crucial to the recruitment and activation of components of adaptive immunity; and (c) many viral proteins are highly immunogenic and act as "helper" signals in the generation of robust cellular immune responses to the target Ag [28]. Viral vectors may be further manipulated to include transgenes for immunostimulants, such as cytokines and costimulatory molecules. Numerous viruses are being developed as therapeutic cancer vaccines taking advantage of these features. They include: poxviruses (vaccinia, MVA, avipox) [114, 168], adenovirus [82], adeno-associated virus, alphaviruses (semliki forest virus, sindbis virus) [193], paramyxoviruses (measles, newcastle disease virus) [141, 145] and herpesviruses [99]. Tables 1 and Tables 2 list representative viral species that have been used therapeutically for the treatment of various cancers both preclinically and in clinical trials, respectively.

Poxvirus Vectors

One of the most studied groups of all viral vectors for cancer vaccines is the poxvirus group. Vaccinia virus, which was derived from a benign pox disease in cows, has been administered to more than 1 billion people and is responsible for the worldwide eradication of smallpox [40]. As a result, smallpox vaccinations in

Table 1. Selected Viral Vectors for the Immunotherapy of Cancer - Preclinical

Virus	Strain	Target Ag/Therapeutic Gene Product	Additional Immunomodulators/Combination Therapy	Cancer Model	Response	Ref.
Poxvirus	Vaccinia	CEA	B7-1, ICAM-1, LFA-3, GM-CSF, IL-2/Radiation	multiple	CD4, CD8 T cell responses; Antigen cascade; tumor prevention; tumor clearance	[19, 49, 63, 86]
	Vaccinia	HPV E6, E7, L1 Capsid	None	Cervical Carcinoma	CD4, CD8 T cell responses; tumor prevention; tumor clearance	[9]
	Vaccinia	Gp100, Mart-1, tyrosinase, TRP-1, TRP-2	None	Melanoma	Humoral responses to TRP-1; tumor prevention; Auto-immune vitiligo	[131]
	MVA	CEA	B7-1, ICAM-1, LFA-3, GM-CSF, IL-2	Peripancreatic CEA+	CD4, CD8 T cells responses; tumor therapy	[64]
	MVA	5T4	None	5T4+ Model lung metastases	Humoral responses;Tumor protection	[115]
	MVA	LacZ/Beta-galactosidase	None	LacZ+ model lung metastases	CD8 T cell responses; Tumor protection; tumor therapy	[17]
	MVA	MUC-1	IL-2	RMA-MUC-1	Tumor preventionTumor therapy	[94]
	Fowlpox/ Canarypox	CEA	B7-1, ICAM-1, LFA-3, GM-CSF, IL-2, radiation	multiple	CD4, CD8 T cell responses; Tumor protection; tumor therapy;	[19, 49, 63, 86]
	Fowlpox	None	GM-CSF	Multiple	Enhanced recruitment of APC to vaccine site; enhanced anti-tumor immunity	[49, 77]
	Fowlpox	LacZ/Beta-galactosidase	None	LacZ+ model lung metastases	T cell responses to LacZ; humoral responses to LacZ; tumor therapy	[71]

Adenovirus	AD5	P53	None		CD8 T cell responses	[85]
	AD5	HER-2	None	HER-2 transgenic spontaneous mammary tumor	Humoral responses to HER-2; prevention of spontaneous tumors	[138]
	AD2	Gp100, TRP-2	None	B16-F10 melanoma model	CD8 T cell responses, Tumor protection	[142]
	ONYX-015	None	Tumor selective replication	Various human/mouse xenograft models	Tumor enriched replication of virus Regression of tumors in several models	[59]
Alphavirus	Sindbis virus-based DNA replicon	TRP-1	PKR activation via dsRNA intermediates	B16.F10	Humoral responses to TRP-1, Tumor protection	[89]
Measles virus	Edmonston B	CEA (used only as a marker for infection)	Tumor selective replication	Various human/mouse xenograft models	Tumor enriched replication of virus Regression of subcutaneous and intracranial tumors. Prolonged survival	[145]
Newcastle Disease Virus	73-T	None	Tumor selective replication following systemic or intratumoral injection	Various human/mouse xenograft models	Regression of tumors following intratumoral or systemic injection	[144]
Herpesvirus	HSV-1 (numerous derivatives)	None	Tumor selective replication following deletion of ribonucleotide reductase genes	Various, primarily gliomas	Tumor enriched replication of virus Enhanced efficacy when used as a suicide gene therapy vector in combination with gancyclovir or acyclovir	[99]

Table 2. Selected Viral Vectors for the Immunotherapy of Cancer - Clinical

Virus	Strain	Target Ag	Additional Immunomodulators/Combination Therapy	Cancer	Comments	Response	Ref.
Poxvirus	Vaccinia/ FowlpoxPrime and Boost	CEA	B7-1, ICAM-1, LFA-3, GM-CSF, IL-2	CEA+ carcinomas	Phase 1	Increase in tumor antigen-specific T cell precursor frequency, 1 complete response, Partial responses	[105]
	Vaccinia/ FowlpoxPrime and Boost	CEA	Low-dose IL-2Local GM-CSF	Advanced CEA+ carcinomas	Phase I	Increase in tumor antigen-specific T cell precursor frequency. Vaccinia priming followed by fowlpox boosting most efficacious	[104]
	Vaccinia/ FowlpoxPrime and Boost	PSA	IL-2GM-CSFB7-1 (in the prime vaccination) Nilutamide	Prostate Cancer (pts with ↑ PSA, resistant to horm. therapy, no radiographic evidence of disease	Phase II	Well-tolerated 12/21 pts on vaccine alone with decreases/stabilization in serum PSA Increases in PSA-specific T cell precursor frequencies	[5]
	Vaccinia/ FowlpoxPrime and Boost	PSA	IL-2GM-CSFB7-1 (in the prime vaccination) Radiation	Prostate Cancer (clinically localized disease)	Phase II	Well-tolerated 13/19 pts receiving combination therapy with increases in PSA-specific T cell precursor frequencies De novo generation of T cell responses to prostate antigens not found in the vaccine	[52]
	Vaccinia	CEA	None	Advanced colorectal cancer	Phase I	Well-tolerated	[106]
	Vaccinia	PSA	None	Hormone-insensitive prostate cancer	Phase 1	CD8 T cell responses,	[51]
	Vaccinia	PSA	GM-CSF	Advanced/metastatic prostate cancer	Phase 1	CD8 T cell responses to PSA, 14/33 patients with stable PSA $\geq$ 6 months, 6/33 patients with progression-free survival for 11 to 25 months	[37]

Vaccinia	HPV E6/E7	None	Cervical cancer	Phase II	CD8 T cell responses to HPV Ags Serological responses to HPV Ags	[1, 80]
Vaccinia	MUC-1	IL-2	Advanced prostate cancer	Phase 1	Objective clinical response in 1 patient,	[134]
Vaccinia	None	B7-1	Melanoma	Phase I 12pts Intralesional injection	Well-tolerated 1 pt partial response 2 pts with disease stabilization T cell responses to melanoma Ags	[79]
UV-inactivated Vaccinia	Melan-A/MART-1 (27–35), gp100 (280–288), tyrosinase (1–9) epitopes	B7-1, B7-2, GM-CSF	Metastatic melanoma	Phase I/II	15/18 evaluable patients with increasing T cell precursor frequency, 3/18 patients with regression of individual metastases, 7/18 with stable disease, 7/18 with progressive disease	[197]
MVA	Tyrosinase	None	Stage II Melanoma	Phase 1	No T cell responses to tyrosinase,	[109]
MVA	Multiple melanoma-associated CTL epitopes (HLA-A2)	None	Surgically treated melanoma (adjuvant setting)	Phase I Used in a DNA/ MVA prime and boost Or as a single agent	2/6 patients generated CTL responses to a single epitope after DNA/MVA prime and boost 4/7 patients developed CTL responses to a single epitope when MVA used alone	[163]
Canarypox (ALVAC)	CEA	None	Advanced CEA+Carcinomas	Phase I	Increased CEA-specific T cell precursor frequency	[103]
Canarypox (ALVAC)	CEA	B7-1	CEA+ adenocarcinomas	Phase I	3/18 pts with stable disease correlating with increase in CEA-specific T cell precursor frequency	[66]
Canarypox (ALVAC)	CEA	B7-1	Various advanced CEA+(Majority are colorectal)	Phase 1	No objective clinical responses Increase in CTL precursor frequency (CD8 responses) to CEA Disease stabilization in some patients Decline in serum CEA levels in some patients	[182]

(*Continued*)

Table 2. (Continued)

Virus	Strain	Target Ag	Additional Immunomodulators/Combination Therapy	Cancer	Comments	Response	Ref.
Adenovirus	Ad5	P53	None	Various advanced stage cancers	Pilot Study	Humoral and cellular responses to adenoviral vector No cellular or humoral responses to p53	[85]
	Ad5	PSMA	B7-2, GM-CSF	Prostate Cancer	Phase 1 Used in prime and boost strategy with DNA	DTH responses to PSMA Some local responses, effects on PSA levels	[111]
	Ad5	MART-1Gp100	IL-2	Metastatic Melanoma	Phase 1	1 complete response High neutralizing Ab to adenovirus No consistent cellular responses to vectored Ag	[152]
	ONYX-015	None	Tumor selective replication	Various advanced sarcomas	Phase I/II Used in combination with mitomycin C doxorubicin and cisplatin	Well-tolerated Evidence of anti-tumor activity in 1 of 6 patients	[45]
Herpesvirus	HSV-1 G207	None	Tumor selective replication	Gliomas	Phase I Phase II	Well-tolerated	[78]
Newcastle Disease virus	Ulster	None	Autologous tumor cells infected with NDV	Head and neck squamous cell carcinomas, glioblastomas	2 pilot studies	DTH reaction to tumor cells CTL responses to tumor cells	[76, 165]
	PV701	None	None	Advanced solid cancers	Phase I Administered by the i.v. route	1 pt complete response 1 pt partial response 7 pts with measurable tumor reduction 14 pts with progression-free survival for 4-30+ months	

the United States and most Western countries were halted over 30 years ago. As it relates to therapeutic vaccination though, most adult cancer patients are over the age of 30 and, therefore, likely have some level of pre-existing immunity to vaccinia virus that may limit the efficacy of the experimental vaccine – a consideration addressed below. One of the major advantages in using vaccinia virus and/or replication incompetent poxviruses, however, is that large amounts of foreign DNA (up to 25 kb) can be inserted into the vector [114]. Another major advantage is that proteins expressed in vaccinia virus tend to be more immunogenic than the native protein, which is most likely due to the inflammatory responses triggered against highly immunogenic vaccinia virus proteins [28]. Other advantages of poxviruses include: (a) wide host range; (b) stable recombinants; (c) authentic replication; and (d) efficient post-translational processing of the inserted gene [114]. It should be noted that while vaccinia virus is an extremely efficient vaccine vector, there are safety concerns with its use [146]. Other poxvirus vectors with better safety profiles are becoming increasingly prevalent in vaccine studies. Modified vaccinia Ankara (MVA) is an example of one such vector [114, 166]. MVA has been attenuated by serial passage in avian cells resulting in the deletion of large portions of its genome. It retains many of the attractive features of vaccinia virus but lacks toxicity because it cannot replicate in mammalian cells. Similarly, other replication-defective members of the poxvirus family are the avipox vectors (e.g., fowlpox and canarypox/ALVAC) [135, 168]. Clinical studies have shown that avipox-based vectors can be given numerous times to patients with a resulting increase in Ag-specific T cell responses [103]. Thus, it appears that in addition to an enhanced safety profile, its repeated use as a booster vaccine is not limited by the host anti-vector response, most likely because it is replication-incompetent.

Early studies of recombinant vaccinia viruses containing HIV transgenes showed that vaccinia virus-immune patients could not mount as potent an immune response as vaccinia virus-naive patients [23]. Subsequent studies have shown that when higher doses of recombinant vaccinia viruses are used, even vaccinia virus-immune patients can mount a vigorous response to the transgene after vaccination. However, this response is greatly diminished at the second and third vaccination [178]. Thus, preclinical [49] and recent clinical [104, 105] studies have shown that the optimal use of recombinant vaccinia viruses is to prime the immune response, followed by boost vaccinations with other vectors (such as replication-defective avipox vectors), peptides or proteins. Several clinical trials involving vaccinia virus recombinants expressing TAA, such as CEA [105], PSA [5,52], MUC-1 [134], human papilloma virus E2 [24], E6 and E7 antigens [7], melanoma antigens melan-A/MART-1, gp100, and tyrosinase [109, 153, 163] are actively being engaged. Additional tumor Ag are being evaluated as candidate targets in preclinical studies using recombinant poxvirus vectors. They include p53 [42], 5T4 [115], GA733 [198], and Epstein-Barr viral antigens EBNA1, LMP1 and LMP2 to name a few [47, 167].

First-generation poxvirus-based cancer vaccines encoded only the TAA and relied solely on the inherent immunogenicity of the virus to overcome tolerance and trigger immune responses to the TAA. Preclinical studies and clinical trial results indicate that while capable of breaking tolerance to the TAA, this is not sufficient to mediate potent antitumor immunity and clearance of established tumors in the majority of animal models [49] or patients [104]. Second- and third-generation poxvirus vaccines have been engineered to not only encode TAA but also cytokines, such as IL-2 [134], IL-12 [20], GM-CSF [77, 176]and TNF-α [48], and costimulatory molecules, such as B7-1, ICAM-1, LFA-3 [63, 91, 105, 176], OX40L [50], and CD40L [39]. Vaccines encoding both TAA and immune stimulatory molecules have been demonstrated to enhance antitumor immunity in both preclinical models and clinical studies [5, 19, 49, 50, 52, 61–66, 75, 77, 86, 105, 182, 195, 196, 199].

Preclinical and clinical studies indicated that immune responses to the TAA were further enhanced by the use of heterologous vaccine vector combinations, such as recombinant vaccinia in the primary vaccination and avipox, in the boost [49, 62, 63, 104, 199]. For example, a vaccine regimen consisting of recombinant vaccinia virus (rV) encoding CEA along with the costimulatory molecules B7-1, ICAM-1 and LFA-3 (termed rV-CEA/TRICOM), was followed by booster vaccinations with a heterologous recombinant fowlpox (rF) encoding the same TAA and costimulatory molecules (termed rF-CEA/TRICOM). Recombinant GM-CSF protein was administered during each vaccine cycle. In animal models, this approach has been proven to be far superior to vaccination with viruses encoding only the TAA, or repeated vaccinations with a single agent, resulting in both enhanced immune responses to the TAA and tumor clearance [49, 63].

A clinical trial [105] following this regimen reported that 23 of 58 patients had stable disease for at least 4 months, 14 had prolonged (6 months or more) stable disease, 11 had decreases in serum CEA levels from baseline and 1 patient had a pathologic complete response. Furthermore, enhanced CEA-specific $CD8^+$ T cells responses were generated in 10 of 13 patients analyzed. Overall, these findings indicated that the vaccine induced TAA-specific T cell responses and, in some patients, prolonged progression-free survival.

Adenovirus Vectors

Adenoviruses are ubiquitous human respiratory pathogens. Typically in humans, adenoviruses cause transient mild disease symptoms including fever, chills, joint and abdominal pain, and fatigue when acquired through normal respiratory routes of infection. Most adults have pre-existing immunity to adenoviruses. The immune response to adenovirus includes a rapid innate immune reaction involving the release of inflammatory cytokines leading to the activation of adaptive immunity [10].

Adenovirus has also been proposed as an attractive vector for application in recombinant vaccine design because its viral genome can be altered to accept foreign genes that are stably integrated. Furthermore, to produce recombinant adenovectors, endogenous viral DNA sequences are typically deleted from replication-competent regions, which results in an attenuated form of the virus with potentially improved safety. In some adenoviral vectors, the entire genome has been "gutted" – essentially removing all viral sequences and replacing them with irrelevant DNA (to maintain genome size) in addition to therapeutic genes of interest. This serves as an additional safety feature but also results in prolonged transgene expression since infected cells do not express foreign adenoviral genes that potentially could be a target for immune clearance.

Recombinant adenoviruses have been widely used in gene therapy protocols, and a number of vaccine protocols for the induction of immune responses have already been conducted [21, 74, 152, 192]. Recombinant adenoviruses have been employed in immunotherapy, both in preclinical models and in clinical trials of patients with metastatic melanoma [152]. In preclinical studies, immunization of mice with a recombinant adenovirus expressing a model TAA led to the induction of an Ag-specific CTL response and regression of established pulmonary metastases. In clinical trials, recombinant adenoviruses encoding MART-1 or gp100 genes were administered to patients with malignant melanoma. The vaccine, given at multiple routes, doses and frequencies, did not produce significant adverse effects. However, immunologic findings did not reveal a consistent pattern of induction of TAA-specific T cell responses, as determined by IFN-γ production in response to MART-1 or gp100-associated peptides, presumably because of the high levels of pre-existing and/or inducible neutralizing antibodies found in this patient population. Thus, recombinant adenoviruses may eventually be more appropriate in diversified prime and boost protocols.

Additional proposed strategies to enhance adenovirus-based vaccines include (a) general suppression of the anti-vector immune response using immunomodulatory molecules such as IL-10 or CTLA4-Ig (b) genetic modification of the capsid protein genes and other immunogenic genomic elements (c) use of different human serotypes for boosting (d) polymer coating of viruses (e) use in a prime-boost strategy with other vectors and (f) redirected targeting to dendritic cells via modification of proteins involved in viral binding and penetration [8].

Alphavirus Vectors/Replicons

One experimental approach for improving the immunogenicity of polynucleotide or genetic vaccines is to endow them with "self-replicating" ability. To achieve this effect, a gene encoding a RNA replicase, an enzyme produced from alphaviruses, is introduced into the RNA vector [88, 156]. Alphaviruses are members of the Togaviridae family and include Semliki Forest virus, Sindbis virus, and Venezuelan equine encephalitis virus. They have a single-stranded (+)-sense RNA genome in that the viral genome serves as an mRNA molecule upon infection. Following infection, the mRNA genome is translated to produce non-structural proteins (replicase/transcriptase) involved in genome replication. The replication of the genome is highly efficient, producing up to 200,000 copies of the genome per infected cell. Replication takes place entirely in the cytosol with no DNA intermediate and no integration into the host genome. As such, recombinant alphaviruses are capable of high levels of transient protein expression in a broad range of host cells. Replication deficient (requiring "helper" vectors for packaging) as well as replication-competent vectors have been developed [8, 200].

In preclinical studies using model TAA, RNA viral vectors have been shown to be strongly immunogenic for the induction of Ag-specific Ab and CTL responses, and effective in tumor prevention and tumor-therapy settings in vivo [88]. Additional studies revealed that cells infected with self-replicating RNA vectors transiently synthesize large amounts of antigenic materials before undergoing apoptotic cell death. Apoptosis is thought to result from the formation of double-stranded RNA intermediates, which, interestingly, may also have a secondary consequence and promote activation of resident DC [88]. Thus, the pro-inflammatory effects of such RNA intermediates may play a role in further potentiating immunogenicity, over and above what is observed with conventional plasmids.

To date, no clinical trials using alphavirus vectors to induce therapeutic antitumor immune responses have been reported although several animal studies have been described [6].

Oncolytic Viruses/in situ Vaccination

The recombinant viral vaccines described above are designed to elicit tumor-specific immune responses via viral-mediated expression of recombinant proteins. This approach undoubtedly holds great promise in the field of cancer immunotherapy, but makes some general assumptions: First, that the target Ag is appropriately specific or highly selective for immune recognition; second, that the Ag presentation pathways of the neoplastic cell remain functionally intact providing sufficient expression of the relevant MHC/peptide ligand complexes for recognition by the vaccine-induced T cell response; and third, that an immune response directed against the target Ag will be sufficiently robust as to overcome tolerance, immunosuppressive mechanisms and escape phenomena, such as "immunoediting". It may be argued that a failure in any one of these assumptions will not necessarily lead to loss of vaccine efficacy though.

An immune response to a single TAA likely results in the cytolytic destruction of a number of tumor cells. The cellular debris from these killed tumor cells would then be scavenged by phagocytic APC. This would result in the presentation of potentially numerous tumor Ag, not part of the original vaccine, to the immune system, triggering "antigenic cascade" or a broadening of the specificity of the immune response from a single Ag to many other Ag expressed by the tumor cell. That this does indeed occur is supported by various lines of experimental evidence in both preclinical models [19, 86] and in clinical trials [15, 18, 149, 150]. Robust immune responses directed against a single TAA result in the generation of immune responses to other TAA not part of the original vaccine. Current vaccine strategies are likely to exploit this immunologic principle in order to enhance the repertoire of immune effector cells engaged against neoplastic lesions. It remains to be determined, however, whether the anticancer reactivity seen in patients with chemotherapeutic agents and/or radiation therapy also involves or is accompanied by such an antigenic cross-priming or cascade mechanism.

By its very nature, oncolytic viruses may also contribute to this phenomenon. Oncolytic viruses preferentially target and/or replicate in tumor tissue [4,57,92,117]. For example, ONYX-015 is a genetically engineered adenovirus with a deleted E1B 55k gene. The viral E1B 55k gene product normally suppresses cellular p53 function allowing viral replication without induction of apoptosis. In normal cells, whereby p53 function is intact, ONYX-015 replication is severely inhibited due to the inability of the virus to block induction of apoptosis. Many cancer cells are defective for p53 function; thus, ONYX-015 is capable of replication in cancer cells. An additional factor enhancing the tumor specificity of this virus is the availability of the viral receptor on cancer cells. While normal cells express the receptor, it may be sequestered from viral binding by tight cell-cell junctions. Many cancer cells up-regulate the receptor and also fail to form tight cell-cell junctions, thus making them a better target of infection. Preclinical and clinical studies demonstrate preferential replication of ONYX-015 in, and destruction of, tumor tissue relative to normal surrounding tissues [58, 59, 107]. Tumor-specific immune responses following treatment with ONYX-015 have not been characterized. Humoral immune responses to the virus limit its efficacy and efforts are being considered to circumvent this roadblock [177].

The oncolytic properties of two paramyxoviruses are also being studied both preclinically and clinically [117, 164]. The Edmonston B measles vaccine strain exhibits potent tumor-specific cytolytic activity in human tumor xenografts. The altered tropism (and a contributor to attenuation) of the vaccine strain relative to wild-type measles virus is a result of receptor preference. Wild-type strains of measles preferentially bind to and infect cells expressing signaling lymphocyte activation molecule (SLAM), normally expressed by T and B lymphocytes. The Edmonston vaccine strain preferentially binds to and infects cells expressing CD46. CD46 is expressed on all nucleated cells and regulates complement activation [154]. As a mode of evading complement-mediated lysis, many tumor cells up-regulate CD46 and, in so doing, become preferential targets for Edmonston strains of measles virus. Tumor specificity is not assured due to the ubiquitous expression of CD46, and efforts are being taken to modify the virus further to enhance specificity [118]. Currently, no clinical trials have been carried out using measles virus for cancer therapy.

Newcastle Disease Virus (NDV) has a storied and sometimes controversial record of use for the treatment of many types of cancer in humans. NDV is an avian paramyxovirus causing severe disease in chickens but only mild and short-lived disease symptoms in humans [120]. Anecdotal accounts in humans and numerous preclinical studies have demonstrated that NDV preferentially infects and kills human tumors cells of many types [120]. NDV vaccines for the treatment of cancer are used in two ways: 1) direct injection of the virus alone or 2) the virus is used to infect a patient's autologous tumor cells *ex vivo* and then re-injected either as a whole tumor cell vaccine or as an oncolysate. Three mechanisms have been proposed to explain the role of the virus in promoting antitumor responses: 1) lytic strains simply target, infect and kill tumor cells, 2) infection results in the insertion of viral proteins into the membranes of tumor cells making them better targets of immune attack, or 3) the virus may stimulate the host to produce pro-inflammatory cytokines (e.g, , interferons or tumor necrosis factor) thus activating both innate and adaptive immune responses.

In xenograft and syngeneic tumor models, local administration of virus (peri-tumoral or intra-tumoral) was found to be more efficacious than systemic viral administration (intraperitoneal or intravenous) in the clearance of tumors; albeit the response to systemic administration was still meaningful [144]. In clinical trials, NDV has been administered by intravenous infusion but is most often used as a component of autologous whole-tumor cell vaccines. There are a number of clinical trials and case reports in which complete or partial regressions were observed, and progression-free survival and overall survival were prolonged following treatment with NDV-modified whole tumor cell vaccines [76, 98, 141]. In one Phase I trial in advanced solid tumors in which NDV was administered intravenously to 79 patients (62 patients available for response assessment), the following clinical findings were observed: a complete response in one patient, a partial response in another, measurable tumor reduction in 7 other patients, and progression-free survival of 4 – 30+ months in 14 patients [141].

Herpes viruses are also being developed as oncolytic therapeutics for cancer [99, 147]. Herpes simplex virus (HSV) is an enveloped, double-stranded DNA virus with a 152 kb genome. HSV produces many of its own enzymes necessary for nucleotide metabolism, thus making it independent of host cell function in some aspects of these pathways. This facilitates replication in various cell types in which the host nucleotide metabolism is near stasis. Mutants of HSV have been constructed in which one or more of these genes have been altered, thus rendering them dependent on the host for its nucleotide pool and limits the number of cells in which the virus can replicate due to limiting nucleotide resources in most cells. Tumor cells are characterized by dysregulated metabolic processes, which often include rapid replication, and requiring abundant precursors for DNA and RNA synthesis. This is managed by the upregulation of numerous enzymes involved in nucleotide metabolism. This is frequently a target of chemotherapeutic agents. It also facilitates the replication of HSV mutants in which genes such as ribonucleotide reductase or thymidine kinase are deleted or otherwise inactive.

Numerous clinical trials (Phase I and II) have been conducted with tumor-selective oncolytic HSV [78]. In one such trial, a mutant HSV (G207), in which both genomic copies of ICP34.5, a gene involved in neurovirulence, and the gene for ribonucleotide reductase have been deleted, has been used for the treatment of malignant gliomas. In that trial there was radiographic and neuropathologic evidence of antitumor activity. Animal models in which this vaccine was employed showed evidence of viral-mediated tumor eradication. Interestingly, this virus was also shown to induce antitumor immunity *in vivo* via the induction of tumor-specific

CTL responses and may also have stimulated immunity by enhancing the expression of costimulatory molecules.

Other oncolytic viruses under consideration for cancer therapy include vaccinia virus and reovirus [125, 161]. Efforts are underway to enhance the antitumor effect of oncolytic viruses through further modification of the viral genome or by the addition of other treatment modalities. These include engineering the viruses to encode immunostimulatory molecules such as cytokines or costimulatory molecules, or combination with radiotherapy or cyclophosphamide.

BACTERIAL VECTORS

More than a hundred years ago observations of cancer remission following bacterial infection was made, leading researchers to suggest bacterial infection may induce anticancer properties. [119]. Since that time, areas in which bacteria have been used in tumor therapeutics involve direct oncolytic activity, due to preferential replication in tumor tissue, nonspecific immunostimulatory effects, and as vectors for protein and/or gene delivery. Tables 3 and Tables 4 list representative bacterial species that have been used therapeutically for the treatment of various cancers both preclinically and in clinical trials, respectively.

Bacteria as Immunostimulants/Adjuvants

Bacille Calmette Guérin (BCG) is a non-anaerobic *Mycobacterium*. The non-specific immunotherapy of bladder cancer using BCG likely represents a significant advance in immunotherapy in the last 25 years [3]. Intravesical therapy of bladder cancer using BCG was pioneered by Morales in 1976 and has been clinically approved. Superficial papillary bladder cancer is treatable by surgery but often recurs and at times progresses to potentially lethal invasive disease. Historically, adjuvant intravesical chemotherapy has been used to reduce recurrences and prevent progression, but this has been shown to be ineffective in numerous clinical trials [140]. In this setting (post surgical adjuvant treatment) BCG has been demonstrated to be the most efficacious treatment to prevent recurrence and progression to invasive cancer. The precise mechanism by which BCG acts to induce its anti-cancer effect is not entirely clear, but there is ample evidence that it is immune-mediated with possible roles for CD4, CD8, and NK cells as well as BCG-induced IFN-γ production (reviewed in [3]).

In addition to its use as an immunoprophylactic agent, BCG has been widely used as an adjuvant for modified cancer cell vaccines for several different types of tumors [180]. For example, it is used in combination with CancerVax, a polyvalent tumor cell vaccine that has been shown to improve overall survival in stage II melanoma patients and in patients treated after curative resection of distant melanoma [67,68]. The combination of BCG with an allogeneic vaccine for prostate cancer has also demonstrated promising results [110]. Beneficial effects following BCG treatment of lung cancers have not been observed.

Table 3. Selected Bacterial Vectors for the Immunotherapy of Cancer - Preclinical

Bacterium	Strain	Target Ag/Therapeutic Gene Product	Additional Immunomodulators/Modifications	Cancer Model	Responses to Vaccine	Ref.
Salmonella typhimurium	SL7207	gp100, TRP-2	Genetic fusion of ubiquitin to antigen peptide-minigenes	Melanoma	CD8 response & protection from tumor challenge	[188]
	SL7207	TRP-2, gp100	Targeting of IL-2 to tumor tissues by coupling to a tumor-specific antibody	Melanoma	CD8 and CD4 responses, DC activation & protection from tumor challenge	[123]
	SL7207	TRP-2, gp100	Targeting of the antigen to the MHCII presentation pathway of APC	Melanoma	CD8 and CD4 responses & protection from tumor challenge	[184]
	SL7207	gp100	None	Melanoma	CD8 response, DC activation & protection from tumor challenge	[22]
	SL7207	Model antigen β-gal	None	Fibrosarcoma	CD8 response & protection from tumor challenge	[133]
	RE88	Fos-related antigen 1	Genetic fusion of the tumor antigen to polyubiquitin. Cotransformation of the bacterial carrier with a second plasmid encoding secretory IL-18	Breast Cancer	CD8 and CD4 responses, DC activation & protection from tumor challenge	[100]
	SL3261	MG7-Ag	Genetic fusion of the antigen with helper T cell epitope PADRE	Gastric Cancer	Protection from tumor challenge	[53]
	SL7202	Tyrosine hydroxylase	Genetic fusion of computational predicted MHCI-epitope-minigenes to ubiquitin	Neuroblastoma	CD8, CD4 responses & protection from tumor challenge	[96]
	SL7207	Tyrosine hydroxylase	Boosts with IL-2 targeted to tumor tissue by coupling to a tumor-specific antibody and enhanced DNA vaccine encoding the WPRE sequence	Neuroblastoma	CD8 response & protection from tumor challenge	[143]
	SL7207	CEA	Boosts with an antibody specific for a second tumor antigen coupled to IL-2	Colon carcinoma	CD8 response, DC activation & protection from tumor challenge	[190]
	SL7207	CEA	CD40L Dual-function DNA vaccine. Boosts with IL-2 coupled to a tumor-specific antibody	Colon carcinoma	CD8 response, DC activation & protection from tumor challenge	[189]

	SL7207	CEA	Boosts with IL-2 fused to a tumor-specific antibody	Lung carcinoma	CD8 response, DC activation & protection from tumor challenge	[122]
	SL7207	Model antigen lacZ	None	Renal cell carcinoma	CD8, CD4 responses & protection from tumor challenge	[201]
	SL5000	None	CD40L expression in the intestinal immune system	Lymphoma, Solid Tumor	Protection from tumor challenge	[179]
	SL7202	VEGFR-2	Targeting of proliferating endothelial cells in the tumor vasculature	Melanoma, colon carcinoma, lung carcinoma	CD8 response, negative CD4 response & protection from tumor challenge	[124]
	TAPET-CD(VNP20009)	CDase suicide gene	None	Solid Tumor	Increase response and survival in animal model & protection from tumor challenge	[81, 87]
Clostridium	acetobutylicum	CDase suicide gene,	TNF-a	Solid Tumor	Increase tumor cell kill by 500-fold and enhanced kill with angiogenesis inhibition	[171]
	beijerinckii	E. coli nitroreductase suicide gene	None	Solid Tumor	Increase tumor cell killing by 22-fold	[90]
	sporogenes, acetobutylicum	CDaseTranscriptional control by radio-inducible promoters	TNFα	Solid Tumor	Demonstrated radio-induced tumor-specific gene expression	[126–128]
Listeria monocyto-genes	XFL-7	HPV-16 E7	None	HNSCC, cervical	Tumor regressionCD8 T cell responses	[159]
E. coli	BM2710	DeoD plasmid GB2Ω inv-hly	None	Solid Tumor	Enhanced sensitization to 6-MPDR prodrug Tumor necrosis and growth inhibition	[25]
Mycobacterium	BCG	TNFα	Solid Tumor	ICAM-1 and HLA-DR cytokine induction	[54]	
Bifodobacterium Longum	105-A	CDase	None	Solid Tumor	Selective CDase expressionLocalized 5-FC to 5-FU conversion	[116]

Table 4. Selected Bacterial Vectors for the Immunotherapy of Cancer – Clinical*

Bacterium	Strain	Target AgThera-peutic Gene Product	Additional Immunomodu-lators/Combination Therapy	Cancer	Comments	Response	Ref.
Salmonella typhimurium	TAPET-CD(VNP 20009)	CDase	Tumor localized expression of CDase + 5-FC	Refractory cancer patients1 pt. Squamous cell carcinoma – head and neck 2 pts. adeno-carcinomaesophageal	Pilot Trial 3 patients	Tumor colonization in 2/3 patients localized conversion of 5-FC to 5-FU	[121]
	VNP20009	None	Tumor enriched replication of bacteria	AdvancedMelanoma	Phase I Hypoxic tumor environment targeted by anaerobic bacterium	Tumor colonization in 3/25 patients Induction of pro-inflammatory cytokinesNo objective anti-tumor responses	[175]

* Note: Although Clostridia have been used historically for the treatment of cancer, it is not currently used clinically nor are there recent published clinical trials. BCG is not listed although it is clinically approved for adjuvant therapy of surgically treated superficial bladder cancer. Clinical trials with BCG are numerous.

Live Bacterial Vectors

Live bacterial vectors designed to elicit a specific antitumor immune response may be categorized as (a) protein delivery vehicles or (b) DNA delivery vehicles (reviewed in [29, 83, 97]). In the first category, bacteria are transformed with plasmid-borne genes or are genomically modified to express foreign genes under the control of bacterial transcription and translation regulatory elements. As such, "therapeutic" proteins are delivered to the immune system by phagocytic cells that either take up the bacterial secreted protein or engulf the entire bacterium followed by bacteria-mediated secretion of the protein into the cytosol of the phagocytic cell. Either mechanism results in the processing and presentation of peptide Ag to T cells. This method, however, has limited efficacy for two reasons; (a) bacterial secreted proteins that are taken up by phagocytic APC are primarily processed through the MHC class II pathway and result in $CD4^+$ T cell activation and humoral immune responses but not necessarily $CD8^+$ T cell activation, and (b) intracellular bacteria, appropriately attenuated for vaccine use, have a limited capacity to produce proteins under the control of bacterial transcription and translation due to reduced replication efficiency and host-limiting anti-vector immune responses.

Currently an attractive mode of live bacterial vector gene delivery is being developed in which bacteria are transformed with plasmid-borne therapeutic genes under the control of mammalian promoters. For example, following orogastric vaccine delivery, bacteria are engulfed by phagocytic APC present in the mucosal lining of the gut or, alternatively, inherently target certain APC during normal infection. Attenuations limit bacterial intracellular replication and cell-to-cell spread and enhance safety. This results in the intracellular breakdown of the bacteria and subsequent release of plasmids to the cytosol of the mammalian host cell. Following nuclear localization, therapeutic genes are then expressed under mammalian promoter control resulting in both MHC class I and class II processing and presentation to $CD4^+$ and $CD8^+$ T cells. The exact mechanism of DNA transfer from the bacterial vector into the mammalian host is not yet completely known. Undoubtedly, further characterization of this phenomenon should lead to advances in live bacterial vector development and potentially numerous clinical applications. Candidate vaccines employing both of these modes of therapeutic protein delivery include *Shigella flexneri*, *Salmonella typhi*, *Salmonella typhimurium* and *Listeria monocytogenes*.

Bacteria are entirely capable of independently completing transcription and translation and, as such, are sometimes called "protein delivery vehicles" following therapeutic gene insertion. Thus, bacteria can be used to deliver cancer-therapeutic genes, not only to the cytoplasm of cells, but also to the extracellular space. Viral species, on the other hand, are dependent on the host nucleotides for DNA to be transcribed then translated into protein.

The use of live bacterial vectors holds promise for the targeted delivery of therapeutic genes/proteins to mammalian cells and tissues via the mucosal route. Depending on particular bacterial species, their specific virulence mechanisms and inherent metabolic preferences, bacteria infect various tissues/cells where they consequently deliver their cargo. In contrast to *Clostridia* (see below) or BCG, live bacterial vectors such as *Salmonella* are facultative anaerobes that grow well in both oxygen-rich and oxygen-depleted conditions. Facultative intracellular bacteria are particularly ideal carriers for potential immune therapeutic approaches involving Ag expression, due to their ability to access intracellular spaces in APC. Other facultative anaerobes such as *Shigella* and *Listeria* replicate in the cytosol and spread directly from one cell to another.

There is much preclinical data, but little recent clinical data demonstrating that live bacterial vectors can potentially be attenuated genetically and utilized for the cancer-therapeutic delivery of DNA and/or proteins [13, 81, 139, 148, 191]. DNA delivery in infectious disease models with live bacterial vectors has demonstrated remarkable safety and successful delivery of functional genes, particularly in the induction of immune responses and protection against bacterial, viral and parasitic infections [46, 151, 158].

Oncolytic Bacteria

Several bacterial species have been demonstrated to selectively replicate in and as a result, destroy tumor tissue [93, 174]. For example, in 1927, antitumor activity was observed with *Clostridium*, a spore-forming anaerobic bacteria that grows under hypoxic conditions (reviewed in [93]). Germination of Clostridial spores will only occur under anaerobic conditions. Large tumors typically have hypoxic/necrotic centers suggesting that the tumor-selective growth of anaerobic bacteria is due to a favorable environment.

The first experiments to demonstrate tumor-selective germination of Clostridial spores were carried out by Malmgren and Flanigan [102] in 1955, who injected mice i.v. with spores of *C. tetani*. The animals were unaffected unless they had tumors, in which case spores germinated, released tetanus toxin, resulting in death within 48 hours. Furthermore, they did not find vegetative organisms in the healthy tissues of mice carrying colonized tumors. Mose and Mose [113] treated Ehrlich-carcinoma bearing mice with a non-pathogenic strain of *C. butyricum* M-55, demonstrating that it retained its oncolytic effect following i.v. infection with spores, resulting in the destruction of large parts of the tumor. Further exploration with attenuated *Clostridium* species in murine models has revealed extensive tumor lysis with no adverse effect on normal tissue [2, 11, 27, 172]. In recent years, non-pathogenic strains that have no association with human disease, such as *C. acetobutylicum* and *C. beijerinckii*, have been examined as potential delivery system for therapeutic agents [43, 90, 112, 174].

Clostridium spore treatment was first tested in cancer patients in 1935. In more recent clinical trials, glioma patients were i.v. injected with up to 10^{10} *C. oncolyticum* spores [60]. These injections were well tolerated, and the only treatment-associated toxicities involved low-grade fever. The presence of the bacteria resulted in partial lysis of the tumor. Animal and human experiments demonstrate that Clostridial spore treatment is remarkably well tolerated and that growth of the organism frequently leads to the destruction of large parts of the tumor. Invariably, however, an outer viable rim remains from which tumor re-growth frequently occurs. From these observations it may be concluded that treatment of wild-type Clostridia spores is not sufficient to affect complete tumor regression. Combining Clostridia with other treatment modalities, such as radiation [11, 126, 127], targeting vascular components of tumors [27, 172], or tumoricidal gene therapy [43, 95, 128, 170, 173, 174] enhances the efficacy of Clostridia tumor therapy. It has been demonstrated in animals that Clostridial spore treatment may be repeated and that the host anti-Clostridial immune response does not hinder tumor colonization [172]. This suggests the possibility of long-term colonization of tumors with Clostridia gene therapy vectors.

As a result of advances in genetic engineering, Clostridium can now be genetically modified to produce anti-tumor agents. In addition, vector systems have been developed for the introduction of heterologous DNA into a number of strains [170]. This should allow for the generation of safer strains, improvements in tumor targeting, and importantly, the tumor-localized expression of therapeutic molecules. In animal models for cancer, Clostridia vectors are now being used to deliver drugs that exert a direct cytotoxic effect, such as the cytokine tumor necrosis factor (TNF)-α and proteins such as cytosine deaminase (CDase) or nitroreductase, that convert a non-toxic prodrug into a toxic therapeutic drug [90, 126, 128, 170, 171]. Anti-cancer effects of the Clostridia/CDase/5-FC system have been observed in a number of animal models [174]. Transfection of less than 4% of cells with CDase proved to be sufficient to achieve a 60% cure rate following 5-FC treatment. While promising in animal models, to date no clinical trials have been conducted with Clostridial gene therapy vectors.

CONCLUSIONS

In human neoplasia numerous TAA have now been defined, which has facilitated the development and application of diverse immunotherapies in the clinic, including those outlined in this chapter. Effective immunotherapy will likely result from the integration of innovative strategies that optimize both quantitative and qualitative elements of the innate and adaptive immune responses in the face of constant genetic and epigenetic alterations regulating tumor development, survival and progression.

Perhaps, combination therapies, which are described elsewhere, involving vaccination with other oncological treatments, such as radiation [16, 19], chemotherapy [32, 101], cytokines (e.g., IFN, IL-2, IL-12, IL-15) [32, 183, 185], passive administration of tumor-specific monoclonal antibodies [186], or non-steroidal anti-inflammatory drugs (e.g., cyclooxygenase-2 inhibitors) [55, 199] may prove even more effective to promote longer-term clinical responses concurrent with a lower risk toward the generation of aggressive tumor escape variants. Future directions will be faced with several major questions, such as: [1] which combination therapies involving recombinant viral or bacterial-based cancer vaccines and conventional therapies, such as radiation or chemotherapy should be more actively pursued in clinical trials? [2] will such clinical strategies be more effective in prevention settings, in patients with high risk of disease development or recurrence or in patients with minimal disease, as compared to those with advanced or metastatic disease? and [3] for such immunotherapy approaches to be effective, could these interventions serve to maintain cancer as a chronic condition in much the same way that diabetes, arthritis and other autoimmune diseases are treated?

REFERENCES

1. Adams M, Borysiewicz L, Fiander A, Man S, Jasani B, Navabi H, Lipetz C, Evans AS, Mason M (2001) Clinical studies of human papilloma vaccines in pre-invasive and invasive cancer. Vaccine 19(17–19): 2549–2556
2. Agrawal N, Bettegowda C, Cheong I, Geschwind JF, Drake CG, Hipkiss EL, Tatsumi M, Dang LH, Diaz LA, Jr., Pomper M, Abusedera M, Wahl RL, Kinzler KW, Zhou S, Huso DL, Vogelstein B (2004) Bacteriolytic therapy can generate a potent immune response against experimental tumors. Proc Natl Acad Sci U S A 101(42): 15172–15177
3. Alexandroff AB, Jackson AM, O'Donnell MA, James K (1999) BCG immunotherapy of bladder cancer: 20 years on. Lancet 353(9165): 1689–1694
4. Anderson BD, Nakamura T, Russell SJ, Peng KW (2004) High CD46 receptor density determines preferential killing of tumor cells by oncolytic measles virus. Cancer Res 64(14): 4919–4926
5. Arlen PM, Gulley JL, Todd N, Lieberman R, Steinberg SM, Morin S, Bastian A, Marte J, Tsang KY, Beetham P, Grosenbach DW, Schlom J, Dahut W (2005) Antiandrogen, Vaccine And Combination Therapy In Patients With Nonmetastatic Hormone Refractory Prostate Cancer. J Urol 174(2): 539–546
6. Atkins GJ, Smyth JW, Fleeton MN, Galbraith SE, Sheahan BJ (2004) Alphaviruses and their derived vectors as anti-tumor agents. Curr Cancer Drug Targets 4(7): 597–607
7. Baldwin PJ, van der Burg SH, Boswell CM, Offringa R, Hickling JK, Dobson J, Roberts JS, Latimer JA, Moseley RP, Coleman N, Stanley MA, Sterling JC (2003) Vaccinia-expressed human papillomavirus 16 and 18 e6 and e7 as a therapeutic vaccination for vulval and vaginal intraepithelial neoplasia. Clin Cancer Res 9(14): 5205–5213
8. Basak SK, Kiertscher SM, Harui A, Roth MD (2004) Modifying adenoviral vectors for use as gene-based cancer vaccines. Viral Immunol 17(2): 182–196
9. Berry JM, Palefsky JM (2003) A review of human papillomavirus vaccines: from basic science to clinical trials. Front Biosci 8(s333–345)
10. Bessis N, GarciaCozar FJ, Boissier MC (2004) Immune responses to gene therapy vectors: influence on vector function and effector mechanisms. Gene Ther 11 Suppl 1(S10–17)
11. Bettegowda C, Dang LH, Abrams R, Huso DL, Dillehay L, Cheong I, Agrawal N, Borzillary S, McCaffery JM, Watson EL, Lin KS, Bunz F, Baidoo K, Pomper MG, Kinzler KW, Vogelstein B, Zhou S (2003) Overcoming the hypoxic barrier to radiation therapy with anaerobic bacteria. Proc Natl Acad Sci U S A 100(25): 15083–15088
12. Blattman JN, Greenberg PD (2004) Cancer immunotherapy: a treatment for the masses. Science 305(5681): 200–205
13. Brockstedt DG, Giedlin MA, Leong ML, Bahjat KS, Gao Y, Luckett W, Liu W, Cook DN, Portnoy DA, Dubensky TW, Jr. (2004) Listeria-based cancer vaccines that segregate immunogenicity from toxicity. Proc Natl Acad Sci U S A 101(38): 13832–13837
14. Burnet FM (1970) The concept of immunological surveillance. Prog Exp Tumor Res 13(1–27)
15. Butterfield LH, Ribas A, Dissette VB, Amarnani SN, Vu HT, Oseguera D, Wang HJ, Elashoff RM, McBride WH, Mukherji B, Cochran AJ, Glaspy JA, Economou JS (2003) Determinant spreading associated with clinical response in dendritic cell-based immunotherapy for malignant melanoma. Clin Cancer Res 9(3): 998–1008

16. Cao ZA, Daniel D, Hanahan D (2002) Sub-lethal radiation enhances anti-tumor immunotherapy in a transgenic mouse model of pancreatic cancer. BMC Cancer 2(1): 11
17. Carroll MW, Overwijk WW, Chamberlain RS, Rosenberg SA, Moss B, Restifo NP (1997) Highly attenuated modified vaccinia virus Ankara (MVA) as an effective recombinant vector: a murine tumor model. Vaccine 15(4): 387–394
18. Cavacini LA, Duval M, Eder JP, Posner MR (2002) Evidence of determinant spreading in the antibody responses to prostate cell surface antigens in patients immunized with prostate-specific antigen. Clin Cancer Res 8(2): 368–373
19. Chakraborty M, Abrams SI, Coleman CN, Camphausen K, Schlom J, Hodge JW (2004) External beam radiation of tumors alters phenotype of tumor cells to render them susceptible to vaccine-mediated T-cell killing. Cancer Res 64(12): 4328–4337
20. Chen B, Timiryasova TM, Andres ML, Kajioka EH, Dutta-Roy R, Gridley DS, Fodor I (2000) Evaluation of combined vaccinia virus-mediated antitumor gene therapy with p53, IL-2, and IL-12 in a glioma model. Cancer Gene Ther 7(11): 1437–1447
21. Chen PW, Wang M, Bronte V, Zhai Y, Rosenberg SA, Restifo NP (1996) Therapeutic antitumor response after immunization with a recombinant adenovirus encoding a model tumor-associated antigen. J Immunol 156(1): 224–231
22. Cochlovius B, Stassar MJ, Schreurs MW, Benner A, Adema GJ (2002) Oral DNA vaccination: antigen uptake and presentation by dendritic cells elicits protective immunity. Immunol Lett 80(2): 89–96
23. Cooney EL, Collier AC, Greenberg PD, Coombs RW, Zarling J, Arditti DE, Hoffman MC, Hu SL, Corey L (1991) Safety of and immunological response to a recombinant vaccinia virus vaccine expressing HIV envelope glycoprotein. Lancet 337(8741): 567–572
24. Corona Gutierrez CM, Tinoco A, Navarro T, Contreras ML, Cortes RR, Calzado P, Reyes L, Posternak R, Morosoli G, Verde ML, Rosales R (2004) Therapeutic vaccination with MVA E2 can eliminate precancerous lesions (CIN 1, CIN 2, and CIN 3) associated with infection by oncogenic human papillomavirus. Hum Gene Ther 15(5): 421–431
25. Critchley RJ, Jezzard S, Radford KJ, Goussard S, Lemoine NR, Grillot-Courvalin C, Vassaux G (2004) Potential therapeutic applications of recombinant, invasive E. coli. Gene Ther 11(15): 1224–1233
26. Curiel TJ, Coukos G, Zou L, Alvarez X, Cheng P, Mottram P, Evdemon-Hogan M, Conejo-Garcia JR, Zhang L, Burow M, Zhu Y, Wei S, Kryczek I, Daniel B, Gordon A, Myers L, Lackner A, Disis ML, Knutson KL, Chen L, Zou W (2004) Specific recruitment of regulatory T cells in ovarian carcinoma fosters immune privilege and predicts reduced survival. Nat Med 10(9): 942–949
27. Dang LH, Bettegowda C, Agrawal N, Cheong I, Huso D, Frost P, Loganzo F, Greenberger L, Barkoczy J, Pettit GR, Smith AB, 3rd, Gurulingappa H, Khan S, Parmigiani G, Kinzler KW, Zhou S, Vogelstein B (2004) Targeting vascular and avascular compartments of tumors with C. novyi-NT and anti-microtubule agents. Cancer Biol Ther 3(3): 326–337
28. Demkowicz WE, Maa JS, Esteban M (1992) Identification and characterization of vaccinia virus genes encoding proteins that are highly antigenic in animals and are immunodominant in vaccinated humans. J Virol 66(1): 386–398
29. Dietrich G, Spreng S, Favre D, Viret JF, Guzman CA (2003) Live attenuated bacteria as vectors to deliver plasmid DNA vaccines. Curr Opin Mol Ther 5(1): 10–19
30. Dranoff G (2004) Cytokines in cancer pathogenesis and cancer therapy. Nat Rev Cancer 4(1): 11–22
31. Dudley ME, Wunderlich JR, Robbins PF, Yang JC, Hwu P, Schwartzentruber DJ, Topalian SL, Sherry R, Restifo NP, Hubicki AM, Robinson MR, Raffeld M, Duray P, Seipp CA, Rogers-Freezer L, Morton KE, Mavroukakis SA, White DE, Rosenberg SA (2002) Cancer regression and autoimmunity in patients after clonal repopulation with antitumor lymphocytes. Science 298(5594): 850–854
32. Dudley ME, Wunderlich JR, Yang JC, Hwu P, Schwartzentruber DJ, Topalian SL, Sherry RM, Marincola FM, Leitman SF, Seipp CA, Rogers-Freezer L, Morton KE, Nahvi A, Mavroukakis SA, White DE, Rosenberg SA (2002) A phase I study of nonmyeloablative chemotherapy and

adoptive transfer of autologous tumor antigen-specific T lymphocytes in patients with metastatic melanoma. J Immunother 25(3): 243–251
33. Dudley ME, Rosenberg SA (2003) Adoptive-cell-transfer therapy for the treatment of patients with cancer. Nat Rev Cancer 3(9): 666–675
34. Dudley ME, Wunderlich JR, Shelton TE, Even J, Rosenberg SA (2003) Generation of tumor-infiltrating lymphocyte cultures for use in adoptive transfer therapy for melanoma patients. J Immunother 26(4): 332–342
35. Dunn GP, Old LJ, Schreiber RD (2004) The three Es of cancer immunoediting. Annu Rev Immunol 22(329–360)
36. Dunn GP, Old LJ, Schreiber RD (2004) The immunobiology of cancer immunosurveillance and immunoediting. Immunity 21(2): 137–148
37. Eder JP, Kantoff PW, Roper K, Xu GX, Bubley GJ, Boyden J, Gritz L, Mazzara G, Oh WK, Arlen P, Tsang KY, Panicali D, Schlom J, Kufe DW (2000) A phase I trial of a recombinant vaccinia virus expressing prostate-specific antigen in advanced prostate cancer. Clin Cancer Res 6(5): 1632–1638
38. Emens LA, Jaffee EM (2003) Cancer vaccines: an old idea comes of age. Cancer Biol Ther 2(4 Suppl 1): S161–168
39. Feder-Mengus C, Schultz-Thater E, Oertli D, Marti WR, Heberer M, Spagnoli GC, Zajac P (2005) Nonreplicating recombinant vaccinia virus expressing CD40 ligand enhances APC capacity to stimulate specific CD4+ and CD8+ T cell responses. Hum Gene Ther 16(3): 348–360
40. Fenner F (1980) The global eradication of smallpox. Med J Aust 1(10): 455–455
41. Finn OJ (2003) Cancer vaccines: between the idea and the reality. Nat Rev Immunol 3(8): 630–641
42. Fodor I, Timiryasova T, Denes B, Yoshida J, Ruckle H, Lilly M (2005) Vaccinia virus mediated p53 gene therapy for bladder cancer in an orthotopic murine model. J Urol 173(2): 604–609
43. Fox ME, Lemmon MJ, Mauchline ML, Davis TO, Giaccia AJ, Minton NP, Brown JM (1996) Anaerobic bacteria as a delivery system for cancer gene therapy: in vitro activation of 5-fluorocytosine by genetically engineered clostridia. Gene Ther 3(2): 173–178
44. Gabrilovich D (2004) Mechanisms and functional significance of tumour-induced dendritic-cell defects. Nat Rev Immunol 4(12): 941–952
45. Galanis E, Okuno SH, Nascimento AG, Lewis BD, Lee RA, Oliveira AM, Sloan JA, Atherton P, Edmonson JH, Erlichman C, Randlev B, Wang Q, Freeman S, Rubin J (2005) Phase I-II trial of ONYX-015 in combination with MAP chemotherapy in patients with advanced sarcomas. Gene Ther 12(5): 437–445
46. Gentschev I, Dietrich G, Spreng S, Pilgrim S, Stritzker J, Kolb-Maurer A, Goebel W (2002) Delivery of protein antigens and DNA by attenuated intracellular bacteria. Int J Med Microbiol 291(6–7): 577–582
47. Gottschalk S, Edwards OL, Sili U, Huls MH, Goltsova T, Davis AR, Heslop HE, Rooney CM (2003) Generating CTLs against the subdominant Epstein-Barr virus LMP1 antigen for the adoptive immunotherapy of EBV-associated malignancies. Blood 101(5): 1905–1912
48. Griffith TS, Kawakita M, Tian J, Ritchey J, Tartaglia J, Sehgal I, Thompson TC, Zhao W, Ratliff TL (2001) Inhibition of murine prostate tumor growth and activation of immunoregulatory cells with recombinant canarypox viruses. J Natl Cancer Inst 93(13): 998–1007
49. Grosenbach DW, Barrientos JC, Schlom J, Hodge JW (2001) Synergy of vaccine strategies to amplify antigen-specific immune responses and antitumor effects. Cancer Res 61(11): 4497–4505
50. Grosenbach DW, Schlom J, Gritz L, Gomez Yafal A, Hodge JW (2003) A recombinant vector expressing transgenes for four T-cell costimulatory molecules (OX40L, B7–1, ICAM-1, LFA-3) induces sustained CD4+ and CD8+ T-cell activation, protection from apoptosis, and enhanced cytokine production. Cell Immunol 222(1): 45–57
51. Gulley J, Chen AP, Dahut W, Arlen PM, Bastian A, Steinberg SM, Tsang K, Panicali D, Poole D, Schlom J, Michael Hamilton J (2002) Phase I study of a vaccine using recombinant vaccinia virus expressing PSA (rV-PSA) in patients with metastatic androgen-independent prostate cancer. Prostate 53(2): 109–117

52. Gulley JL, Arlen PM, Bastian A, Morin S, Marte J, Beetham P, Tsang KY, Yokokawa J, Hodge JW, Menard C, Camphausen K, Coleman CN, Sullivan F, Steinberg SM, Schlom J, Dahut W (2005) Combining a recombinant cancer vaccine with standard definitive radiotherapy in patients with localized prostate cancer. Clin Cancer Res 11(9): 3353–3362
53. Guo CC, Ding J, Pan BR, Yu ZC, Han QL, Meng FP, Liu N, Fan DM (2003) Development of an oral DNA vaccine against MG7-Ag of gastric cancer using attenuated salmonella typhimurium as carrier. World J Gastroenterol 9(6): 1191–1195
54. Haley JL, Young DG, Alexandroff A, James K, Jackson AM (1999) Enhancing the immunotherapeutic potential of mycobacteria by transfection with tumour necrosis factor-alpha. Immunology 96(1): 114–121
55. Haller DG (2003) COX-2 inhibitors in oncology. Semin Oncol 30(4 Suppl 12): 2–8
56. Hanahan D, Weinberg RA (2000) The hallmarks of cancer. Cell 100(1): 57–70
57. Hawkins LK, Lemoine NR, Kirn D (2002) Oncolytic biotherapy: a novel therapeutic plafform. Lancet Oncol 3(1): 17–26
58. Heise C, Sampson-Johannes A, Williams A, McCormick F, Von Hoff DD, Kirn DH (1997) ONYX-015, an E1B gene-attenuated adenovirus, causes tumor-specific cytolysis and antitumoral efficacy that can be augmented by standard chemotherapeutic agents. Nat Med 3(6): 639–645
59. Heise CC, Williams AM, Xue S, Propst M, Kirn DH (1999) Intravenous administration of ONYX-015, a selectively replicating adenovirus, induces antitumoral efficacy. Cancer Res 59(11): 2623–2628
60. Heppner F (1982) New technologies to combat malignant tumours of the brain. Anticancer Res 2(1–2): 101–109
61. Hodge JW, Sabzevari H, Yafal AG, Gritz L, Lorenz MG, Schlom J (1999) A triad of costimulatory molecules synergize to amplify T-cell activation. Cancer Res 59(22): 5800–5807
62. Hodge JW, Grosenbach DW, Schlom J (2002) Vector-based delivery of tumor-associated antigens and T-cell co-stimulatory molecules in the induction of immune responses and anti-tumor immunity. Cancer Detect Prev 26(4): 275–291
63. Hodge JW, Grosenbach DW, Aarts WM, Poole DJ, Schlom J (2003) Vaccine therapy of established tumors in the absence of autoimmunity. Clin Cancer Res 9(5): 1837–1849
64. Hodge JW, Poole DJ, Aarts WM, Gomez Yafal A, Gritz L, Schlom J (2003) Modified vaccinia virus ankara recombinants are as potent as vaccinia recombinants in diversified prime and boost vaccine regimens to elicit therapeutic antitumor responses. Cancer Res 63(22): 7942–7949
65. Hodge JW, Greiner JW, Tsang KY, Sabzevari H, Kudo-Saito C, Grosenbach DW, Gulley JL, Arlen PM, Marshall JL, Panicali D, Schlom J (2006) Costimulatory molecules as adjuvants for immunotherapy. Front Biosci 11(788–803)
66. Horig H, Lee DS, Conkright W, Divito J, Hasson H, LaMare M, Rivera A, Park D, Tine J, Guito K, Tsang KW, Schlom J, Kaufman HL (2000) Phase I clinical trial of a recombinant canarypoxvirus (ALVAC) vaccine expressing human carcinoembryonic antigen and the B7.1 co-stimulatory molecule. Cancer Immunol Immunother 49(9): 504–514
67. Hsueh EC, Gupta RK, Qi K, Morton DL (1998) Correlation of specific immune responses with survival in melanoma patients with distant metastases receiving polyvalent melanoma cell vaccine. J Clin Oncol 16(9): 2913–2920
68. Hsueh EC, Essner R, Foshag LJ, Ye W, Morton DL (2002) Active immunotherapy by reinduction with a polyvalent allogeneic cell vaccine correlates with improved survival in recurrent metastatic melanoma. Ann Surg Oncol 9(5): 486–492
69. Hurwitz AA, Foster BA, Kwon ED, Truong T, Choi EM, Greenberg NM, Burg MB, Allison JP (2000) Combination immunotherapy of primary prostate cancer in a transgenic mouse model using CTLA-4 blockade. Cancer Res 60(9): 2444–2448
70. Ikeda H, Old LJ, Schreiber RD (2002) The roles of IFN gamma in protection against tumor development and cancer immunoediting. Cytokine Growth Factor Rev 13(2): 95–109
71. Irvine KR, Chamberlain RS, Shulman EP, Surman DR, Rosenberg SA, Restifo NP (1997) Enhancing efficacy of recombinant anticancer vaccines with prime/boost regimens that use two different vectors. J Natl Cancer Inst 89(21): 1595–1601

72. Iwasaki A, Medzhitov R (2004) Toll-like receptor control of the adaptive immune responses. Nat Immunol 5(10): 987–995
73. Jahrsdorfer B, Weiner GJ (2003) CpG oligodeoxynucleotides for immune stimulation in cancer immunotherapy. Curr Opin Investig Drugs 4(6): 686–690
74. Juillard V, Villefroy P, Godfrin D, Pavirani A, Venet A, Guillet JG (1995) Long-term humoral and cellular immunity induced by a single immunization with replication-defective adenovirus recombinant vector. Eur J Immunol 25(12): 3467–3473
75. Kalus RM, Kantor JA, Gritz L, Gomez Yafal A, Mazzara GP, Schlom J, Hodge JW (1999) The use of combination vaccinia vaccines and dual-gene vaccinia vaccines to enhance antigen-specific T-cell immunity via T-cell costimulation. Vaccine 17(7–8): 893–903
76. Karcher J, Dyckhoff G, Beckhove P, Reisser C, Brysch M, Ziouta Y, Helmke BH, Weidauer H, Schirrmacher V, Herold-Mende C (2004) Antitumor vaccination in patients with head and neck squamous cell carcinomas with autologous virus-modified tumor cells. Cancer Res 64(21): 8057–8061
77. Kass E, Panicali DL, Mazzara G, Schlom J, Greiner JW (2001) Granulocyte/macrophage-colony stimulating factor produced by recombinant avian poxviruses enriches the regional lymph nodes with antigen-presenting cells and acts as an immunoadjuvant. Cancer Res 61(1): 206–214
78. Kasuya H, Takeda S, Nomoto S, Nakao A (2005) The potential of oncolytic virus therapy for pancreatic cancer. Cancer Gene Ther
79. Kaufman HL, Deraffele G, Mitcham J, Moroziewicz D, Cohen SM, Hurst-Wicker KS, Cheung K, Lee DS, Divito J, Voulo M, Donovan J, Dolan K, Manson K, Panicali D, Wang E, Horig H, Marincola FM (2005) Targeting the local tumor microenvironment with vaccinia virus expressing B7.1 for the treatment of melanoma. J Clin Invest 115(7): 1903–1912
80. Kaufmann AM, Stern PL, Rankin EM, Sommer H, Nuessler V, Schneider A, Adams M, Onon TS, Bauknecht T, Wagner U, Kroon K, Hickling J, Boswell CM, Stacey SN, Kitchener HC, Gillard J, Wanders J, Roberts JS, Zwierzina H (2002) Safety and immunogenicity of TA-HPV, a recombinant vaccinia virus expressing modified human papillomavirus (HPV)-16 and HPV-18 E6 and E7 genes, in women with progressive cervical cancer. Clin Cancer Res 8(12): 3676–3685
81. King I, Bermudes D, Lin S, Belcourt M, Pike J, Troy K, Le T, Ittensohn M, Mao J, Lang W, Runyan JD, Luo X, Li Z, Zheng LM (2002) Tumor-targeted Salmonella expressing cytosine deaminase as an anticancer agent. Hum Gene Ther 13(10): 1225–1233
82. Kirn D, Martuza RL, Zwiebel J (2001) Replication-selective virotherapy for cancer: Biological principles, risk management and future directions. Nat Med 7(7): 781–787
83. Kochi SK, Killeen KP, Ryan US (2003) Advances in the development of bacterial vector technology. Expert Rev Vaccines 2(1): 31–43
84. Krieg AM (2000) Immune effects and mechanisms of action of CpG motifs. Vaccine 19(6): 618–622
85. Kuball J, Schuler M, Antunes Ferreira E, Herr W, Neumann M, Obenauer-Kutner L, Westreich L, Huber C, Wolfel T, Theobald M (2002) Generating p53-specific cytotoxic T lymphocytes by recombinant adenoviral vector-based vaccination in mice, but not man. Gene Ther 9(13): 833–843
86. Kudo-Saito C, Schlom J, Hodge JW (2005) Induction of an antigen cascade by diversified subcutaneous/intratumoral vaccination is associated with antitumor responses. Clin Cancer Res 11(6): 2416–2426
87. Lee KC, Zheng LM, Margitich D, Almassian B, King I (2001) Evaluation of the acute and subchronic toxic effects in mice, rats, and monkeys of the genetically engineered and Escherichia coli cytosine deaminase gene-incorporated Salmonella strain, TAPET-CD, being developed as an antitumor agent. Int J Toxicol 20(4): 207–217
88. Leitner WW, Ying H, Restifo NP (1999) DNA and RNA-based vaccines: principles, progress and prospects. Vaccine 18(9–10): 765–777
89. Leitner WW, Hwang LN, deVeer MJ, Zhou A, Silverman RH, Williams BR, Dubensky TW, Ying H, Restifo NP (2003) Alphavirus-based DNA vaccine breaks immunological tolerance by activating innate antiviral pathways. Nat Med 9(1): 33–39

90. Lemmon MJ, van Zijl P, Fox ME, Mauchline ML, Giaccia AJ, Minton NP, Brown JM (1997) Anaerobic bacteria as a gene delivery system that is controlled by the tumor microenvironment. Gene Ther 4(8): 791–796
91. Levy B, Panicalli D, Marshall J (2004) TRICOM: enhanced vaccines as anticancer therapy. Expert Rev Vaccines 3(4): 397–402
92. Lin E, Nemunaitis J (2004) Oncolytic viral therapies. Cancer Gene Ther 11(10): 643–664
93. Lin J, Lin E, Nemunaitis J (2004) Bacteria in the treatment of cancer. Curr Opin Mol Ther 6(6): 629–639
94. Liu M, Acres B, Balloul JM, Bizouarne N, Paul S, Slos P, Squiban P (2004) Gene-based vaccines and immunotherapeutics. Proc Natl Acad Sci U S A 101 Suppl 2(14567–14571
95. Liu SC, Minton NP, Giaccia AJ, Brown JM (2002) Anticancer efficacy of systemically delivered anaerobic bacteria as gene therapy vectors targeting tumor hypoxia/necrosis. Gene Ther 9(4): 291–296
96. Lode HN, Pertl U, Xiang R, Gaedicke G, Reisfeld RA (2000) Tyrosine hydroxylase-based DNA-vaccination is effective against murine neuroblastoma. Med Pediatr Oncol 35(6): 641–646
97. Loessner H, Weiss S (2004) Bacteria-mediated DNA transfer in gene therapy and vaccination. Expert Opin Biol Ther 4(2): 157–168
98. Lorence RM, Pecora AL, Major PP, Hotte SJ, Laurie SA, Roberts MS, Groene WS, Bamat MK (2003) Overview of phase I studies of intravenous administration of PV701, an oncolytic virus. Curr Opin Mol Ther 5(6): 618–624
99. Lou E (2003) Oncolytic herpes viruses as a potential mechanism for cancer therapy. Acta Oncol 42(7): 660–671
100. Luo Y, Zhou H, Mizutani M, Mizutani N, Reisfeld RA, Xiang R (2003) Transcription factor Fos-related antigen 1 is an effective target for a breast cancer vaccine. Proc Natl Acad Sci U S A 100(15): 8850–8855
101. Machiels JP, Reilly RT, Emens LA, Ercolini AM, Lei RY, Weintraub D, Okoye FI, Jaffee EM (2001) Cyclophosphamide, doxorubicin, and paclitaxel enhance the antitumor immune response of granulocyte/macrophage-colony stimulating factor-secreting whole-cell vaccines in HER-2/neu tolerized mice. Cancer Res 61(9): 3689–3697
102. Malmgren RA, Flanigan CC (1955) Localization of the vegetative form of Clostridium tetani in mouse tumors following intravenous spore administration. Cancer Res 15(7): 473–478
103. Marshall JL, Hawkins MJ, Tsang KY, Richmond E, Pedicano JE, Zhu MZ, Schlom J (1999) Phase I study in cancer patients of a replication-defective avipox recombinant vaccine that expresses human carcinoembryonic antigen. J Clin Oncol 17(1): 332–337
104. Marshall JL, Hoyer RJ, Toomey MA, Faraguna K, Chang P, Richmond E, Pedicano JE, Gehan E, Peck RA, Arlen P, Tsang KY, Schlom J (2000) Phase I study in advanced cancer patients of a diversified prime-and-boost vaccination protocol using recombinant vaccinia virus and recombinant nonreplicating avipox virus to elicit anti-carcinoembryonic antigen immune responses. J Clin Oncol 18(23): 3964–3973
105. Marshall JL, Gulley JL, Arlen PM, Beetham PK, Tsang KY, Slack R, Hodge JW, Doren S, Grosenbach DW, Hwang J, Fox E, Odogwu L, Park S, Panicali D, Schlom J (2005) Phase I study of sequential vaccinations with fowlpox-CEA(6D)-TRICOM alone and sequentially with vaccinia-CEA(6D)-TRICOM, with and without granulocyte-macrophage colony-stimulating factor, in patients with carcinoembryonic antigen-expressing carcinomas. J Clin Oncol 23(4): 720–731
106. McAneny D, Ryan CA, Beazley RM, Kaufman HL (1996) Results of a phase I trial of a recombinant vaccinia virus that expresses carcinoembryonic antigen in patients with advanced colorectal cancer. Ann Surg Oncol 3(5): 495–500
107. McCormick F (2003) Cancer-specific viruses and the development of ONYX-015. Cancer Biol Ther 2(4 Suppl 1): S157–160
108. Melani C, Chiodoni C, Forni G, Colombo MP (2003) Myeloid cell expansion elicited by the progression of spontaneous mammary carcinomas in c-erbB-2 transgenic BALB/c mice suppresses immune reactivity. Blood 102(6): 2138–2145

109. Meyer RG, Britten CM, Siepmann U, Petzold B, Sagban TA, Lehr HA, Weigle B, Schmitz M, Mateo L, Schmidt B, Bernhard H, Jakob T, Hein R, Schuler G, Schuler-Thurner B, Wagner SN, Drexler I, Sutter G, Arndtz N, Chaplin P, Metz J, Enk A, Huber C, Wolfel T (2005) A phase I vaccination study with tyrosinase in patients with stage II melanoma using recombinant modified vaccinia virus Ankara (MVA-hTyr). Cancer Immunol Immunother 54(5): 453–467
110. Michael A, Ball G, Quatan N, Wushishi F, Russell N, Whelan J, Chakraborty P, Leader D, Whelan M, Pandha H (2005) Delayed disease progression after allogeneic cell vaccination in hormone-resistant prostate cancer and correlation with immunologic variables. Clin Cancer Res 11(12): 4469–4478
111. Mincheff M, Tchakarov S, Zoubak S, Loukinov D, Botev C, Altankova I, Georgiev G, Petrov S, Meryman HT (2000) Naked DNA and adenoviral immunizations for immunotherapy of prostate cancer: a phase I/II clinical trial. Eur Urol 38(2): 208–217
112. Minton NP, Mauchline ML, Lemmon MJ, Brehm JK, Fox M, Michael NP, Giaccia A, Brown JM (1995) Chemotherapeutic tumour targeting using clostridial spores. FEMS Microbiol Rev 17(3): 357–364
113. Mose JR, Mose G, Propst A, Heppner F (1967) [Oncolysis of malignant tumors by Clostridium strain M 55]. Med Klin 62(5): 189–193
114. Moss B (1996) Genetically engineered poxviruses for recombinant gene expression, vaccination, and safety. Proc Natl Acad Sci U S A 93(21): 11341–11348
115. Mulryan K, Ryan MG, Myers KA, Shaw D, Wang W, Kingsman SM, Stern PL, Carroll MW (2002) Attenuated recombinant vaccinia virus expressing oncofetal antigen (tumor-associated antigen) 5T4 induces active therapy of established tumors. Mol Cancer Ther 1(12): 1129–1137
116. Nakamura T, Sasaki T, Fujimori M, Yazawa K, Kano Y, Amano J, Taniguchi S (2002) Cloned cytosine deaminase gene expression of Bifidobacterium longum and application to enzyme/pro-drug therapy of hypoxic solid tumors. Biosci Biotechnol Biochem 66(11): 2362–2366
117. Nakamura T, Russell SJ (2004) Oncolytic measles viruses for cancer therapy. Expert Opin Biol Ther 4(10): 1685–1692
118. Nakamura T, Peng KW, Harvey M, Greiner S, Lorimer IA, James CD, Russell SJ (2005) Rescue and propagation of fully retargeted oncolytic measles viruses. Nat Biotechnol 23(2): 209–214
119. Nauts HC, McLaren JR (1990) Coley toxins–the first century. Adv Exp Med Biol 267(483–500)
120. Nelson NJ (1999) Scientific interest in Newcastle disease virus is reviving. J Natl Cancer Inst 91(20): 1708–1710
121. Nemunaitis J, Cunningham C, Senzer N, Kuhn J, Cramm J, Litz C, Cavagnolo R, Cahill A, Clairmont C, Sznol M (2003) Pilot trial of genetically modified, attenuated Salmonella expressing the E. coli cytosine deaminase gene in refractory cancer patients. Cancer Gene Ther 10(10): 737–744
122. Niethammer AG, Primus FJ, Xiang R, Dolman CS, Ruehlmann JM, Ba Y, Gillies SD, Reisfeld RA (2001) An oral DNA vaccine against human carcinoembryonic antigen (CEA) prevents growth and dissemination of Lewis lung carcinoma in CEA transgenic mice. Vaccine 20(3–4): 421–429
123. Niethammer AG, Xiang R, Ruehlmann JM, Lode HN, Dolman CS, Gillies SD, Reisfeld RA (2001) Targeted interleukin 2 therapy enhances protective immunity induced by an autologous oral DNA vaccine against murine melanoma. Cancer Res 61(16): 6178–6184
124. Niethammer AG, Xiang R, Becker JC, Wodrich H, Pertl U, Karsten G, Eliceiri BP, Reisfeld RA (2002) A DNA vaccine against VEGF receptor 2 prevents effective angiogenesis and inhibits tumor growth. Nat Med 8(12): 1369–1375
125. Norman KL, Lee PW (2005) Not all viruses are bad guys: the case for reovirus in cancer therapy. Drug Discov Today 10(12): 847–855
126. Nuyts S, Theys J, Landuyt W, van Mellaert L, Lambin P, Anne J (2001) Increasing specificity of anti-tumor therapy: cytotoxic protein delivery by non-pathogenic clostridia under regulation of radio-induced promoters. Anticancer Res 21(2A): 857–861
127. Nuyts S, Van Mellaert L, Theys J, Landuyt W, Lambin P, Anne J (2001) The use of radiation-induced bacterial promoters in anaerobic conditions: a means to control gene expression in clostridium-mediated therapy for cancer. Radiat Res 155(5): 716–723

128. Nuyts S, Van Mellaert L, Theys J, Landuyt W, Lambin P, Anne J (2002) Clostridium spores for tumor-specific drug delivery. Anticancer Drugs 13(2): 115–125
129. Okamoto M, Sato M (2003) Toll-like receptor signaling in anti-cancer immunity. J Med Invest 50(1–2): 9–24
130. Ostrand-Rosenberg S (2004) Animal models of tumor immunity, immunotherapy and cancer vaccines. Curr Opin Immunol 16(2): 143–150
131. Overwijk WW, Lee DS, Surman DR, Irvine KR, Touloukian CE, Chan CC, Carroll MW, Moss B, Rosenberg SA, Restifo NP (1999) Vaccination with a recombinant vaccinia virus encoding a "self" antigen induces autoimmune vitiligo and tumor cell destruction in mice: requirement for CD4(+) T lymphocytes. Proc Natl Acad Sci U S A 96(6): 2982–2987
132. Overwijk WW, Theoret MR, Finkelstein SE, Surman DR, de Jong LA, Vyth-Dreese FA, Dellemijn TA, Antony PA, Spiess PJ, Palmer DC, Heimann DM, Klebanoff CA, Yu Z, Hwang LN, Feigenbaum L, Kruisbeek AM, Rosenberg SA, Restifo NP (2003) Tumor regression and autoimmunity after reversal of a functionally tolerant state of self-reactive CD8+ T cells. J Exp Med 198(4): 569–580
133. Paglia P, Medina E, Arioli I, Guzman CA, Colombo MP (1998) Gene transfer in dendritic cells, induced by oral DNA vaccination with Salmonella typhimurium, results in protective immunity against a murine fibrosarcoma. Blood 92(9): 3172–3176
134. Pantuck AJ, van Ophoven A, Gitlitz BJ, Tso CL, Acres B, Squiban P, Ross ME, Belldegrun AS, Figlin RA (2004) Phase I trial of antigen-specific gene therapy using a recombinant vaccinia virus encoding MUC-1 and IL-2 in MUC-1-positive patients with advanced prostate cancer. J Immunother 27(3): 240–253
135. Paoletti E (1996) Applications of pox virus vectors to vaccination: an update. Proc Natl Acad Sci U S A 93(21): 11349–11353
136. Pardoll D (2003) Does the immune system see tumors as foreign or self? Annu Rev Immunol 21(807–839)
137. Pardoll DM (1998) Cancer vaccines. Nat Med 4(5 Suppl): 525–531
138. Park JM, Terabe M, Sakai Y, Munasinghe J, Forni G, Morris JC, Berzofsky JA (2005) Early role of CD4+ Th1 cells and antibodies in HER-2 adenovirus vaccine protection against autochthonous mammary carcinomas. J Immunol 174(7): 4228–4236
139. Paterson Y, Ikonomidis G (1996) Recombinant Listeria monocytogenes cancer vaccines. Curr Opin Immunol 8(5): 664–669
140. Pawinski A, Sylvester R, Kurth KH, Bouffioux C, van der Meijden A, Parmar MK, Bijnens L (1996) A combined analysis of European Organization for Research and Treatment of Cancer, and Medical Research Council randomized clinical trials for the prophylactic treatment of stage TaT1 bladder cancer. European Organization for Research and Treatment of Cancer Genitourinary Tract Cancer Cooperative Group and the Medical Research Council Working Party on Superficial Bladder Cancer. J Urol 156(6): 1934–1940, discussion 1940–1931
141. Pecora AL, Rizvi N, Cohen GI, Meropol NJ, Sterman D, Marshall JL, Goldberg S, Gross P, O'Neil JD, Groene WS, Roberts MS, Rabin H, Bamat MK, Lorence RM (2002) Phase I trial of intravenous administration of PV701, an oncolytic virus, in patients with advanced solid cancers. J Clin Oncol 20(9): 2251–2266
142. Perricone MA, Claussen KA, Smith KA, Kaplan JM, Piraino S, Shankara S, Roberts BL (2000) Immunogene therapy for murine melanoma using recombinant adenoviral vectors expressing melanoma-associated antigens. Mol Ther 1(3): 275–284
143. Pertl U, Wodrich H, Ruehlmann JM, Gillies SD, Lode HN, Reisfeld RA (2003) Immunotherapy with a posttranscriptionally modified DNA vaccine induces complete protection against metastatic neuroblastoma. Blood 101(2): 649–654
144. Phuangsab A, Lorence RM, Reichard KW, Peeples ME, Walter RJ (2001) Newcastle disease virus therapy of human tumor xenografts: antitumor effects of local or systemic administration. Cancer Lett 172(1): 27–36
145. Phuong LK, Allen C, Peng KW, Giannini C, Greiner S, TenEyck CJ, Mishra PK, Macura SI, Russell SJ, Galanis EC (2003) Use of a vaccine strain of measles virus genetically engineered to

produce carcinoembryonic antigen as a novel therapeutic agent against glioblastoma multiforme. Cancer Res 63(10): 2462–2469
146. Poland GA, Grabenstein JD, Neff JM (2005) The US smallpox vaccination program: a review of a large modern era smallpox vaccination implementation program. Vaccine 23(17–18): 2078–2081
147. Post DE, Fulci G, Chiocca EA, Van Meir EG (2004) Replicative oncolytic herpes simplex viruses in combination cancer therapies. Curr Gene Ther 4(1): 41–51
148. Reisfeld RA, Niethammer AG, Luo Y, Xiang R (2004) DNA vaccines suppress tumor growth and metastases by the induction of anti-angiogenesis. Immunol Rev 199(181–190)
149. Ribas A, Timmerman JM, Butterfield LH, Economou JS (2003) Determinant spreading and tumor responses after peptide-based cancer immunotherapy. Trends Immunol 24(2): 58–61
150. Ribas A, Glaspy JA, Lee Y, Dissette VB, Seja E, Vu HT, Tchekmedyian NS, Oseguera D, Comin-Anduix B, Wargo JA, Amarnani SN, McBride WH, Economou JS, Butterfield LH (2004) Role of dendritic cell phenotype, determinant spreading, and negative costimulatory blockade in dendritic cell-based melanoma immunotherapy. J Immunother 27(5): 354–367
151. Roland KL, Tinge SA, Killeen KP, Kochi SK (2005) Recent advances in the development of live, attenuated bacterial vectors. Curr Opin Mol Ther 7(1): 62–72
152. Rosenberg SA, Zhai Y, Yang JC, Schwartzentruber DJ, Hwu P, Marincola FM, Topalian SL, Restifo NP, Seipp CA, Einhorn JH, Roberts B, White DE (1998) Immunizing patients with metastatic melanoma using recombinant adenoviruses encoding MART-1 or gp100 melanoma antigens. J Natl Cancer Inst 90(24): 1894–1900
153. Rosenberg SA, Yang JC, Schwartzentruber DJ, Hwu P, Topalian SL, Sherry RM, Restifo NP, Wunderlich JR, Seipp CA, Rogers-Freezer L, Morton KE, Mavroukakis SA, Gritz L, Panicali DL, White DE (2003) Recombinant fowlpox viruses encoding the anchor-modified gp100 melanoma antigen can generate antitumor immune responses in patients with metastatic melanoma. Clin Cancer Res 9(8): 2973–2980
154. Russell S (2004) CD46: a complement regulator and pathogen receptor that mediates links between innate and acquired immune function. Tissue Antigens 64(2): 111–118
155. Sakai Y, Morrison BJ, Burke JD, Park JM, Terabe M, Janik JE, Forni G, Berzofsky JA, Morris JC (2004) Vaccination by genetically modified dendritic cells expressing a truncated neu oncogene prevents development of breast cancer in transgenic mice. Cancer Res 64(21): 8022–8028
156. Schlesinger S, Dubensky TW (1999) Alphavirus vectors for gene expression and vaccines. Curr Opin Biotechnol 10(5): 434–439
157. Schneeberger A, Luhrs P, Kutil R, Steinlein P, Schild H, Schmidt W, Stingl G (2003) Granulocyte-macrophage colony-stimulating factor-based melanoma cell vaccines immunize syngeneic and allogeneic recipients via host dendritic cells. J Immunol 171(10): 5180–5187
158. Schoen C, Stritzker J, Goebel W, Pilgrim S (2004) Bacteria as DNA vaccine carriers for genetic immunization. Int J Med Microbiol 294(5): 319–335
159. Sewell DA, Douven D, Pan ZK, Rodriguez A, Paterson Y (2004) Regression of HPV-positive tumors treated with a new Listeria monocytogenes vaccine. Arch Otolaryngol Head Neck Surg 130(1): 92–97
160. Shankaran V, Ikeda H, Bruce AT, White JM, Swanson PE, Old LJ, Schreiber RD (2001) IFNgamma and lymphocytes prevent primary tumour development and shape tumour immunogenicity. Nature 410(6832): 1107–1111
161. Shen Y, Nemunaitis J (2005) Fighting cancer with vaccinia virus: teaching new tricks to an old dog. Mol Ther 11(2): 180–195
162. Siegel PM, Massague J (2003) Cytostatic and apoptotic actions of TGF-beta in homeostasis and cancer. Nat Rev Cancer 3(11): 807–821
163. Smith CL, Dunbar PR, Mirza F, Palmowski MJ, Shepherd D, Gilbert SC, Coulie P, Schneider J, Hoffman E, Hawkins R, Harris AL, Cerundolo V (2005) Recombinant modified vaccinia Ankara primes functionally activated CTL specific for a melanoma tumor antigen epitope in melanoma patients with a high risk of disease recurrence. Int J Cancer 113(2): 259–266
164. Stanziale SF, Fong Y (2003) Novel approaches to cancer therapy using oncolytic viruses. Curr Mol Med 3(1): 61–71

165. Steiner HH, Bonsanto MM, Beckhove P, Brysch M, Geletneky K, Ahmadi R, Schuele-Freyer R, Kremer P, Ranaie G, Matejic D, Bauer H, Kiessling M, Kunze S, Schirrmacher V, Herold-Mende C (2004) Antitumor vaccination of patients with glioblastoma multiforme: a pilot study to assess feasibility, safety, and clinical benefit. J Clin Oncol 22(21): 4272–4281
166. Sutter G, Wyatt LS, Foley PL, Bennink JR, Moss B (1994) A recombinant vector derived from the host range-restricted and highly attenuated MVA strain of vaccinia virus stimulates protective immunity in mice to influenza virus. Vaccine 12(11): 1032–1040
167. Taylor GS, Haigh TA, Gudgeon NH, Phelps RJ, Lee SP, Steven NM, Rickinson AB (2004) Dual stimulation of Epstein-Barr Virus (EBV)-specific CD4+- and CD8+-T-cell responses by a chimeric antigen construct: potential therapeutic vaccine for EBV-positive nasopharyngeal carcinoma. J Virol 78(2): 768–778
168. Taylor J, Paoletti E (1988) Fowlpox virus as a vector in non-avian species. Vaccine 6(6): 466–468
169. Terabe M, Berzofsky JA (2004) Immunoregulatory T cells in tumor immunity. Curr Opin Immunol 16(2): 157–162
170. Theys J, Nuyts S, Landuyt W, Van Mellaert L, Dillen C, Bohringer M, Durre P, Lambin P, Anne J (1999) Stable Escherichia coli-Clostridium acetobutylicum shuttle vector for secretion of murine tumor necrosis factor alpha. Appl Environ Microbiol 65(10): 4295–4300
171. Theys J, Landuyt AW, Nuyts S, Van Mellaert L, Lambin P, Anne J (2001) Clostridium as a tumor-specific delivery system of therapeutic proteins. Cancer Detect Prev 25(6): 548–557
172. Theys J, Landuyt W, Nuyts S, Van Mellaert L, Bosmans E, Rijnders A, Van Den Bogaert W, van Oosterom A, Anne J, Lambin P (2001) Improvement of Clostridium tumour targeting vectors evaluated in rat rhabdomyosarcomas. FEMS Immunol Med Microbiol 30(1): 37–41
173. Theys J, Landuyt W, Nuyts S, Van Mellaert L, van Oosterom A, Lambin P, Anne J (2001) Specific targeting of cytosine deaminase to solid tumors by engineered Clostridium acetobutylicum. Cancer Gene Ther 8(4): 294–297
174. Theys J, Barbe S, Landuyt W, Nuyts S, Van Mellaert L, Wouters B, Anne J, Lambin P (2003) Tumor-specific gene delivery using genetically engineered bacteria. Curr Gene Ther 3(3): 207–221
175. Toso JF, Gill VJ, Hwu P, Marincola FM, Restifo NP, Schwartzentruber DJ, Sherry RM, Topalian SL, Yang JC, Stock F, Freezer LJ, Morton KE, Seipp C, Haworth L, Mavroukakis S, White D, MacDonald S, Mao J, Sznol M, Rosenberg SA (2002) Phase I study of the intravenous administration of attenuated Salmonella typhimurium to patients with metastatic melanoma. J Clin Oncol 20(1): 142–152
176. Triozzi PL, Aldrich W, Allen KO, Lima J, Shaw DR, Strong TV (2005) Antitumor activity of the intratumoral injection of fowlpox vectors expressing a triad of costimulatory molecules and granulocyte/macrophage colony stimulating factor in mesothelioma. Int J Cancer 113(3): 406–414
177. Tsai V, Johnson DE, Rahman A, Wen SF, LaFace D, Philopena J, Nery J, Zepeda M, Maneval DC, Demers GW, Ralston R (2004) Impact of human neutralizing antibodies on antitumor efficacy of an oncolytic adenovirus in a murine model. Clin Cancer Res 10(21): 7199–7206
178. Tsang KY, Zaremba S, Nieroda CA, Zhu MZ, Hamilton JM, Schlom J (1995) Generation of human cytotoxic T cells specific for human carcinoembryonic antigen epitopes from patients immunized with recombinant vaccinia-CEA vaccine. J Natl Cancer Inst 87(13): 982–990
179. Urashima M, Suzuki H, Yuza Y, Akiyama M, Ohno N, Eto Y (2000) An oral CD40 ligand gene therapy against lymphoma using attenuated Salmonella typhimurium. Blood 95(4): 1258–1263
180. Vermorken JB, Claessen AM, van Tinteren H, Gall HE, Ezinga R, Meijer S, Scheper RJ, Meijer CJ, Bloemena E, Ransom JH, Hanna MG, Jr., Pinedo HM (1999) Active specific immunotherapy for stage II and stage III human colon cancer: a randomised trial. Lancet 353(9150): 345–350
181. Vogelstein B, Kinzler KW (2004) Cancer genes and the pathways they control. Nat Med 10(8): 789–799
182. von Mehren M, Arlen P, Tsang KY, Rogatko A, Meropol N, Cooper HS, Davey M, McLaughlin S, Schlom J, Weiner LM (2000) Pilot study of a dual gene recombinant avipox vaccine containing both carcinoembryonic antigen (CEA) and B7.1 transgenes in patients with recurrent CEA-expressing adenocarcinomas. Clin Cancer Res 6(6): 2219–2228
183. Waldmann TA (2003) IL-15 in the life and death of lymphocytes: immunotherapeutic implications. Trends Mol Med 9(12): 517–521

184. Weth R, Christ O, Stevanovic S, Zoller M (2001) Gene delivery by attenuated Salmonella typhimurium: comparing the efficacy of helper versus cytotoxic T cell priming in tumor vaccination. Cancer Gene Ther 8(8): 599–611
185. Wigginton JM, Gruys E, Geiselhart L, Subleski J, Komschlies KL, Park JW, Wiltrout TA, Nagashima K, Back TC, Wiltrout RH (2001) IFN-gamma and Fas/FasL are required for the antitumor and antiangiogenic effects of IL-12/pulse IL-2 therapy. J Clin Invest 108(1): 51–62
186. Wolpoe ME, Lutz ER, Ercolini AM, Murata S, Ivie SE, Garrett ES, Emens LA, Jaffee EM, Reilly RT (2003) HER-2/neu-specific monoclonal antibodies collaborate with HER-2/neu-targeted granulocyte macrophage colony-stimulating factor secreting whole cell vaccination to augment CD8+ T cell effector function and tumor-free survival in Her-2/neu-transgenic mice. J Immunol 171(4): 2161–2169
187. Wooldridge JE, Weiner GJ (2003) CpG DNA and cancer immunotherapy: orchestrating the antitumor immune response. Curr Opin Oncol 15(6): 440–445
188. Xiang R, Lode HN, Chao TH, Ruehlmann JM, Dolman CS, Rodriguez F, Whitton JL, Overwijk WW, Restifo NP, Reisfeld RA (2000) An autologous oral DNA vaccine protects against murine melanoma. Proc Natl Acad Sci U S A 97(10): 5492–5497
189. Xiang R, Primus FJ, Ruehlmann JM, Niethammer AG, Silletti S, Lode HN, Dolman CS, Gillies SD, Reisfeld RA (2001) A dual-function DNA vaccine encoding carcinoembryonic antigen and CD40 ligand trimer induces T cell-mediated protective immunity against colon cancer in carcinoembryonic antigen-transgenic mice. J Immunol 167(8): 4560–4565
190. Xiang R, Silletti S, Lode HN, Dolman CS, Ruehlmann JM, Niethammer AG, Pertl U, Gillies SD, Primus FJ, Reisfeld RA (2001) Protective immunity against human carcinoembryonic antigen (CEA) induced by an oral DNA vaccine in CEA-transgenic mice. Clin Cancer Res 7(3 Suppl): 856s-864s
191. Xiang R, Mizutani N, Luo Y, Chiodoni C, Zhou H, Mizutani M, Ba Y, Becker JC, Reisfeld RA (2005) A DNA vaccine targeting survivin combines apoptosis with suppression of angiogenesis in lung tumor eradication. Cancer Res 65(2): 553–561
192. Xiang ZQ, Yang Y, Wilson JM, Ertl HC (1996) A replication-defective human adenovirus recombinant serves as a highly efficacious vaccine carrier. Virology 219(1): 220–227
193. Yamanaka R (2004) Alphavirus vectors for cancer gene therapy (review). Int J Oncol 24(4): 919–923
194. Yang AS, Monken CE, Lattime EC (2003) Intratumoral vaccination with vaccinia-expressed tumor antigen and granulocyte macrophage colony-stimulating factor overcomes immunological ignorance to tumor antigen. Cancer Res 63(20): 6956–6961
195. Yang S, Hodge JW, Grosenbach DW, Schlom J (2005) Vaccines with Enhanced Costimulation Maintain High Avidity Memory CTL. J Immunol 175(6): 3715–3723
196. Yang S, Tsang KY, Schlom J (2005) Induction of higher-avidity human CTLs by vector-mediated enhanced costimulation of antigen-presenting cells. Clin Cancer Res 11(15): 5603–5615
197. Zajac P, Oertli D, Marti W, Adamina M, Bolli M, Guller U, Noppen C, Padovan E, Schultz-Thater E, Heberer M, Spagnoli G (2003) Phase I/II clinical trial of a nonreplicative vaccinia virus expressing multiple HLA-A0201-restricted tumor-associated epitopes and costimulatory molecules in metastatic melanoma patients. Hum Gene Ther 14(16): 1497–1510
198. Zaloudik J, Li W, Jacob L, Kieny MP, Somasundaram R, Acres B, Song H, Zhang T, Li J, Herlyn D (2002) Inhibition of tumor growth by recombinant vaccinia virus expressing GA733/CO17–1A/EpCAM/KSA/KS1–4 antigen in mice. Cancer Gene Ther 9(4): 382–389
199. Zeytin HE, Patel AC, Rogers CJ, Canter D, Hursting SD, Schlom J, Greiner JW (2004) Combination of a poxvirus-based vaccine with a cyclooxygenase-2 inhibitor (celecoxib) elicits antitumor immunity and long-term survival in CEA.Tg/MIN mice. Cancer Res 64(10): 3668–3678
200. Zhang WW (1999) Development and application of adenoviral vectors for gene therapy of cancer. Cancer Gene Ther 6(2): 113–138
201. Zoller M, Christ O (2001) Prophylactic tumor vaccination: comparison of effector mechanisms initiated by protein versus DNA vaccination. J Immunol 166(5): 3440–3450
202. Zou W (2005) Immunosuppressive networks in the tumour environment and their therapeutic relevance. Nat Rev Cancer 5(4): 263–274

CHAPTER 11

DENDRITIC CELL VACCINES

SYLVIA ADAMS, NINA BHARDWAJ, AND DAVID W. O'NEILL
NYU Cancer Institute Tumor Vaccine Center, New York University School of Medicine, New York, NY (522 First Ave., Smilow Research Building, # 1307, New York, NY 10016)

INTRODUCTION

Dendritic cells (DCs) are professional antigen presenting cells (APCs) central to the induction and regulation of immunity. These specialized immune cells can efficiently acquire antigens in the periphery, process them and present them to cells of the adaptive immune system, inducing antigen-specific immunity. DC-based vaccination therapies against cancer are very promising, since DCs are the most powerful T cell activators. The first part of the following chapter discusses dendritic cell biology pertinent to the design of dendritic cell vaccines (Figure 1), the second part focuses on advances in therapeutic DC cancer vaccination (Figure 2).

BIOLOGY OF DCS

DC Subtypes

DCs represent a small percentage of peripheral white blood cells. They are lineage-negative, Major Histocompatibility Complex (MHC) Class II positive bone marrow-derived mononuclear cells. In human blood, DCs and DC precursors are commonly divided into two populations by staining with antibodies to CD11c and CD123. $CD11c^{+}CD123^{lo}$ blood DCs have a monocytoid appearance and are termed myeloid DCs (MDCs), whereas $CD11c^{-}CD123^{hi}$ DCs have morphological features similar to plasma cells and have thus been termed plasmacytoid DCs (PDCs). PDCs and MDCs differ in many ways, including their tissue distribution, cytokine production and growth requirements. PDCs are important cells in innate anti-viral immunity and autoimmunity and are found primarily in the blood and lymphoid organs. They

H.L. Kaufman and J.D. Wolchok (eds.), General Principles of Tumor Immunotherapy, 251–274.

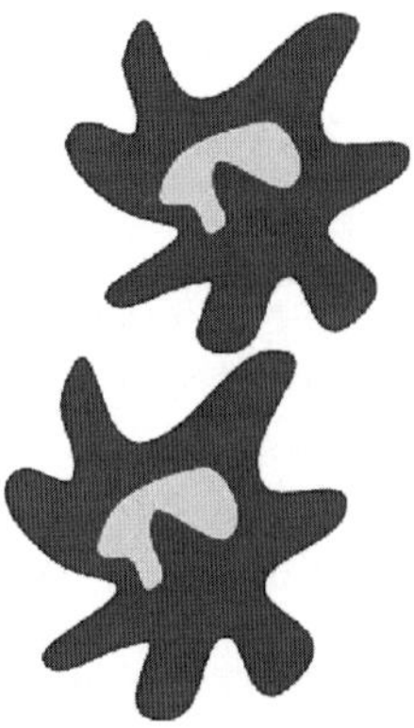

- •Function as sentinels in periphery
- •Several developmental stages (precursor, immature, mature DC)
- •Antigen uptake via several mechanisms and receptors (Fc receptors, Integrins, C-type lectin-like receptors, TLR, Scavenger receptors, CD91)
- •Maturation process with phenotypic and functional changes
- •Antigen processing and presentation via MHC class I and II, Cross-presentation
- •Migration to secondary lymphoid organs
- •Priming of CD4+, CD8+ T cells (effector and memory cells)
- •Interaction with other immune cells (NK cells, NKT cells, B cells, monocytes and macrophages)
- •Induction and skewing of immune response versus induction and maintenance of tolerance

Figure 1. Overview of MDCS and Their Features/Tasks as APCS

are the major interferon α (IFNα) producing cells in the body and can as such induce anti-viral, and in certain circumstances, anti-tumor immune responses [1]. This chapter focuses on MDCs. These are thought to be similar to DCs generated from blood monocytes and constitute the majority of DCs used for vaccination trials.

In tissues, MDCs can be divided into subtypes depending on their anatomic location: Langerhans cells of the epidermis (which express CD1a, langerin and

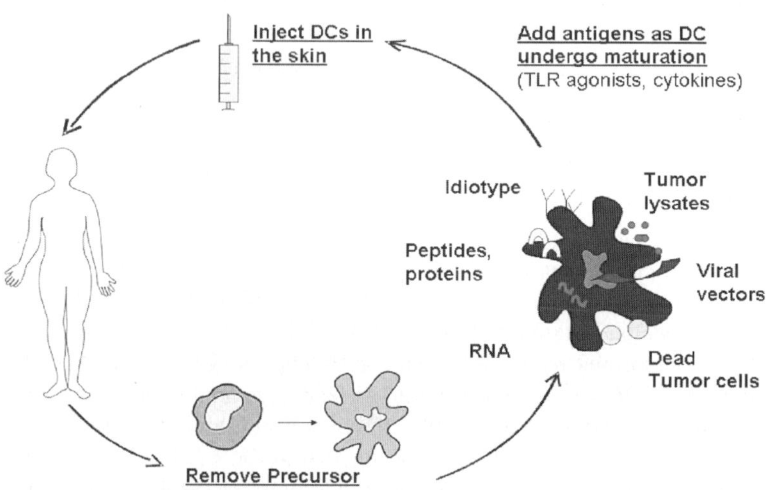

Figure 2. Overview of Dc-Based Vaccination

E-cadherin) and interstitial or mucosal DCs, which express mannose receptor, DC-SIGN and, in the dermis, CD13 [2,3]. DCs directly isolated from blood may not express DC-SIGN.

Antigen Uptake, Processing and Presentation

DCs process antigens acquired both endogenously (i.e., synthesized within the DC cytosol), or exogenously (acquired from the extracellular environment). Exogenous antigen sources include bacteria, viruses, apoptotic or necrotic cells, heat shock proteins, proteins and immune complexes. These are captured through phagocytosis, pinocytosis and endocytosis with the help of cell surface receptors on the DC. Examples include Fc receptors [4], integrins [5], C-type lectins [6], and so-called "scavenger receptors" such as LOX-1 and CD91 [7–9]. Many of these receptors have additional functions such as initiating intracellular signaling or mediating cell-cell interactions. DCs process protein antigens into peptides which are loaded onto MHC I and II molecules and transported to the cell surface for recognition by antigen-specific T cells.

Endogenous protein antigens which are processed onto MHC I are first ubiquitinated and degraded into peptides by the proteasome in the cytosol. These are transported via transporters for antigen presentation (TAP) molecules into the endoplasmic reticulum (ER), where they are loaded onto MHC I. The peptide-MHC I complexes (pMHC I) are then transported from the ER via the trans-Golgi network to the cell surface for presentation to $CD8^+$ T cells.

Exogenously acquired protein antigens, on the other hand, are engulfed and processed in endosomes. Endosomes containing ingested proteins mature and fuse with lysosomes, where proteases degrade the proteins into peptides that are loaded onto MHC II molecules. This requires proteolytic degradation of the MHC II-associated invariant chain (Ii) that normally blocks access to the peptide-binding pocket of MHC II [10]. Peptide-MHC II complexes (pMHC II) are then transported to the cell surface within specialized tubules for presentation to $CD4^+$ T cells [11].

Exogenous antigens may also be processed by DCs onto MHC I [5]. This phenomenon, called "cross-presentation" or "cross-priming," permits DCs to elicit $CD8^+$ as well as $CD4^+$ T cell responses to exogenously acquired antigens [12–14]. Cross-presentation occurs in specialized, self-sufficient, ER-phagosome derived compartments that contain MHC I, Sec61 protein (presumably to translocate antigens into the cytosol for proteosomal processing), TAP (to transport processed peptides from the cytosol), and calreticulin and calnexin (which facilitate loading of peptide onto MHC I) [12,14,15]. While still controversial, one group has shown that MHC class I molecules which lack endosomal signaling motifs in their cytoplasmic tail do not cross-present, suggesting that at least for some antigens, the MHC I must come from the cell surface [16]. Not all antigens are cross-presented efficiently. For example, peptides located in signal sequences are efficiently processed through the endogenous pathway but cross-presentation is markedly impaired [17].

Lipid antigens expressed on pathogens or self tissues are presented on DCs by CD1 molecules, which heterodimerize with β2-microglobulin and are structurally similar to MHC I [18, 19]. Processing of lipid antigens onto the various CD1 molecules is carried out in specialized intracellular compartments, not unlike antigen processing onto MHC II. The CD1d-restricted repertoire includes T cells with substantial TCR diversity as well as relatively invariant NKT cells. The latter, which have the potential to secrete IFNγ, recognize galactosyl ceramides and tumor cell-derived gangliosides and are important mediators of T cell immunity [20].

DC Maturation

Maturation is a complex process by which DCs are transformed from antigen-capturing cells into cells potent for T cell stimulation. This is accompanied by reduced phagocytic uptake, migration to lymphoid tissues, enhanced T cell activation potential and the development of characteristic cytoplasmic extensions or 'dendrites'. Mature DCs express a number of specific markers which distinguish them from immature DCs such as CD83, a cell surface molecule involved in $CD4^+$ T cell development and cell-cell interactions [21,22] and DC-LAMP, a DC-specific lysosomal protein.

Maturation is induced by stimuli ('danger signals') that alert the resting DC to the presence of pathogens, inflammation or tissue injury [23,24]. Maturation signals come from either host-derived inflammatory molecules (such as CD40 ligand, TNFα, IL-1, IL-6 and IFNα), microbial products, or molecules released by damaged host tissues. All of these stimulate Toll-like receptors (TLRs) [25], a group of highly conserved transmembrane receptors found on many types of immune cells including DCs. Matured DCs are highly efficient in antigen processing and presentation. Low levels of lysosomal proteases in DCs as compared with monocytes lead to delayed degradation of internalized antigen resulting in enhanced antigen presentation of several T cell epitopes even after migration to secondary lymphoid organs [29].

Furthermore, MHC II molecules in immature DCs are largely retained in lysosomes and therefore unable to form pMHC II, but maturation enables DCs to form pMHC II through the activation of lysosomal hydrolases, which degrade endocytosed proteins and MHC II-associated Ii. Mature DCs also develop tubules which enhance the transport of pMHC II from lysosomes to the cell surface [11]. In mice, cross-presentation of exogenous antigens on MHC I is tightly controlled by DC maturation induced by CD40 ligation and treatment with TLR agonists such as LPS, poly I:C or immunostimulatory CpG DNA [30, 31].

Maturation is accompanied by increased expression of adhesion molecules and co-stimulatory molecules that are involved in the formation of the immunological synapse (which constitutes the area of contact between T cells and DCs) Up-regulated molecules, such as semaphorins, pMHC and members of the B7, TNF receptor and TNF families, are involved in bidirectional signaling between DCs and T cells, modulating both T cell activation and DC function.

The complexity of these interactions can be illustrated by the B7 family of molecules, of which there are five members described to date. Signaling via pMHC and the T cell receptor (signal 1), and B7-1/B7-2 and CD28 (signal 2) is essential for T cell activation. B7-DC, a molecule primarily found on DCs, synergizes with B7-1 and B7-2 to stimulate $CD4^+$ T cells, enhance DC presentation of pMHC, promote DC survival and increase DC secretion of IL-12p70, a key Th1-promoting cytokine [32, 33]. In contrast, related members of the B7 (B7-H3, B7x) and CD28 (CTLA-4, PD-1) families serve to down-regulate T cell activation. B7-H3 and B7x are broadly expressed on many cell types and may be involved in attenuation of inflammatory responses in peripheral tissues [34, 35]. Triggering receptors expressed by myeloid cells (TREMs) are a unique family of receptors expressed by several cell types including DCs. Triggering of TREM2, expressed on human, immature monocyte-derived DCs promotes their differentiation, whereas absent TREM2 signalling results in functional impairment [36].

Maturation induces DCs to secrete cytokines which determine the type of ensuing immune response. The specific cytokine profile induced depends upon the type of maturation stimulus, the subtype of DC stimulated and the origin of the DC. For example, Listeria monocytogenes induces production of IL-12, IL-23, IL-27 and IL-15 by MDCs [37], whereas cholera toxin generates mature MDCs which do not produce IL-12 [38]. Maturation enables peripheral DCs to migrate from tissues to T cell zones of lymph nodes. This is accomplished through down-regulation of CCR1 and CCR5 and up-regulation of CCR7, which targets DCs to lymphatic vessels and lymph nodes via chemokines CCL19 and CCL21. CCL19-mediated migration is enhanced by local secretion of leukotrienes, perhaps from the DCs themselves [39]. Maturation also induces DCs to secrete chemokines such as TARC, MDC or IP-10 (which recruit various T cell subsets), and RANTES, MIP-1α and MIP-1β (which recruit monocytes and DCs into the local environment). In addition, CCR7 has been identified as essential to the migration of dermal and epidermal DCs into afferent dermal lymphatics, both under inflammatory and steady-state conditions [40].

In the absence of maturation stimuli, DCs function to maintain peripheral tolerance to self antigens. In the steady state, immature DCs delete T cells in the periphery and induce regulatory T cells leading to antigen-specific tolerance [41]. It has been clearly established that injection of immature DCs induces suppressor or anergic responses [42, 43], providing the basis for the design of vaccine trials utilizing matured DCs [44].

T Cell Priming

Dendritic cells play a central role in the regulation of innate and adaptive immunity and directly interact with T cells, natural killer (NK) cells, natural killer T (NKT) cells and B lymphocytes. Our focus here is on T cell activation only. DCs prime T cell responses in secondary lymphoid organs such as lymph nodes, spleen or mucosal lymphoid tissues. Interactions between T cell receptors (TCRs) on T cells and specific pMHC occur in the specialized T cell-APC junction termed immunological synapse which occupy the central supramolecular activation cluster (C-SMAC) region. The spatial organization of C-SMAC directly regulates TCR signaling [45]. Real-time imaging of murine DCs and naive T cells in intact explanted lymph nodes reveals that a DC interacts with as many as 500 T cells/hour [21, 46, 47]. In the presence of antigen, stable and durable DC-T cell contacts form, with antigen-bearing DCs engaging more than 10 T cells at a time.

Effective priming of naive T cells results in their clonal expansion and differentiation into cytokine-secreting effector cells and memory cells, which subsequently exit through efferent lymphatics. The ensuing T cell response is dependent on many factors, including the concentration of antigen on the DC, the affinity of the T cell receptor for the pMHC, the duration of the DC-T cell interaction, the state of DC maturation and the type of DC maturation stimulus [48]. T cell stimulation by mature DCs is required for long-term T cell survival and differentiation into memory and effector T cells. This enhanced T cell survival capacity is defined by resistance to cell death in the absence of cytokines, and by responsiveness to IL-7 and IL-15, which promote T cell survival in the absence of antigen stimulation [48, 49].

Following priming, $CD4^+$ T cells may differentiate towards T helper 1 (Th1) cells which produce IFNγ and support $CD8^+$ cytotoxic T lymphocyte (CTL) responses, or towards T helper 2 (Th2) cells which produce IL-4, IL-5 and IL-13, support humoral immunity and down-regulate Th1 responses. Th17 cells, a new subset secreting the proinflammatory cytokine IL-17, have been recently described in autoimmune diseases, their role in antitumor immunity and involvement of DCs need to be elucidated [50]. The secreted cytokine profile of the stimulating DC determines the direction of this Th polarization. IL-12, IL-18 and IL-27 polarize toward Th1, whereas CCL17, CCL22 or the absence of IL-12 skew the response toward Th2. The DC cytokine profile depends on the DC subtype, the local environment and anatomic location of the DC and the type of maturation stimulus [38]. These factors control other characteristics of the T cell response as well, such as tolerance induction [51] or T cell homing [52, 53]. Th3 regulatory cells are a recently identified subset of CD4+ cells associated with oral tolerance. They are preferentially induced by a unique class of dendritic cells in the gut following oral antigen administration and primarily secrete transforming growth factor (TGF)-beta [54].

$CD4^+$ T cell help at the time of priming is required to generate $CD8^+$ T cell memory [53, 55, 56]. It is believed that this T cell help is mediated by CD40-CD40L interactions with DCs, which in turn fully prime the $CD8^+$ T cell response [57]. Other T cell surface molecules are also involved in the generation of memory [58, 59]. In the absence of this help, the $CD8^+$ T cells can upon restimulation, act as effectors, but do not undergo a second round of clonal expansion. They acquire program death 1 (PD-1) receptor and tumor necrosis factor-related apoptosis-inducing ligand (TRAIL) and undergo activation-induced cell death [60].

CLINICAL APPLICATIONS

Preparation of Autologous DCs

Several methods have been described to prepare human DC vaccines ex vivo. The most commonly used approach is the differentiation of DCs from blood or leukapheresis derived monocytes with GM-CSF and IL-4[61, 62]. Other methods include GM-CSF and TNFα-mediated differentiation of $CD34^+$ hematopoietic stem cells into mixtures of cells resembling interstitial DCs and Langerhans cells [43], or by direct isolation of DCs from leukapheresis products by density gradient centrifugation [63] or selection with immunomagnetic beads. Direct isolation from peripheral blood yields low numbers, therefore pre-stimulation with subcutaneous granulocyte-macrophage colony- stimulating factor (GM-CSF) and IL-4 might be necessary [64]. Although no direct comparisons have been performed in clinical trials, all three types of DC preparation can stimulate antigen-specific T cell responses and have been associated with occasional clinical responses. DC cultured in GM-CSF with IFN alpha or GM-CSF with IL-15 might be more potent T cell stimulators and are undergoing clinical testing (personal communication).

Maturing DCs prior to vaccination is critical, as immature DCs are weak immunogens and can be even tolerogenic. Injection of normal volunteers with antigen-loaded immature DCs induces tolerogenic responses [42], and a randomized trial in patients with metastatic melanoma comparing peptide-pulsed immature DCs to peptides administered with adjuvant demonstrated significantly lower immunogenicity in patients receiving the DC vaccine [44,65]. In a trial from another group, a direct comparison of peptide-loaded immature and mature DCs in patients with metastatic melanoma showed that only mature DCs induced antigen-specific CTL responses [66]. It remains critical to compare matured DCs in a randomized trial to other vaccine adjuvants and to explore the clinical efficacy of DCs matured in situ.

Many laboratories induce maturation of monocyte-derived DCs by the addition of a "cocktail" of IL-1β, IL-6, TNFα and prostaglandin E_2 (PGE_2) [67]. DCs matured in this manner do not secrete IL-12, but still potently induce cytotoxic T lymphocytes (CTL) responses and express CCR7. Other maturation approaches such as ligation of TLRs might be superior and induce IL-12 secretion by DCs. IL-12 skews naive T cells towards the Th1 phenotype (IFNγ producing cells), which are critical for exerting anti-tumor effects in addition to maintaining effective CD8 memory responses.

Antigen Sources and Loading

The discovery of many tumor antigens allows active immunotherapy with defined antigens. This is particularly attractive since the adaptive immune system can eradicate tumors via antigen-specific T and B lymphocytes. The magnitude of tumor infiltrating lymphocytes (TIL) for instance is an independent positive prognostic factor for a variety of malignancies. For instance, improved survival was demonstrated for patients with pancreatic cancer, ovarian cancer and follicular lymphoma, respectively, if tumor-infiltrated immune cells were present [68, 69].

Tumor antigens can be divided into several categories 1) Antigens unique to the tumor (due to altered gene products, eg. amplified, aberrantly expressed, overexpressed or mutated genes, splice variants, gene fusion products), 2) Lineage-specific antigens (eg., tyrosinase expressed in the melanocyte lineage), 3) Cancer-testis antigens (which are normally expressed by gametes and trophoblasts and aberrantly expressed in several tumors) and 4) Antigens derived from oncogenic viruses (eg., human papilloma virus E6 and E7 proteins in cervical cancer). 'Cryptic epitopes' which represent non-contiguous peptide sequences created by posttranslational protein splicing add to the complex task of identifying antigenic peptides. [70–72]. Preferred tumor antigens for vaccination protocols would be those consistently expressed by tumors, absent from normal tissues and critical to tumor but not somatic cell growth. Cancer-testis antigens are of interest due to their expression pattern, but also because these proteins might play a role in oncogenesis. They could mark cells with stem-cell-like properties within tumors representing an exciting therapeutic target [73].

MHC-restricted peptide antigens are frequently used for DC vaccines, including altered or enhanced peptides which boost immunity to less immunogenic self antigens, or which improve antigen presentation or T cell receptor affinity [43, 74–79]. Several MHC class I and II epitopes have been used, however the HLA restriction in patient selection is a major disadvantage. Alternatively, DCs may be loaded with purified or recombinant proteins, transfected with RNA or transduced with non-replicating viral vectors encoding an antigen of interest [80–83] These methods allow the host's HLA molecules to select epitopes from an antigen's entire amino acid sequence. The immunogenicity of these vaccines may be enhanced by using antigens coupled or fused with other more immunogenic molecules such as foreign proteins or cytokine sequences, costimulatory molecules or chemokines that attract other DCs into the local environment.

The use of the entire antigenic repertoire of the tumor is also of interest, since the use of only a few defined antigens may select for tumor variants with loss of the antigen. In addition, whole tumor cell approaches allow for immunization with unknown antigens and cryptic epitopes. Therefore, DCs have been loaded with whole tumor cells or tumor cell lysates, transfected with whole tumor RNA, or fused with tumor cells, permitting vaccination with the complete antigenic content of the tumor [84–86]. Potential disadvantages are the laborious preparation of patient's tumor if autologous approaches are employed, the limited availability of immune monitoring tools and the possibility of inducing autoimmunity to self antigens.

Vaccination Logistics with DCs

Dendritic cell vaccines are typically injected intradermally, subcutaneously or intravenously, but other routes such as intranodal, intralymphatic or intratumoral injections have been described. Intravenous injection of DCs leads to their transient lung uptake before being redistributed to the liver, spleen and bone marrow [87, 88], whereas subcutaneous or intradermal vaccination leads to improved migration of DCs to lymph nodes [89] and enhanced Th1 polarization [90].

Migration of injected DCs to draining nodes might be a limiting factor in DC vaccination. In one study, only 1% or less of injected DCs were eventually detected in the draining lymph nodes via technetium- or indium labeling [91]. Maturation of DCs and intradermal injection is likely the most effective approach, since migration is threefold higher for intradermal versus subcutaneous administration and six- to eightfold higher when mature DC were compared with immature DC [91]. Alternatives to improve DC migration are the in situ activation through injection of immature DCs into adjuvant treated skin [92] or the in situ activation and maturation of DCs through TLR agonists (such as Imiquimod) applied to the skin [93].

There is no consensus concerning the optimal DC dose, DC subset or the frequency of boosters. Continued vaccination is now feasible due to the fact that DC vaccines may be stored frozen prior to vaccination [74, 85]. Vaccination of mice with matured, peptide-loaded DCs showed a rapid induction of memory cells. These cells then underwent vigorous secondary expansion in response to a variety of booster vaccinations, leading to protective immunity toward pathogens [94]. This observed accelerated generation of immunological memory compared to infection as well as its amplification through boosters is crucial for the development of effective anti-cancer vaccines. Clinical benefit with tumor regressions has been clearly shown in patients after adoptive transfer of tumor antigen-specific T cells, indicating the importance of inducing adequate numbers of high affinity CTL and memory cells. In addition, adjunctive cytokine therapy may be needed for continued memory T cell support.

Results of DC Vaccination Trials

DC vaccination is at a relatively early stage of clinical development. Greater understanding of DC biology and of mechanisms to enhance DC immunogenicity should permit improvement of current strategies. More than 1000 patients with a variety of tumor types have been treated with DC vaccines to date [95]. Feasibility has been established as well as a non-toxic profile. Fever, injection site reactions, adenopathy, and fatigue are commonly mild and transient. Although these initial trials were not designed to evaluate clinical responses (and therefore often lack confirmatory scans for responders), complete responses were reported for 15/168 melanoma patients. Larger controlled trials are now underway to objectively assess the clinical efficacy of DC vaccines by documenting responses according to World Health Organization (WHO) or Response Evaluation Criteria in Solid Tumors Group (RECIST) guidelines [96]. A randomized phase III trial comparing peptide loaded, matured MDCs with Dacarbacine (approved front-line chemotherapy) given to patients with metastatic melanoma was prematurely halted for low efficacy of therapies in both arms. Response rate and progression-free survival were not significantly different between DC vaccination and chemotherapy [97]. We believe that trials to optimize the use of DCs and to determine their efficacy should be done before comparing DCs to other therapies.

Among several DC vaccine trials published to date, the most impressive objective clinical responses have been associated with the use of whole antigens (whole proteins, killed whole tumor cells or whole tumor lysates) as opposed to peptide antigens. This may be because these are exogenous antigens which can target MHC II to generate $CD4^+$ T cell help but also target MHC I via cross-presentation to generate $CD8^+$ CTLs. In a study using tumor-specific idiotype immunoglobulin-pulsed DCs in patients with follicular lymphoma, Timmerman et al reported two long-lasting complete responses and one partial response among 10 patients with measurable disease in the pilot phase of the study [80]. An additional 25 patients were vaccinated after their best clinical response was achieved by chemotherapy, and objective tumor regression was seen in 4 of 18 patients with residual disease. In another study, Holtl et al treated 35 patients with metastatic renal cell carcinoma with monthly injections of autologous, mature monocyte-derived DCs loaded with tumor cell lysates [98]. Of 27 evaluable patients, two had objective complete responses (per WHO criteria), one had a partial response and 7 had stable disease. Objective responses and stabilization of disease were long-lasting, ranging from 6 months to 3 years.

Durable complete clinical responses were also reported by O'Rourke et al in a trial of 17 patients with metastatic melanoma [99]. Patients received mature monocyte-derived DCs loaded with autologous irradiated tumor cells. By WHO criteria there were 3 complete responses (with durable disease remissions of over 3 years) and 3 partial responses among 12 patients who completed the vaccinations. One patient with progressive disease was treated with vaccinations every 6 weeks for over 3 years, indicating that maintenance vaccinations may be useful even for patients with slowly progressive disease. Another promising trial utilizing autologous tumor lysate pulsed DC was reported by Maier et al, who showed partial and complete responses in patients with refractory cutaneous T-cell lymphoma after intranodal vaccination. Interestingly, responses could be reinduced in progressing patients if DC vaccination was reinstituted using tumor lysates from progressing lesions [100].

Several DC-based vaccination trials in solid and hematological cancers recently published have confirmed the feasibility and safety of this approach and demonstrated the ability to induce immunological and clinical responses in a subset of patients [101–112]. NK cell and NK T cell activation might also contribute to the antitumor effects of DC-based vaccination. Increased NK cell activity was observed in patients with clinical benefit after DC vaccination [113].

Multi-modal approaches, as discussed in the following section, will likely be necessary to achieve effective, durable, anti-tumor immune responses in a larger proportion of patients. In addition, it seems plausible that patients with low tumor burden such as in the adjuvant setting might derive a greater benefit from active immunotherapy than patients with large volume disease.

Novel Strategies/Multimodality

Provision of CD4$^+$ T cell help for CD8$^+$ T cells

Since the induction of CD4$^+$ T helper cells at the time of priming is critical to the development of long-lived CD8$^+$ CTL responses, DC vaccines should incorporate antigens targeting both types of T cells. This can be achieved by utilizing peptide epitope combinations which bind MHC I and II or using full length protein antigens, but a more practical approach may be to target cross-presentation. For example, targeting of antigen to Fc receptors on DCs using antibody-antigen complexes has been shown to activate both CD4 and CD8 effector responses and tumor immunity in mice [4]. Cross-presentation can also be enhanced by targeting DC surface receptors such as DEC-205, loading DCs with killed cells or cell lysates, and by stimulating DCs with TLR agonists that up-regulate cross presentation [31]. However, it was observed in mice that cross-presentation can be impaired after DC maturation with several TLR agonists [114]. Vaccination protocols should therefore avoid providing DC activation signals prior to antigen exposure to prevent premature inactivation of DCs. One must also carefully choose the TLR agonist, since ligation of TLR2 and dectin-1 for instance, regulates cytokine secretion in DCs (such as IL-10) and macrophages inducing immunological tolerance [115]. RNA transcripts as antigen sources (which primarily target MHC I) may also be targeted to both MHC I and II. MHC II presentation of RNA-encoded antigens can be improved using fusion constructs carrying an endosomal/lysosomal sorting signal of a lysosome-associated protein (LAMP-1) [116].

Strategies to target DCs in situ

Novel approaches to simultaneously recruit, mature and load DCs with antigens in vivo are being explored. They offer the potential advantage of being less labor-intensive, less expensive as well as inducing superior DC maturation, viability, migration and antigen-presenting capacity. One approach to manipulate DCs in situ is the ligation of TLRs. DNA based vaccines which target TLR9 are the best known example of this approach. CpG containing oligodeoxynucleotides (CpG-ODNs) are excellent vaccines in animal models of cancer and chronic virus infection. For example, simple vaccines in mice using CpG motif DNA conjugated to a protein antigen have been shown to stimulate DC maturation, cross-priming and protective CTL immunity against challenge with antigen-expressing tumors [117, 118].

CpG motifs introduced into the backbone are useful adjuvants for plasmid-based DNA (pDNA) vaccines. They enhance the antigen-specific T cell response and provide protection against a subsequent challenge with melanoma cells in a murine model [119]. Using the particulate Hepatitis B surface antigen (HBbsAg) as a model antigen, CpG ODNs were strong stimulators of in vitro splenocytes, superior to R-848 (which ligates TLR7/8) including a dramatically stronger IL-12 induction, with CpG being 250 times more potent than R-848 and augmented cellular and humoral immune responses against HBsAg when mice were immunized with CpG as adjuvant [120]. Superiority of CpG ODNs as a vaccine adjuvant over R-848 was also shown in mice immunized with HIV gag protein [121]. Using the soluble antigen chicken ovalbumin (OVA) vaccination with CpG / incomplete Freund's adjuvant (IFA) led to superior CTL responses in mice as compared with Imiquimod (TLR7 agonist) as adjuvant [122]. Activation of plasmacytoid DCs in draining lymph nodes was observed in mice immunized with TERT peptide and CpG ODN. Protective CD8+ immunity leading to longer survival in an induced tumor model was demonstrated. CpG-ODNs have been tested in cancer patients and are shown to be safe, well-tolerated and to increase vaccine-induced immune responses [123]. The addition of CpG to a peptide/Montanide vaccine increased the magnitude and duration of antigen-specific T cell responses in melanoma patients [124].

DNA vaccines encoding tumor antigens may also be used, although this approach has not yet been compared with simply adding CpG to an antigen as adjuvant. These DNA vaccines can be engineered to encode survival factors such as Bcl-xL or to use DC-specific promoters to augment vaccine potency by enhancing DC survival in vivo [125] or by specifically targeting antigen expression to DCs, respectively [126]. Gene gun techniques to deliver plasmid DNA into the skin may be particularly useful for this approach [127].

Imiquimod, an imidazoquinoline, is a synthetic compound available as a topical preparation due to its licensed use as immune response modifier in HPV-related anogenital warts. It ligates TLR7, which is found on DC subsets, Langerhans cells and several epithelial tissues. TLR7 ligation promotes DC maturation and migration to draining lymph nodes, a desirable feature given that most ex vivo-derived DCs are retained at the injection site. A topical preparation of the TLR7 agonist Imiquimod matures DCs injected locally into the treated skin and enhances migratory and LN homing capacity [92]. This approach may be preferable to ex vivo DC maturation since important proinflammatory cytokines such as IL-12 are expressed only briefly after exposure to a maturation stimulus. Local production of cytokines and chemokines induced by Imiquimod application alone may promote DC viability and DC migration to draining lymph nodes. Indeed, murine models indicate that DC migration is enhanced by pre-conditioning the subcutaneous injection site with either DCs themselves or with IL-1 or TNFα [128]. Sequence and timing of TLR agonist administration are important to prevent impairment of cross-presentation [114].

Certain microbes (eg Influenza virus, Listeria) directly induce MDC or PDC maturation, even in non-replicating form, and are being tested as recombinant vaccine vectors. In mouse models, adenoviral, retroviral and pox vectors have been used. When engineered to express adhesion molecules, costimulatory molecules or cytokines, these vectors can induce high avidity T cell responses [79]. The advantages of this approach are the feasibility of combining compounds that promote DC survival (eg TRANCE, CD40L or Bcl-2) together with factors that direct Th polarization and promote T cell activation and longevity.

Vaccination with Heat shock protein-peptide complexes provides another method for maturing DCs in situ, and has been shown to induce immunologic and clinical responses in melanoma patients [129]. Finally, membrane-permeable proteins such as HIV tat or herpes simplex virus VP22 ligated to antigens offer a novel way to deliver these antigens to DCs in an immunogenic form [130].

Enhancers of dendritic cell differentiation and function may be exploited as well. Retinoids such as all-trans retinoic acid have been shown to skew monocyte differentiation to IL-12 producing DCs in vitro [131]. PT-100, a small molecule dipeptidyl peptidase inhibitor, exerts its antitumor effects through the induction of cytokines and chemokines known to enhance innate and adaptive immune responses against the tumor including DC function [132]. Selective inhibition of Jak2/STAT3 was shown to enhance DC function and overcome the differentiation block induced by tumor-derived factors in vitro [133]. In addition, silencing of suppressor of cytokine signaling (SOCS) 1, which is a negative regulator of JAK/STAT, by small interfering RNA (siRNA) has been shown to enhance DC function in a model of HIV DNA vaccination [134].

Combination with targeted therapies

Anti-tumor vaccination in combination with therapies that target the tumor's vascular supply are under consideration. The incorporation of RNA encoding VEGF, VEGFR-2, Tie-2 and tumor antigens into DC vaccines as well as anti-VEGF antibodies administered in combination with DC vaccines have been shown to be synergistic in inhibiting tumor growth in mice [135,136]. A recombinant humanized monoclonal antibody to VEGF (Bevacizumab) is now available due to its approval for the treatment of metastatic colorectal cancer. Its antitumor effect is likely due to the decrease in interstitial pressure allowing better penetration of chemotherapeutic drugs into the tumor. This mechanism might be utilized in synergy with active immunotherapies. Therapeutic effects might also be due to the inhibition of tumor-produced VEGF which may contribute to defective DC function and an immunosuppressive tumor microenvironment. Preliminary results in patients with prostate cancer treated with Bevacizumab and an autologous APC vaccine are encouraging [137]. Other promising agents for combination therapies are small molecule inhibitors of kinases and receptor kinases involved in angiogenesis and intracellular signaling. Sunitinib and Sorafinib are approved selective, multi-targeted inhibitors of RAF kinase, VEGFR, stem cell factor receptor (KIT), Fms-like tyrosine kinase-3 (FLT-3) and the glial cell line–derived neurotrophic factor receptor (RET). Imatinib mesylate (Gleevac), an inhibitor of c-KIT is another attractive compound to use in combination with vaccines. It enhances NK cell activation, counteracting the T reg induced NK cell inhibition, as observed in patients with gastrointestinal stromal tumors [138,139].

Inhibition of tolerogenic co-stimulatory molecules

Vaccine efficacy may be enhanced by blocking inhibitory co-stimulatory signals. For example, tumor lymphocytic infiltration and necrosis can be induced in previously vaccinated cancer patients by administering an inhibitory antibody to CTLA-4

[140]. Synergy of CTLA-4 blockade and concomitant gp100 tumor antigen vaccination has been shown in patients with metastatic melanoma [141]. However, significant multi-organ autoimmunity is associated with the use of Ipilimumab (MDX-010), often correlating with tumor regressions in metastatic melanoma and clear cell renal cell carcinoma [142, 143]. Blockade of another inhibitory co-stimulatory molecule, B7-H1, improves DC-mediated T cell dependent anti-tumor immunity in mice [144], possibly through up-regulation of IL-12 and concomitant down-regulation of IL-10 in DCs. Other B7/CD28 family members that down-regulate immune responses and which could be targeted for blockade include B7x, B7-H3 and BTLA [34, 35, 145, 146].

Regulatory T cell inhibition

CD25+CD4+ T regulatory cells (Tr) cells constitute 5 to 10% of peripheral CD4+ T cells and are critically important in the maintenance of peripheral immune tolerance [147, 148]. In addition, patients with epithelial malignancies have increased numbers of functional regulatory T-cells in peripheral blood and among tumor-infiltrating lymphocytes [149, 150], which strongly correlates with poor survival [151].

Depletion of Tr through the use of cytotoxic anti-CD25 antibodies or IL-2 coupled to cytotoxic molecules seems a logical approach to enhance immunotherapies. Synergy was shown when antigen-pulsed mature DCs were administered to CD 25 depleted mice [152]. The development of MHC class I and II–restricted IFNγ-producing cells was consistently enhanced in the absence of Tr, as was their cytotoxic activity. Effective Tr depletion by Denileukin diftitox (cytotoxic fusion protein binding to IL-2 receptor on Tr) was shown in cancer patients, resulting in enhanced immunity to a subsequently administered DC vaccine [153].

Vaccination after Bone Marrow Transplantation

The induction of antitumor immunity may be more effective in the lymphopenic host following bone marrow transplant (BMT). In pre-clinical studies examining this approach in mice, tumor lysate-pulsed DCs given during early lymphoid recovery elicited an effective and long-lasting anti-tumor immune response [154]. After total body irradiation, mice received a syngeneic BMT followed by weekly DC vaccinations starting 7 days following the transplant. Tumor regression was observed in mice with tumors established prior to BMT, and protection from subsequent tumor challenge was seen in DC-immunized mice. Although infectious disease vaccines are routinely administered following allogeneic BMT, no studies have been reported for anti-tumor vaccines in humans after BMT. It has been shown that infusion of *in vivo* primed autologous T cells immediately after auto transplant restored immune readiness to pneumococcal vaccination in myeloma patients [155], which typically demonstrate significant deficits in immune responsiveness after auto transplant. Therefore, therapeutic anticancer vaccines could be administered pre-transplant followed by adoptive cell transfer after BMT.

Combinations of vaccination and adoptively transferred T cells

Adoptively transferred, tumor antigen-specific T cells have demonstrated significant anti-tumor activity in patients with metastatic melanoma, especially after non-myeloablative lymphodepleting chemotherapy [156]. Lymphodepletion enhances antitumor activity of transferred lymphocytes by removal of 'cellular sinks', cells competing for the homeostatic cytokines IL-7 and IL-15 [157]. Adoptive cell transfer with MART-1 TCR transduced autologous lymphocytes, co-administered with high dose IL-2 also showed durable engraftment and tumor regressions in 2/17 of patients with advanced melanoma [158].

Such an approach may also enhance the activity of tumor vaccines. In a murine model with large, pre-established tumors, adoptively transferred tumor-infiltrating T cells alone had no significant effect on tumor growth, whereas the combination of adoptively transferred T cells, vaccination with an altered peptide ligand and administration of IL-2 induced tumor regression and long term cures [159].

Combined modality with radiotherapy

Currently there is no clear evidence that single modality radiotherapy induces anti-tumor immunity. Radiotherapy alone can achieve local control but distant failure is common. The addition of cytotoxic chemotherapy in the adjuvant setting improves clinical outcomes due to systemic protection. The combination of radiation therapy with immunotherapies such as dendritic cell vaccines to induce systemic anti-tumor immunity could prove to be another successful approach in treating cancers. The desired biological effect of ionizing radiation therapy here is the induction of tumor cell apoptosis and/or necrosis, causing a release of tumor antigens and 'danger signals' such as heat shock proteins and proinflammatory cytokines. Intratumorally injected dendritic cells would then capture released antigens and receive a strong maturation stimulus simultaneously, leading to effective migration, to draining nodes and T cell priming. In addition, radiotherapy can upregulate MHC, costimulatory molecules and death receptors such as Fas (CD95) on tumor cells (reviewed in [160]), which might render them more susceptible to CTL recognition and lysis.

Synergy of radiotherapy and a DC vaccine was shown in a murine model. Effective phagocytosis of apoptotic tumor and migration of DCs was observed when DCs were injected into pre-established tumor nodules 24 hours after local irradiation. 8.4% of nodal DCs were detected to have phagocytosed tumor cells; in contrast to 0% if no irradiation was delivered, or 0.8% if radiation but no DCs were administered (detected DCs were then derived from endogenous tumors). The combined approach resulted in enhanced CTL responses, fewer metastatic tumors, and increased survival [161]. An early study in cancer patients has shown safety and induction of tumor-specific immunity when radiotherapy was combined with intratumoral injections of immature DCs [162].

Combined modality with chemotherapy

Several mechanisms allow chemotherapy to synergize with active immunotherapy (reviewed in [163]). Chemotherapy-induced cell death leads to release of a broad range of antigens in increasing amounts. Induction of apoptosis increases antigen cross-presentation, and sensitizes APC to CD 40 signaling, which drives T cell priming, expansion and circulation. Chemotherapy might sensitize tumor cells to lysis by low-avidity CTL via up-regulation of death receptors. Cytotoxic reduction of the tumor bulk could also decrease tumor-derived immune suppression as well as the chance for escape variants and leaves smaller target volumes for immunotherapy.

Chemotherapy can induce cell death by apoptosis. This mechanism has been regarded as non-immune stimulatory, but in the context of cellular stress, secondary necrosis or ligation of death receptors such as Fas (CD95) a pro-inflammatory milieu can be induced. Although few chemotherapeutic agents cause cell death through non-apoptotic pathways, it is well-established that necrosis causes DC maturation necessary for T cell priming. In addition, chemotherapy can impact lymphocyte subsets themselves. Cytoxan for instance preferentially eliminates Tr, but does not affect other populations. A homeostatic proliferative response following lymphopenia may allow for expansion of tumor-specific T cells. A clinical trial of adoptive TIL transfer therapy following non-myeloablative but lymphodepleting chemotherapy with Cytoxan and Fludarabine resulted in long term clonal persistence of TILs in blood [156]. Specific T cells comprised 66% of CD8+ cells over a year after treatment in one patient. Clinical responses were promising in this group of IL2-refractory metastatic melanoma patients; they were seen in 51% of patients and occurred in bulky metastases and several organs including the brain. Recurrent lesions showed loss of HLA-A2 and/or MART-1 protein suggesting a strong selection pressure in this subset. It is thought that the effectiveness of this approach is due to two potential mechanisms: [1] elimination of regulatory T cells and [2] the decreased competition by endogenous lymphocytes for homeostatic regulatory cytokines such as IL-7 and IL-15.

Intratumoral applications of TLR agonists

Dysregulation of DC maturation and function have been reported in cancer patients and is thought to contribute to ineffective anti-tumor immunity [164, 165]. CpG-ODN ligate TLR 9 and, when injected intratumorally can overcome tumor-mediated DC inhibition, enable DCs to cross-present tumor-derived antigens to naïve CD8+ T cells, result in tumor necrosis and prolong survival of treated animals [166–168]. In a malignant glioma model, combined modality treatment with sequential radiotherapy and CpG-ODN immunotherapy further increased the percentages of animals with complete tumor remissions [169]. Interestingly, TLR 9 expression as well as immune cell infiltration in tumors were not affected by radiation.

CONCLUDING REMARKS

Recent advances in DC biology make the exploitation of these cells for immunotherapies an exciting new opportunity. Several DC-based clinical trials have shown safety and feasibility as well as very dramatic antitumor responses in some instances. Current efforts are focused on optimizing vaccination strategies and selecting the right patient population.

ACKNOWLEDGEMENTS

Supported by grants from the National Institutes of Health (CA-84512, AI-44628), the Cancer Research Institute, the Burroughs Wellcome Fund, the Doris Duke Charitable Foundation and the Elizabeth Glaser Pediatric AIDS Foundation. S.A. is supported in part by the Cancer Research Institute, an NYU Cancer Institute Pilot Grant and a Career Development Award from the American Society of Clinical Oncology.

REFERENCES

1. McKenna, K., A.S. Beignon, and N. Bhardwaj, *Plasmacytoid dendritic cells: linking innate and adaptive immunity*. J Virol, 2005. 79(1): p. 17–27.
2. Shortman, K. and Y.J. Liu, *Mouse and human dendritic cell subtypes*. Nat Rev Immunol, 2002. 2(3): p. 151–61.
3. Ebner, S., et al., *Expression of C-type lectin receptors by subsets of dendritic cells in human skin*. Int Immunol, 2004. 16(6): p. 877–87.
4. Rafiq, K., A. Bergtold, and R. Clynes, *Immune complex-mediated antigen presentation induces tumor immunity*. J Clin Invest, 2002. 110(1): p. 71–9.
5. Albert, M.L., et al., *Immature dendritic cells phagocytose apoptotic cells via alphavbeta5 and CD36, and cross-present antigens to cytotoxic T lymphocytes*. J Exp Med, 1998. 188(7): p. 1359–68.
6. Bonifaz, L., et al., *Efficient targeting of protein antigen to the dendritic cell receptor DEC-205 in the steady state leads to antigen presentation on major histocompatibility complex class I products and peripheral CD8+ T cell tolerance*. J Exp Med, 2002. 196(12): p. 1627–38.
7. Peiser, L., S. Mukhopadhyay, and S. Gordon, *Scavenger receptors in innate immunity*. Curr Opin Immunol, 2002. 14(1): p. 123–8.
8. Basu, S., et al., *CD91 is a common receptor for heat shock proteins gp96, hsp90, hsp70, and calreticulin*. Immunity, 2001. 14(3): p. 303–13.
9. Delneste, Y., et al., *Involvement of LOX-1 in dendritic cell-mediated antigen cross-presentation*. Immunity, 2002. 17(3): p. 353–62.
10. Guermonprez, P., et al., *Antigen presentation and T cell stimulation by dendritic cells*. Annu Rev Immunol, 2002. 20: p. 621–67.
11. Chow, A., et al., *Dendritic cell maturation triggers retrograde MHC class II transport from lysosomes to the plasma membrane*. Nature, 2002. 418(6901): p. 988–94.
12. Guermonprez, P., et al., *ER-phagosome fusion defines an MHC class I cross-presentation compartment in dendritic cells*. Nature, 2003. 425(6956): p. 397–402.
13. Fonteneau, J.F., M. Larsson, and N. Bhardwaj, *Interactions between dead cells and dendritic cells in the induction of antiviral CTL responses*. Curr Opin Immunol, 2002. 14(4): p. 471–7.
14. Ackerman, A.L., et al., *Early phagosomes in dendritic cells form a cellular compartment sufficient for cross presentation of exogenous antigens*. Proc Natl Acad Sci U S A, 2003. 100(22): p. 12889–94.

15. Houde, M., et al., *Phagosomes are competent organelles for antigen cross-presentation*. Nature, 2003. 425(6956): p. 402–6.
16. Lizee, G., et al., *Control of dendritic cell cross-presentation by the major histocompatibility complex class I cytoplasmic domain*. Nat Immunol, 2003. 4(11): p. 1065–73.
17. Wolkers, M.C., et al., *Antigen bias in T cell cross-priming*. Science, 2004. 304(5675): p. 1314–7.
18. Moody, D.B. and S.A. Porcelli, *Intracellular pathways of CD1 antigen presentation*. Nat Rev Immunol, 2003. 3(1): p. 11–22.
19. Joyce, S. and L. Van Kaer, *CD1-restricted antigen presentation: an oily matter*. Curr Opin Immunol, 2003. 15(1): p. 95–104.
20. Fujii, S., et al., *Prolonged IFN-gamma-producing NKT response induced with alpha-galactosylceramide-loaded DCs*. Nat Immunol, 2002. 3(9): p. 867–74.
21. Fujimoto, Y., et al., *CD83 expression influences CD4+ T cell development in the thymus*. Cell, 2002. 108(6): p. 755–67.
22. Lechmann, M., et al., *CD83 on dendritic cells: more than just a marker for maturation*. Trends Immunol, 2002. 23(6): p. 273–5.
23. Matzinger, P., *The danger model: a renewed sense of self*. Science, 2002. 296(5566): p. 301–5.
24. Skoberne, M., A.S. Beignon, and N. Bhardwaj, *Danger signals: a time and space continuum*. Trends Mol Med, 2004. 10(6): p. 251–7.
25. Cheng, F., et al., *A critical role for Stat3 signaling in immune tolerance*. Immunity, 2003. 19(3): p. 425–36.
26. Kadowaki, N., et al., *Subsets of human dendritic cell precursors express different toll-like receptors and respond to different microbial antigens*. J Exp Med, 2001. 194(6): p. 863–9.
27. Hornung, V., et al., *Quantitative expression of toll-like receptor 1–10 mRNA in cellular subsets of human peripheral blood mononuclear cells and sensitivity to CpG oligodeoxynucleotides*. J Immunol, 2002. 168(9): p. 4531–7.
28. Jarrossay, D., et al., *Specialization and complementarity in microbial molecule recognition by human myeloid and plasmacytoid dendritic cells*. Eur J Immunol, 2001. 31(11): p. 3388–93.
29. Delamarre, L., et al., *Differential lysosomal proteolysis in antigen-presenting cells determines antigen fate*. Science, 2005. 307(5715): p. 1630–4.
30. Delamarre, L., H. Holcombe, and I. Mellman, *Presentation of exogenous antigens on major histocompatibility complex (MHC) class I and MHC class II molecules is differentially regulated during dendritic cell maturation*. J Exp Med, 2003. 198(1): p. 111–22.
31. Datta, S.K., et al., *A subset of Toll-like receptor ligands induces cross-presentation by bone marrow-derived dendritic cells*. J Immunol, 2003. 170(8): p. 4102–10.
32. Shin, T., et al., *Cooperative B7–1/2 (CD80/CD86) and B7-DC costimulation of CD4+ T cells independent of the PD-1 receptor*. J Exp Med, 2003. 198(1): p. 31–8.
33. Nguyen, L.T., et al., *Cross-linking the B7 family molecule B7-DC directly activates immune functions of dendritic cells*. J Exp Med, 2002. 196(10): p. 1393–8.
34. Suh, W.K., et al., *The B7 family member B7-H3 preferentially down-regulates T helper type 1-mediated immune responses*. Nat Immunol, 2003. 4(9): p. 899–906.
35. Zang, X., et al., *B7x: a widely expressed B7 family member that inhibits T cell activation*. Proc Natl Acad Sci U S A, 2003. 100(18): p. 10388–92.
36. Colonna, M., *TREMs in the immune system and beyond*. Nat Rev Immunol, 2003. 3(6): p. 445–53.
37. Kolb-Maurer, A., et al., *Production of IL-12 and IL-18 in human dendritic cells upon infection by Listeria monocytogenes*. FEMS Immunol Med Microbiol, 2003. 35(3): p. 255–62.
38. Dzionek, A., et al., *BDCA-2, a novel plasmacytoid dendritic cell-specific type II C-type lectin, mediates antigen capture and is a potent inhibitor of interferon alpha/beta induction*. J Exp Med, 2001. 194(12): p. 1823–34.
39. Randolph, G.J., G. Sanchez-Schmitz, and V. Angeli, *Factors and signals that govern the migration of dendritic cells via lymphatics: recent advances*. Springer Semin Immunopathol, 2004.
40. Ohl, L., et al., *CCR7 governs skin dendritic cell migration under inflammatory and steady-state conditions*. Immunity, 2004. 21(2): p. 279–88.

41. Steinman, R.M. and M.C. Nussenzweig, *Avoiding horror autotoxicus: the importance of dendritic cells in peripheral T cell tolerance.* Proc Natl Acad Sci U S A, 2002. 99(1): p. 351–8.
42. Dhodapkar, M.V., et al., *Antigen-specific inhibition of effector T cell function in humans after injection of immature dendritic cells.* J Exp Med, 2001. 193(2): p. 233–8.
43. Banchereau, J., et al., *Immune and clinical responses in patients with metastatic melanoma to CD34(+) progenitor-derived dendritic cell vaccine.* Cancer Res, 2001. 61(17): p. 6451–8.
44. Adams, S., D. O'Neill, and N. Bhardwaj, *Maturation matters: importance of maturation for antitumor immunity of dendritic cell vaccines.* J Clin Oncol, 2004. 22(18): p. 3834–5; author reply 3835.
45. Mossman, K.D., et al., *Altered TCR signaling from geometrically repatterned immunological synapses.* Science, 2005. 310(5751): p. 1191–3.
46. Stoll, S., et al., *Dynamic imaging of T cell-dendritic cell interactions in lymph nodes.* Science, 2002. 296(5574): p. 1873–6.
47. Bousso, P. and E. Robey, *Dynamics of CD8+ T cell priming by dendritic cells in intact lymph nodes.* Nat Immunol, 2003. 4(6): p. 579–85.
48. Gett, A.V., et al., *T cell fitness determined by signal strength.* Nat Immunol, 2003. 4(4): p. 355–60.
49. van Stipdonk, M.J., et al., *Dynamic programming of CD8+ T lymphocyte responses.* Nat Immunol, 2003. 4(4): p. 361–5.
50. Tato, C.M., A. Laurence, and J.J. O'Shea, *Helper T cell differentiation enters a new era: le roi est mort; vive le roi!* J Exp Med, 2006. 203(4): p. 809–12.
51. Akbari, O., R.H. DeKruyff, and D.T. Umetsu, *Pulmonary dendritic cells producing IL-10 mediate tolerance induced by respiratory exposure to antigen.* Nat Immunol, 2001. 2(8): p. 725–31.
52. Mora, J.R., et al., *Selective imprinting of gut-homing T cells by Peyer's patch dendritic cells.* Nature, 2003. 424(6944): p. 88–93.
53. Hoebe, K., et al., *Identification of Lps2 as a key transducer of MyD88-independent TIR signalling.* Nature, 2003. 424(6950): p. 743–8.
54. Weiner, H.L., *The mucosal milieu creates tolerogenic dendritic cells and T(R)1 and T(H)3 regulatory cells.* Nat Immunol, 2001. 2(8): p. 671–2.
55. Shedlock, D.J. and H. Shen, *Requirement for CD4 T cell help in generating functional CD8 T cell memory.* Science, 2003. 300(5617): p. 337–9.
56. Karsunky, H., et al., *Flt3 ligand regulates dendritic cell development from Flt3+ lymphoid and myeloid-committed progenitors to Flt3+ dendritic cells in vivo.* J Exp Med, 2003. 198(2): p. 305–13.
57. Schoenberger, S.P., et al., *T-cell help for cytotoxic T lymphocytes is mediated by CD40-CD40L interactions.* Nature, 1998. 393(6684): p. 480–3.
58. Croft, M., *Co-stimulatory members of the TNFR family: keys to effective T-cell immunity?* Nat Rev Immunol, 2003. 3(8): p. 609–20.
59. Rogers, P.R., et al., *OX40 promotes Bcl-xL and Bcl-2 expression and is essential for long-term survival of CD4 T cells.* Immunity, 2001. 15(3): p. 445–55.
60. Janssen, E.M., et al., *CD4+ T-cell help controls CD8+ T-cell memory via TRAIL-mediated activation-induced cell death.* Nature, 2005. 434(7029): p. 88–93.
61. Thurner, B., et al., *Generation of large numbers of fully mature and stable dendritic cells from leukapheresis products for clinical application.* J Immunol Methods, 1999. 223(1): p. 1–15.
62. O'Neill, D. and N. Bhardwaj, *Generation of autologous peptide- and protein-pulsed dendritic cells for patient-specific immunotherapy.* Methods Mol Med, 2005. 109: p. 97–112.
63. Hsu, F.J., et al., *Vaccination of patients with B-cell lymphoma using autologous antigen- pulsed dendritic cells.* Nat Med, 1996. 2(1): p. 52–8.
64. Kiertscher, S.M., et al., *Granulocyte/macrophage-colony stimulating factor and interleukin-4 expand and activate type-1 dendritic cells (DC1) when administered in vivo to cancer patients.* Int J Cancer, 2003. 107(2): p. 256–61.
65. Slingluff, C., et al., *Clinical and Immunologic Results of a Randomized Phase II Trial of Vaccination Using Four Melanoma Peptides Either Administered in Granulocyte-Macrophage*

Colony-Stimulating Factor in Adjuvant or Pulsed on Dendritic Cells. J. Clin. Oncol., 2003(November): p. 4016–4026.

66. Jonuleit, H., et al., *A comparison of two types of dendritic cell as adjuvants for the induction of melanoma-specific T-cell responses in humans following intranodal injection*. Int J Cancer, 2001. 93(2): p. 243–51.
67. Jonuleit, H., et al., *Pro-inflammatory cytokines and prostaglandins induce maturation of potent immunostimulatory dendritic cells under fetal calf serum-free conditions*. Eur J Immunol, 1997. 27(12): p. 3135–42.
68. Sato, E., et al., *Intraepithelial CD8+ tumor-infiltrating lymphocytes and a high CD8+/regulatory T cell ratio are associated with favorable prognosis in ovarian cancer*. Proc Natl Acad Sci U S A, 2005. 102(51): p. 18538–43.
69. Dave, S.S., et al., *Prediction of survival in follicular lymphoma based on molecular features of tumor-infiltrating immune cells*. N Engl J Med, 2004. 351(21): p. 2159–69.
70. Hanada, K., J.W. Yewdell, and J.C. Yang, *Immune recognition of a human renal cancer antigen through post-translational protein splicing*. Nature, 2004. 427(6971): p. 252–6.
71. Vigneron, N., et al., *An antigenic peptide produced by peptide splicing in the proteasome*. Science, 2004. 304(5670): p. 587–90.
72. Warren, E.H., et al., *An antigen produced by splicing of noncontiguous peptides in the reverse order*. Science, 2006. 313(5792): p. 1444–7.
73. Simpson, A.J., et al., *Cancer/testis antigens, gametogenesis and cancer*. Nat Rev Cancer, 2005. 5(8): p. 615–25.
74. Schuler-Thurner, B., et al., *Rapid induction of tumor-specific type 1 T helper cells in metastatic melanoma patients by vaccination with mature, cryopreserved, peptide- loaded monocyte-derived dendritic cells*. J Exp Med, 2002. 195(10): p. 1279–88.
75. Nestle, F.O., et al., *Vaccination of melanoma patients with peptide- or tumor lysate-pulsed dendritic cells*. Nat Med, 1998. 4(3): p. 328–32.
76. Dhodapkar, M.V., et al., *Rapid generation of broad T-cell immunity in humans after a single injection of mature dendritic cells*. J Clin Invest, 1999. 104(2): p. 173–80.
77. Fong, L., et al., *Altered peptide ligand vaccination with Flt3 ligand expanded dendritic cells for tumor immunotherapy*. Proc Natl Acad Sci U S A, 2001. 98(15): p. 8809–14.
78. Wang, R.F. and H.Y. Wang, *Enhancement of antitumor immunity by prolonging antigen presentation on dendritic cells*. Nat Biotechnol, 2002. 20(2): p. 149–54.
79. Berzofsky, J.A., J.D. Ahlers, and I.M. Belyakov, *Strategies for designing and optimizing new generation vaccines*. Nat Rev Immunol, 2001. 1(3): p. 209–19.
80. Timmerman, J.M., et al., *Idiotype-pulsed dendritic cell vaccination for B-cell lymphoma: clinical and immune responses in 35 patients*. Blood, 2002. 99(5): p. 1517–26.
81. Heiser, A., et al., *Autologous dendritic cells transfected with prostate-specific antigen RNA stimulate CTL responses against metastatic prostate tumors*. J Clin Invest, 2002. 109(3): p. 409–17.
82. Engelmayer, J., et al., *Mature dendritic cells infected with canarypox virus elicit strong anti- human immunodeficiency virus CD8+ and CD4+ T-cell responses from chronically infected individuals*. J Virol, 2001. 75(5): p. 2142–53.
83. Dietz, A.B. and S. Vuk-Pavlovic, *High efficiency adenovirus-mediated gene transfer to human dendritic cells*. Blood, 1998. 91(2): p. 392–8.
84. Su, Z., et al., *Immunological and clinical responses in metastatic renal cancer patients vaccinated with tumor RNA-transfected dendritic cells*. Cancer Res, 2003. 63(9): p. 2127–33.
85. Thumann, P., et al., *Antigen loading of dendritic cells with whole tumor cell preparations*. J Immunol Methods, 2003. 277(1–2): p. 1–16.
86. Parkhurst, M.R., et al., *Hybrids of dendritic cells and tumor cells generated by electrofusion simultaneously present immunodominant epitopes from multiple human tumor-associated antigens in the context of MHC class I and class II molecules*. J Immunol, 2003. 170(10): p. 5317–25.
87. Morse, M.A., et al., *Migration of human dendritic cells after injection in patients with metastatic malignancies*. Cancer Res, 1999. 59(1): p. 56–8.

88. Mackensen, A., et al., *Homing of intravenously and intralymphatically injected human dendritic cells generated in vitro from CD34+ hematopoietic progenitor cells.* Cancer Immunol Immunother, 1999. 48(2–3): p. 118–22.
89. Mullins, D.W., et al., *Route of Immunization with Peptide-pulsed Dendritic Cells Controls the Distribution of Memory and Effector T Cells in Lymphoid Tissues and Determines the Pattern of Regional Tumor Control.* J Exp Med, 2003. 198(7): p. 1023–34.
90. Fong, L., et al., *Dendritic cells injected via different routes induce immunity in cancer patients.* J Immunol, 2001. 166(6): p. 4254–9.
91. Ridolfi, R., et al., *Evaluation of in vivo labelled dendritic cell migration in cancer patients.* J Transl Med, 2004. 2(1): p. 27.
92. Nair, S., et al., *Injection of immature dendritic cells into adjuvant-treated skin obviates the need for ex vivo maturation.* J Immunol, 2003. 171(11): p. 6275–82.
93. Suzuki, H., et al., *Imiquimod, a topical immune response modifier, induces migration of Langerhans cells.* J Invest Dermatol, 2000. 114(1): p. 135–41.
94. Badovinac, V.P., et al., *Accelerated CD8+ T-cell memory and prime-boost response after dendritic-cell vaccination.* Nat Med, 2005. 11(7): p. 748–56.
95. Ridgway, D., *The first 1000 dendritic cell vaccinees.* Cancer Invest, 2003. 21(6): p. 873–86.
96. Therasse, P., et al., *New guidelines to evaluate the response to treatment in solid tumors. European Organization for Research and Treatment of Cancer, National Cancer Institute of the United States, National Cancer Institute of Canada.* J Natl Cancer Inst, 2000. 92(3): p. 205–16.
97. Schadendorf, D., et al., *Dacarbazine (DTIC) versus vaccination with autologous peptide-pulsed dendritic cells (DC) in first-line treatment of patients with metastatic melanoma: a randomized phase III trial of the DC study group of the DeCOG.* Ann Oncol, 2006. 17(4): p. 563–70.
98. Holtl, L., et al., *Immunotherapy of metastatic renal cell carcinoma with tumor lysate-pulsed autologous dendritic cells.* Clin Cancer Res, 2002. 8(11): p. 3369–76.
99. O'Rourke, M.G., et al., *Durable complete clinical responses in a phase I/II trial using an autologous melanoma cell/dendritic cell vaccine.* Cancer Immunol Immunother, 2003. 52(6): p. 387–95.
100. Maier, T., et al., *Vaccination of patients with cutaneous T-cell lymphoma using intranodal injection of autologous tumor-lysate-pulsed dendritic cells.* Blood, 2003. 102(7): p. 2338–44.
101. Antonia, S.J., et al., *Combination of p53 cancer vaccine with chemotherapy in patients with extensive stage small cell lung cancer.* Clin Cancer Res, 2006. 12(3 Pt 1): p. 878–87.
102. Arnould, L., et al., *Trastuzumab-based treatment of HER2-positive breast cancer: an antibody-dependent cellular cytotoxicity mechanism?* Br J Cancer, 2006. 94(2): p. 259–67.
103. Babatz, J., et al., *Induction of cellular immune responses against carcinoembryonic antigen in patients with metastatic tumors after vaccination with altered peptide ligand-loaded dendritic cells.* Cancer Immunol Immunother, 2006. 55(3): p. 268–76.
104. Di Pucchio, T., et al., *Immunization of stage IV melanoma patients with Melan-A/MART-1 and gp100 peptides plus IFN-alpha results in the activation of specific CD8(+) T cells and monocyte/dendritic cell precursors.* Cancer Res, 2006. 66(9): p. 4943–51.
105. Fuessel, S., et al., *Vaccination of hormone-refractory prostate cancer patients with peptide cocktail-loaded dendritic cells: results of a phase I clinical trial.* Prostate, 2006. 66(8): p. 811–21.
106. Lou, E., et al., *A phase II study of active immunotherapy with PANVAC or autologous, cultured dendritic cells infected with PANVAC after complete resection of hepatic metastases of colorectal carcinoma.* Clin Colorectal Cancer, 2006. 5(5): p. 368–71.
107. Loveland, B.E., et al., *Mannan-MUC1-pulsed dendritic cell immunotherapy: a phase I trial in patients with adenocarcinoma.* Clin Cancer Res, 2006. 12(3 Pt 1): p. 869–77.
108. Perambakam, S., et al., *Induction of specific T cell immunity in patients with prostate cancer by vaccination with PSA146–154 peptide.* Cancer Immunol Immunother, 2006. 55(9): p. 1033–42.
109. Thomas-Kaskel, A.K., et al., *Vaccination of advanced prostate cancer patients with PSCA and PSA peptide-loaded dendritic cells induces DTH responses that correlate with superior overall survival.* Int J Cancer, 2006.

110. Trakatelli, M., et al., *A new dendritic cell vaccine generated with interleukin-3 and interferon-beta induces CD8+ T cell responses against NA17-A2 tumor peptide in melanoma patients.* Cancer Immunol Immunother, 2006. 55(4): p. 469–74.
111. Tuettenberg, A., et al., *Induction of strong and persistent MelanA/MART-1-specific immune responses by adjuvant dendritic cell-based vaccination of stage II melanoma patients.* Int J Cancer, 2006. 118(10): p. 2617–27.
112. Wierecky, J., M. Mueller, and P. Brossart, *Dendritic cell-based cancer immunotherapy targeting MUC-1.* Cancer Immunol Immunother, 2006. 55(1): p. 63–7.
113. Osada, T., et al., *NK cell activation by dendritic cell vaccine: a mechanism of action for clinical activity.* Cancer Immunol Immunother, 2006. 55(9): p. 1122–31.
114. Wilson, N.S., et al., *Systemic activation of dendritic cells by Toll-like receptor ligands or malaria infection impairs cross-presentation and antiviral immunity.* Nat Immunol, 2006. 7(2): p. 165–72.
115. Dillon, S., et al., *Yeast zymosan, a stimulus for TLR2 and dectin-1, induces regulatory antigen-presenting cells and immunological tolerance.* J Clin Invest, 2006. 116(4): p. 916–28.
116. Su, Z., et al., *Enhanced induction of telomerase-specific CD4(+) T cells using dendritic cells transfected with RNA encoding a chimeric gene product.* Cancer Res, 2002. 62(17): p. 5041–8.
117. Merad, M., et al., *In vivo manipulation of dendritic cells to induce therapeutic immunity.* Blood, 2002. 99(5): p. 1676–82.
118. Cho, H.J., et al., *Immunostimulatory DNA-based vaccines induce cytotoxic lymphocyte activity by a T-helper cell-independent mechanism.* Nat Biotechnol, 2000. 18(5): p. 509–14.
119. Schneeberger, A., et al., *CpG motifs are efficient adjuvants for DNA cancer vaccines.* J Invest Dermatol, 2004. 123(2): p. 371–9.
120. Weeratna, R.D., et al., *TLR agonists as vaccine adjuvants: comparison of CpG ODN and Resiquimod (R-848).* Vaccine, 2005. 23(45): p. 5263–70.
121. Wille-Reece, U., et al., *Immunization with HIV-1 Gag protein conjugated to a TLR7/8 agonist results in the generation of HIV-1 Gag-specific Th1 and CD8+ T cell responses.* J Immunol, 2005. 174(12): p. 7676–83.
122. Itoh, T. and E. Celis, *Transcutaneous immunization with cytotoxic T-cell peptide epitopes provides effective antitumor immunity in mice.* J Immunother, 2005. 28(5): p. 430–7.
123. Klinman, D.M., et al., *Use of CpG oligodeoxynucleotides as immune adjuvants.* Immunol Rev, 2004. 199: p. 201–16.
124. Speiser, D.E., et al., *Rapid and strong human CD8+ T cell responses to vaccination with peptide, IFA, and CpG oligodeoxynucleotide 7909.* J Clin Invest, 2005. 115(3): p. 739–46.
125. Kim, T.W., et al., *Enhancing DNA vaccine potency by combining a strategy to prolong dendritic cell life with intracellular targeting strategies.* J Immunol, 2003. 171(6): p. 2970–6.
126. Sudowe, S., et al., *Transcriptional targeting of dendritic cells in gene gun-mediated DNA immunization favors the induction of type 1 immune responses.* Mol Ther, 2003. 8(4): p. 567–75.
127. Garg, S., et al., *Genetic tagging shows increased frequency and longevity of antigen-presenting, skin-derived dendritic cells in vivo.* Nat Immunol, 2003. 4(9): p. 907–12.
128. MartIn-Fontecha, A., et al., *Regulation of dendritic cell migration to the draining lymph node: impact on T lymphocyte traffic and priming.* J Exp Med, 2003. 198(4): p. 615–21.
129. Belli, F., et al., *Vaccination of metastatic melanoma patients with autologous tumor-derived heat shock protein gp96-peptide complexes: clinical and immunologic findings.* J Clin Oncol, 2002. 20(20): p. 4169–80.
130. Wang, H.Y., et al., *Induction of CD4(+) T cell-dependent antitumor immunity by TAT-mediated tumor antigen delivery into dendritic cells.* J Clin Invest, 2002. 109(11): p. 1463–70.
131. Mohty, M., et al., *All-trans retinoic acid skews monocyte differentiation into interleukin-12-secreting dendritic-like cells.* Br J Haematol, 2003. 122(5): p. 829–36.
132. Adams, S., et al., *PT-100, a small molecule dipeptidyl peptidase inhibitor, has potent antitumor effects and augments antibody-mediated cytotoxicity via a novel immune mechanism.* Cancer Res, 2004. 64(15): p. 5471–80.
133. Nefedova, Y., et al., *Hyperactivation of STAT3 is involved in abnormal differentiation of dendritic cells in cancer.* J Immunol, 2004. 172(1): p. 464–74.

134. Song, X.T., et al., *An alternative and effective HIV vaccination approach based on inhibition of antigen presentation attenuators in dendritic cells*. PLoS Med, 2006. 3(1): p. e11.
135. Nair, S., et al., *Synergy between tumor immunotherapy and antiangiogenic therapy*. Blood, 2003. 102(3): p. 964–71.
136. Gabrilovich, D.I., et al., *Antibodies to vascular endothelial growth factor enhance the efficacy of cancer immunotherapy by improving endogenous dendritic cell function*. Clin Cancer Res, 1999. 5(10): p. 2963–70.
137. Rini, B.I., et al., *Combination immunotherapy with prostatic acid phosphatase pulsed antigen-presenting cells (provenge) plus bevacizumab in patients with serologic progression of prostate cancer after definitive local therapy*. Cancer, 2006. 107(1): p. 67–74.
138. Borg, C., et al., *Novel mode of action of c-kit tyrosine kinase inhibitors leading to NK cell-dependent antitumor effects*. J Clin Invest, 2004. 114(3): p. 379–88.
139. Ghiringhelli, F., et al., *CD4+CD25+ regulatory T cells inhibit natural killer cell functions in a transforming growth factor-beta-dependent manner*. J Exp Med, 2005. 202(8): p. 1075–85.
140. Hodi, F.S., et al., *Biologic activity of cytotoxic T lymphocyte-associated antigen 4 antibody blockade in previously vaccinated metastatic melanoma and ovarian carcinoma patients*. Proc Natl Acad Sci U S A, 2003. 100(8): p. 4712–7.
141. Phan, G.Q., et al., *Cancer regression and autoimmunity induced by cytotoxic T lymphocyte-associated antigen 4 blockade in patients with metastatic melanoma*. Proc Natl Acad Sci U S A, 2003. 100(14): p. 8372–7.
142. Attia, P., et al., *Autoimmunity correlates with tumor regression in patients with metastatic melanoma treated with anti-cytotoxic T-lymphocyte antigen-4*. J Clin Oncol, 2005. 23(25): p. 6043–53.
143. Beck, K.E., et al., *Enterocolitis in patients with cancer after antibody blockade of cytotoxic T-lymphocyte-associated antigen 4*. J Clin Oncol, 2006. 24(15): p. 2283–9.
144. Curiel, T.J., et al., *Blockade of B7-H1 improves myeloid dendritic cell-mediated antitumor immunity*. Nat Med, 2003. 9(5): p. 562–7.
145. Watanabe, N., et al., *BTLA is a lymphocyte inhibitory receptor with similarities to CTLA-4 and PD-1*. Nat Immunol, 2003. 4(7): p. 670–9.
146. Carreno, B.M. and M. Collins, *BTLA: a new inhibitory receptor with a B7-like ligand*. Trends Immunol, 2003. 24(10): p. 524–7.
147. Francois Bach, J., *Regulatory T cells under scrutiny*. Nat Rev Immunol, 2003. 3(3): p. 189–98.
148. Jonuleit, H. and E. Schmitt, *The regulatory T cell family: distinct subsets and their interrelations*. J Immunol, 2003. 171(12): p. 6323–7.
149. Woo, E.Y., et al., *Regulatory CD4(+)CD25(+) T cells in tumors from patients with early-stage non-small cell lung cancer and late-stage ovarian cancer*. Cancer Res, 2001. 61(12): p. 4766–72.
150. Wolf, A.M., et al., *Increase of regulatory T cells in the peripheral blood of cancer patients*. Clin Cancer Res, 2003. 9(2): p. 606–12.
151. Curiel, T.J., et al., *Specific recruitment of regulatory T cells in ovarian carcinoma fosters immune privilege and predicts reduced survival*. Nat Med, 2004. 10(9): p. 942–9.
152. Oldenhove, G., et al., *CD4+ CD25+ regulatory T cells control T helper cell type 1 responses to foreign antigens induced by mature dendritic cells in vivo*. J Exp Med, 2003. 198(2): p. 259–66.
153. Dannull, J., et al., *Enhancement of vaccine-mediated antitumor immunity in cancer patients after depletion of regulatory T cells*. J Clin Invest, 2005. 115(12): p. 3623–33.
154. Asavaroengchai, W., Y. Kotera, and J.J. Mule, *Tumor lysate-pulsed dendritic cells can elicit an effective antitumor immune response during early lymphoid recovery*. Proc Natl Acad Sci U S A, 2002. 99(2): p. 931–6.
155. Rapoport, A.P., et al., *Restoration of immunity in lymphopenic individuals with cancer by vaccination and adoptive T-cell transfer*. Nat Med, 2005.
156. Dudley, M.E., et al., *Adoptive cell transfer therapy following non-myeloablative but lymphodepleting chemotherapy for the treatment of patients with refractory metastatic melanoma*. J Clin Oncol, 2005. 23(10): p. 2346–57.

157. Gattinoni, L., et al., *Removal of homeostatic cytokine sinks by lymphodepletion enhances the efficacy of adoptively transferred tumor-specific CD8+ T cells*. J Exp Med, 2005. 202(7): p. 907–12.
158. Morgan, R.A., et al., *Cancer Regression in Patients After Transfer of Genetically Engineered Lymphocytes*. Science, 2006.
159. Overwijk, W.W., et al., *Tumor regression and autoimmunity after reversal of a functionally tolerant state of self-reactive CD8+ T cells*. J Exp Med, 2003. 198(4): p. 569–80.
160. Friedman, E.J., *Immune modulation by ionizing radiation and its implications for cancer immunotherapy*. Curr Pharm Des, 2002. 8(19): p. 1765–80.
161. Chen, Z., et al., *Combined radiation therapy and dendritic cell vaccine for treating solid tumors with liver micro-metastasis*. J Gene Med, 2005. 7(4): p. 506–17.
162. Chi, K.H., et al., *Combination of conformal radiotherapy and intratumoral injection of adoptive dendritic cell immunotherapy in refractory hepatoma*. J Immunother, 2005. 28(2): p. 129–35.
163. Lake, R.A. and B.W. Robinson, *Immunotherapy and chemotherapy–a practical partnership*. Nat Rev Cancer, 2005. 5(5): p. 397–405.
164. Gabrilovich, D.I., et al., *Production of vascular endothelial growth factor by human tumors inhibits the functional maturation of dendritic cells*. Nat Med, 1996. 2(10): p. 1096–103.
165. Gabrilovich, D.I., et al., *Decreased antigen presentation by dendritic cells in patients with breast cancer*. Clin Cancer Res, 1997. 3(3): p. 483–90.
166. Furumoto, K., et al., *Induction of potent antitumor immunity by in situ targeting of intratumoral DCs*. J Clin Invest, 2004. 113(5): p. 774–83.
167. Sharma, S., et al., *Cytokines and chemokines are expressed at different levels in small and large murine colon-26 tumors following intratumoral injections of CpG ODN*. Neoplasia, 2004. 6(5): p. 523–8.
168. Carpentier, A.F., et al., *Successful treatment of intracranial gliomas in rat by oligodeoxynucleotides containing CpG motifs*. Clin Cancer Res, 2000. 6(6): p. 2469–73.
169. Meng, Y., et al., *Successful combination of local CpG-ODN and radiotherapy in malignant glioma*. Int J Cancer, 2005. 116(6): p. 992–7.

CHAPTER 12

WHOLE CELL VACCINES

MARK B. FARIES* AND DONALD L. MORTON

From the Sonya Valley Ghidossi Vaccine Laboratory of the Roy E. Coats Research Laboratories of the John Wayne Cancer Institute at Saint John's Health Center, Santa Monica, CA.

INTRODUCTION

A great deal of progress has been made in recent decades in identifying and characterizing tumor-specific antigens that can be used as targets in immunotherapy. However, there are undoubtedly a large number of antigens that remain undiscovered. An alternative strategy to defined antigens is the use of tumor cells themselves as the source of antigen. This approach includes the broadest array of antigens but presents additional challenges that are not seen in vaccines using purified antigens such as peptides or proteins. This chapter will discuss vaccine therapy using whole tumor cells as antigen sources including not only whole cell vaccines, but also tumor cell lysate and shed antigen vaccines.

HISTORY

Efforts to develop cancer vaccines predate identification of tumor-specific antigens. One of the earliest examples is that of William Bradford Coley, a New York surgeon who noted spontaneous regression of a sarcoma after the patient developed erysipelas adjacent to the tumor. He subsequently attempted to induce such responses by injecting derivatives of bacterial cultures ("Coley's toxins") into the tumors of other patients [1,2]. He did see several additional episodes of regression, but was unable to engender such responses consistently.

*2200 Santa Monica Blvd. Santa Monica, CA 90404 fariesm@jwci.org

H.L. Kaufman and J.D. Wolchok (eds.), General Principles of Tumor Immunotherapy, 275–295.

Early in the twentieth century, murine models of tumor vaccination were developed that utilized irradiated, whole tumor cells injected as vaccine. The mice developed protective immunity to subsequent tumor challenge. However, these studies, and others using tumor cell lysates, were performed before an understanding of histocompatibility and transplantation antigens was developed. As such a distinction between rejection of alloantigens, and tumor-specific responses could not be made.

By the middle of the century, experiments using inbred mouse strains established the immunogenicity of tumors [3]. This led to significant efforts to identify the particular tumor antigens that were recognized in these immune responses and to use these antigens in immunotherapy. The appeal of using whole tumor cells as antigen sources has remained, and several such vaccines have come into large-scale trials.

STRATEGIES: SOURCE OF ANTIGEN

The cellular source of vaccine antigens can be derived individually from each patient (autologous) or from pre-existing tumor cell lines (allogeneic). These tumor cells can be used whole, used after processing (e.g. by lysis) or used to produce antigens through shedding into culture supernatants. All these approaches (Figure 1) have in common a diverse array of potential epitopes for presentation to the patient's system. Diversity may decrease the likelihood that tumors will escape immune recognition through loss of expression of vaccine epitopes. Such antigen loss has been reported with peptide-based immunotherapy [4, 5].

Vaccinated individuals also may not respond equally well to all epitopes, even when properly matched by HLA type. As an example, Reynolds et al [6] studied the spectrum of peptides to which patients vaccinated with a polyvalent, shed antigen vaccine responded. They found that, while 59% of patients responded to at least one epitope, no more than 14% of patients responded to any given specific peptide. In other words, most patients were successfully immunized, but the epitopes that the patients' immune systems selected from the polyvalent vaccine were heterogeneous and unpredictable. This heterogeneous immune response, while probably clinically beneficial, makes monitoring of immune responses to vaccination more complex than is the case for simpler vaccine antigens.

Live Whole Cell: Autologous

The antigen source of a vaccine must share epitopes with those of a patient's tumor in order to be effective. Use of the patient's own tumor cells as the antigen source ensures optimal HLA-type matching and may maximize the number of tumor-specific antigen matches for that individual. Because of heterogeneity among metastatic lesions, it is possible that the spectrum of antigens present in the vaccine will be somewhat different from that present in the patient's residual tumor, but, in principle this difference is least significant with autologous tumor.

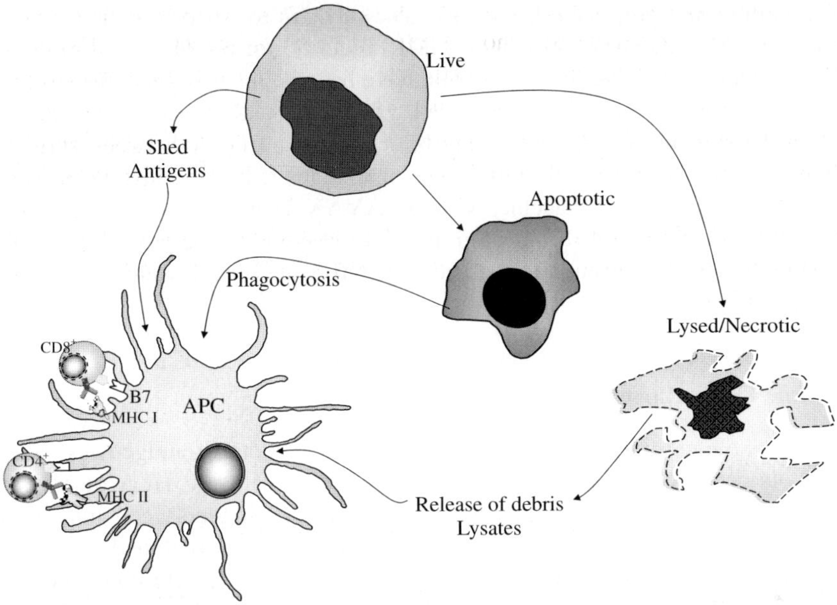

Figure 1. A wide variety of strategies exist to use whole cells as antigen sources. These include live whole cells, apoptotic whole cells, antigens shed by whole cells, and debris derived from lysed whole cells. These antigens can be combined with adjuvants such as dendritic cells or cytokines before or after administration to patients

Autologous tumor specimens can be processed in several ways to obtain an antigenic vaccine. Such methods include use of tumor cells directly (with modification to increase antigenicity), [7] interval expansion of cells in tissue culture, [8] and processing of tumor specimens to obtain a desired portion of the cells, such as RNA or antigens bound to heat shock proteins (HSP) [9].

Production of autologous vaccines is complex and difficult. In order to obtain sufficient material for vaccine production, patients must have at least a moderate tumor burden. Harvesting this tumor requires some type of surgical intervention, and ensuring sterility of the specimen may be challenging, depending on its anatomic location. This difficulty has been recognized from the earliest autologous tumor vaccines, which were chemically sterilized [10]. Different techniques of vaccine manufacture require varying volumes of tumor in order to generate vaccine, but there is always a limit to the amount of vaccine that can be produced. For example, an autologous vaccine developed by Berd and colleagues requires at least 2.5 grams of tumor for vaccine production [11]. The number of doses that these patients can receive may also be limited by the amount of available tumor. In addition, many patients with significant risk of recurrence have only limited accessible tumor, for example those with positive sentinel lymph nodes. These patients are not candidates for autologous vaccines.

Tissue culture and processing ex vivo is also difficult to perform in accordance with the Good Manufacturing Practices (GMP) required for production of biologic agents. As techniques of vaccine production have become more refined, the success rate for generating vaccines has increased. However, with the requirement for in vitro processing or culture, there may be a significant delay between surgical treatment and vaccine administration. These challenges led to the halting of trials of an autologous melanoma vaccine, M-Vax (AVAX Technologies, Philadelphia, PA), by the Food and Drug Administration to improve lot release procedures. This halt appears to have contributed to the end of significant clinical evaluation of this promising vaccine.

Live Whole Cell: Allogeneic

Allogeneic whole-cell tumor vaccines offer a similar breadth of antigens as autologous whole cells. They are not matched to individual patients' HLA or antigen spectrum in the same way as autologous cells are, but allogeneic cell lines may be selected for high levels of tumor antigen expression and combined so that at least a partial HLA match is present for most of the potential patient population. A panel of 150 cell lines were tested at the John Wayne Cancer Institute, and three (M10VACC, M24VACC, and M101VACC) were selected for use as vaccine that expressed relatively high levels of melanoma antigens [12]. Over 20 melanoma- and tumor-associated antigens have since been identified in these lines. These lines comprise the Canvaxin vaccine (CancerVax Corp., Carlsbad, CA), and express a spectrum of HLA types with a partial match for approximately 95% of melanoma patients. Such matching may be important for the generation of effective immunity.

Production of allogeneic vaccines is more straightforward than that of autologous vaccines, since a new vaccine does not need to be individually produced for each patient. Because the patient's tumor is not the source of vaccine cells, small tumor burden is not limiting, and the vaccine can be immediately available for administration. In addition, since the cells are maintained in tissue culture over a longer time period, sterility of the specimens is easier to ensure and maintain than is the case with vaccines derived more directly from surgical specimens. However, GMP issues are still complex with live whole cell allogeneic vaccines. Canvaxin was placed on partial clinical hold after the FDA requested that previously acceptable lot release assays be revised. Though this process revealed no safety issues with the vaccine, the hold delayed clinical evaluation of the vaccine by approximately one year.

Lysate and Shed Antigens

Lysates of whole tumor cells may also be used as an antigen source. Cell lysis simplifies vaccine production in two ways. First, since the cellular material is not viable after lysis, replication incompetence is assured. Second, live cell vaccines require significant care to maintain the viability of cells including cryopreservation using liquid nitrogen. This care is not needed for lysate vaccines, which may be lyophilized or frozen at higher temperatures. Although lysates retain much of the antigenic diversity of whole cells, some epitopes are lost thorough separation of the nuclear fraction and degradation of messenger RNA. Proteins that are secreted by live tumor cells are also diminished (Figure 2). Lysate antigens may be taken up by APC and are classically presented to $CD4^+$ T cells in the context of major histocompatibility complex (MHC) class II. In order for these antigens to be presented to $CD8^+$ T cells, they must be processed through a non-classical path known as cross-presentation [13]. This process is now well described, but requires certain conditions in order to occur. These conditions are probably easiest to achieve in vitro, and some current lysate vaccine strategies apply lysate to APC in vitro and then administer these loaded cells as the vaccine.

Cells used for lysis can be obtained either from autologous tumor or from established cells lines. The choice of antigen source is determined by similar issues to those in live cell vaccines. The most thoroughly evaluated mechanical lysate vaccine

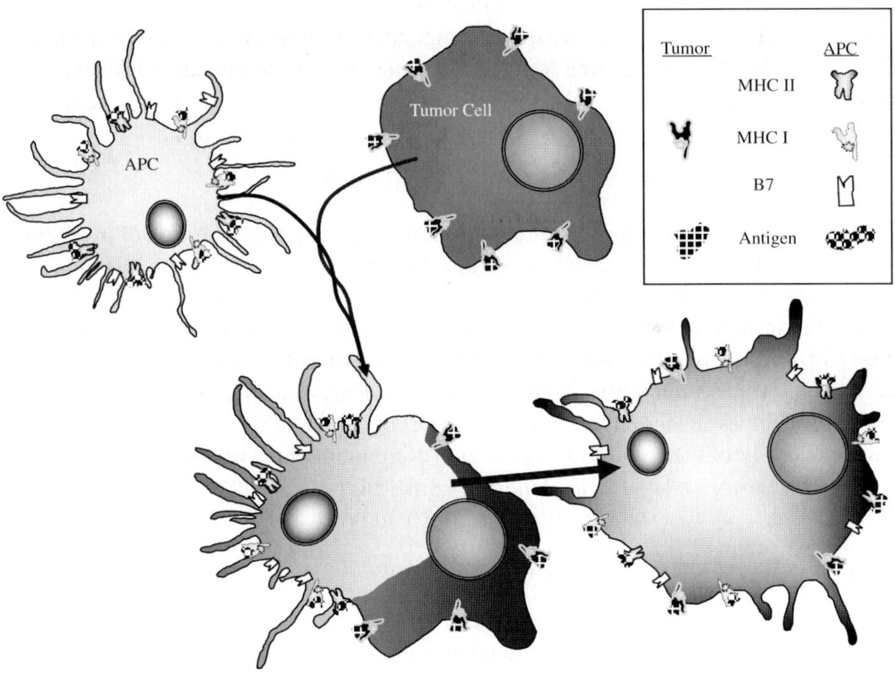

Figure 2. Tumour cells present antigens to the immune system only through components of their cell membranes such as gangliosides. However, the internal processes of the cell are represented on the surface through peptide antigens. Peptides that result from abnormal DNA, RNA, or proteins of cancer cells may serve as effective immunogens for vaccine therapy. Whole cell vaccines provide all of these sources of antigen, antigens shown in white font may be lost in preparation of cell lysates.

is Melacine (Corixa Corp., Seattle, WA), an allogeneic preparation developed by Mitchell and colleagues [14] for patients with melanoma, but mechanical lysates have also been used in breast cancer, renal cell cancer, and other malignancies. Protocols for lysate preparation can be varied to include or remove cellular components such as cell membranes [15].

Tumor cells can also be lysed through application of viruses including vaccinia and influenza A. The earliest application of this strategy in animal models by Lindenmann and Klein in 1967 showed that while simple mixtures of virus and tumor cell lysates could not produce a protective immune response, viral lysates did [16]. The process of viral infection of cells led to production of highly immunogenic foreign antigens or xenogenization of the vaccine. The enhanced response to viral antigens may therefore serve as an adjuvant and strengthen the immune response to relatively poorly immunogenic tumor antigens.

Tumor cells in culture rapidly shed antigenic material into the supernatant. These shed antigens encompass a wide variety of potential tumor-related targets [17]. They are considered partially purified relative to live cell and lysate vaccines, as cellular components retained in the cytoplasm and nucleus are not included. Proponents of these vaccines suggest that the shed antigens may be particularly important since they are generally expressed on the cell surface and are readily available to immune recognition. They have been shown to engender immune responses to a variety of antigens. Like lysates, shed-antigen vaccines are relatively straightforward to produce.

STRATEGIES: INDUCING IMMUNE RESPONSE

Tumor antigen content is only one factor determining the effectiveness of a vaccine. Just as important is the context in which the antigen interacts with the immune system. The same antigen, presented in different contexts, may lead to effective anti-tumor immunity, ineffective immune response, or even tolerance. A wide variety of approaches has been developed to help stimulate a strong and effective anti-tumor immune response. These include modification of the antigens such as with the hapten dinitrophenyl, application of exogenous adjuvants with the vaccine, provision of cytokines with vaccines, and combination of vaccine antigens with antigen presenting cells such as dendritic cells (DC).

Exogenous Adjuvants and Immunomodulators

Many antigens, particularly tumor antigens, are insufficiently immunogenic to induce a beneficial immune response when given in isolation. Adjuvants that non-specifically stimulate the immune system can strengthen immune responses to the target antigen. For example, chemical preparations such as aluminum salts (alum), oil and water emulsions, and bacteria- or plant-derived compounds change the rate and mechanism of antigen absorption and processing. Other adjuvants bind with receptors of the innate immune system, for example toll-like receptors (TLR), inducing cellular activation, maturation of DC and cytokine secretion by immune cells. This changes the environment in which vaccine antigens encounter APC and effector cells leading to stronger immune responses.

Aluminum salts have been used in relatively few tumor vaccine trials and were thought to lead to a predominantly humoral, rather than cellular immune response. However, trials using alum have shown evidence of specific, cellular immune responses to tumor antigens [6]. DETOX is a combination of two bacterial components (monophosphoryl lipid A and mycobacterial cell wall skeleton) in an oil-in-water emulsion. In animal models, injection of these bacterial components into growing tumors led to eradication of regional micrometastases, and it is thought to engender both humoral and cellular immunity. Bacille Calmette-Guerin (BCG), an attenuated mycobacterium used in immunotherapy for superficial bladder cancer, has been used in several vaccine trials. Cellular and humoral immunity are stimulated by BCG.

Until very recently development of adjuvants has been largely empiric. As knowledge of the immune system has increased, new adjuvants and immunomodulators have become available for testing with vaccines. Of particular interest are ligands for the toll-like receptors (TLR). CpG oligonucleotides bind to TLR9 and induce a strong immune response with characteristics thought to be favorable in cancer immunity [18]. These are now under evaluation in immunotherapy trials, though not with any whole cell vaccine. Imidazoquinolines such as imiquimod bind TLR7 and 8 and lead to APC maturation and cytokine secretion, [19] and have been evaluated with DNA- and peptide-based vaccines demonstrating enhanced immune responses.

A number of cytokines are also available for immunomodulation of responses. Granulocyte-macrophage-colony stimulating factor (GM-CSF) and flt-3 ligand increase activation and quantity of APC [20]. Interferon-$\alpha$and interleukin-2 increase or modify vaccine responses. Such adjuvants and cytokines can be administered at the site of vaccination or systemically.

Dendritic Cells

Dendritic cells (DC), first described by Steinman and Cohn in 1973, [21] are the most "professional" antigen presenting cells. These cells are responsible for sensitizing naïve T cells, and are therefore principally responsible for development of new immune responses. They have been evaluated in many vaccine strategies, and can be used with almost all antigen types. The immunostimulatory capacity of DC depend heavily on their lineage and the culture conditions in which they are grown [22]. They are commonly pulsed with antigen and then administered as a vaccine. The most important characteristics of DC used in a vaccine are their maturity and cytokine/chemokine expression profile. Effective cellular antitumor immune responses most likely require three signals. First is the antigen itself, presented in the context of an MHC molecule. However, if this signal is presented in isolation, tolerance rather than recognition is produced. The second signal comes from costimulatory molecules on the surface of APC. These molecules are present on the surface of activated and mature DC. A third signal is provided by the cytokines present during sensitization of the T cells and determines the character of the response [23]. For example, interleukin-12 steers responses toward an interferon-γ-dominated type 1 response that is thought to be more effective in anti-tumor immunity.

Numerous DC-based tumor vaccine trials have been conducted, many using DC pulsed with peptide antigens and a number of others pulsing with proteins or tumor lysates [24, 25]. The important nuances of these types of DC vaccines are outside the scope of this chapter. Lysate and shed antigen vaccines could be used with DC in very similar fashion to purified protein or peptide antigens. Other uses of DC are specifically applicable to whole cell vaccines and will be discussed below.

Whole Cell-only Strategies: Genetic Modification

Several strategies are specifically tailored for use with whole cells, including genetic modification of tumor cells to improve immunogenicity, pulsing of DC with apoptotic whole tumor cells and fusion of tumor cells with DC.

The earliest form of genetic modification of tumor cells was by infection of cells with viruses, such as influenza. This led to incorporation of viral proteins into the cells which increased their immunogenicity, as described above. Several methods of tumor cell transfection are available. The choice of methodology impacts transfection efficiency, and may also have an impact on immunogenicity. Both viral and non-viral methods have been evaluated. Viral vectors include adenovirus, ALVAC (a canary pox virus), fowlpox, vaccinia, Epstein-Barr virus, and retroviruses [26]. Viruses that are able to replicate in mammalian cells, such as adenovirus, may be modified to render them replication incompetent. Gene therapy trials using in vivo infection of cancer or normal cells are subject to a vigorous immune response, limiting transfection of target cells beyond the first vaccination. This type of response probably affects in vitro transfection less. Non-viral methods include the use of electroporation and liposomes. These methods have been compared without consistent demonstration of superior transfection efficiency [27, 28]. Viral and non-viral vectors have also been compared and similar levels of transfection efficiency were seen, [29] though the clinical efficacy and immunogenicity of viral and non-viral vectors have not been directly compared.

Genetic modifications seek to change either the surface antigens or co-stimulatory molecules of tumor cells or the environment in which tumor cells interact with the immune system. Pre-clinical studies examined the introduction of MHC molecules into tumor cells. However, transfer of MHC class I often let to increased tumor growth in these models, possible due to loss of natural killer cell recognition of tumors [30]. Co-transfection of MHC class I molecules with co-stimulatory molecules has been used in early clinical trials with measured immune responses, but without comparison to non-MHC transfected lines. Transfer of MHC class II has been associated with improved immunogenicity, but this has not yet been used in clinical studies.

The best studied approach in clinical trials has been transfection of co-stimulatory molecules such as B7.1 and B7.2 into tumor cells [31]. Co-stimulation is normally provided by antigen presenting cells that have taken up and presented antigens. This vaccine approach genetically modifies tumor cells to look and act more like antigen presenting cells. In addition, B7 expression on transfected tumor cells render them susceptible to killing by natural killer cells. This killing then releases additional antigens for uptake by host APC.

Clinical trials have utilized this strategy in several malignancies. $CD8^+$ lymphocyte immune responses were engendered using transfection of either allogeneic or autologous tumor. There has not been a definitive demonstration that tumor cells transfected with co-stimulatory molecules produce superior immunologic responses than non-transfected cells in clinical trials, though this has been suggested based upon non-cellular vaccine trials [32, 33]. Depending on the vector used, these vaccines can incorporate co-stimulatory molecules and tumor antigens.

Tumor cells may also be transduced with genes encoding various immunostimulatory cytokines. These include interleukin-2 (IL-2) [34–36], IL-4 [37–39], IL-6 [40], IL-7 [41], IL-12 [42], IL-18 [43], interferon-γ [44] and granulocyte-macrophage-colony stimulating factor (GM-CSF) [45–47]. Both allogeneic and autologous tumor cells have been used. Because of the complexity of in vitro culture and transfection of autologous tumor cells, a third method mixes autologous tumor cells with transfected allogeneic tumor or fibroblast cells [40]. The principle of these modifications is enhancement of recruiting, activation, proliferation, or immunophenotype of responding leukocytes in order to boost the magnitude and effectiveness of anti-tumor immunity. The most thoroughly studied of these cytokines are IL-2 and GM-CSF.

GM-CSF leads to recruitment and differentiation of dendritic cells. In animal studies, immunization with tumors transduced with the gene for GM-CSF led to long-lasting systemic immunity. This immunity required participation of both $CD4^+$ and $CD8^+$ T cells. In clinical studies it has been used in melanoma, ovarian cancer, and non-small cell lung cancer. An evaluation of autologous melanoma cells transduced with the gene for GM-CSF demonstrated lymphocytic infiltrates of the vaccine site (19 of 26), resected metastases (10 of 16), and delayed-type hypersensitivity (DTH) skin test responses (17 of 25) to non-transduced tumor cells in vaccinated patients [46]. Despite the complexity of vaccine preparation in this trial, 97% of patients were able to have vaccine successfully produced. The same investigators demonstrated similar results in patients with non-small cell lung cancer [47].

IL-2 is a growth factor for lymphocytes and has been shown to restore responsiveness in anergic or unresponsive T cells. It is approved for use in patients with metastatic melanoma, and in a minority of cases induces dramatic and durable regressions of tumors. Cellular vaccines transduced with the gene for IL-

2 have been tested, largely in melanoma. Trials using allogeneic cell vaccines have demonstrated increases cytotoxic lymphocyte (CTL) responses [39]. Others have used autologous tumor as vaccine. In an example of the potential difficulties of generating a transfected vaccine from autologous tumors, one such study was able to produce vaccine in only 54% of patients, and only 37% actually received vaccine. Among 15 vaccinated patients in this trial, though, over half demonstrated increased DTH responses (8/15), and 3 patients showed evidence of autoimmunity (vitiligo) [36]. Others have demonstrated increased tumor-reactive CTL [48].

Whole Cell-only Strategies: Dendritic Cell Combinations

Other vaccine types that require whole cells as an antigen source are DC loaded with apoptotic tumor cells and DC-tumor fusions. Uptake by DC of cells undergoing programmed cell death (apoptosis) is quite efficient and can generate both $CD4^+$ and $CD8^+$ T cell responses. The nature of the immune response to DC loaded with apoptotic cells is affected by the stage of apoptosis. Apoptosis of non-malignant cells is a normal part of physiologic homeostasis and should not engender an immune response. Not surprisingly, investigators have shown that tumor cells in early apoptosis frequently do not generate an effective immune response. Conversely, cells in late apoptosis do generate immune responses; these responses are characterized by interferon-γ-dominated type 1 cytokines and may therefore be more effective against malignant cells [50].

It has also been suggested that uptake of apoptotic or necrotic tumor cells leads to maturation of the DC, [51–54] though the methodology leading to some of these results has been questioned [55]. Uptake of dying or necrotic cells appears to be best accomplished by myeloid lineage DC and at the immature stage of DC development [56]. In a recent trial, 16 patients with non-small cell lung cancer received DC loaded with irradiated apoptotic allogeneic cells. Six patients developed antigen-specific immune responses [49].

A patient's DC may also be physically fused with autologous or allogeneic tumor cells. Fusion may be accomplished using polyethyleneglycol [57, 58] or by electrofusion [59]. The latter appears to be a more efficient process [60]. The fusion product is a hybrid cell which possesses the immunostimulatory characteristics of APC and presents the antigens of tumor cells (Figure 3). Hybrid cells express MHC molecules of the DC and the tumor cells. Proteins from the tumor cells are processed by the antigen presentation machinery of the DC and are presented in both MHC class I and MHC class I of the patient [59].

The majority of reported data are preclinical, but a few small clinical trials have been reported with apparent safety, but limited efficacy. These were polyethylene glycol fusions tested in patients with glioma, breast cancer, renal cell cancer and melanoma [57, 58, 61]. Additionally, the methods of vaccine production by electrofusion have been reported for use in colon cancer and melanoma patients [62, 63].

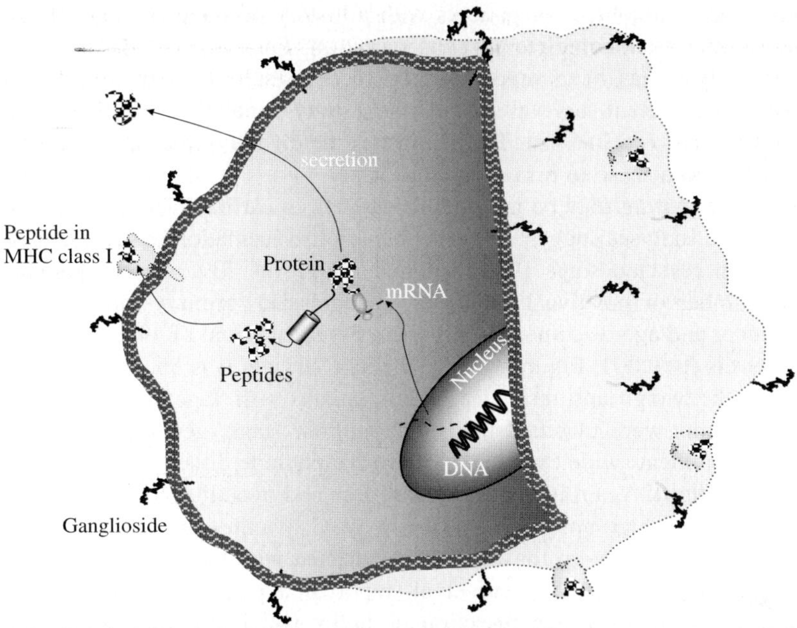

Figure 3. Dendritic cells can be physically fused with tumor cells to produce hybrid vaccine cells. These hybrids have the antigen presentation and co-stimulatory ability of antigen presenting cells, and the antigens of tumor cells. Tumor antigens derived from allogeneic vaccine cell lines can be presented in patient-derived MHC molecules

WHOLE CELL VACCINE TRIALS: CLINICAL RESULTS

Of the clinical trials of using whole tumor cells as the antigen source, many have been small trials examining immunologic endpoints, but several have been large enough to provide data regarding clinical efficacy.

Clinical Results: Live Whole Cells

The most thoroughly tested allogeneic live whole cell vaccine is Canvaxin, developed by Morton and colleagues and under clinical evaluation since 1985. Its three melanoma cell lines were selected from a panel of more than 150 lines based on their antigenic profile with expression of more than 20 immunogenic melanoma- or tumor-associated antigens [64]. The Tice strain of BCG is given as adjuvant with the first two vaccine doses.

Canvaxin has been tested extensively in phase II trials at the John Wayne Cancer Institute (JWCI). In 40 stage IV patients with evaluable disease, a 23% response rate was seen after vaccination (8% complete response, 15% partial response), primarily in patients with metastatic lesions less than 2 cm in diameter [65]. In the adjuvant treatment setting, the vaccine has also shown promising results. Such analyses have been completed for patients with a history of stage II, stage III, or stage IV melanoma after complete surgical resection. For stage IV disease, this matched-pair analysis has been superceded by recent results of a phase III trial that demonstrated excellent survival for the entire study population, but no overall survival benefit in the vaccine arm. This illustrates the difficulty matching patients with fairly advanced disease to historical controls.

Such prognostic pairing may be more representative in earlier stage disease, and the results of these analyses suggest a clinical benefit to vaccination in those stages. For patients with resected stage III melanoma a study of 739 pairs of patients matched for number of positive lymph nodes, nodal size, primary tumor stage, ulceration, gender and age, vaccine patients had a 5-year survival of 49% compared to 37% in controls (p<0.001, Figure 4) [65]. Median survival was 55.3 months and 31.6 months for the two groups, respectively. For patients with stage Ib/II melanoma 315 pairs of patients were matched for primary tumor stage, gender, ulceration, age, and initial treatment (wide excision, elective lymph node dissection or sentinel lymph node dissection). Again increased disease free and overall survival was seen (p=0.03) in the vaccine group. A phase III trial of Canvaxin has now completed accrual and sufficient follow-up for analysis is expected with the next 1–2 years.

Using an autologous vaccine, Berd et al. reported a phase II trial in which 214 patients who had undergone resection of bulky (>2.5 cm) melanoma in a single lymph node basin. Patients received an autologous tumor cells modified with the hapten dinitrophenol (DNP) [11]. Low-dose cyclophosphamide (300 mg/m^2)

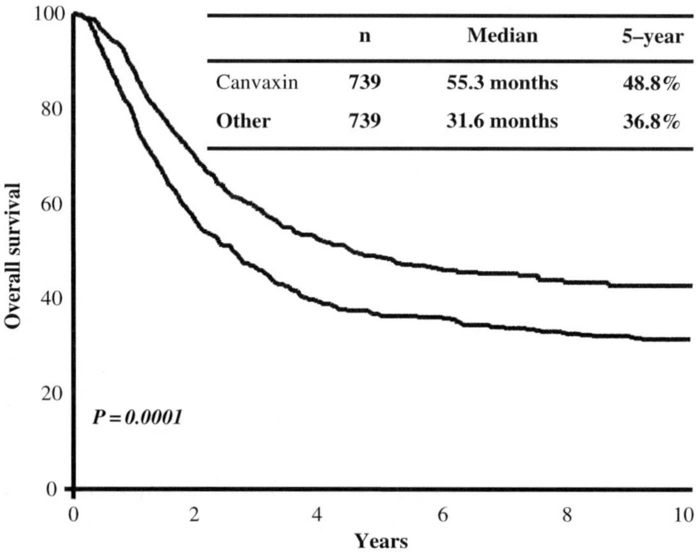

Figure 4. Overall survival of 739 patients with resected stage III melanoma who received Canvaxin and 739 patients matched for prognostic factors who did not (from [65])

was given in an attempt to deplete suppressor T cells, and was followed by multiple intradermal injections of autologous tumor cells mixed with BCG. Four vaccine schedules were examined. Five-year overall survival was 44%. Patients who developed DTH responses to unmodified tumor cells had a much greater overall survival than those who did not (59.3% vs. 29.3%; $P<0.001$). A comparison of patients treated with different schedules showed a significantly higher rate of DTH responses when baseline skin testing was performed 3 to 8 days prior to cyclophosphamide administration rather than on the same day or the day after. A significant difference was also seen in overall survival and the impact remained significant in a multivariate analysis that included the number of positive nodes, presence of extracapsular extension and gender.

This technology was being developed by AVAX technologies under the brand name of M-Vax™. However, due to a combination of financial and regulatory issues this development has stalled. These issues are indicative of the significant challenge associated with preparing autologous cellular vaccines. It is not yet clear whether this vaccine will resume testing.

Two randomized trials have also been conducted using an autologous colon cancer cell vaccine. One was conducted in Belgium and included 254 patients randomized to receive vaccine or no adjuvant treatment [66]. The first dose of the vaccine was given with BCG four weeks after surgical resection. After a median follow-up of 5.3 years, a significant reduction in risk of recurrence was seen for the vaccine group ($p=0.023$). There was no survival benefit seen for patients with stage III disease, but there was a trend approaching significance for stage II patients.

A second study was conducted by the Eastern Cooperative Oncology Group in 412 patients with resected colon cancer [67]. BCG was given with the first two vaccine doses. After 7.6 years of median follow-up, there was no survival benefit in the vaccine arm. However, in patients who were able to have adequate vaccine prepared and administered, and who developed DTH responses ($n=106$), there was a trend toward improved overall ($p=0.12$) and recurrence-free survival ($p=0.078$). When only stage II patients were analyzed, those with positive DTH responses had a significantly better overall survival ($p=0.032$). Taken together, lower tumor burden (stage II compared to III) sets a favorable immunological setting for induction of anti-tumor immunity by vaccination.

A randomized trial was performed using autologous tumor cells of patients with renal cell cancer [68]. The vaccine was given with BCG as an adjuvant. Patients received either hormonal therapy alone or hormonal therapy plus vaccine. After 3 years of follow-up, overall survival was 65% in the vaccine group and 52% in controls. This difference did not achieve statistical significance ($p<0.07$). Positive DTH skin tests correlated with improved survival.

Clinical Results: Tumor Lysate Vaccines

Although lysate-based vaccines have been investigated in patients with breast cancer, colon cancer, ovarian cancer, leukemia, renal cell cancer, lung cancer, sarcoma, and medullary thyroid cancer [69–75]. The largest trials have been conducted in melanoma. Two viral lysates and one mechanical lysate have been evaluated. Vaccinia melanoma oncolysate (VMO) was evaluated by Wallack and colleagues [76]. Four melanoma cell lines (Mel-2, Mel-3, Mel-4, and Mel-B) were infected with vaccinia and lysed by sonication. Two hundred seventeen eligible patients at eleven institutions were randomized to either VMO or vaccinia virus alone in this double-blind study. Overall survival in the vaccine group was 10% greater than in the controls, but this difference did not reach statistical significance. Retrospective subset analysis suggested male patients between 44 and 57 years old with one to five positive lymph nodes had a 21% improvement in survival. However, this benefit has not been prospectively validated.

A larger randomized lysate vaccine trial including 700 patients with stage IIB and III melanoma was conducted by Hersey and colleagues in Australia [77]. The vaccinia melanoma cell lysate (VMCL) used in this trial was an oncolysate of a single melanoma cell line, MM200. With a median follow-up of 8 years, survival vaccine and control groups were 61% and 55% respectively at five years, and 53% and 44% respectively at ten years. The differences in survival did not achieve statistical significance (p=0.17).

The Southwest Oncology Group performed another large (n=689) randomized trial using Melacine (Corixa Corp., Seattle, WA), a mechanical lysate of the MSM-M-2 and MSM-M-1 cell lines developed by Mitchell and colleagues [78]. Patients had clinically localized melanoma with primary tumors 1.5–4.0 mm in thickness or Clark's level IV. Vaccine was given with the DETOX adjuvant. With a median follow-up of 5.6 years there was no overall survival benefit; estimated 5-year survival rates were 65% for vaccine patients and 63% for controls (p=0.51).

Earlier phase II studies of Melacine in patients with measurable disease had shown objective response rates of 12% (3% complete, 5% partial, 4% minor) and stable disease in 23%. A randomized trial in patients with stage IV disease did not show a survival benefit versus chemotherapy [79] but suggested that patients with HLA types that matched those of the vaccine cell lines had improved clinical outcomes. Therefore, for the randomized trial in clinically localized melanoma, a planned subgroup analysis examined the survival of patients who expressed one or two of several HLA types (A2, A28, B44, B45, and C3) [80]. In these patients 5-year relapse-free survival was 83% for vaccine patients (n=97) versus 59% in controls (n=78)(p=0.0002). Much of this benefit came from patients who were HLA-A2$^+$ and/or HLA-C3$^+$: 5-year relapse-free survival of 77% for vaccine versus 63% for controls (p=0.004). A prospective validation trial for this finding was planned, but has not yet been conducted.

Clinical Results: Shed-antigen Vaccines

A vaccine consisting of shed antigens from melanoma cell lines has been evaluated in a randomized clinical trial. This vaccine, developed by Bystryn and colleagues, consists of material shed into culture supernatants of four melanoma cell lines, three allogeneic and one xenogeneic. Thirty-eight patients were randomized to receive either vaccine or placebo [81]. After a median follow-up of 2.5 years, the vaccine patients had a significantly longer time to disease progression (1.6 years versus 0.6 years, p=0.03). Median overall survival was 3.8 years in the treatment group and 2.7 years in the placebo group. Estimated 3-year survival was also higher in the treatment group than the control group (53% vs. 33%). However, the study was insufficiently powered to demonstrate statistical significance at this level of overall survival difference.

MONITORING WHOLE CELL VACCINE-INDUCED IMMUNE RESPONSES

The polyvalent nature of whole cell-based vaccines increases the likelihood of inclusion of relevant epitopes, and decreases the potential for tumor escape through antigen loss. However, immune responses to a polyvalent formulation are more difficult to monitor. Two approaches are possible: use of immune testing using the entire vaccine as a stimulus (e.g. DTH testing to vaccine cells), and selection of a "representative" antigen for monitoring.

The first approach has yielded significant correlations with clinical outcome in vaccine trials. Monitoring of Berd's autologous melanoma vaccine demonstrated that DTH responsiveness (>5mm) to unmodified tumor cells (but not DNP-modified cells) predicted improved overall survival (p<0.001) [11]. Immune responses to Canvaxin have also been evaluated with DTH testing to the entire vaccine. A examination of responses in patients with resected stage IV melanoma showed that patients with a positive (>10mm) DTH response to vaccine cells had significantly prolonged overall survival (p=0.018)(Figure 5) [82].

Humoral responses can also be evaluated without reference to a specific antigen. Hsueh and colleagues using a complement-dependent cytotoxicity assay to monitor immune responses to Canvaxin. Vaccine cells were incubated with pre- or post-vaccination patient serum and then complement. Increased lysis by post-vaccination serum suggested increased complement fixing antibody, and correlated with significantly better 5-year disease-free survival (54% versus 14%, p=0.0001) [83].

Alternatively, immune responses to specific antigens may be monitored. This allows for monitoring by a wide variety of assays including humoral responses monitored by ELISA, cellular responses monitored by ELISPOT, intracellular cytokine secretion, cytotoxicity assays, and MHC tetramer flow cytometry [84]. Serum IgM responses to the TA90 tumor-associated antigen have been correlated with overall survival in patients receiving vaccine for stage III and stage IV melanoma. When the results of the TA90 antibody assay are combined with the results of DTH testing, there is a dramatic correlation between immune response and survival: 5-year OS rate is 75% with both an elevated level of anti-TA90 IgM and a strong DTH response, 36% with either an elevated IgM response or a strong DTH response, and only 8% with neither response (p<0.001, figure 6) [85]. Survival did not correlate with responses to the BCG adjuvant as determined by purified protein derivative (PPD) testing, suggesting that the benefit is not a measure of

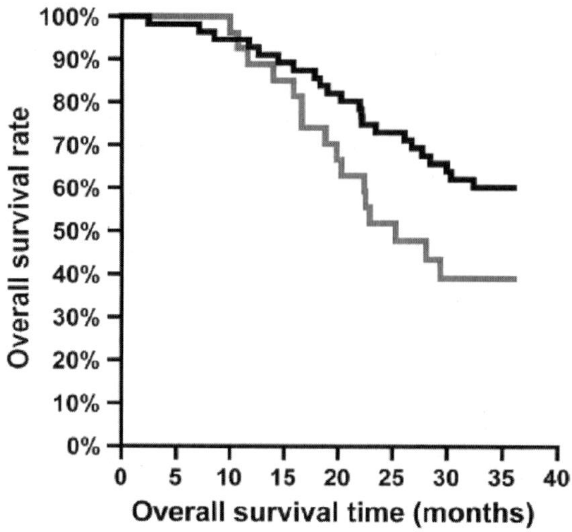

Figure 5. Overall survival of patients with stage IV melanoma treated with Canvaxin according to positive (>10 mm induration, n = 56) or negative (n=38, p = 0.0178) DTH response (from [82])

simple immune competence. This association remains significant in multivariate analysis (p=0.03).

One difficulty with choosing a particular defined antigen is that the selection of antigens for response by patient's immune system is impossible to predict.

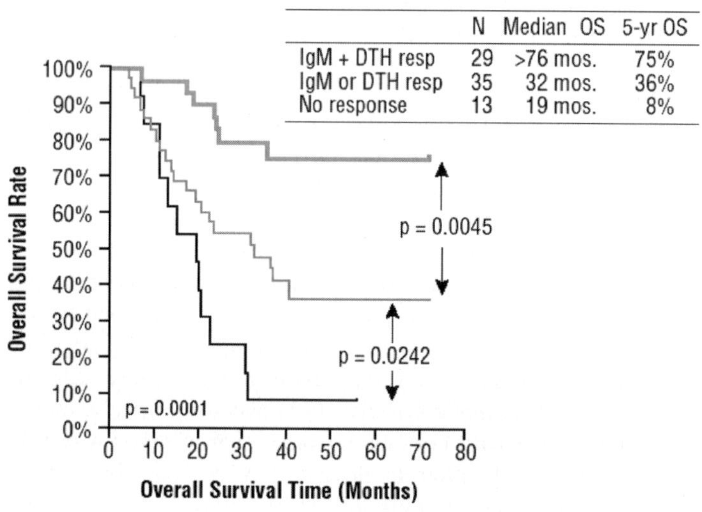

Figure 6. Overall survival of patients with stage IV melanoma treated with Canvaxin according to immune (DTH and anti-TA90 IgM) responses (from [85]).

Responses may be generated to a wide variety of protein and carbohydrate antigens. As described above, Reynolds et al examined the variety of epitopes from several melanoma-associated proteins to which patients vaccinated with a polyvalent shed antigen vaccine responded [6]. They found that no more than 14% of individuals responded to any given peptide epitope. Thus, selecting a "representative" peptide epitope for cellular immune response monitoring may be impossible for highly polyvalent antigens. Development of high-throughput monitoring assays may improve investigators' ability to measure responses to numerous antigens and derive a more accurate assessment of the immunologic results of vaccination.

CONCLUSION

Whole tumor cells are an attractive source of tumor antigens for use in immunotherapy. They provide the broadest array of antigens and presumably the best chance for matching vaccine antigens with patients' tumor cells. A wide variety of active specific immunotherapy strategies use whole cells as antigen sources. A great deal of evidence now suggests that these vaccines can provide clinical benefit to patients, particularly those who generate a strong immune response to vaccination. One current challenge is to improve the frequency, magnitude, and character of immune responses using new, more effective adjuvants and immune response modifiers. The practical challenges of preparing these complex biologic agents has slowed the development of several promising vaccines, but large trials of whole cell and other vaccines are currently underway, and hold promise for wider and more effective use of these agents.

ACKNOWLEDGEMENT

Supported in part by grants CA12582 and CA76489 from the National Cancer Institute and by funding from the Wayne and Gladys Valley Foundation (Oakland, CA) and the Harold McAlister Charitable Foundation (Los Angeles, CA).

REFERENCES

1. Coley W. Treatment of inoperable malignant tumors with the toxins of erysipelas and the bacillus prodigiosus. Trans Am Surg Assoc 1894; 12:183.
2. Coley W. The therapeutic value of the mixed toxins of the streptococcus of erysipelas and the bacillus prodigiousus. Am J Med Sci 1896; 112:251–281.
3. Gross L. Intradermal immunization of C3H mice against sarcoma that originated in an animal of the same line. Cancer Res 1943; 3:326–33.
4. Riker A, Cormier J, Panelli M, et al. Immune selection following antigen specific immunotherapy of melanoma. Surgery 1999; 126(2):112–20.
5. Dudley M, Wunderlich J, Yang J, et al. Adoptive cell transfer therapy following non-myeloablative but lymphodepleting chemotherapy for the treatment of patients with refractory metastatic melanoma. J Clin Oncol 2005; 23(10):2346–57.
6. Reynolds S, Celis E, Sette A, et al. HLA-independent heterogeneity of CD8+ T cell responses to MAGE-3, Melan-A/MART-1, gp100, tyrosinase, MC1R, and TRP-2 in vaccine-treated melanoma patients. J Immunol 1998; 161:6970–6976.

7. Berd D. M-Vax: an autologous, hapten-modified vaccine for human cancer. Expert Opin Biol Ther 2002; 2(3):335–42.
8. Dillman R, Weimann M, Nayak S, et al. Interferon-gamma or granulocyte-macrophage colony-stimulating factor adminstered as adjuvants with a vaccine of irradiated autologous tumor cells from short-term cell line cultures: a randomized phase 2 trial of the cancer biotherapy research group. J Immunother 2003; 26(4):367–73.
9. Mazzaferrro V, Coppa J, Carrabba M, et al. Vaccination with autologous tumor-derived heat-shock protein gp96 after liver resection for metastatic colorectal cancer. Clin Cancer Res 2003; 9(9):3235–45.
10. Coca A, Dorrance G, Lebredo M. Vaccination in cancer: a report of the results of vaccination therapy as applied to seventy-nine cases of human cancer. Journal of Immunology and Experimental Therapeutics 1912; 13:543–51.
11. Berd D, Sato T, Maguire H, et al. Immunopharmacologic analysis of an autologous, hapten-modified human melanoma vaccine. J Clin Oncol 2004; 22(3):403–15.
12. Morton D, Barth A. Vaccine therapy for malignant melanoma. CA Cancer J Clin 1996; 46(4):225–44.
13. Ackerman A, Cresswell P. Cellular mechanisms governing cross-presentation of exogenous antigens. Nat Immunol 20004; 5(7):678–84.
14. Mitchell M. Perspective on allogeneic melanoma lysates in active specific immunotherapy. Semin Oncol 1998; 25(6):623–35.
15. Marcove R, Southam C, Levin A, al e. A clinical trial of autogenous vaccine in osteogenic sarcoma in patients under the age of twenty-five. *In* Mathe G, Weiner R, eds. Investigation and stimulation of immunity in cancer patients. New York: Springer-Verlag, 1974.
16. Lindenmann J, Klein P. Viral oncolysis: increased immunogenicity of host cell antigen associated with influenza virus. J Exp Med 1967; 126:93.
17. Bystryn J. Shedding and degradation of cell-surface macromolecules and tumor-associated antigens by human melanoma. *In* Reisfeld R, Ferrone S, eds. Melanoma antigens and antibodies. New York: Plenum Press, 1982. pp. 37–52.
18. Lore K, Betts M, Brenchley J, et al. Toll-like recpetor ligands modulate dendritic cells to augment Cytomegalovirus- and HIV-1-specific T cell responses. J Immunol 2003; 171:4320–8.
19. Dockrell D, Kinghorn G. Imiquimod and resiquimod as novel immunomodulators. J Antimicrob Chemother 2001; 48:751–5.
20. Pulendran B, Bancheereau J, Burkeholder S, et al. Flt3-ligand and granulocyte colony-stimulating factor mobilize distinct human dendritic cell subsets in vivo. J Immunol 2000; 165(1):566–72.
21. Steinman R, Cohn Z. Identification of a novel cell type in peripheral lymphoid organs of mice: Morphology, quantitation, tissue distribution. J Exp Med 1973; 137(5):1142–62.
22. Czerniecki B, Cohen P, Faries M, et al. Diverse functional activity of CD83+ monocyte-derived dendritic cells and the implications for cancer vaccines. Critical Rev Immunol 2001; 21(1–3):157–78.
23. Faries M, Bedrosian I, Xu S, et al. Calcium signaling inhibits interleukin-12 production and activates CD83+ dendritic cells that induce Th2 cell development. Blood 2001; 98:2489–2497.
24. Bedrosian I, Mick R, Xu S, et al. Intranodal administration of peptide-pulsed mature dendritic cell vaccines results in superior CD8+ T-cell function in melanoma patients. J Clin Oncol 2003; 21(20):3826–3835.
25. Nestle F, Alijagic S, Gilliet M, et al. Vaccination of melanoma patients with peptide or tumor lysate-pulsed dendritic cells. Nat Med 1998; 4(3):269–70.
26. Dranoff G, Mulligan R. Gene transfer as cancer therapy. Adv Immunol 1995; 58(417–54).
27. Mascarenhas L, Stripecke R, Case S, et al. Gene delivery to human B-precursor acute lymphoblastic leukemia cells. Blood 1998; 92(10):3537–45.
28. Micka B, Trojaneck B, Niemitz S, et al. Comparison of non-viral transfection methods in melanoma primary cell cultures. Cytokine 2000; 12(6):828–33.
29. Lundqvist A, Noffz G, Pavlenko M, et al. Nonviral and viral gene transfer into different subsets of human dendritic cells yield comparable efficiency of transfection. J Immunother 2003; 25(6):445–54.

30. Karre K, Ljunggren H, Piontek G, Kiessling R. Selective rejection of h-2-deficient lymphoma variants suggests alternative defense strategy. Nature 1986; 391(6055):675–8.
31. Huang A, Bruce A, Pardoll D, Levitsky H. Does B7–1 expression confer antigen-presenting cell capacity to tumors in vivo? J Exp Med 1996; 183(3):769–76.
32. Horig H, Lee D, Conkright W, et al. Phase I clinical trial of a recombinant canarypoxvirus (ALVAC) vaccine expressing human carcinoembryonic antigen and the B7.1 co-stimulatory molecule. Cancer Immunol Immunother 2000; 49(9):504–14.
33. vonMehren M, Arlen P, Tsang K, et al. Pilot study of a dual gene recombinant avipox vaccine containing both carcinoembryonic antigen (CEA) and B7.1 transgenes in patients with recurrent CEA-expressing adneocarcinomas. Clin Cancer Res 2000; 6(6):2219–28.
34. Belli F, Arienti F, Sule-Suso J, et al. Active immunization of metastatic melanoma patients with interleukin-2-transduced allogeneic melanoma cells: evaluation of efficacy and tolerability. Cancer Immunol Immunother 1997; 44(4):197–203.
35. Osanto S, Brouwenstyn N, Vaessen N, et al. Immunization with interleukin-2 transfected melanoma cells. A phase I-II study in patients with metastatic melanoma. Hum Gene Ther 1993; 4(3):323–30.
36. Schreiber S, Kampgen E, wagner E, et al. Immunotherapy of metastatic malignant melanoma by a vaccine consisting of autologous interleukin-2-transfected cancer cells: outcome of a phase I study. Hum Gene Ther 1999; 10(6):983–93.
37. Arienti F, Belli F, Napolitano F, et al. Vaccination of melanoma patients with interleukin 4 gene-transduced allogeneic melanoma cells. Hum Gene Ther 2000; 10(18):2907–16.
38. Suminami Y, Elder E, Lotze M, Whiteside T. In situ interleukin-4 gene expression in cancer patients treated with genetically modified tumor vaccine. J Immunother Emphasis Tumor Immunol 1995; 17(4):238–48.
39. Maio M, Fonsatti E, Lamaj E, et al. Vaccination of stage IV patients with allogeneic IL-4- or IL-2-transduced melanoma cells generates functional antibodies against vaccinating and autologous melanoma cells. Cancer Immunol Immunother 2002; 51(1):9–14.
40. Mackiewicz A, Gorny A, Laciak M, et al. Gene therapy of human melanoma. Immunization of patients with autologous tumor cells secreting interleukin-6 and soluable interleukin-6 receptor. Hum Gene Ther 1995; 6:805–11.
41. Moller P, Sun Y, Dorbic T, et al. Vaccination with IL-7 gene-modified autologous melanoma cells can enhance the anti-melanoma lytic activity in peripheral blood of patients with good clinical performance status: a phase I clinical study. Br J Cancer 1998; 77(11):1907–16.
42. Sun Y, Jurgovsky K, Moller P, et al. Vaccination with IL-12 gene-modified autologous melanoma cells: preclinical results and a first clinical phase I study. Gene Ther 1998; 5(4):481–90.
43. Asada H, Kishida T, Hirai H, et al. Significant antitumor effects obtained by autologous tumor cell vaccine engineered to secrete interleukin (IL)-12 and IL-18 by means of the EBV/lipoplex. Mol Ther 2002; 5(5):609–16.
44. Abdel-Wahab Z, Weltz C, Hester D, et al. A phase I clinical trial of immunotherapy with interferon-gamma gene-modified autologous melnaoma cells: monitoring the humoral immune response. Cancer 1997; 80(3):401–12.
45. Ellem K, O'Rourke M, Johnson G, et al. A case report: immune responses and clinical course of the first human use of granulocyte/macrophage-colony-stimulating factor-transduced autologous melanoma cells for immunotherapy. Cancer Immunol Immunother 1997; 44(1):10–20.
46. Soiffer R, Hodi F, Haluska F, et al. Vaccination with irradiated, autologous melanoma cells engineered to secrete granulocyte-macrophage colony-stimulating factor by adenoviral-mediated gene transfer augments antitumor immunity in patients with metastatic melanoma. J Clin Oncol 2003; 21(17):3343–50.
47. Salgia R, Lynch T, Skarin A, et al. Vaccination with irradiated autologous tumor cells engineered to secrete granulocyte-macrophage colony-stimulating factor augments antitumor immunity in some patients with metastatic non-small-cell lung carcinoma. J Clin Oncol 2003; 21(4):624–30.
48. Palmer K, Moore J, Everard M, et al. Gene therapy with autologous, interleukin 2-secreting tumor cells in patients with malignant melanoma. Hum Gene Ther 1999; 10(8):1261–8.

49. Hirschowitz E, Foody T, Kryscio R, et al. Autologous dendritic cell vaccines for non-small-cell lung cancer. J Clin Oncol 2004; 22(14):2808–15.
50. Ip W, Lau Y. Distinct maturation of, but not migration between, human monocyte-derived dendritic cells upon ingestion of apoptotic cells of early or late phases. J Immunol 2004; 173(1):189–96.
51. Kacani L, Wurm M, Schwentner I, et al. Maturation of dendritic cells in the presence of living, apoptotic and necrotic tumour cells derived from squamous cell carcinoma of head and neck. Oral Oncol 2005; 41(1):17–24.
52. Chen Z, Moyana T, Saxena A, et al. Efficient antitumor immunity derived from maturation of dendritic cells that had phagocytosed apoptotic/necrotic tumor cells. Int J Cancer 2001; 93(4):539–48.
53. Pietra G, Mortarini R, Parmiani G, Anichini A. Phases of apoptosis of melanoma cells, but not of normal melanocytes differently affect maturation of myeloid dendritic cells. Cancer Res 2001; 61(22):8218–26.
54. Hirao M, Onai N, Hiroishi K, et al. CC chemokine receptor-7 on dendritic cells is induced after interaction with apoptotic tumor cells: critical role in migration from the tumor site to draining lymph nodes. Cancer Res 2000; 60(8):2209–17.
55. Salio M, Cerundolo V, Lanzavecchia A. Dendritic cell maturation is induced by mycoplasma infection but not by necrotic cells. Eur J Immunol 2000; 30(2):705–8.
56. Dalgaard J, Beckstrom K, Jahnsen F, Brinchmann J. Differential capability for phagocytosis of apoptotic and necrotic leukemia cells by human peripheral blood dendritic cells subsets. J Leukoc Biol 2005; Epub ahead of print.
57. Krause S, Neumann C, Soruri A, et al. The treatment of patients with disseminated malignant melanoma by vaccination with autologous cell hybrids of tumor cells and dendritic cells. J Immunother 2002; 25(5):421–8.
58. Kikuchi T, Akasaki Y, Irie M, et al. Results of a phase I clinical trial of vaccination of glioma patients with fusions of dendritic and glioma cells. Cancer Immunol Immunother 2001; 50(7):337–44.
59. Parkhurst M, DePan C, Riley J, et al. Hybrids of dendritic cells and tumor cells generated by electrofusion simultaneously present immunodominant epitopes from multiple human tumor-associated antigens in the context of MHC class I and class II molecules. J Immunol 2003; 170(10):5317–25.
60. Kuriyama H, Shimizu K, Lee W, et al. Therapeutic vaccine generated by electrofusion of dendritic cells and tumour cells. Dev Biol 2004; 116:169–78.
61. Avigan D, Vasir B, Gong J, et al. Fusion cell vaccination of patients with metastatic breast and renal cell cancer induces immunological and clinical responses. Clin Cancer Res 2004; 10(14):4699–708.
62. Trevor K, Cover C, Ruiz Y, et al. Generation of dendritic cell-tumor cell hybrids by electrofusion for clinical vaccine application. Cancer Immunol Immunother 2004; 53(8):705–14.
63. Shimizu K, Kuriyama H, Kjaergaard J, et al. Comparative analysis of antigen loading strategies of dendritic cells for tumor immunotherapy. J Immunother 2004; 27(4):265–72.
64. Faries M, Morton D. Melanoma: Is immunotherapy of benefit? Advances in Surgery 2003; 37:139–169.
65. Morton DL, Hsueh EC, Essner R, et al. Prolonged survival of patients receiving active immunotherapy with Canvaxin therapeutic polyvalent vaccine after complete resection of melanoma metastatic to regional lymph nodes. Ann Surg 2002; 236: 438–48.
66. Vermorken J, Claessen A, vanTinteren H, et al. Active specific immunotherapy for stage II and stage III human colon cancer: a randomised trial. Lancet 1999; 353(9150):345–50.
67. Harris J, Ryan L, Hoover H, et al. Adjuvant active specific immunotherapy for stage II and III colon cancer with an autologous tumor cell vaccine: Eastern Cooperative Oncology Group study E5283. J Clin Oncol 2000; 18(1):148–57.
68. Adler A, Gillon G, Lurie H, et al. Active specific immunotherapy of renal cell carcinoma patients: a prospective randomized study of hormono-immuno-versus hormonotherapy. Preliminary report of immunological and clinical aspects. J Biol Response Mod 1987; 6(6):610–24.
69. Lytle G, McGee J, Yamanashi W, et al. Five-year survival in breast cancer treated with adjuvant immunotherapy. Am J Surg 1994; 168(1):19–21.

70. Hollinshead A. Active specific immunotherapy and immunochemotherapy in the treatment of lung and colon cancer. Semin Surg Oncol 1991; 7(4):199–210.
71. Hernando J, Park T, Kubler K, et al. Vaccination with autologous tumour antigen-pulsed dendritic cells in advanced gynecologic malignancies: clinical and immunological evaluation of a phase I trial. Cancer Immunol Immunother 2002; 51(1):45–52.
72. Kaminski E, Goddard R, Prentice A. Dendritic cells and their potential therapeutic role in haemoatological malignancy. Leuk Lymphoma 2003; 44(10):1657–66.
73. Alth G, Denck H, Fischer M, et al. Aspects of the immunologic treatment of lung cancer. Cancer Chemother Rep [3] 1973; 4(2):271–4.
74. Geiger J, Hutchinson R, Hohenkirk L, et al. Vaccination of pediatric solid tumor patients with tumor lysate-pulsed dendritic cells can expand specific T cells and mediate tumor regression. Cancer Res 2001; 61(23):8513–9.
75. Stift A, Sachet M, Yagubian R, et al. Dendritic cell vaccination in medullary thyroid carcinoma. Clin Cancer Res 2004; 10(9):2944–53.
76. Wallack M, Sivanandham M, Balch C, et al. Surgical adjuvant active specific immunotherapy for patients with stage III melanoma: the final analysis of data from a phase III, randomized, double-blind, multicenter vaccinia melanoma oncolysate trial. J Am Coll Surg 1998; 187(1):69–77.
77. Hersey P, Coates A, McCarthy W, et al. Adjuvant immunotherapy of patients with high-risk melanoma using vaccinia viral lysates of melanoma: results of a randomized trial. J Clin Oncol 2002; 20:4148–4190.
78. Sondak V, Liu P, Tuthill R, et al. Adjuvant immunotherapy or resected, intermediate-thickness, node-negative melanoma with an allogeneic tumor vaccine: overall results of a randomized trial of the Southwest Oncology Group. J Clin Oncol 2002; 20:2058–2066.
79. Vaishampayan U, Abrams J, Darrah D, et al. Active immunotherapy of metastatic melanoma with allogeneic melanoma lysates and interferon alpha. Clin Cancer Res 2002; 8(12):3696–701.
80. Sosman J, Unger J, Liu P, et al. Adjuvant immunotherapy of resected, intermediate-thickness, node-negative melanoma with an allogeneic tumor vaccine: Impact of HLA class I antigen epression on outcome. J Clin Oncol 2002; 20(8):2067–2075.
81. Bystryn J, Zeleniuch-Jacquotte A, Oratz R, et al. Double-blind trial of a polyvalent, shed-antigen melanoma vaccine. Clin Cancer Res 2001; 7:1882.
82. Hsueh E, Essner R, Foshag L, et al. Active immunotherapy by reinduction with a polyvalent allogeneic cell vaccine correlates with improved survival in recurrent metastatic melanoma. Ann Surg Oncol 2002; 9(5):486–92.
83. Hsueh E, Famatiga E, Gupta R, et al. Enhancement of complement-dependent cytotoxicity by polyvalent melanoma cell vaccine (CancerVax): correlation with survival. Ann Surg Oncol 1998; 5(7):595–602.
84. Keiholz U, Weber J, Finke J, et al. Immunologic monitoring of cancer vaccine therapy: results of a workshop sponsored by the Society for Biological Therapy. J Immunother 2002; 25(2):97–138.
85. Hsueh EC, Gupta RK, Qi K, et al. Correlation of specific immune responses with survival in melanoma patients with distant metastases receiving polyvalent melanoma cell vaccine. J Clin Oncol 1998; 16: 2913–20.

CHAPTER 13

CARBOHYDRATE VACCINES AGAINST CANCER

PHILIP O. LIVINGSTON* AND GOVIND RAGUPATHI

Laboratory of Tumor Vaccinology, Department of Medicine
Memorial Sloan-Kettering Cancer Center
1275 York Avenue
New York, NY 10021

Keywords: polyvalent, cancer, vaccine, antibody, conjugate, ganglioside, mucin, adjuvant

THE RATIONALE FOR CANCER VACCINES AGAINST CARBOHYDRATE ANTIGENS

Carbohydrate cell surface antigens have proved to be unexpectedly potent targets for immune recognition and attack against cancers [1]. Of the many tumor-restricted monoclonal antibodies derived by immunization of mice with human tumor cells, most have been directed against carbohydrate antigens expressed at the cell surface as glycolipids or mucins [2–4]. Antibodies against cell surface antigens such as these are ideally suited for eradication of free tumor cells and micrometastases. In adjuvant immunization trials, the primary targets are individual tumor cells or early micrometastases which may persist for long periods after apparent resection of all residual tumor [5–7]. After surgery and completion of chemotherapy is the ideal time for immune intervention, and in particular for administration of cancer vaccines aimed at instructing the immune system to identify and kill these few remaining cancer cells. If antibodies of sufficient titer can be induced against tumor antigens to eliminate tumor cells from the blood and lymphatic systems, and to eradicate micrometastases (making establishment of new metastases no longer possible) this

*E-mail: livingsp@mskcc.org

Consultant and shareholder for Progenics Pharmaceuticals Inc. (GM2) and Australian Cancer Technologies. (GPI-0100)

H.L. Kaufman and J.D. Wolchok (eds.), General Principles of Tumor Immunotherapy, 297–317.

would dramatically change our approach to treating the cancer patient. Aggressive local therapies, including surgery, radiation therapy and intralesional treatments might result in long term control of even metastatic cancers.

In fact, antibodies have demonstrated antitumor efficacy *in vivo*:

1 There are many preclinical models demonstrating that passively administered or actively induced antibodies (generally against carbohydrate antigens) can prevent tumor recurrence (reviewed in [8–10]) .
2 There are an increasing number of clinical trials where passively administered monoclonal antibodies (mAb) have demonstrated clinical efficacy, and
3 Naturally acquired or vaccine induced antibodies against cancer cell surface antigens, especially carbohydrate antigens, have correlated with improved prognosis in several different clinical settings (reviewed in [11–16]).

BIOLOGICAL ROLES OF CELL SURFACE CARBOHYDRATES

The great majority of the molecules on the mammalian plasma membrane are glycosylated such that glycan structures form a dense forest covering the cell surface. These glycan chains are found on glycolipids and integral membrane glycoproteins as well as on more specialized glycoproteins such as mucins and proteoglycans. To some extent these carbohydrates serve structural, protective and stabilizing roles but it is becoming increasingly recognized that they can have information-bearing functions as selectins and adhesins in cell-cell recognition and adhesion as well (reviewed in [3]). Carbohydrate structures on glycoproteins and glycolipids have been implicated in such normal cell functions as proliferation, interaction with endothelial cells, leukocytes and platelets, embryogenesis, neural cell adhesion, and the biology and metastatic potential of tumor cells. All tumors studied have changes in the expression of carbohydrate structures which are characteristic of the tissue of origin of the tumor. As a general rule, tumors of neural crest origin (e.g. melanoma, sarcoma and neuroblastoma) exhibit over-expression of gangliosides (sialylated glycolipids) whereas epithelial cancers (carcinomas) have altered fucosylated structures (Le^y and Globo H) and mucin core structures (TF, Tn, sTn) as their characteristic antigens. Numerous studies have shown a correlation between high expression of certain carbohydrate specificities (including Le^y, sTn and Tn blood group antigens) and metastatic potential and decreased patient survival.

EFFECTOR MECHANISMS OF ANTIBODIES AGAINST CELL SURFACE CARBOHYDRATE ANTIGENS

Mechanisms of Tumor Elimination Some antibodies may have direct effects such as by inhibiting tumor cell attachment or inhibiting growth hormone receptors, but in general the interaction of antibody and antigen is without consequence unless Fc-mediated secondary effector mechanisms are activated. Binding of antibody to antigen results in a functional change in the Fc portion of the antibody and activation of several effector mechanisms. For cancer carbohydrate antigens, IgM bound to antigen is the most active complement activator in the intravascular space and in humans IgG1 and IgG3 are the most important complement activators extravascularly. IgG antibodies of these subclasses are also known to induce antibody dependent cell mediated cytotoxicity (ADCC). Complement activation mediates inflammatory reactions, opsonization for phagocytosis, clearance of antigen antibody complexes from the circulation and complement-dependent cytotoxicity (CDC) mediated by membrane attack complex (CDC). Opsonization for ingestion and destruction by phagocytosis or cytotoxic mechanism can occur through complement activation but also can occur directly as a consequence of Fc receptors on phagocytic cells (ADCC).

Serological analysis of the series of clinical trials described below has suggested that the six vaccines containing carbohydrate antigens expressed as glycolipids induced antibodies mediating CDC whereas the four vaccines containing carbohydrate or peptide epitopes carried by mucin molecules induced antibodies that were not capable of mediating CDC. To determine whether this dichotomy was a result of the properties of the induced antibodies (ie. class and effector functions), the different target cells used, or the nature of the target antigens, we compared the cell surface reactivity (assayed by FACS), complement-fixing ability (using the immune adherence assay) and the CDC activity of a panel of monoclonal antibodies and immune sera from these trials on the same two tumor cell lines. Antibodies against carbohydrates expressed on glycolipids (GM2, globo H and Le^Y) or on mucins (Tn, sTn and TF) all reacted with these antigens expressed on tumor cells and all fixed and activated complement [17]. CDC, however, was mediated by antibodies against the glycolipids and a globular protein (KSA), but not by antibodies against the mucin antigens. The inability of antibodies against mucin antigens to induce CDC is attributed to the great distance from the cell surface that complement activation is occurring [17].

It must be emphasized that although we showed that mucins are poor targets for complement-mediated lysis of tumor cells, studies have shown that induction of antibodies against either glycolipid or mucin antigens results in protection from tumor recurrence in several different preclinical mouse models (reviewed in [8,9]). Also, antibodies against either glycolipid or mucin epitopes correlate with a more favorable prognosis in patients [11–15]. It does not appear that the inability of antibodies against mucin antigens to induce complement-mediated lysis is necessarily detrimental to the anti-tumor response. Consequently, complement-mediated inflammation, opsonization and antibody dependent cellular cytotoxicity but not CDC are likely mechanisms for the prolonged survival seen in the preclinical experiments targeting mucin antigens and suggested in the clinical trials with passively administered and actively induced antibodies against mucin antigens. With regard to bacterial infections, this is supported by the severe consequences of hereditary deficiency states involving either the classical or alternate complement pathways and the comparatively trivial consequences to deficiencies of the complement membrane attack complex [18].

TREATMENT IN THE ADJUVANT SETTING

The basis for emphasis on vaccination in the adjuvant setting is best demonstrated in preclinical models. The syngeneic murine tumor models involving EL4 lymphoma are particularly informative in terms of trial design [9]. EL4 lymphoma naturally expresses GD2 ganglioside which is recognized by mAb 3F8. Vaccines containing GD2 covalently conjugated to KLH and mixed with immunological adjuvant QS21 are optimal for vaccination against GD2. Relatively higher levels of mAb administered two or four days after intravenous tumor challenge or moderate titers induced by vaccine that were present by day four after tumor challenge were able to eradicate disease in most mice. If mAb administration was deferred until day seven or ten after *i.v* challenge, little or no benefit could be demonstrated. If the number of cells in the EL4 challenge was decreased, giving a longer window of opportunity, the vaccinations could be initiated after tumor challenge and good protection seen [9]. These results are consistent with the need to initiate immunization with vaccines inducing antibodies in the adjuvant setting, when the targets are circulating tumor cells and micrometastases.

Comparable benefit is also seen when a subcutaneous foot-pad tumor challenge model which more closely mirrors the clinical setting is used. Vaccination or mAb administration after amputation of the foot-pad primary tumor results in cure of most mice. There are comparable syngeneic models demonstrating the anti-tumor efficacy of mAbs or vaccines against other glycolipids (GD3, GM3), mucin antigens (Tn, TF and MUC1) and a protein antigen (gp75) (reviewed in [1, 8, 9]). These trials all share one thing in common, benefit is seen primarily in minimal disease settings, comparable to the adjuvant setting in the clinic.

SELECTION OF CELL SURFACE CARBOHYDRATE ANTIGENS AS TARGETS FOR IMMUNE ATTACK AGAINST CANCER

Carbohydrate cell surface cancer antigens the MSKCC experience We have screened a variety of malignancies and normal tissues with a series of 40 monoclonal antibodies against 25 antigens which were potential target antigens for immunotherapy [19–22]. Twelve defined antigens were expressed strongly in 50% or more of biopsy specimens of breast, ovary, prostate cancer, melanoma, sarcoma and small cell lung cancer (SCLC). With the exception of the mucin MUC1 peptide backbone and the protein KSA, the widely expressed antigens were carbohydrates. The prevalence of these ten carbohydrate antigens on these cancers is summarized in Table 1. The 13 excluded antigens (including CEA and HER2/neu) were expressed in 0-2 of the 5-10 specimens.

Our results are consistent with those from other centers with one exception, we did not find increased levels of GD2 or GD3 in most SCLC specimens. There is a striking similarity in expression of these 12 antigens among tumors of similar embryologic background (ie. epithelial versus neuroectodermal). Epithelial cancers (breast, ovary, prostate colon, etc) but not cancers of neuroectodermal origin (melanomas,

Table 1. Proportion of Tumor Specimens with 50% or more of Cells Positive by Immunohistology

	Cell Surface Carbohydrate Antigens									
Antigen	STn	Tn	TF	Globo H	Le^Y	GM2	GD2	GD3	FUC GM1	Polysialic acid
mAb	CC49	IE3	49H.8	MBr1	BR96	696	3F8	R24	F12	735
Tumor										
Breast	5/10*	5/10	6/10	4/5	7/10	5/5	0/5	0/5	0/5	0/6
Ovary	4/5	1/5	5/5	3/5	5/5	5/5	0/5	0/5	0/5	0/5
Prostate	6/11	10/11	10/11	2/11	4/11	11/11	0/5	0/5	0/5	0/5
Melanoma	0/5	0/5	0/5	0/10	0/5	10/10	6/10	8/10	0/10	0/6
Sarcoma	0/5	0/5	0/5	0/5	0/5	8/9	5/9	4/9	0/0	1/5
Small cell lung cancer	0/5	0/5	0/5	4/6	2/5	6/6	0/6	0/6	4/6	6/6

*Number of tumor specimens positive/number of tumor specimens tested.

sarcomas, neuroblastomas) expressed MUC1, Tn, sTn, TF, globo H and Lewis^y (Le^y) while only the neuroectodermal cancers expressed GD2 and GD3. Small cell lung cancer shared some characteristics of each and in addition expressed fucosyl GM1 and long chains of poly-α2,8-sialic acid which were not expressed in other cancers of either background.

Gangliosides GM2, GD2, GD3 and Fucosyl GM1 Gangliosides are sialic acid containing glycolipids that are expressed at the cell surface with their lipid (ceramide) moiety incorporated into the cell surface lipid bilayer. Most gangliosides considered as potential targets for cancer therapy are expressed primarily in tissues and tumors of neuroectodermal origin. This is true for the melanoma, sarcoma and neuroblastoma antigens GM2, GD2 and GD3, and the SCLC antigen fucosyl GM1. The structures of these antigens as they appear on the cell surface lipid bilayer are shown in Figure 1. Surprisingly, however, GM2 has also recently been identified in a number of epithelial cancers [23, 24] and at the luminal surfaces of a variety of normal epithelial tissues.

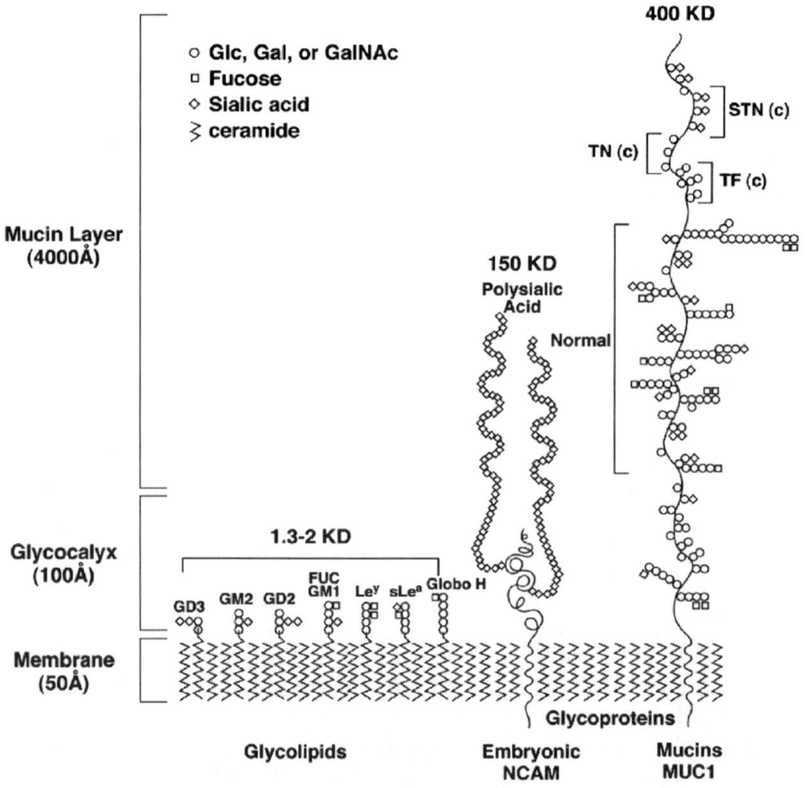

Figure 1. Carbohydrate epitopes on cell membrane glycoconjugates. Glc, glucose, Gal, galactose; GalNAc, N-acetyl galactosamine; NCAM neural cell adhesion molecule

Neutral glycolipids Lewis^y and Globo H Le^y and Globo H antigens are found at the cell surface of epithelial cancers primarily expressed as glycolipids attached to the lipid bilayer by hydrophobic forces through the ceramide, but they are also O-linked via -OH groups of serine or threonine to mucins and N-linked via the NH_2 group of asparagine in other proteins [2,4,20]. Whether expressed as glycolipids or glycoproteins, the immune response against these antigens is predominantly against the carbohydrate moiety. The expression of Le^y and Globo H on various types of cancer cells has been well documented [25–28]. They are expressed in lesser amounts on a variety of normal tissues, again at the lumen border of ducts and in secretions as described for TF and sTn [4]. Monoclonal antibodies against each have shown good localization to human cancers *in vivo* [29, 30]. The structures of Le^y and Globo H in their glycolipid form at the cell surface are suggested in Figure 1.

TF, Tn and sTn antigens Mucins are major cell surface antigens on most epithelial cancers. They are proteins that contain multiple copies of highly glycosylated serine and threonine rich tandem repeats that extend thousands of angstroms above the cell surface lipid bilayer [31, 32]. Though mucins (including carbohydrate and peptide epitopes) are also expressed on some normal tissues they have proved to be excellent targets for anti-cancer attack for two reasons: 1) Expression on normal tissues is largely restricted to the ductal border of secretory cells [21, 31, 32], a site largely inaccessible to the immune system. Cancer cells, on the other hand, have no patent ducts and so accumulate mucins over the entire cell surface. 2) Peptide backbones of cancer mucins are not fully glycosylated and glycosylation that does occur is not complete. Glycosylation of cancer mucins with mono- or di-saccharides such as Tn, sTn or TF O-linked to serines or threonines is especially common. Thomsen-Friedenreich antigen (TF; Galβ1-3GalNAcα-O-serine/threonine), Tn (GalNAcα1-O-serine/threonine) and sialylated Tn (sTn; NeuAcα2-6GalNAcα1-O-serine/threonine) are monosaccharide or disaccharide antigens expressed O-linked to mucins in a variety of epithelial cancers [33,34] (see Figure 1) Expression of these mono- and disaccharides correlates with a more aggressive phenotype and a more ominous prognosis [35, 36].

TF, Tn and sTn are expressed in 50–80% of various epithelial cancers [37–39]. STn trimer (cluster) is the epitope recognized by monoclonal antibody B72.3, and TF and sTn are, or are closely associated with the clustered epitope recognized by monoclonal antibody CC49 [40, 41]. Clinical trials of radiolabeled CC49 administered *i.p* in patients with breast cancer [41] and ovarian cancer [42] at this center and elsewhere have shown excellent targeting. TF has also been used successfully as a target for cancer imaging [43]. TF, Tn and sTn are expressed to a lesser extent on a variety of normal tissues, where they are expressed predominately as occasional monomers at luminal surfaces [20,44]. Immunohistology performed with mAbs identifying these trimers react strongly with a variety of epithelial cancers but only minimally with normal tissues, suggesting that focusing on the trimers of Tn, sTn and TF further increases the tumor specificity of the immune response. Immunization with TF and Tn has been shown to protect mice from subsequent challenge with syngeneic cancer cell lines expressing these antigens [10,45]. Hence both active and passive immunotherapy trials have identified TF, Tn and sTn antigens as uniquely effective targets for cancer targeting and immunotherapy.

Polysialic acid The neural cell adhesion molecule (N-CAM) is expressed on the cell surface of embryonic tissues, neuroendocrine cells and a variety of neuroendocrine tumors including SCLC, neuroblastomas and carcinoids [46, 47]. N-CAM undergoes a series of post-translational modifications, with the acquisition of α2,8-linked sialic acid residues as long polysialic acid chains (20–100 residues) in the embryo and these cancers. In most adult normal tissues, however, N-CAM contains polysialic acid chains of fewer than 10 residues. Several monoclonal antibodies, including mAb 735 and NP-4 [48] recognize these long polysialic acid chains (but not the shorter chains) and have allowed characterization of this antigen in both normal and malignant tissue. Zhang et al, has demonstrated that 6 of 6 SCLC tumor specimens were reactive by immunohistochemistry using mAb 735, and 5 of 6 tested SCLC tumor specimens were positive using mAb NP-4 [19]. This confirms previous results of Kimminoth [46], and suggests that polysialic acid may serve as a useful target for immune attack against SCLC. Polysialic acid is also expressed in the gray matter of the brain, bronchial epithelia and pneumocytes, epithelia of the colon, stomach, and pancreas, and capillary endothelial cells and ganglion neurons in the colon. The reactivity of these antibodies in epithelia is restricted to the luminal surfaces of glandular tissues, where access to the immune system is restricted. Two to five percent of normal donors have high levels of antibody against polysialic acid as a consequence of exposure to bacteria such as *Neisseria meningitidis* group B (MenB) and *Escherichia coli* K1 that also express polysialic acid. This has not been associated with any signs of autoimmunity [48]. Consequently, vaccines against polysialic acid are being tested to combat these infections. However, polysialic acid has proven to be poorly immunogenic.

With few exceptions (MUC1, CEA and KSA on a variety of epithelial cancers, CA125 on ovarian cancers and PSMA on prostate cancers), non-carbohydrate antigens are not as abundantly expressed, nor are they expressed with the same high frequency on cancers from different patients as are the carbohydrate antigens described above. In addition, antigens such as the cancer-testis antigens and p53 are not cell surface

Table 2. Carbohydrate cancer cell-surface targets for vaccine construction

Tumor	Antigens*
Melanoma	GM2, GD2, GD3
Neuroblastoma	GM2, GD2, GD3, polysialic acid
Sarcoma	GM2, GD2, GD3
Small-cell lung cancer	GM2, fucosyl GM1, polysialic acid, globo H, sialyl Le^a
Breast	GM2, globo H, Le^y, TF, Tn, sTn, sialyl Le^a
Prostate	GM2, Tn, sTn, TF, Le^y
Ovary	GM2, globo H, sTn, TF, Le^y

*Antigens present on at least 50% of cancer cells in at least 50% of biopsy specimens.

antigens, which may restrict the relevant immune response to a T-cell response. This complicates vaccine design and the analysis of immunogenicity in vaccine trials. Consequently, we have focused on antibody inducing polyvalent vaccines targeting primarily the carbohydrate antigens listed in Table 2 plus a few glycoprotein antigens such as MUC1 and KSA (also termed EpCAM) [49–53] in epithelial cancers, PSMA in prostate cancers, and CA125 (now termed MUC16) in ovarian cancers [54].

IMMUNOGENICITY OF CELL SURFACE CARBOHYDRATES IN CANCER PATIENTS

Selection of KLH conjugate plus GPI-0100 vaccines We have explored a variety of approaches for increasing the antibody response against carbohydrate cancer antigens, including the use of different immunological adjuvants [55–60], chemical modification of gangliosides to make them more immunogenic [61–64] and conjugation to various immunogenic carrier proteins [55, 65]. The conclusion from these studies is that the use of a carrier protein plus an immunological adjuvant is the optimal approach. The optimal immunological adjuvant in each case was one or more purified saponin fractions (QS-21 or GPI-0100) obtained from the bark of *Quillaja saponaria* [58, 66]. The optimal carrier protein was in each case keyhole limpet hemocyanin (KLH). This approach (covalent attachment of the carbohydrate to KLH and administration mixed with QS-21 or GPI-0100) has proved optimal for antibody induction in mice and cancer patients for each of the antigens in Table 2, except for sLe^a which has not been tested yet. The role of carrier protein in these conjugate vaccines is to induce potent T-lymphocyte help against the carrier (KLH) which also provides help for the antibody response against any covalently attached molecules such as these tumor antigens. Potent immunological adjuvants can greatly magnify this response. For instance, antibody titers induced against GD3 and MUC1 after immunization with GD3-KLH and MUC1-KLH increased from 0 to over $1/10^4$ and $1/10^7$ respectively with the use of the saponin adjuvant GPI-0100 [58, 67].

Two additional variables have proved critical for increasing antibody titers, the method of conjugation and the epitope ratio of antigen molecules per KLH molecule. The optimal conjugation approach has varied with the antigen. Gangliosides are best conjugated using ozone cleavage of the ceramide double bond and introducing an aldehyde group followed by coupling to aminolysyl groups of KLH by reductive amination. This approach was not as effective for conjugation of Tn, sTn, TF clusters or Globo H to KLH where an M2C2H linker arm has proved most efficient [68] or for MUC1 or MUC2 where an MBS linker group was optimal [69] . We have demonstrated that covalent conjugation of antigen (ganglioside GD3) to KLH is required, simply mixing the two is of little benefit [65] . Based on our experience with GM2 and GD3 conjugate vaccines, it is our impression that within the restrictions imposed by current conjugation methods, higher epitope ratios result in higher immunogenicity. Consequently considerable effort is devoted to optimizing this ratio with each vaccine.

We have also performed a series of Phase I dosing trials to determine the impact of dose of conjugate on antibody response in vaccinated patients, and a series of experiments to determine the impact of treatments designed to decrease suppressor cell reactivity in mice. The lowest dose of antigen in the KLH conjugates resulting in optimal antibody titers for each antigen is listed in Table 3. The lowest optimal doses range from 1 μg for TF to 30 μg for some glycolipids. Decreasing suppressor cell activity using low dose cyclophosphamide or anti-CTLA4 mAb had no impact on antibody titers induced by these vaccines [70].

Ganglioside vaccines We have been refining our ability to induce antibodies against GM2 in melanoma patients for fifteen years, since it was first demonstrated that patients immunized with irradiated melanoma cells occasionally produced antibodies against GM2, and that vaccines containing purified GM2 could be more immunogenic than vaccines containing tumor cells expressing GM2 [71]. Initially GM2 adherent to BCG was selected as optimal, inducing IgM antibody responses in 85% of patients. Antibody responses are defined here as an ELISA titer of 1/40 or greater (or at least 8 fold above baseline) confirmed by reactivity against cancer cells by immune thin layer chromatography or flow cytometry. Though these antibodies and monoclonal antibodies against GM2 were only able to kill 25% of melanoma cell lines by CDC, patients with natural or vaccine-induced antibodies had significantly longer disease free and overall survival [12]. This was the basis for a randomized trial comparing immunization with BCG to immunization with GM2/BCG in 122 patients with AJCC Stage 3 melanoma [13]. While the difference was not statistically significant, the GM2/BCG treated patients had a 12% improvement in survival and 15% improvement in disease free survival compared to the BCG patients after a minimum follow-up of 70 months. The IgM antibodies had a median titer of 1/160 and were short lived (8–12 weeks). IgG antibody induction was rare. We explored a variety of approaches to further improve this antibody response [65]. The use of GM2 conjugated to KLH and mixed with immunological adjuvant QS-21 was consistently optimal, inducing higher titer IgM antibodies (median titer 1/640-1/1280) in all patients and IgG antibodies in most patients. Reactivity against GM2 positive melanoma cells and complement mediated lysis was seen in over 90% of patients, and the antibody duration was 3–6 months after each vaccination [56, 59, 71]. Antibody titers have been maintained for over three years by administration of repeated booster immunizations at 3–4 month intervals. Antibody titers could not be further increased by pretreatment with a low dose of cyclophosphamide (300mg/M^2) to decrease suppressor cell reactivity. As with the other carbohydrate antigen vaccines described below, no evidence of T-cell immunity detected by delayed type hypersensitivity skin test reactivity (DTH) against GM2 was found.

This GM2-KLH plus QS-21 vaccine has been tested in a Phase III randomized trial in melanoma patients in this country compared to high dose interferon alpha. The trial was stopped because after a median followup of 16 months, patients receiving interferon had a significantly longer disease free and over all survival. Longer follow-up will be required to determine the long term impact, but the results to date indicate that induction of antibodies against GM2 in Stage III melanoma

Table 3. Summary of Median Serological Results in Patients Vaccinated with Monovalent Vaccines Against Carbohydrates

		ELISA				FACS			Median IA	CDC	
Antigen	Total # of pts	% pts pos	IgM Pre/post	IgG* Pre/post	IgG Subclass	% pts pos	IgM Pre/post	IgG Pre/Post	post	%pts pos	Pre/post
GM2	12	100	0/640	0/320	IgG1+3	90	11/65	10/41	++	90	2/44
GD2L	12	80	0/320	0/160		60	10/38	11/11		50	0/30
GD3L	12	70	0/40	0/160		50	9/30	10/30	+	40	2/54
FucGM1	18	100	0/320	0/320	IgG1	90	10/84	11/33		90	9/73
Globo H	30	90	0/640	0/40	IgG1+3	75	10/41	10/13	++	55	4/36
Lewis Y	18	60	0/80	0		30	7/23	10/12	+	40	3/26
PolySA	6	100	0/640	0/20		80	10/48	10/12		0	-
Tn(c)	15	100	0/1280	0/1280		60	10/44	10/10	+	0	-
STn(c)	27	100	0/1280	0/160	IgG3	90	10/85	10/8	+	0	-
TF(c)	15	60	0/320	0/10		60	11/41	10/25	+	0	-

* 0 = titer less than 1/10.
- = not detected in patient.
blank = not tested.

patients is not associated with demonstrable benefit [72]. This may be because while essentially all melanomas express some GM2, only a minority expresses enough GM2 to permit cell lysis with mAbs or immune sera.

Fucosyl GM1, like GM2, is highly immunogenic. Essentially all patients vaccinated with fucosyl GM1-KLH plus QS-21 produced IgM antibodies and most produced IgG antibodies against fucosyl GM1 that also reacted with the SCLC cell surface as demonstrated by FACS and CDC [73, 74].

Trials of GD2 and GD3 conjugated to KLH in melanoma patients induced only low (GD2) or no (GD3) antibodies reactive with the immunizing ganglioside or antigen positive melanoma cells. GD2 and GD3 are clearly less immunogenic than GM2. Based on early work from Nores and colleagues [75], we have demonstrated that conversion of these two gangliosides to lactones by treatment with acid after conjugation to KLH resulted in more immunogenic vaccines [76, 77]. Increased antibody titers against the native gangliosides and against tumor cells were induced in the majority of patients (see results in Table 3).

Le^y and Globo H vaccines: The development of Le^y and Globo H vaccines was previously limited by the lack of sufficient quantities of antigen for vaccine construction and testing. Over the last six years, Dr. Samuel Danishefsky in our group has successfully synthesized both antigens [16, 78–80]. We have immunized groups of mice with Globo H-ceramide plus or minus adjuvants QS-21 and Salmonella minnesota mutant R595, and with Globo H covalently attached to KLH or BSA plus immunological adjuvants QS-21 or GPI-0100. The highest antibody titers against both synthetic antigen and MCF7 cells expressing Globo H were induced by the Globo H-KLH plus QS-21 (or GPI-0100) vaccine [79]. The antibody titer induced against synthetic Globo H was 1/120,000 by ELISA, the titer induced against MCF7 was 1/320, and potent complement mediated cytotoxicity was seen as well. Le^y-BSA and Le^y-KLH vaccines have also been tested in the mouse. High titer antibody responses against the synthetic epitope of Le^y and against tumor cells expressing Le^y have been observed in the majority of mice immunized [80]. Based on these results, clinical trials with Globo H-KLH plus QS-21 and Le^y–KLH plus QS21 have been initiated in patients with breast, prostate or ovary cancer. The results are summarized in Table 3. Antibodies against the purified antigens and against tumor cells expressing these antigens were induced in most patients immunized with globo H [80, 82, 83] but only occasional patients immunized with Le^y [84].

TF, Tn and sTn vaccines: Patients with various epithelial cancers have been immunized with unclustered TF-KLH and sTn-KLH vaccines plus various adjuvants [85]. High titer IgM and IgG antibodies against TF and sTn antigens were induced. In our hands the majority of the reactivity was against antigenic epitopes present in the vaccine which were not present on naturally expressed mucins (porcine or ovine submaxillary mucins (PSM or OSM)) or tumor cells [85]. Based on previous studies with Tn antigen [86], Kurosaka and Nakada et al. hypothesized that MLS102, a monoclonal antibody against sTn, might preferentially recognize clusters ((c)) of sTn [87]. Studies with monoclonal antibody B72.3 and with sera raised against

TF-KLH and sTn-KLH conjugate vaccines in mice and in patients reached the same conclusion [40, 85, 88]. The availability of synthetic TF, Tn and sTn clusters consisting of 3 epitopes covalently linked to 3 consecutive serines or threonines has permitted proof of this hypothesis. In both direct tests and inhibition assays, B72.3 recognized sTn clusters exclusively, and sera from mice immunized with sTn(c)-KLH reacted strongly with both natural mucins and tumor cells expressing sTn [40]. Based on these studies, we initiated trials with the TF(c)-KLH, Tn(c)-KLH and sTn(c)-KLH conjugate vaccines in patients with breast cancer [89–91]. Antibodies of relevant high titer and specificity, including against OSM or PSM and cancer cells expressing TF, Tn or sTn, were induced for the first time in our experience (Table 3). Based on these results, we plan to include clustered Tn, sTn and TF in the polyvalent vaccines against epithelial cancers.

Several trials with TF, Tn and sTn vaccines have been reported from other centers, and a large multicenter Phase III trial with an sTn vaccine has recently been completed. George Springer's pioneering trials in breast cancer patients with vaccines containing TF and Tn purified from natural sources and mixed with typhoid vaccine (as adjuvant) began in the mid 1970s [15, 34, 92]. DTH and IgM responses against the immunizing antigens and prolonged survival compared to historical controls were reported. MacLean immunized ten ovarian cancer patients with synthetic TF conjugated to KLH plus immunological adjuvant Detox (monophosphoryl Lipid A plus BCG cell wall skeletons) and described augmentation of IgG and IgM antibodies against synthetic TF in 9 of 10 patients [93]. Lower levels of antibody reactivity against TF from natural sources were detected in some of these cases. MacLean has also immunized patients with breast and other adenocarcinomas with sTn-KLH plus Detox [14, 94, 95]. Induction of IgM and IgG antibodies against synthetic and natural sources of sTn was seen in essentially all patients and this response was further increased by pretreatment of patients with a low dose of cyclophosphamide. Reactivity of these sera with natural mucins and tumor cells despite the use of an unclustered sTn vaccine is probably explained by the 4-fold higher sTn/KLH epitope ratio achieved in the MacLean vaccine compared to our previous unclustered vaccine. Overall survival appeared to be improved compared to historical controls, and patients who responded with high antibody titers survived longer than those with lower titers. Reactivity with breast cancer cells, including complement dependent cytotoxicity, was described. However, a multicenter Phase III randomized trial of sTn-KLH plus the immunological adjuvant Detox versus KLH alone plus Detox in breast cancer patients with stable disease or clinical response to chemotherapy was recently completed. This trial has been closed because it demonstrated no difference in recurrence free and overall survival between the two groups.

Polysialic acid vaccines: Initial attempts at preparing a vaccine against polysialic acid for use in military recruits who are at risk of group B meningococcus infection were unsuccessful. We have completed analysis of a clinical trial with polysialic acid conjugated to KLH plus QS-21 and found that no antibody responses were induced in the 5 vaccinated patients. Consequently, we tested a second polysialic acid vaccine that had been modified (N-propionylated) to increase its immunogenicity in collaboration with Dr. Harold Jennings who pioneered the use of N-propionylation for this purpose [96]. This induced an antibody response against unmodified polysialic acid in six of six patients immunized [97]. These vaccine-induced antibodies also reacted with small cell lung cancer cells (and were cytotoxic for antigen positive bacteria). This N-propionylated polysialic acid vaccine is suitable for inclusion in our polyvalent vaccine against SCLC and possibly for trials in students and military recruits for prevention of group B meningococcus infections.

POLYVALENT VACCINES

The basis for emphasis on polyvalent vaccines is tumor cell heterogeneity, heterogeneity of the human immune response and the correlation between overall antibody titer against tumor cells and effector mechanisms such as complement dependent cytotoxicity (CDC) or antibody dependent cell mediated cytotoxicity (ADCC). For example, using a series of 14 tumor cell lines and mAbs against 3 gangliosides, we have shown that significant cell surface reactivity analyzed by flow cytometry and CDC increased from 2 to 8 of the cell lines by using one of three mAbs to all 14 of the cell lines when the 3 mAbs were pooled. The median CDC increased 4 fold with the pooled mAbs compared to the best single mAb [98].

SUMMARY

A variety of carbohydrate cell surface antigens are over-expressed on cancer cells and have proved to be unexpectedly potent targets for immune recognition and attack against these cancers. The majority of cancer patients can initially be rendered free of detectable disease by surgery and/or chemotherapy. Adjuvant chemotherapy or radiation therapy at this point are in general only minimally beneficial, so there is a real need for additional methods to eliminate residual circulating cancer cells and micrometastases. This is the ideal setting for treatment with antibody inducing cancer vaccines which primarily target carbohydrate antigens. The immune response induced is critically dependent on both vaccine design and the antigenic epitope. For antibody induction there is one best vaccine design, conjugation of the antigen to an immunogenic protein such as KLH and the use of a potent adjuvant such as the saponins QS-21 and GPI-0100. This approach alone induced strong antibody responses against the glycolipids GM2, fucosyl GM1 and globo H and cancer cells expressing these glycolipids. Other carbohydrate antigens require additional modifications to augment relevant immunogenicity. GD2 and GD3 lactones, N-propionylated polysialic acid, Tn, sTn and TF trimers (clusters) were significantly more effective at inducing antibodies against the naturally expressed antigens on tumor cells.

Antibodies are ideally suited for eradicating pathogens from the bloodstream and from early tissue invasion. Passively administered and vaccine induced antibodies have accomplished this, eliminating circulating tumor cells and systemic or intraperitoneal micrometastases in a variety of preclinical models, so antibody-inducing vaccines offer real promise in the adjuvant setting. Polyvalent vaccines will probably be required due to tumor cell heterogeneity, heterogeneity of the human immune response and the correlation between overall antibody titer against tumor cells and antibody effector mechanisms. Over the next several years, Phase II clinical trials designed to determine the clinical impact of a series of polyvalent conjugate vaccines that target primarily carbohydrate antigens will be initiated. The target populations will be patients with SCLC, melanoma, neuroblastoma, ovarian cancer and breast cancer who are in complete or partial remission after optimal surgery and/or chemotherapy.

REFERENCES

1. G. Ragupathi and P.O. Livingston. Antibody-inducing cancer vaccines against cell-surface carbohydrate antigens. 11: p. 137–155, (2003).
2. T. Feizi. Demonstration by monoclonal antibodies that carbohydrate structures of glycoproteins and glycolipids are onco-developmental antigens. *Nature*. 314(6006): p. 53–7, (1985).
3. S. Hakomori. Tumor-associated carbohydrate antigens. *Annu Rev Immunol*. 2: p. 103–26, (1984).
4. K.O. Lloyd, Molecular characteristic of tumor antigens. Vol. 10. 1990. 765–779.
5. P. Brossart, U. Keilholz, M. Willhauck, C. Scheibenbogen, T. Mohler, and W. Hunstein. Hematogenous spread of malignant melanoma cells in different stages of disease. *J Invest Dermatol*. 101(6): p. 887–9, (1993).
6. R.A. Ghossein, H.I. Scher, W.L. Gerald, W.K. Kelly, T. Curley, A. Amsterdam, Z.F. Zhang, and J. Rosai. Detection of circulating tumor cells in patients with localized and metastatic prostatic carcinoma: clinical implications. *J Clin Oncol*. 13(5): p. 1195–200, (1995).
7. D.S. Hoon, Y. Wang, P.S. Dale, A.J. Conrad, P. Schmid, D. Garrison, C. Kuo, L.J. Foshag, A.J. Nizze, and D.L. Morton. Detection of occult melanoma cells in blood with a multiple-marker polymerase chain reaction assay. *J Clin Oncol*. 13(8): p. 2109–16, (1995).
8. P. Livingston, The case for melanoma vaccines that induce antibodies. Kirkwood JM ed. Molecular Diagnosis Prevention and Treatment of Melanoma ed. 1998: Marcel Dekker, Inc. 139–157.
9. H. Zhang, S. Zhang, N.K. Cheung, G. Ragupathi, and P.O. Livingston. Antibodies against GD2 ganglioside can eradicate syngeneic cancer micrometastases. *Cancer Res*. 58(13): p. 2844–9, (1998).
10. P.Y. Fung, M. Madej, R.R. Koganty, and B.M. Longenecker. Active specific immunotherapy of a murine mammary adenocarcinoma using a synthetic tumor-associated glycoconjugate. *Cancer Res*. 50(14): p. 4308–14, (1990).
11. P.C. Jones, L.L. Sze, P.Y. Liu, D.L. Morton, and R.F. Irie. Prolonged survival for melanoma patients with elevated IgM antibody to oncofetal antigen. *J Natl Cancer Inst*. 66(2): p. 249–54, (1981).
12. P.O. Livingston, G. Ritter, P. Srivastava, M. Padavan, M.J. Calves, H.F. Oettgen, and L.J. Old. Characterization of IgG and IgM antibodies induced in melanoma patients by immunization with purified GM2 ganglioside. *Cancer Res*. 49(24 Pt 1): p. 7045–50, (1989).
13. P.O. Livingston, G.Y. Wong, S. Adluri, Y. Tao, M. Padavan, R. Parente, C. Hanlon, M.J. Calves, F. Helling, G. Ritter, and et al. Improved survival in stage III melanoma patients with GM2 antibodies: a randomized trial of adjuvant vaccination with GM2 ganglioside. *J Clin Oncol*. 12(5): p. 1036–44, (1994).
14. G.D. MacLean, M.A. Reddish, R.R. Koganty, and B.M. Longenecker. Antibodies against mucin-associated sialyl-Tn epitopes correlate with survival of metastatic adenocarcinoma patients undergoing active specific immunotherapy with synthetic STn vaccine. *J Immunother Emphasis Tumor Immunol*. 19(1): p. 59–68, (1996).

15. G.F. Springer. Immunoreactive T and Tn epitopes in cancer diagnosis, prognosis, and immunotherapy. *J Mol Med.* 75(8): p. 594–602, (1997).
16. J. Dalmau, H.S. Gultekin, and J.B. Posner. Paraneoplastic neurologic syndromes: pathogenesis and physiopathology. *Brain Pathol.* 9(2): p. 275–84, (1999).
17. G. Ragupathi, N.X. Liu, S. Cappello, C. Musselli, and P.O. Livingston. Complement activation by antibodies against cancer cell surface glycolipids and proteins, but not mucins, results in cell lysis. *J Immunol.* (2005).
18. H.R. Colten and F.S. Rosen. Complement deficiencies. *Annu Rev Immunol.* 10: p. 809–34, (1992).
19. S. Zhang, C. Cordon-Cardo, H.S. Zhang, V.E. Reuter, S. Adluri, W.B. Hamilton, K.O. Lloyd, and P.O. Livingston. Selection of tumor antigens as targets for immune attack using immunohistochemistry: I. Focus on gangliosides. *Int J Cancer.* 73(1): p. 42–9, (1997).
20. S. Zhang, H.S. Zhang, C. Cordon-Cardo, V.E. Reuter, A.K. Singhal, K.O. Lloyd, and P.O. Livingston. Selection of tumor antigens as targets for immune attack using immunohistochemistry. II. Blood group-related antigens. *Int. J. Cancer.* 73: p. 50–56, (1997).
21. S. Zhang, H.S. Zhang, C. Cordon-Cardo, G. Ragupathi, and P.O. Livingston. Selection of tumor antigens as targets for immune attack using immunohistochemistry: III protein antigens. *Clin. Cancer Res.* 4: p. 2669–2676, (1998).
22. S. Zhang, H.S. Zhang, V.E. Reuter, K.O. Lloyd, H. Scher, and P.O. Livingston. Expression of potential target antigens for immunotherapy on primary and metastatic prostate cancers. *Clin Cancer Res.* 4: p. 295–302, (1998).
23. K. Nakamura, M. Koike, K. Shitara, Y. Kuwana, K. Kiuragi, S. Igarashi, M. Hasegawa, and N. Hanai. Chimeric anti-ganglioside GM2 antibody with antitumor activity. *Cancer Res.* 54: p. 1511–1516, (1994.).
24. Y. Nishinaka, M.N.H. Ravindranath, and R.F. Ire. Development of a human monoclonal antibody to ganglioside GM2 with potential for cancer treatment. *Cancer Res.* 56: p. 5666–5671, (1996).
25. S. Canevari, G. Fossati, A. Balsari, S. Sonnino, and M.I. Colnaghi. Immunochemical analysis of the determinant recognized by a monoclonal antibody (MBr1) which specifically binds to human mammary epithelial cells. *Cancer Res.* 43(3): p. 1301–5, (1983).
26. I. Hellström, H.J. Garrigues, U. Garrigues, and K.E. Hellström. Highly tumor-reactive, internalizing, mouse monoclonal antibodies to Ley-related cell surface antigens. *Cancer Res.* 50: p. 2183–2190, (1990).
27. S. Menard, E. Tagliabue, S. Canevari, G. Fossati, and M.I. Colnaghi. Generation of monoclonal antibodies reacting with normal and cancer cells of human breast. *Cancer Res.* 43(3): p. 1295–300, (1983).
28. F. Perrone, S. Menard, S. Canevari, M. Calabrese, P. Boracchi, R. Bufalino, S. Testori, M. Baldini, and M.I. Colnaghi. Prognostic significance of the CaMBr1 antigen on breast carcinoma: relevance of the type of recognised glycoconjugate. *Eur J Cancer.* 29A(15): p. 2113–7, (1993).
29. M.I. Colnaghi, S. Menard, J.G. Da Dalt, R. Agresti, G. Cattoretti, S. Andreola, G. Di Fronzo, M. Del Vecchio, L. Verderio, N. Cascinelli, and F. Rilke. A multiparametric study by monoclonal antibodies in breast cancer., (1987).
30. P.A. Trail, D. Willner, S.J. Lasch, A.J. Henderson, S. Hofstead, A.M. Casazza, R.A. Firestone, I. Hellstrom, and K.E. Hellstrom. Cure of xenografted human carcinomas by BR96-doxorubicin immunoconjugates. *Science.* 261(5118): p. 212–5, (1993).
31. S.J. Gendler, A.P. Spicer, E.-N. Lalani, T. Duhig, N. Peat, J. Burchell, L. Pemberton, M. Boshell, and J. Taylor-Papadimitriou. Structure and biology of a carcinoma-associated mucin, MUC1. *Am. Rev. Respir. Dis.* 144: p. S42-S47, (1991).
32. L. Perez, D.F. Hayes, P. Maimonis, M. Abe, C. O'Hara, and D.W. Kufe. Tumor selective reactivity of a monoclonal antibody prepared against a recombinant peptide derived from the DF3 human breast carcinoma-associated antigen. *Cancer Res.* 52: p. 2563–2568, (1992).
33. K.O. Lloyd. Blood group antigens as markers for normal differentiation and malignant change in human tissues. *Amer. J. Clin. Pathol.* 87: p. 129–139, (1987).
34. G.F. Springer. T and Tn, general carcinoma autoantigens. *Science.* 224: p. 1198–1206, (1984).

35. S.-H. Cho, A. Sahin, G.N. Hortobagyi, W.N. Hittelman, and K. Dhingra. Sialyl-Tn antigen expression occurs early during human mammary carcinogenesis and is associated with high nuclear grade and aneuploidy. *Cancer Res.* 54: p. 6302–6305, (1994).
36. S. Itzkowitz, E.J. Bloom, W.A. Kokal, G. Modin, S.-I. Hakomori, and Y.S. Kim. Sialosyl Tn: A novel mucin antigen associated with prognosis in colorectal carcinoma patients. *Cancer.* 66: p. 1960–1966, (1990).
37. A. Thor, N. Ohuchi, C.A. Szpak, W.W. Johnston, and J. Schlom. Distribution of oncofetal antigen tumor-associated glycoprotein-72 defined by monoclonal antibody B72.3. *Cancer Res.* 46(6): p. 3118–24, (1986).
38. A. Contegiacomo, M. Alimandi, R. Muraro, C. Pizzi, R. Calderopoli, L. De Marchis, A. Sgambato, G. Pettinato, G. Petrella, M.R. De Filippo, and et al. Expression of epitopes of the tumour-associated glycoprotein 72 and clinicopathological correlations in mammary carcinomas. *Eur J Cancer.* 30A(6): p. 813–20, (1994).
39. B.M. Longenecker, D.J. Willans, G.D. MacLean, S. Selvaraj, M.R. Suresh, and A.A. Noujaim. Monoclonal antibodies and synthetic tumor-associated glycoconjugates in the study of the expression of Thomsen-Friedenreich-like and Tn-like antigens on human cancers. *J Natl Cancer Inst.* 78(3): p. 489–96, (1987).
40. S. Zhang, L.A. Walberg, S. Ogata, S.H. Itzkowitz, R.R. Koganty, M. Reddish, S.S. Gandhi, B.M. Longenecker, K.O. Lloyd, and P.O. Livingston. Immune sera and monoclonal antibodies define two configurations for the sialyl Tn tumor antigen. *Cancer Res.* 55(15): p. 3364–8, (1995).
41. L. Kostakoglu, C.R. Divgi, T. Gilewski, M. Theodoulou, J. Schlom, and S.M. Larson. Phase II radioimmunotherapy (RIT) trial with I-131 labeled monoclonal antibody CC49 in Tag-72 expressing breast cancer. *J Nucl Med (Suppl).* 35: p. 234, (1994).
42. S.M. Larson, J.A. Carrasquillo, D.C. Colcher, K. Yokoyama, J.C. Reynolds, S.A. Bacharach, A. Raubitchek, L. Pace, R.D. Finn, M. Rotman, and et al. Estimates of radiation absorbed dose for intraperitoneally administered iodine-131 radiolabeled B72.3 monoclonal antibody in patients with peritoneal carcinomatoses. *J Nucl Med.* 32(9): p. 1661–7, (1991).
43. G.D. MacLean, McEwan A., Noujaim A., Sykes T.R., Suresch M.R., Catz Z., H. H.R., and L. B.M. A novel strategy for cancer immunoscinitgrapy. *Antibody Immunoconj Radiopharmaceut.* 2: p. 15, (1989).
44. S.H. Itzkowitz, M. Yuan, C.K. Montgomery, T. Kjeldsen, H.K. Takahashi, W.L. Bigbee, and Y.S. Kim. Expression of Tn, sialosyl-Tn, and T antigens in human colon cancer. *Cancer Res.* 49(1): p. 197–204, (1989).
45. G.D. MacLean, M.A. Reddish, M.B. Bowen-Yacyshyn, S. Poppema, and B.M. Longenecker. Active specific immunotherapy against adenocarcinomas. *Cancer Invest.* 12(1): p. 46–56, (1994).
46. P. Kimminoth, J. Roth, P.M. Lackie, D. Bitter-Suermann, and P.U. Heintz. Polysialic acid of the neural cell adhesion melecule distinquishes small cell lung carcinoma from carcinoids. *Am J Pathol.* 139: p. 297–304, (1991).
47. P.M. Lackie, C. Zuber, and J. Roth. Polysialic acid of the neural cell adhesion molecule (N-CAM) is widely expressed during organogenesis in mesodermal and endodermal derivatives. *Differentiation.* 57(2): p. 119–31, (1994).
48. J. Hayrinen, H. Jennings, H.V. Raff, G. Rougon, N. Hanai, R. Gerardy-Schahn, and J. Finne. Antibodies to polysialic acid and its N-propyl derivative: binding properties and interaction with human embryonal brain glycopeptides. *Journal of Infectious Diseases.* 171: p. 1481–90, (1995).
49. H.G. Gottlinger, I. Funke, J.P. Johnson, J.M. Gokel, and G. Riethmuller. The epithelial cell surface antigen 17–1A, a target for antibody-mediated tumor therapy: its biochemical nature, tissue distribution and recognition by different monoclonal antibodies. *Int J Cancer.* 38(1): p. 47–53, (1986).
50. A.F. LoBuglio, M.N. Saleh, J. Lee, M.B. Khazaeli, R. Carrano, H. Holden, and R.H. Wheeler. Phase I trial of multiple large doses of murine monoclonal antibody CO17–1A. I. Clinical aspects. *J Natl Cancer Inst.* 80(12): p. 932–6, (1988).
51. G. Riethmuller, E. Schneider-Gadicke, G. Schlimok, W. Schmiegel, R. Raab, K. Hoffken, R. Gruber, H. Pichlmaier, H. Hirche, R. Pichlmayr, and et al. Randomised trial of monoclonal antibody for

adjuvant therapy of resected Dukes' C colorectal carcinoma. German Cancer Aid 17–1A Study Group. *Lancet*. 343(8907): p. 1177–83, (1994).
52. R. Somasundaram, J. Zaloudik, L. Jacob, A. Benden, M. Sperlagh, E. Hart, G. Marks, M. Kane, M. Mastrangelo, and D. Herlyn. Induction of Antigen-Specific Tand B Cell Immunity in Colon Carcinoma Patients by Anti-Idiotypic Antibody. *Journal of Immunology*. p. 3253–3261, (1995).
53. S. Szala, M. Froehlich, M. Scollon, Y. Kasai, Z. Steplewski, H. Koprowski, and A.J. Linnenbach. Molecular cloning of cDNA for the carcinoma-associated antigen GA733–2. *Proc Natl Acad Sci U S A*. 87(9): p. 3542–6, (1990).
54. W.T. Yin, A. Dnistrian, and K. Lloyd. Ovarian cancer antigen CA125 is encoded by the MUC16 mucin gene. *International Journal of Cancer*. 98: p. 737–740, (2002).
55. S. Zhang, L.A. Graeber, F. Helling, G. Ragupathi, S. Adluri, K.O. Lloyd, and P.O. Livingston. Augmenting the immunogenicity of synthetic MUC1 peptide vaccines in mice. *Cancer Res*. 56(14): p. 3315–9, (1996).
56. P. Livingston, S. Zhang, S. Adluri, T.J. Yao, L. Graeber, G. Ragupathi, F. Helling, and M. Fleisher. Tumor cell reactivity mediated by IgM antibodies in sera from melanoma patients vaccinated with GM2 ganglioside covalently linked to KLH is increased by IgG antibodies. *Cancer Immunol Immunother*. 43(6): p. 324–30, (1997).
57. F. Helling, A. Zhang, A. Shang, S. Adluri, M. Calves, R. Koganty, B.M. Longenecker, H.F. Oettgen, and P.O. Livingston. GM2-KLH conjugate vaccine: Increased immunogenicity in melanoma patients after administration with immunological adjuvant QS-21. *Cancer Res*. 55: p. 2783–2788, (1995).
58. S.-K. Kim, G. Ragupathi, S. Cappello, E. Kagan, and P.O. Livingston. Effect of immunological adjuvant combinations on the antibody and T-cell response to vaccination with MUC1-KLH and GD3-KLH conjugates. *Vaccine*. 19: p. 530–537, (2000).
59. P.O. Livingston, S. Adluri, F. Helling, T.-J. Yao, C.R. Kensil, M.J. Newman, and D. Marciani. Phase I trial of immunological adjuvant QS-21 with a GM2 ganglioside-KLH conjugate vaccine in patients with malignant melanoma. *Vaccine*. 12: p. 1275–1280, (1994).
60. P.O. Livingston, M.J. Calves, and E.J. Natoli, Jr. Approaches to augmenting the immunogenicity of the ganglioside GM2 in mice: purified GM2 is superior to whole cells. *J Immunol*. 138(5): p. 1524–9, (1987).
61. G. Ritter, E. Boosfeld, M.J. Calves, H.F. Oettgen, L.J. Old, and P.O. Livingston. Antibody response to immunization with purified GD3 ganglioside and GD3 derivatives (lactones, amide and gangliosidol) in the mouse. *Immunobiology*. 182(1): p. 32–43, (1990).
62. G. Ritter, E. Boosfeld, E. Markstein, R.K. Yu, S.L. Ren, W.B. Stallcup, H.F. Oettgen, L.J. Old, and P.O. Livingston. Biochemical and serological characteristics of natural 9-O-acetyl GD3 from human melanoma and bovine buttermilk and chemically O-acetylated GD3. *Cancer Res*. 50(5): p. 1403–10, (1990).
63. G. Ritter, E. Boosfeld, R. Adluri, M. Calves, H.F. Oettgen, L.J. Old, and P. Livingston. Antibody response to immunization with ganglioside GD3 and GD3 congeners (lactones, amide and gangliosidol) in patients with malignant melanoma. *Int J Cancer*. 48(3): p. 379–85, (1991).
64. G. Ritter, E. Ritter-Boosfeld, R. Adluri, M. Calves, S. Ren, R.K. Yu, H.F. Oettgen, L.J. Old, and P.O. Livingston. Analysis of the antibody response to immunization with purified O-acetyl GD3 gangliosides in patients with malignant melanoma. *Int J Cancer*. 62(6): p. 668–72, (1995).
65. F. Helling, A. Shang, M. Calves, S. Zhang, S. Ren, R.K. Yu, H.F. Oettgen, and P.O. Livingston. GD3 vaccines for melanoma: superior immunogenicity of keyhole limpet hemocyanin conjugate vaccines. *Cancer Res*. 54(1): p. 197–203, (1994).
66. C.R. Kensil, U. Patel, M. Lennick, and D. Marciani. Separation and characterization of saponins with adjuvant activity fro Quillaja saponaria molina cortex. *J. Immunology*. 146: p. 431, (1991).
67. S.-K. Kim, G. Ragupathi, C. Musselli, and P.O. Livingston. Comparison of the effect of different immunological adjuvants on the antibody and T cell response to immunization with MUC1-KLH and GD3-KLH conjugate vaccines. *Vaccine*. 18: p. 597–603, (1999).
68. G. Ragupathi, R.R. Koganty, D. Qui, K.O. Lloyd, and P.O. Livingston. A novel and efficient method for synthetic carbohydrate vaccine preparation: Synthesis of sialyl Tn-KLH conjugate using a

(4-N-maleimido methyl) cyclohexane-1-carboxyl hydrazide (MMCCH) linker arm. *Glycoconjugate J.* 15: p. 217–221, (1998).
69. G. Ragupathi, L. Howard, S. Cappello, R.R. Koganty, D. Qiu, B.M. Longenecker, M.A. Reddish, K.O. Lloyd, and P.O. Livingston. Vaccines prepared with sialyl-Tn and sialyl-Tn trimers using the 4-(4-maleimidomethyl) cyclohexane-1-carboxyl hydrazide linker group result in optimal antibody titers against ovine submaxillary mucin and sialyl-Tn-positive tumor cells. *Can Immunol Immunother.* 48: p. 1–8, (1999).
70. G. Ragupathi, F. Koide, N. Sathyan, E. Kagan, M. Spassova, W. Bornmann, P. Gregor, C.A. Reis, H. Clausen, S.J. Danishefsky, and P.O. Livingston. A preclinical study comparing approaches for augmenting the immunogenicity of a heptavalent KLH-conjugate vaccine against epithelial cancers. *Cancer Immunol Immunother.* 52(10): p. 608–16, (2003).
71. P.O. Livingston, E.J. Natoli, M.J. Calves, E. Stockert, H.F. Oettgen, and L.J. Old. Vaccines containing purified GM2 ganglioside elicit GM2 antibodies in melanoma patients. *Proc Natl Acad Sci U S A.* 84(9): p. 2911–5, (1987).
72. J.M. Kirkwood, J.G. Ibrahim, J.A. Sosman, V.K. Sondak, S.S. Agarwala, M.S. Ernstoff, and U. Rao. High-dose interferon alfa-2b significantly prolongs relapse-free and overall survival compared with the GM2-KLH/QS-21 vaccine in patients with resected stage IIB-III melanoma: results of intergroup trial E1694/S9512/C509801. *J Clin Oncol.* 19(9): p. 2370–80, (2001).
73. M.N. Dickler, G. Ragupathi, N.X. Liu, C. Musselli, D.J. Martino, V.A. Miller, M.G. Kris, F.T. Brezicka, P.O. Livingston, and S.C. Grant. Immunogenicity of the fucosyl-GM1-keyhole limpet hemocyanin (KLH) conjugate vaccine in patients with small cell lung cancer. *Cancer Res.* 5: p. 2773–2779, (1999).
74. L.M. Krug, G. Ragupathi, C. Hood, M.G. Kris, V.A. Miller, J.R. Allen, S.J. Keding, S.J. Danishefsky, J. Gomez, L. Tyson, B. Pizzo, V. Baez, and P.O. Livingston. Vaccination of patients with small-cell lung cancer with synthetic fucosyl GM-1 conjugated to keyhole limpet hemocyanin. *Clin Cancer Res.* 10(18 Pt 1): p. 6094–100, (2004).
75. G.A. Nores, T. Dohi, M. Taniguchi, and S. Hakomori. Density-dependent recognition of cell surface GM3 by a certain anti-melanoma antibody, and GM3 lactone as a possible immunogen: requirements for tumor-associated antigen and immunogen. *J Immunol.* 139(9): p. 3171–6, (1987).
76. G. Ragupathi, M. Meyers, S. Adluri, L. Howard, R.K. Yu, G. Ritter, and P.O. Livingston. Phase I trial with GD3-lactone-KLH conjugate and immunological adjuvant QS-21 vaccine with malignant melanoma. *Int. J. Cancer.* 85: p. 659–666, (2000).
77. G. Ragupathi, P.O. Livingston, C. Hood, J. Gathuru, S.E. Krown, P.B. Chapman, J.D. Wolchok, L.J. Williams, R.C. Oldfield, and W.J. Hwu. Consistent antibody response against ganglioside GD2 induced in patients with melanoma by a GD2 lactone-keyhole limpet hemocyanin conjugate vaccine plus immunological adjuvant QS-21. *Clin Cancer Res.* 9(14): p. 5214–20, (2003).
78. V. Behar and S. Danishefsky. A highly convergent synthesis of the Lewis-y blood group determinant in conjugatable form. *Angew Chem Int Ed Engl.* 33: p. 1468–1470, (1994).
79. G. Ragupathi, T.K. Park, S. Zhang, I.J. Kim, K. Graeber, S. Adluri, K.O. Lloyd, S.J. Danishefsky, and P.O. Livingston. Immunization of mice with the synthetic hexasaccharide Globo H results in antibodies against human cancer cells. *Angewandte. Chemie.* 36: p. 125–128, (1997).
80. G. Ragupathi, S. Slovin, S. Adluri, D. Sames, I.-J. Kim, H.M. Kim, M. Spassova, W.G. Bornmann, K. Lloyd, H.I. Scher, P.O. Livingston, and S.J. Danishefsky. A fully synthetic globo H carbohydrate vaccine induces a focused humoral response in prostate cancer patients. *Angewandte. Chemie.* 38(A proof of Principle.): p. 563–566, (1999).
81. V. Kudryashov, H.M. Kim, G. Ragupathi, S.J. Danishefsky, P.O. Livingston, and K.O. Lloyd. Immunogenicity of synthetic conjugates of Lewis^y oligosaccharide with protein in mice: towards the design of anticancer vaccines. *Cancer Immunol. Immunother.* 45: p. 281, (1998).
82. T. Gilewski, G. Ragupathi, S. Bhuta, L.J. Williams, C. Musselli, X.F. Zhang, K.P. Bencsath, K.S. Panageas, J. Chin, L. Norton, A.N. Houghton, P.O. Livingston, and S.J. Danishefsky. Immunization of metastatic breast cancer patients with a fully synthetic globo H conjugate: a phase I trial. *Proc Natl Acad Sci USA.* 98: p. 3270–3275, (2001).

83. S.F. Slovin, G. Ragupathi, S. Adluri, G. Ungers, K. Terry, S. Kim, M. Spassova, W.G. Bornmann, M. Fazzari, L. Dantis, K. Olkiewicz, K.O. Lloyd, P.O. Livingston, S.J. Danishefsky, and H.I. Scher. Carbohydrate vaccines in cancer: immunogenicity of a fully synthetic globo H hexasaccharide conjugate in man. *Proc Natl Acad Sci U S A*. 96(10): p. 5710–5, (1999).
84. P. Sabbatini, V. Kudryashov, S. Danishefsky, P.O. Livingston, G. Ragupathi, W. Bornmann, M. Spassova, D. Spriggs, C. Aghajanian, S. Soignet, M. Peyton, C. O'Flaherty, J. Curtin, and K.O. Lloyd. Immunization of ovarian cancer patients with a synthetic LewisY - protein conjugate vaccine: clinical and serological results. *Int. J. Cancer*. 87: p. 79–85, (2000).
85. S. Adluri, F. Helling, M.J. Calves, K.O. Lloyd, and P.O. Livingston. Immunogenicity of synthetic TF- and sTn-KLH conjugates in colorectal carcinoma patients. *Cancer Immunol. Immunother*. 41: p. 185–192, (1995).
86. H. Nakada, M. Inoue, Y. Numata, N. Tanaka, I. Funakoshi, S. Fukui, A. Mellors, and I. Yamashina. Epitopic structure of Tn glycophorin A for an anti-Tn antibody (MLS 128). *Proc Natl Acad Sci U S A*. 90(6): p. 2495–9, (1993).
87. A. Kurosaka, H. Kitagawa, S. Fukui, Y. Numata, H. Nakada, I. Funakoshi, T. Kawasaki, T. Ogawa, H. Iijima, and I. Yamashina. A monoclonal antibody that recognizes a cluster of a disaccharide, NeuAc alpha(2—-6)GalNAc, in mucin-type glycoproteins. *J Biol Chem*. 263(18): p. 8724–6, (1988).
88. P.O. Livingston, R.R. Koganty, B.M. Longenecker, K.O. Lloyd, and M. Calves. Studies on the immunogencity of synthetic and natural Thomsen-Friedenreich (TF) antigens in mice: Augmentation of the response by Quil A and SAF-m adjuvants and analysis of the specificity of the responses. *Vaccine Res*. 1: p. 99–109, (1992).
89. T. Gilewski, G. Ragupathi, S. Powell, S. Bhuta, K. Panageas, J. Chin, L. Norton, A.N. Houghton, and P.O. Livingston. Vaccination of high risk breast cancer patients with sTn (clustered)-keyhole limpet hemocyanin conjugate plus the immunological adjuvant QS-21. *Clin Cancer Res*. p. In Press, (2005).
90. S.F. Slovin, G. Ragupathi, C. Musselli, C. Fernandez, M. Diani, D. Verbel, S. Danishefsky, P.O. Livingston, and H.I. Scher. Thomsen-Friedendreich (TF) antigen as a target for prostate cancer vaccine: Results of a phase I trial with TF cluster (c)-KLH-QS-21 conjugate vaccine in biochemically relapsed prostate cancer. *Can Imm Immuno*. p. In Press, (2005).
91. S.F. Slovin, G. Ragupathi, C. Musselli, K. Olkiewicz, D. Verbel, S.D. Kuduk, J.B. Schwarz, D. Sames, S. Danishefsky, P.O. Livingston, and H.I. Scher. Fully synthetic carbohydrate-based vaccines in biochemically relapsed prostate cancer: clinical trial results with alpha-N-acetylgalactosamine-O-serine/threonine conjugate vaccine. *J Clin Oncol*. 21(23): p. 4292–8, (2003).
92. G.F. Springer, P.R. Desai, H. Tegtmeyer, B.D. Spencer, and E.F. Scanlon. Pancarcinoma T/Tn antigen detects human carcinoma long before biopsy does and its vaccine prevents breast carcinoma recurrence. *Ann N Y Acad Sci*. 690: p. 355–7, (1993).
93. G.D. MacLean, M.B. Bowen-Yacyshyn, J. Samuel, A. Meikle, G. Stuart, J. Nation, S. Poppema, M. Jerry, R. Koganty, T. Wong, and et al. Active immunization of human ovarian cancer patients against a common carcinoma (Thomsen-Friedenreich) determinant using a synthetic carbohydrate antigen. *J Immunother*. 11(4): p. 292–305, (1992).
94. G.D. MacLean, D.W. Miles, R.D. Rubens, M.A. Reddish, and B.M. Longenecker. Enhancing the effect of THERATOPE STn-KLH cancer vaccine in patients with metastatic breast cancer by pretreatment with low-dose intravenous cyclophosphamide. *J Immunother Emphasis Tumor Immunol*. 19(4): p. 309–16, (1996).
95. G.D. MacLean, M. Reddish, R.R. Koganty, T. Wong, S. Gandhi, M. Smolenski, J. Samuel, J.M. Nabholtz, and B.M. Longenecker. Immunization of breast cancer patients using a synthetic sialyl-Tn glycoconjugate plus Detox adjuvant. *Cancer Immunol Immunother*. 36(4): p. 215–22, (1993).
96. R.A. Pon, M. Lussier, Q.-L. Yang, and H.J. Jennings. N-Propionylated group B meningococcal polysaccharide mimics a Unique bactericidal capsular epitope in group B Neisseria menigitidis. *J. Exp. Med*. 185(11): p. 1929–1938, (1997).

97. L.M. Krug, G. Ragupathi, K.K. Ng, C. Hood, H.J. Jennings, Z. Guo, M.G. Kris, V. Miller, B. Pizzo, L. Tyson, V. Baez, and P.O. Livingston. Vaccination of small cell lung cancer patients with polysialic acid or N-propionylated polysialic acid conjugated to keyhole limpet hemocyanin. *Clin Cancer Res*. 10(3): p. 916–23, (2004).
98. S. Zhang, F. Helling, K.O. Lloyd, and P.O. Livingston. Increased tumor cell reactivity and complement-dependent cytotoxicity with mixtures of monoclonal antibodies against different gangliosides. *Cancer Immunol Immunother*. 40(2): p. 88–94, (1995).

PART 3

PASSIVE IMMUNOTHERAPY APPROACHES

CHAPTER 14

MONOCLONAL ANTIBODY THERAPY OF CANCER

JOSEPH G. JURCIC, DEBORAH A. MULFORD,
AND DAVID A. SCHEINBERG

Memorial Sloan-Kettering Cancer Center and
Weill Medical College of Cornell University
New York, NY 10021

INTRODUCTION

After two decades of preclinical and clinical trials, monoclonal antibodies (mAbs) are now used routinely in the treatment of cancer. The development of hybridoma technology, first described by Köhler and Milstein in 1975, allowed the therapeutic potential of mAbs to be explored [1]. With the promise to target and destroy malignant cells selectively, mAbs were initially seen as "magic bullets." Early studies, however, revealed various physical, biological, and immunological limitations to their clinical use. Advances in immunology and molecular biology allowed many obstacles to the effective use of mAbs to be surmounted. Genetically engineered chimeric, humanized, and fully human antibodies have been developed to overcome the lack of intrinsic antitumor activity of many murine mAbs. Because host effector mechanisms are not required for tumor killing, radioimmunotherapy and antibody-drug conjugates have also become promising approaches.

IMMUNOGLOBULIN STRUCTURE

Immunoglobulins are separated into five classes or isotypes based on structure and biologic properties. IgM is the primordial antibody whose expression by B cells represents the commitment to a particular recognition space that subsequently narrows during maturation induced by antigen interactions [2]. IgD is normally

H.L. Kaufman and J.D. Wolchok (eds.), General Principles of Tumor Immunotherapy, 321–342.

co-expressed with IgM on B cells. IgE, IgA, and IgG are mature immunoglobulins that are expressed after maturation of response and class switch. IgE participates in immediate-type hypersensitivity reactions and parasite immunity; IgA, in mucosal immunity, and IgG, in humoral immunity. IgA is further divided into two subclasses, and IgG, into four subclasses. Most mAbs used clinically belong to the IgG isotype.

The basic structural elements of all antibodies are heavy chains of 55 to 75 kDa and light chains of 22 kDa. The μ, δ, γ, ε, and α heavy chains correspond to IgM, IgD, IgG, IgE, and IgA isotypes, respectively. Light chains, distributed among all immunoglobulin subclasses, are either κ or λ. The amino-terminal domain of each chain is the variable (V_H or V_L) region, composed of subdomains consisting of framework regions interdigitated with complementarity-determining regions (CDRs), or hypervariable regions, that make primary contact with antigens [3]. Each heavy and light chain has three CDRs that may participate in antigen binding. The remaining domains are constant regions designated C_L for light chain and C_H1, C_H2, and C_H3 for heavy chain (and C_H4 for μ and ε). The smallest

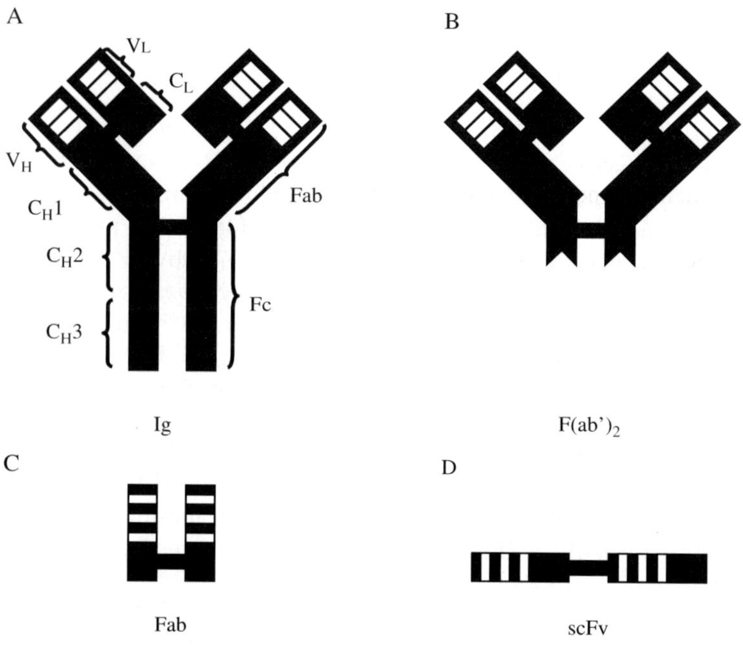

Figure 1. Structure of antibody fragments. (A) The immunoglobulin G (IgG) molecule consists of four polypeptide chains, two heavy chains (V_H, C_H1, C_H2, and C_H3) and two light chains (V_L and C_L). The hypervariable sequences, shown in white, are found with the V_H and V_L regions and are responsible for antigen binding. The Fc portion within the constant regions C_H1, C_H2, C_H3, and C_L, shown in black, mediates effector functions. (B) The F(ab()$_2$ fragment contains both Fab(domains linked by a disulfide bond. (C) The Fab contains V_H and C_H1 along with the entire light chain. (D) V_H and V_L domains can be joined by a synthetic peptide linker to make a single-chain antibody fragment

stable unit consists of two pairs of heavy and light chains, $(HL)_2$. IgE and IgG are composed of a single $(HL)_2$ unit, but IgM exists as a pentamer of $(HL)_2$ units joined by disulfide bonds with a third J-chain component. IgA exists mainly as a monomer in serum and as a dimer plus trimer in secretions.

The IgG antibody has been defined in terms of susceptibility to proteases that cleave in the exposed, unfolded regions of the antibody (Figure 1). The Fab contains the V region and the first constant domain of the heavy chain and the entire light chain. Fab´ also includes a portion of the H chain hinge region and one or more free cysteines. $(Fab')_2$ is a dimer of Fab´ linked by a disulfide bond. Fv is a semi-stable fragment including one V_H and V_L. Genetically engineered products include C_H2 deletion constructs that lack the second C domain of the heavy chain, resulting in more rapid serum clearance, and single-chain Fv (scFv), an Fv with a peptide linkage engineered to join the C-terminus of one chain to the N-terminus of the other. More advanced products have been designed that conceptually represent the antigen-binding domain in a single peptide product [4].

STRATEGIES FOR MONOCLONAL ANTIBODY THERAPY OF CANCER

Immune-Mediated Cytotoxicity

MAbs can be used to focus an inflammatory response against a tumor cell. The binding of mAbs to a target cell can result in complement activation, leading to a number of biologically important effects that include chemotaxis for phagocytic cells and production of the membrane attack complex. Additionally, cells with antibody and complement on their surfaces may also be engulfed, or opsonized, by macrophages. Another important mechanism for tumor cell killing by is antibody-dependent cell-mediated cytotoxicity (ADCC), in which an effector cell expressing an Fc receptor binds to a cell-bound mAb and is triggered to kill the target cell. Monocytes, macrophages, natural killer (NK) cells, and neutrophils can mediate ADCC.

Chimeric and humanized antibodies have been constructed to overcome the weak antitumor activity and immunogenicity of many murine mAbs (Figure 2). These antibodies retain the binding specificity of the original rodent antibody determined by the variable region but can potentially activate the human immune system through their human constant region. Bispecific mAbs represent another approach to enhance ADCC. Created by joining antibodies that react with specific tumors and mAbs directed against immune effector cells, these constructs can potentially direct cytotoxic cells to targeted tumor cells [5]. Among the most effective bispecific mAbs are those which activate T cells by binding to the CD3-T-cell receptor (TCR) complex and NK cells by binding to the CD16-FcγRIII receptor, as well as other lymphocyte activation proteins such as CD28. Although this approach is promising in experimental systems, clinical trials have been limited.

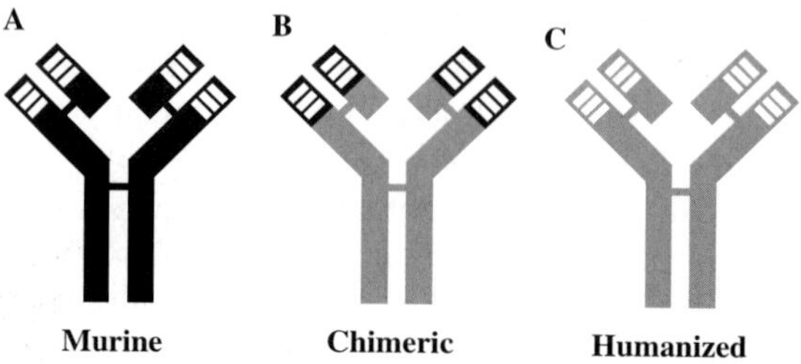

Figure 2. Structure of murine, murine-human chimeric, and humanized mAbs. The chimeric antibody consists of human antibody sequences shown in gray with rodent V_H and V_L domains shown in black and white. The humanized antibody is composed of the orginal rodent hypervariable sequences, shown in white within a human immunoglobulin framework and constant region shown in gray

Anti-idiotypic Antibodies

Recognizing unique idiotypic structure in the variable region of immunoglobulin molecules, anti-idiotypic mAbs were first used in the treatment of follicular lymphomas, with the goal of targeting the idiotype expressed by the transformed B-cell clone [6]. Several mechanisms of action have been postulated, including complement-mediated cytotoxicity (CMC), ADCC, downregulation of the malignant clone through the idiotypic network, inhibition of cell proliferation, and induction of apoptosis. In another approach, "mirror-image" anti-idiotypic mAbs that structurally resemble the antigen recognized by the original immunoglobulin can be used as surrogate immunogens to induce protective immunity against various malignancies.

Interference with Cell Growth and Regulation

MAbs can exert cytostatic or cytotoxic effects by binding to growth factors or cellular receptors needed for tumor survival. Antibodies directed against cytokines, such as interleukin-2 (IL-2), tumor necrosis factor-α (TNF-α) and IL-6, and growth factor receptors, such as the IL-2 receptor, vascular endothelial growth factor (VEGF) and epidermal growth factor receptor (EGFR) have been studied. The most clinically useful mAbs may operate by several mechanisms. For example, in addition to mediating cytotoxic effects by complement and cellular mechanisms, rituximab, a chimeric mAb targeting the B-cell surface antigen CD20, can directly induce apoptosis *in vitro* in lymphoma cells.

Delivery of Cytotoxic Agents

Because of the lack of potency of many unconjugated mAbs, they have been used to deliver radioisotopes, chemotherapeutic agents, and toxins directly to tumor cells. Since radioisotopes emit particles capable of inducing lethal DNA damage to cells lying within a fixed range, radioimmunoconjugates may allow the killing of antigen-negative tumor variants or tumor cells not reached by mAbs.

Chemotherapeutic agents such as doxorubicin, calicheamicin, methotrexate, and vinca alkaloids have been conjugated to various mAbs. To increase drug concentrations at tumor sites and avoid nonspecific cytotoxic effects, antibody-dependent enzyme-prodrug therapy (ADEPT) has been developed [7]. In this approach, an enzyme-conjugated mAb is administered followed by injection of a low-molecular-weight prodrug after antigen saturation is achieved. The prodrug rapidly penetrates tumor and is converted to active drug. To reduce the conversion of prodrug outside the tumor further, unbound antibody may be cleared from circulation by a second antibody [8].

Toxins used clinically have been derived from either bacterial products, such as diphtheria toxin (DT) and *Pseudomonas* exotoxin A (PE), or plant products, such as ricin, pokeweed antiviral protein (PAP), and gelonin. Ricin, DT, and PE each have molecular domains responsible for binding to the target cell, translocating the toxin into the cytosol, and inhibiting protein synthesis through inactivation of elongation factor 2 [9]. Modifications to these toxins can eliminate or block the adherence domain, leading to a marked reduction in nonspecific toxicity. Other toxins, such as PAP, gelonin, and saporin, lack specific binding domains and may be less toxic to intact cells. The immunotoxin BL22, composed of an anti-CD22 Fv and truncated PE has shown significant activity in patients with cladribine-refractory hairy-cell leukemia [10]. Other toxin constructs include B4 (anti-CD19)-blocked ricin for lymphoma [11], and HuM195 (anti-CD33)-gelonin for acute myeloid leukemia (AML) [12, 13].

ANTIBODY PHARMACOKINETICS

Tumor Characteristics

Various physical and biological factors can prevent the delivery of mAbs to tumor. Because of their large size and high molecular weight (typically 150–180 kDa), mAbs may have difficulty diffusing to sites of bulky disease. In early lymphoma trials, impaired tumor targeting was reported in patients with bulky adenopathy or massive splenomegaly [14, 15]. Additionally, variations in tumor vasculature can limit the distribution of mAbs to only well-perfused areas of tumor. Endothelial integrity and interstitial back-pressure can also affect mAb delivery. Interstitial pressure is consistently higher in solid tumors than in normal tissues, which partly explains the nonuniform distribution of antibody in solid tumors and the increased antibody uptake in smaller tumor cell clusters [16].

A further obstacle to mAb penetration of a cluster of antigen-positive cells is the binding-site barrier phenomenon [17]. The binding-site barrier results from a low antibody concentration in the tumor interstitial space relative to the local antigen concentration, thereby preventing mAb diffusion into the interior of the solid tumor until the antigen sites in the periphery are occupied [18]. The use of antibody fragments potentially offers improved tumor penetration because of their smaller size and lower molecular weight. The utility of these constructs, however, may be limited by rapid serum clearance, decreased binding avidity, and decreased molecular stability and activity when conjugated to radioisotopes.

Antigen Characteristics

The number of available antigen sites will alter antibody pharmacokinetics and biodistribution. In a dose-escalation trial of trace-labeled ^{131}I-anti-CD33 mAb M195 for myeloid leukemias, for example, superior targeting to sites of disease as determined by gamma camera imaging was seen with a comparatively small dose. This may be explained in part by the relatively low number of binding sites (approximately 10,000–20,000) on each leukemia cell [19]. Circulating antigenic targets can also prevent delivery of mAbs to the tumor, as first reported with anti-idiotypic mAbs directed against surface Ig on B-cell lymphomas [6]. Secreted idiotype prevented access of antibody to the idiotype on tumor cells, effectively neutralizing the drug unless high doses were given. Pre-infusions of unlabeled antibodies have been used to saturate circulating target cells and to increase delivery of therapeutically radiolabeled mAbs to tumors in several systems, including ^{131}I-p67 (anti-CD33) for AML [20] and ^{131}I-tositumomab (anti-CD20) for lymphoma [15, 21].

The influence of antigenic modulation on mAb-based treatments relates to specific therapeutic applications. Differences in the rates of endocytosis, intracellular degradation, and cell surface shedding can affect the selection of mAbs for therapy. Tumors in which antigen-antibody complexes remain on the cell surface may be better suited to treatments dependent upon immune-mediated cytotoxicity or delivery of radioisotopes with long-ranged emissions, such as ^{131}I. Internalization of the antigen-antibody complex after binding can optimize delivery of some radioisotopes, such as short-ranged α particle-emitters, chemotherapeutic agents, and toxins.

Antibody Characteristics

Most studies suggest that high-affinity mAbs confer a therapeutic advantage, particularly for small tumors. The affinity of an antibody for substrate relates to the particular amino acid sequence and spatial presentation of the CDRs. In many cases, CDR manipulation in humanization causes loss of affinity due to changes in single, critical residues or carbohydrates [22–24]. Phage display technology, however, offers a powerful technique to improve affinities by mutating the CDRs. Fab molecules are expressed on the surface of phage, selected against immobilized antigen, and enriched in proportion to their affinity [25].

The catabolic rate of an antibody will influence the dose and schedule necessary to maintain therapeutic blood levels. The Brambell receptor (FcRB, also known as FcRn), located in endosomes of endocytically active tissues, particularly the vascular endothelium is a key factor in the regulation of IgG catabolism [26]. The FcRB binds IgG, recycling it to the cell surface and diverting it from the pathway to lysosomes and catabolism that is the fate of other proteins.

Because most mAbs used clinically are derived from mice, they can generate a HAMA (human antimouse antibody) response. HAMA has been implicated in poor therapeutic results by neutralizing mAb on repeated doses and enhancing clearance of mAb. Usually no additional toxicities are seen; however, with large mAb doses circulating immune complexes can lead to serum sickness. The use of immunosuppressive agents to prevent the development of HAMA has met with variable results. The use of chimeric and humanized mAbs remains the most promising strategy to avoid HAMA responses. Additionally, fully "human" IgG have been produced *in vivo* in transgenic mice [27,28]. For some humanized mAbs, however, a prolonged biological half-life may result in nonspecific dose deposition and toxicity when used to deliver radioisotopes or chemotherapeutic agents.

RADIOIMMUNOTHERAPY

Isotope Selection and Radiolabeling

Targeted radiotherapy offers a promising strategy to increase the potency of mAbs and overcome tumor antigen heterogeneity. The choice of an appropriate isotope depends on various factors, including the physical and biological half-life of the radionuclide and its emission characteristics, and the labeling efficiency of the isotope and pharmacology of the immunoconjugate (Table 1). The α and β particles emitted by these isotopes have different properties that confer theoretical advantages and disadvantages to each. Since the range of β-emissions extends for several millimeters, radioimmunotherapy with β-emitters can create a "crossfire effect," destroying tumor cells to which the radioimmunoconjugate is not directly bound. Therefore, therapy with β-emitters is likely to be useful in the setting of bulky tumors and as conditioning for hematopoietic stem cell transplantation. Alpha particles are positively charged helium nuclei that have a short range in tissue (50–80 μm) and a high linear energy transfer (LET) (~100 keV/μm) compared to β particles. Because the range of an α particle measures only a few cell diameters, the use of α-emitting isotopes may result in more specific tumor cell kill and less damage to surrounding normal tissue. These characteristics make α particles ideal for the treatment of small-volume or minimal residual disease.

Most clinical studies to date have used the β particle-emitters iodine-131 (^{131}I) or yttrium-90 (^{90}Y). The γ emissions from iodine-131 (^{131}I) allow biodistribution and dosimetry studies to be performed easily using γ camera imaging, but treatment at high doses requires patient isolation. Radiolabeling with ^{131}I can also cause loss of biological function, particularly at high specific activities. This decrease in immunoreactivity is directly related to the number of tyrosine residues in the hypervariable region of the mAb to which radioiodine attaches [29]. ^{90}Y is a pure β-emitter; its lack of gamma emissions allows outpatient administration of high

Table 1. Characteristics of Selected Radioisotopes for Therapy

Isotope	Particle(s) emitted	Half-Life	Particulate energy (KeV)	Mean range of emission (mm)
β-emitters				
Iodine-131	β, γ	8.1 days	610	0.8
Yttrium-90	β	2.5 days	2280	2.7
Copper-67	β, γ	2.6 days	580	0.9
Rhenium-186	β, γ	3.7 days	1100	1.1
Rhenium-188	β, γ	17 hours	2100	2.4
α-emitters				
Bismuth-212	1 α, 1 β, 1 γ	1 hour	7800	0.04–0.10
Bismuth-213	1 α, 2 β, 1 γ	46 minutes	8400	0.05–0.08
Astatine-211	1 α, 1 γ	7.2 days	6800	0.04–0.10
Actinium-225	4 α, 2 β, 2 γ	10 days	6000–8400	0.04–0.08
Radium-223	4 α, 2 β, 3 γ	11.4 days	6000–7000	0.04–0.08
Lead-212	1α, 2 β, 1 γ	10.6 hours	7800	0.04–0.10

doses. The high-energy, long-range β-emissions of ^{90}Y result in a lower effective dose than ^{131}I [30]. Moreover, if the targeted antigen undergoes modulation, ^{90}Y is more likely to be retained intracellularly than ^{131}I [31]. Therapy with ^{90}Y, however, poses several difficulties. Unlike ^{131}I, ^{90}Y must be linked to a mAb by a bifunctional chelator, and because of the absence of γ emissions, biodistribution and dosimetry studies require administration of mAb trace-labeled with a second isotope, usually indium-111 (^{111}In). The use of quantitative positron emission tomography (PET) following the administration of ^{86}Y-labeled mAb may permit more precise dose estimates, thereby maximizing the antitumor effect and minimizing toxicity [32]. Other radiometals, such as rhenium-186 (^{86}Re), rhenium-188 (^{188}Re), and copper-67 (^{67}Cu), have been studied.

Alpha particle-emitting isotopes, such as bismuth-212 (^{212}Bi), bismuth-213 (^{213}Bi), and astatine-211 (^{211}At), have also displayed potent antitumor effects [33]. Finding a suitable approach for labeling these radioisotopes to carrier molecules has often been a limiting factor in the development of radiolabeled molecules for therapeutic use. For a labeling technique to be useful, it must produce the immunoconjugate in high yield in a time compatible with the half-life of the radioisotope. Furthermore, it must not alter the specificity and affinity of the carrier molecule for the target antigen. Finally, the radioimmunoconjugate must be stable *in vivo*. The most effective chelator for bismuth has been the cyclohexylbenzyl derivative of diethylenetriamine pentaacetic acid (CHX-A-DTPA). The safety and feasibility of α-particle immunotherapy was first demonstrated using the humanized anti-CD33 mAb HuM195 labeled with ^{213}Bi in patients with AML [34]. Fourteen of the 18 patients had a reduction in the percentage of bone marrow blasts after therapy; however, there were no complete remissions, demonstrating the difficulty of targeting one or two ^{213}Bi atoms to each leukemic blast at the specific activities used in this trial. Subsequently, remissions have been seen in some patients treated with ^{213}Bi-HuM195 after partial cytoreduction with cytarabine [35].

Produced by the bombardment of bismuth with α particles in a cyclotron, the halogen ^{211}At emits two α particles in its decay to stable ^{107}Pb [36]. Due to its long 7.2 hr half-life, ^{211}At-labeled constructs can be used even when the targeting molecule does not gain immediate access to tumor cells. Additionally, its daughter, polonium-211 (^{211}Po), emits K x-rays that allow photon counting of samples and external imaging for biodistribution studies. Investigators at Duke University have studied ^{211}At-labeled 81C6, a chimeric mAb that targets tenascin, a glycoprotein overexpressed on gliomas relative to normal brain tissue. Early results of a phase I trial suggest that therapy with ^{211}At-81C6 following resection of malignant glioma prolongs survival compared with historical controls [37].

^{225}Ac decays by α-emission with a 10-day half-life through three atoms, each of which also emits an α particle. It can be conjugated to a variety of mAbs using derivatives of the macrocyclic ligand 1,4,7,10-tetraazacyclododecane tetraacetic acid (DOTA). Therefore, ^{225}Ac-DOTA can act as an atomic nanogenerator, delivering an α-particle cascade to a cancer cell when coupled to an internalizing antibody. As a result of these properties, ^{225}Ac-immunoconjugates are approximately 1,000 times more potent than ^{213}Bi-containing conjugates [38]. Although this increased potency could make ^{225}Ac more effective than other α-emitters, the possibility of free daughter radioisotopes in circulation after decay of ^{225}Ac raises concerns about the potential toxicity of this isotope. In nude mice bearing human prostate carcinoma and lymphoma xenografts, single nanocurie doses of ^{225}Ac-labeled tumor specific antibodies prolonged survival compared with controls and cured a substantial proportion of animals.

Dosimetry

Dosimetric studies, usually based on the Medical Internal Radiation Dose model, are performed routinely in most radioimmunotherapy studies [39]. These techniques use serial external imaging after administration of the radioimmunoconjugate, along with measurements of plasma, urine, bone marrow, and occasionally biopsied tumor, to estimate radiation doses to tumor, marrow, and other normal organs. Cumulated activity (the total number of decays) for a region of interest is calculated by integrating the time-activity curve generated from these data over time. The result is then multiplied by the total energy released per radionuclide decay and by a factor that accounts for the fraction of emitted energy that is absorbed within the tissue. This "S factor" depends on the tissue's geometry as well as the energy and range of each radionuclide emission. Dividing by the mass of the target tissue yields the absorbed dose in Grays (energy absorbed per unit mass of tissue). Depending on the range and type of radionuclide emissions, radioactivity in other organs also may contribute to the total absorbed dose of a given target organ. Contributions from other organs are calculated similarly, except that the geometric factor reflects the fraction of emitted energy in a source organ that is absorbed by the given target organ. Models based on dosimetric data may provide information about radiation doses delivered to tissues not directly sampled and may also be used to estimate total tumor burden and tumor burden in individual organs.

Conventional methodologies that estimate mean absorbed dose over a specific organ volume may not always yield biologically meaningful information for short-ranged α particles. Cells targeted by an α-emitter may receive high absorbed radiation doses, while adjacent cells may receive no radiation at all. Therefore, microdosimetric or stochastic analyses that account for the spatial distribution of various cell types and the distribution of α decays within the organ are necessary to estimate the absorbed dose to tumor cells and normal tissues more accurately. Since the geometric relationship between the radionuclide and the target cell is not uniform, α particle hits cannot be assumed to be a Poisson distribution. Several distributions have been modeled, and microdosimetric spectra expressed as specific energy probability densities have been calculated. Based on this work, methods have been developed to perform basic microdosimetric assessments that account for the probability of the number of hits and the mean specific energy from a single hit [40].

Pretargeting Methods

In an effort to reduce radiation doses to normal organs and improve tumor-to-normal organ dose ratios, pretargeted methods of radioimmunotherapy similar to the ADEPT approach discussed earlier have been developed [41]. First, a mAb or engineered targeting molecule conjugated to streptavidin is given. After administration of a biotinylated N-acetylgalactosamine-containing "clearing agent" to remove excess circulating antibody through the liver, therapeutically radiolabeled biotin is infused. The radiolabeled biotin can bind specifically to pretargeted streptavidin at the tumor, while unbound radiolabeled biotin is rapidly excreted in the urine.

This approach has been applied to a xenograft model of adult T-cell leukemia/lymphoma [42]. Following administration of humanized anti-Tac (anti-CD25)-streptavidin and the clearing agent, treatment with ^{213}Bi-labeled biotin improved survival compared with ^{90}Y-labeled biotin. Moreover, mice treated with ^{213}Bi by the pretargeting approach survived longer than those treated with ^{213}Bi labeled directly to anti-Tac. Significant antitumor effects were also seen using an anti-Tac single chain Fv-streptavidin fusion protein followed by ^{213}Bi-biotin in the same xenograft model [43]. Pretargeting methods using an anti-CD20 fusion protein [44] and a CC49 fusion protein [45] followed by ^{90}Y/^{111}In-DOTA-biotin have been applied clinically to the treatment of non-Hodgkin's lymphoma (NHL) and gastrointestinal malignancies, respectively.

CLINICAL TRIALS

Among the many therapeutic trials with mAbs and other immunoconjugates, those that illustrate important aspects of mAb therapy or describe pivotal trials that have altered the standard of care for a certain malignancy will be addressed

(Table 2). We will focus on the eight mAbs that have been approved by the U.S. Food and Drug Administration (FDA) for human use in the treatment of specific malignancies.

Rituximab

Rituximab (Rituxan®, Mabthera®), a chimeric IgG1 anti-CD20 antibody, represents an important advance in the treatment of B-cell NHL. In the phase II licensing trial, the overall response rate to single-agent rituximab among patients with relapsed low-grade lymphoma was 48%, with a 12-month median response duration [46]. Similarly, phase II studies in relapsed or refractory intermediate- and high-grade NHL demonstrated a 32% overall response with rituximab alone. Hainsworth *et al.* studied both the effect of both first-line therapy and maintenance with rituximab for indolent NHL in a randomized phase II trial [47]. Four weekly doses of rituximab produced an overall response rate of 39%. Following initial therapy with rituximab, patients were randomized to receive the same regimen at six month intervals or re-treatment with rituximab at the time of progression. Although progression-free survival was longer in the maintenance group (31 mos. vs. 7 mos.), the duration of rituximab benefit was similar in both groups (31 mos. vs. 27 mos.).

The impressive single-agent activity of rituximab led to the exploration of its use in combination with standard chemotherapy for treatment of indolent and aggressive NHL. Czuczman *et al.* established the safety and efficacy of rituximab when added to cyclophosphamide, doxorubicin, vincristine, and prednisone (CHOP) in a phase II trial of patients with previously treated and newly diagnosed low-grade NHL [48]. In a large, multi-center, randomized phase III trial, the addition of rituximab to cyclophosphamide, vincristine, and prednisone (CVP) significantly improved overall response rate (81% vs. 57%), (CR 40% vs. 10%), and time to treatment failure (27 mos. vs. 7 mos.) [49]. The benefit of rituximab in combination with chemotherapy for elderly patients with untreated, diffuse large B-cell lymphoma was investigated in a randomized phase III trial [50]. With a median follow-up of three years, those patients treated with rituximab and CHOP (R-CHOP) had a significantly better CR rate (76% vs. 63%), event-free survival (53% vs. 35%), and overall survival (62% vs. 51%) than those treated with chemotherapy alone [51]. In another phase III multicenter trial, a similar patient population was randomized to R-CHOP versus CHOP followed by a second randomization for maintenance with rituximab [52]. Although maintenance significantly prolonged time-to-treatment failure in patients who received CHOP alone, there were no statistically significant differences in overall survival among the two groups. In general, the addition of rituximab to standard chemotherapy did not produce an increase in expected toxicities. As a result of these and other studies, rituximab has become a common part of many lymphoma treatment regimens.

A number of studies using rituximab at standard doses of 375 mg/m^2 weekly demonstrated an inferior response rate for patients with small lymphocytic leukemia (SLL) or chronic lymphocytic leukemia (CLL) compared to patients with follicular

Table 2. Monoclonal antibodies for cancer approved by FDA

Drug	Target Antigen	Antibody Type	FDA Indication	Other potential uses
Rituximab	CD20	Chimeric	Relapsed/refractory low-grade B-cell NHL	CLL, WM, upfront DLBCL
Alemtuzumab	CD52	Humanized	CLL after alkylators and fludarabine	T-PLL, HSCT
Trastuzumab	Her2/neu	Humanized	Metastatic breast carcinoma	Adjuvant breast carcinoma
Bevacizumab	VEGF	Humanized	Metastatic colorectal carcinoma with 5-FU-based therapy	RCC, NSCLC
Cetuximab	EGFR	Humanized	Metastatic colorectal carcinoma, refractory to or intolerant of irinotecan	H/N cancer (with RT)
Gemtuzumab ozogamicin	CD33	Humanized	AML over age 60 in first relapse	Upfront AML
^{131}I-tositumomab	CD20	Murine	Relapsed/refractory FL ± transformation	Upfront FL, DLBCL
^{90}Y-ibritumomab tiuxetan	CD20	Murine	Relapsed/refractory FL ± transformation	Upfront FL, DLBCL

Abbreviations: VEGF, vascular endothelia growth factor; EGFR, epithelial growth factor receptor; NHL, non-Hodgkin's lymphoma; CLL, chronic lymphocytic leukemia; 5-FU, 5-fluorouracil; AML, acute myeloid leukemia; FL, follicular lymphoma; WM, Waldenström's macroglobulinemia; DLBCL, diffuse large B-cell lymphoma; T-PLL, T-cell prolymphocytic leukemia; HSCT, hematopoietic stem cell transplantation; RCC, renal cell carcinoma; NSCLC, non-small cell lung carcinoma; H/N, head and neck; RT, radiation therapy.

NHL [46,53]. This may be due in part to the low density of CD20 on CLL cells and to the higher number of circulating tumor cells, resulting in rapid clearance of the drug [54,55]. Rituximab at standard doses three times weekly [56] or a high doses (500–2250 mg/m^2) weekly [57] overcame the pharmacologic disadvantage seen in earlier SLL/CLL studies. Currently, the use of rituximab in combination cyclophosphamide and either fludarabine [58] or pentostatin [59] is under investigation in both upfront and relapsed CLL.

Alemtuzumab

Alemtuzumab (Campath®) is humanized mAb that targets CD52, a glycoprotein expressed on CLL cells, normal B- and T-cells, and monocytes. Initial studies demonstrated that this agent was effective at clearing tumor cells from the blood and bone marrow of patients with NHL but did not result in significant reductions of bulky lymphadenopathy [60]. Additional studies, therefore, were undertaken in CLL, since it is primarily a malignancy of the peripheral blood and bone marrow. In a pivotal, multicenter phase II trial, alemtuzumab, given intravenously three times weekly for 12 weeks, produced responses in 33% of patients with fludarabine-refractory CLL; however, the CR rate was only 2%. Grade 3–4 infections were seen in 26% of patients [61]. Subsequently, previously untreated, symptomatic CLL patients were treated with alemtuzumab subcutaneously in a phase II trial [62]. The overall response and CR rates were 87% and 19%, respectively. Although significant clearance of tumor cells was noted in the blood, bone marrow and non-bulky lymphadenopathy, no patient with lymphadenopathy measuring greater than 5 cm achieved a CR. In an attempt to increase response rates and ultimately improve survival of CLL patients, investigators at the M.D. Anderson Cancer Center have examined the use of alemtuzumab in combination therapy with fludarabine, cyclophosphamide, and rituximab (CFAR) [63]. In a preliminary report, the overall response and CR rates among 21 patients with relapsed or refractory CLL were 52% and 17%, respectively. Grade 3–4 neutropenia was seen in 62% of patients, and 24% had CMV reactivation, illustrating the immunosuppressive effects of this agent.

Alemtuzumab has shown significant activity in other clinical settings. In a retrospective analysis of 76 patients with heavily pretreated T cell-prolymphocytic leukemia (T-PLL), Keating *et al.* demonstrated a 51% overall response rate and 39.5% CR rate following alemtuzumab [64]. In a prospective phase II trial, alemtuzumab produced an overall response rate of 76% and a CR rate of 60% in patients with relapsed T-PLL [65]. Because of its generalized immunosuppressive effects, alemtuzumab has shown promise in various preparative regimens for non-myeloablative allogeneic stem cell transplantation [66] and in *ex vivo* depletion of T cells before stem cell transplantation [67].

Trastuzumab

Trastuzumab (Herceptin®) is a humanized IgG1 mAb that targets the her2/neu antigen, which is overexpressed in 25–30% of breast carcinomas. Trastuzumab appears to act through multiple mechanisms, including down-regulation of her-2/neu expression, induction of G1 arrest, initiation of ADCC and complement-dependent cytotoxicity, and promotion of apoptosis [68]. Trastuzumab has single-agent activity in patients whose tumors over-express her-2/neu [69, 70]. In combination with standard chemotherapy, such as paclitaxel, docetaxel, or doxorubicin, response rate, time-to-progression, and overall survival are significantly improved in patients with metastatic breast disease [71,72]. Survival benefit, however, was not observed in patients with her-2/neu-negative tumors assessed by fluorescence in situ hybridization or immunohistochemical analysis. Based on these findings, trastuzumab is being studied in combination with chemotherapy in the adjuvant setting or in conjunction with other targeted therapies. Its use in other her-2/neu-overexpressing epithelial tumors is another area of active research.

Bevacizumab

Bevacizumab (Avastin®), a humanized mAb against VEGF, has shown activity in a variety of solid tumors in early phase I and II trials. It was approved in 2004 for the treatment of metastatic colorectal cancer. VEGF is overexpressed by many solid tumors and hematologic malignancies and is commonly associated with poor prognosis. Antibodies that target the VEGF receptor or neutralize VEGF were developed to block this important regulator of tumor angiogenesis. A randomized, phase III trial showed that the addition of bevacizumab to irinotecan, fluorouracil, and leucovorin (IFL) significantly improved median survival (20.3 mos. vs. 15.6 mos.) and progression-free survival (10.6 mos. vs. 6.2 mos.) in patients with metastatic colorectal cancer [73]. Bevacizumab is under study in a variety of solid tumors and hematologic malignancies as monotherapy and in combination with other cytotoxic agents. A randomized, double-blind, phase II trial demonstrated a significantly longer time to progression in patients with metastatic renal cell carcinoma who received bevacizumab compared to placebo [74]. Other trials are planned or ongoing in head and neck cancer, sarcoma, melanoma, hepatocellular carcinoma, esophageal carcinoma, multiple myeloma, myelodysplastic syndrome (MDS), AML, NHL, and chronic myeloid leukemia (CML).

Cetuximab

Overexpression of the EGFR, a regulator of cellular growth and survival, has been observed in multiple epithelial tumors and is a potential target of the chimeric mAb cetuximab (Erbitux®). In a recent randomized phase III trial, combination irinotecan and cetuximab resulted in a higher response rate (23% vs. 11%) and longer median time to progression (4.1 vs. 1.5 mos.) than cetuximab monotherapy in patients with irinotecan-refractory, EGFR-positive metastatic colorectal cancer [75]. Although the level of EGFR expression did not correlate with response, the previously reported association between skin reactions following cetuximab and higher response rates was confirmed in this study. Based on these data and previous studies [76], cetuximab was FDA-approved for the treatment of irinotecan-refractory metastatic colorectal cancer.

Cetuximab has also displayed activity in advanced head and neck tumors. Among 75 patients with platinum-refractory head and neck cancer, 11% responded when cetuximab was added to the platinum regimen, suggesting that cetuximab can overcome platinum-resistance in some patients [77]. A small randomized study comparing cisplatin alone to cisplatin and cetuximab showed a more than doubling of the response rate but only a modest improvement in time to disease progression in the cetuximab arm [78]. Additionally, a phase III study of radiation with or without cetuximab in patients with advanced head and neck tumors has completed accrual. The use of cetuximab is currently being investigated in other epithelial tumors, including non-small cell lung carcinoma and pancreatic cancer.

Gemtuzumab Ozogamicin

Gemtuzumab ozogamicin (GO, Mylotarg®) consists of a recombinant humanized anti-CD33 mAb conjugated to calicheamicin, a potent antitumor antibiotic. Within the acidic environment of the lysosome following internalization, calicheamicin dissociates from the antibody and migrates to the nucleus, where it causes double-stranded DNA breaks. In a phase I trial, eight of 40 patients with relapsed or refractory AML treated with escalating doses of GO had reductions in marrow blasts to below 5%, and CRs were seen in three patients [79]. Subsequently, 142 patients with AML in first relapse were treated with two doses of GO (9 mg/m^2) two weeks apart in three phase II trials. Patients with secondary AML or prior MDS were excluded. Twenty-three patients (16%) achieved a CR, and 19 patients (13%) had a CRp (CR with incomplete platelet recovery) [80]. Grade 3 or 4 hyperbilirubinemia developed in 23% of patients, and elevated serum transaminases were seen in 17%. Hepatic veno-occlusive disease (VOD) occurred in 4% of patients. Based on this data, GO was approved by the FDA for the treatment of AML patients over age 60 years in first relapse. When used as a single-agent for newly diagnosed AML in older patients, complete response rates of approximately 25% have been reported [81].

VOD remains a major concern with this agent. Among patients who received GO in first relapse and then underwent stem cell transplantation, 17% developed VOD [82]. Another study noted that 11 of 23 patients (48%) treated with GO after stem cell transplantation developed liver injury similar to classical VOD, termed sinusoidal obstruction syndrome [83]. In a series of 119 patients treated with GO at the M.D. Anderson Cancer Center, 14 (12%) developed VOD in the absence of stem cell transplantation. Most of these patients, however, received GO in combination with other agents, including investigational drugs, or at more frequent intervals than originally described [84].

GO-containing combinations are now under investigation for both newly diagnosed and relapsed AML. Because of its toxicity profile, however, administration of full-dose GO with other agents has been difficult. In a study conducted by the Medical Research Council, 86% of patients with newly diagnosed AML achieved remission after receiving one of three standard induction regimens along with GO. The maximum tolerated dose of GO was a single infusion of 3 mg/m^2. Hepatotoxicity and delayed hematopoietic recovery prevented delivery of higher doses duration induction or repeated administration [85]. Preliminary results suggest that GO in combination with ATRA in APL can produce high molecular remission rates as first-line therapy and that its use as consolidation could potentially eliminate the need for standard anthracycline-based consolidation [86].

Radioimmunotherapy for Hematologic Malignancies

Leukemia and lymphoma are well-suited to radioimmunotherapeutic approaches because of the accessibility of malignant cells in the blood, bone marrow, lymph nodes, and spleen, and radiosensitivity of these tumors. Encouraging results in the treatment of AML have been seen when used in conjunction with bone marrow transplantation (BMT). The murine anti-CD33 mAb M195, when therapeutically labeled with ^{131}I, can target leukemia cells and eliminate large leukemic burdens in patients [87]. Based on these findings, ^{131}I-labeled M195 or its humanized counterpart, HuM195, was added to busulfan and cyclophosphamide to intensify conditioning before allogeneic BMT [88]. Three of 16 patients with relapsed or refractory AML remain in remission for over 5 years following transplant. Investigators at the Fred Hutchinson Cancer Research Center have taken a similar approach using ^{131}I-BC8, which targets the pan-leukocyte antigen CD45 [89]. In an ongoing phase I/II trial using a preparative regimen of ^{131}I-BC8, busulfan, and cyclophosphamide in patients with AML in first remission, the disease-free survival is 61% with a median follow-up of 49 months [90]. The use of a murine anti-CD66 mAb labeled with ^{188}Re as part of a preparative regimen before stem cell transplantation has also been examined. Because CD66 is expressed on myeloid cells but not leukemic blasts, the antileukemic effect of this construct must rely on "crossfire" from the long-ranged β particles emitted by ^{188}Re [91]. While these approaches appear promising, randomized trials are required to determine if the addition of radioimmunotherapy to standard preparative regimens improve patient outcomes.

The ^{131}I-labeled murine anti-CD20 mAb tositumomab (Bexxar®) has produced encouraging results in patients with B-cell lymphomas. In initial studies, patients were treated with escalating doses of trace-labeled mAb to determine an optimal dose for tumor targeting before receiving therapeutically labeled mAbs. Therapeutic doses of ^{131}I were escalated based on estimated whole body radiation dose [21]. In a subsequent multicenter trial conducted in patients with relapsed low-grade or transformed lymphoma, 67% of the patients responded after ^{131}I-tositumomab, compared to only 28% of these patients who responded after their last chemotherapy regimen [92]. Based on these data, the FDA approved ^{131}I-tositumomab for the treatment of relapsed, CD20-positive follicular lymphoma. ^{131}I-tositumomab has also produced high complete remission rates when used as first-line therapy for follicular lymphoma [93]. Additional studies using combination or sequential chemotherapy and radioimmunotherapy are now underway [94].

High doses of ^{131}I-tositumomab have also been used in a myeloablative approach. Patients were eligible for a therapeutic infusion of ^{131}I-tositumomab followed by autologous stem cell rescue if biodistribution studies using trace-labeled mAb showed that tumor sites received greater radiation doses than normal tissues. Among 29 patients treated at the maximum tolerated dose of ^{131}I-tositumomab in phase I and II trials, 25 patients had major responses, including 23 complete remissions [95]. Studies combining high-dose ^{131}I-tositumomab with chemotherapy followed by autologous stem cell transplantation have produced encouraging results in patients with relapsed NHL [96], particularly mantle cell lymphoma [97].

Similar results have been seen with ^{90}Y-ibritumomab tiuxetan (Zevalin®). Among 51 patients with relapsed or refractory follicular or relapsed aggressive NHL, 73% responded, including 51% who achieved CR or unconfirmed CR (CRu) [98]. The median time to progression for patients with either a CR or CRu was 28 months. The subset of complete responders who received the maximum tolerated dose of ^{90}Y-ibritumomab tiuxetan (0.4 mCi/kg) had a median time to progression of 45 months. A randomized trial comparing ^{90}Y-ibritumomab tiuxetan to rituximab showed a higher overall response rate (80% vs. 56%) and CR rate (30% vs. 16%) for radioimmunotherapy, but the time to disease progression was similar for both groups [99].

CONCLUSIONS

While mAbs have been proven to be safe and effective anticancer therapies in some clinical settings, they appear most effective when integrated into treatment programs involving chemotherapy, radiation therapy, and other biologic therapies. Early studies showed that single doses rodent mAbs had little antitumor activity and were highly immunogenic. The development of chimeric, humanized, and fully human antibodies has overcome a major obstacle to successful mAb-based therapy. Nevertheless, because of the difficulties in targeting bulky disease, particularly in solid tumors, the use of many mAbs may be most appropriate as adjuvants or in the treatment of minimal residual disease. The conjugation of radioisotopes or toxins to mAbs can enhance the antitumor effects of native antibody. Radioimmunotherapy with β-emitting isotopes may be useful for treatment of bulky tumors and marrow ablation; in contrast, α-particle immunotherapy may be better suited for treatment of minimal residual disease or micrometastases because of the short-range, high-energy emissions. New approaches using mAb fragments or genetically engineered single-chain binding proteins may improve delivery of isotopes or toxins to solid tumors, but the pharmacologic difficulties may still be significant. Additional preclinical and clinical investigations are necessary to define optimal therapeutic targets, antibody constructs, radioisotopes and toxins, chelation chemistry, dosing regimens, and therapeutic strategies in order to take full advantage of this promising therapeutic modality.

REFERENCES

1. Köhler G, Milstein C. Continuous cultures of fused cells secreting antibody of predefined specificity. Nature 1975; 256:495–497.
2. Burrows PD, Cooper MD. B-cell development in man. Curr Opin Immunol 1993; 5:201–206.
3. Petersen JG, Dorrington KJ. An in vitro system for studying the kinetics of interchain disulfide bond formation in immunoglobulin G. J Biol Chem 1974; 249:5633–5641.
4. Welling GW, Geurts T, van Gorkum J, et al. Synthetic antibody fragment as ligand in immunoaffinity chromatography. J Chromatogr 1990; 512:337–343.
5. Segal DM, Wunderlich JR. Targeting of cytotoxic cells with heterocrosslinked antibodies. Cancer Invest 1988; 6:83–92.
6. Meeker TC, Lowder J, Maloney DG, et al. A clinical trial of anti-idiotype therapy for B cell malignancy. Blood 1985; 65:1349–1363.
7. Senter PD. Activation of prodrugs by antibody-enzyme conjugates: a new approach to cancer therapy. FASEB J 1990; 4:188–193.
8. Yuan F, Baxter LT, Jain RK. Pharmacokinetic analysis of two-step approaches using bifunctional and enzyme-conjugated antibodies. Cancer Res 1991; 51:3119–3130.
9. Pastan I, FitzGerald D. Recombinant toxins for cancer treatment. Science 1991; 254:1173–1177.
10. Kreitman RJ, Wilson WH, Bergeron K, et al. Efficacy of the anti-CD22 recombinant immunotoxin BL22 in chemotherapy-resistant hairy-cell leukemia. N Engl J Med 2001; 345:241–247.
11. Grossbard ML, Lambert JM, Goldmacher VS, et al. Anti-B4-blocked ricin: a phase I trial of 7-day continuous infusion in patients with B-cell neoplasms. J Clin Oncol 1993; 11:726–737.
12. Duzkale H, Pagliaro LC, Rosenblum MG, et al. Bone marrow purging studies in acute myelogenous leukemia using the recombinant anti-CD33 immunotoxin HuM195/rGel. Biol Blood Marrow Transplant 2003; 9:364–372.
13. Talpaz M, Kantarjian H, Freireich E, et al. Phase I clinical trial of the anti-CD33-immunotoxin HuM195/rGel. Proc Am Assoc Cancer Res 2003; 44:1228.
14. Scheinberg DA, Straus DJ, Yeh SD, et al. A phase I toxicity, pharmacology, and dosimetry trial of monoclonal antibody OKB7 in patients with non-Hodgkin's lymphoma: effects of tumor burden and antigen expression. J Clin Oncol 1990; 8:792–803.
15. Press OW, Eary JF, Appelbaum FR, et al. Radiolabeled-antibody therapy of B-cell lymphoma with autologous bone marrow support. N Engl J Med 1993; 329:1219–1224.
16. Williams LE, Duda RB, Proffitt RT, et al. Tumor uptake as a function of tumor mass: a mathematic model. J Nucl Med 1988; 29:103–109.
17. Fujimori K, Covell DG, Fletcher JE, et al. A modeling analysis of monoclonal antibody percolation through tumors: a binding-site barrier. J Nucl Med 1990; 31:1191–1198.
18. Juweid M, Neumann R, Paik C, et al. Micropharmacology of monoclonal antibodies in solid tumors: direct experimental evidence for a binding site barrier. Cancer Res 1992; 52:5144–5153.
19. Scheinberg DA, Lovett D, Divgi CR, et al. A phase I trial of monoclonal antibody M195 in acute myelogenous leukemia: specific bone marrow targeting and internalization of radionuclide. J Clin Oncol, 1991;9(3):478–90.
20. Appelbaum FR, Matthews DC, Eary JF, et al. The use of radiolabeled anti-CD33 antibody to augment marrow irradiation prior to marrow transplantation for acute myelogenous leukemia. Transplantation 1992; 54:829–833.

21. Kaminski MS, Zasadny KR, Francis IR, et al. Radioimmunotherapy of B-cell lymphoma with [131I]anti-B1 (anti-CD20) antibody. N Engl J Med 1993; 329:459–465.
22. Caron PC, Co MS, Bull MK, et al. Biological and immunological features of humanized M195 (anti-CD33) monoclonal antibodies. Cancer Res, 1992;52(24):6761–7.
23. Riechmann L, Clark M, Waldmann H, et al. Reshaping human antibodies for therapy. Nature, 1988;332(6162):323–7.
24. Carter P, Presta L, Gorman CM, et al. Humanization of an anti-p185HER2 antibody for human cancer therapy. Proc Natl Acad Sci U S A, 1992;89(10):4285–9.
25. Gram H, Marconi LA, Barbas CF, 3rd, et al. In vitro selection and affinity maturation of antibodies from a naive combinatorial immunoglobulin library. Proc Natl Acad Sci U S A, 1992;89(8):3576–80.
26. Junghans RP. Finally! The Brambell receptor (FcRB). Mediator of transmission of immunity and protection from catabolism for IgG. Immunol Res 1997;16(1):29–57.
27. Green LL, Hardy MC, Maynard-Currie CE, et al. Antigen-specific human monoclonal antibodies from mice engineered with human Ig heavy and light chain YACs. Nat Genet, 1994;7(1):13–21.
28. Ishida I, Tomizuka K, Yoshida H, et al. Production of human monoclonal and polyclonal antibodies in TransChromo animals. Cloning Stem Cells, 2002;4(1):91–102.
29. Nikula TK, Bocchia M, Curcio MJ, et al. Impact of the high tyrosine fraction in complementarity determining regions: measured and predicted effects of radioiodination on IgG immunoreactivity. Mol Immunol 1995; 32:865–872.
30. Jurcic JG, Divgi CR, McDevitt MR, et al. Potential for myeloablation with Yttrium-90-HuM195 (anti-CD33) in myeloid leukemia. Proc Am Soc Clin Oncol, 2000: 19:8a.
31. Scheinberg DA, Strand M. Kinetic and catabolic considerations of monoclonal antibody targeting in erythroleukemic mice. Cancer Res 1983; 43:265–272.
32. Lovqvist A, Humm JL, Sheikh A, et al. PET imaging of ^{86}Y-labeled anti-Lewis Y monoclonal antibodies in a nude mouse model: comparison between ^{86}Y and ^{111}In radiolabels. J Nucl Med 2001; 42:1281–1287.
33. McDevitt MR, Sgouros G, Finn RD, et al. Radioimmunotherapy with alpha-emitting nuclides. Eur J Nucl Med 1998; 25:1341–1351.
34. Jurcic JG, Larson SM, Sgouros G, et al. Targeted alpha particle immunotherapy for myeloid leukemia. Blood 2002; 100:1233–1239.
35. Mulford DA, Pandit-Taskar N, McDevitt MR, et al. Sequential therapy with cytarabine and bismuth-213 (^{213}Bi)-labeled HuM195 (anti-CD33) for acute myeloid leukemia (AML). Blood 2004; 104:496a.
36. Zalutsky MR, Narula AS. Astatination of proteins using an N-succinimidyl tri-n-butylstannyl benzoate intermediate. Int J Rad Appl Instrum [A] 1988; 39:227–232.
37. Zalutksy M, Reardon D, Akabani G, et al. Astatine-211 labeled human/mouse chimeric anti-tenascin monoclonal antibody via surgically created resection davities for patients with recurrent glioma: phase I study. Neuro-oncol 2202; 4(suppl):S103.
38. McDevitt MR, Ma D, Lai LT, et al. Tumor therapy with targeted atomic nanogenerators. Science 2001; 294:1537–1540.
39. Sgouros G. Dosimetry of internal emitters. J Nucl Med 2005; 46:18S-27S.
40. Humm JL, Roeske JC, Fisher DR, Chen GTY. Microdosimetric concepts in radioimmunotherapy. Med Phys 1993; 20:535–543.
41. Axworthy DB, Reno JM, Hylarides MD, et al. Cure of human carcinoma xenografts by a single dose of pretargeted yttrium-90 with negligible toxicity. Proc Natl Acad Sci USA 2000; 97:1802–1807.
42. Zhang M, Zhang Z, Garmestani K, et al. Pretargeting radioimmunotherapy of a murine model of adult T-cell leukemia with the α-emitting radionuclide, bismuth 213. Blood 2002; 100:208–216.
43. Zhang M, Zhang Z, Garmestani K, et al. Pretarget radiotherapy with an anti-CD25 antibody-streptavidin fusion protein was effective in therapy of leukemia/lymphoma xenografts. Proc Natl Acad Sci USA 2003; 100:1891–1895.
44. Forero A, Weiden PL, Vose JM, et al. Phase 1 trial of a novel anti-CD20 fusion protein in pretargeted radioimmunotherapy for B-cell non-Hodgkin lymphoma. Blood 2004; 104:227–236.

45. Shen S, Forero A, LoBulgio AF, et al. Patient-specific dosimetry of pretargeted radioimmunotherapy using CC49 fusion protein in patients with gastrointestinal malignancies. J Nucl Med 2005; 46:642–651.
46. McLaughlin P, Grillo-Lopez AJ, Link BK, et al. Rituximab chimeric anti-CD20 monoclonal antibody therapy for relapsed indolent lymphoma: half of patients respond to a four-dose treatment program. J Clin Oncol 1998; 16:2825–2833.
47. Hainsworth JD, Litchy S, Shaffer DW, et al. Maximizing therapeutic benefit of rituximab: maintenance therapy versus re-treatment at progression in patients with indolent non-Hodgkin's lymphoma—a randomized phase II trial of the Minnie Pearl Cancer Research Network. J Clin Oncol 2005; 23:1088–1095.
48. Czuczman MS, Grillo-Lopez AJ, White CA, et al. Treatment of patients with low-grade B-cell lymphoma with the combination of chimeric anti-CD20 monoclonal antibody and CHOP chemotherapy. J Clin Oncol 1999; 17:268–276.
49. Marcus R, Imrie K, Belch A, et al. An international multi-centre, randomized, open-label, phase III trial comparing rituximab added to CVP chemotherapy to CVP chemotherapy alone in untreated stage III/IV follicular non-Hodgkin's lymphoma. Blood 2003; 102:28a.
50. Coiffier B, Lepage E, Briere J, et al. CHOP chemotherapy plus rituximab compared with CHOP alone in elderly patients with diffuse large-B-cell lymphoma. N Engl J Med 2002; 346:235–242.
51. Coiffier B, Herbrecht R, Tilly H, et al. GELA study comparing CHOP and R-CHOP in elderly patients with DLCL: 3-year median follow-up with an analysis according to co-morbidity factors. Proc Am Soc Clin Oncol, 2003; 22:596.
52. Habermann T, Weller E, Morrison V. Phase III trial of rituximab-CHOP (R-CHOP) vs. CHOP with a second randomization to maintenance rituximab (MR) or observation in patients 60 years of age and older with diffuse large B-cell lymphoma (DLBCL). Blood 2003; 102:6a.
53. Foran JM, Rohatiner AZ, Cunningham D, et al. European phase II study of rituximab (chimeric anti-CD20 monoclonal antibody) for patients with newly diagnosed mantle-cell lymphoma and previously treated mantle-cell lymphoma, immunocytoma, and small B-cell lymphocytic lymphoma. J Clin Oncol 2000; 18:317–324.
54. Berinstein NL, Grillo-Lopez AJ, White CA, et al. Association of serum Rituximab (IDEC-C2B8) concentration and anti-tumor response in the treatment of recurrent low-grade or follicular non-Hodgkin's lymphoma. Ann Oncol 1998; 9:995–1001.
55. Nguyen DT, Amess JA, Doughty H, et al. IDEC-C2B8 anti-CD20 (rituximab) immunotherapy in patients with low-grade non-Hodgkin's lymphoma and lymphoproliferative disorders: evaluation of response on 48 patients. Eur J Haematol 1999; 62:76–82.
56. Byrd JC, Murphy T, Howard RS, et al. Rituximab using a thrice weekly dosing schedule in B-cell chronic lymphocytic leukemia and small lymphocytic lymphoma demonstrates clinical activity and acceptable toxicity. J Clin Oncol 2001; 19:2153–2164.
57. O'Brien SM, Kantarjian H, Thomas DA, et al. Rituximab dose-escalation trial in chronic lymphocytic leukemia. J Clin Oncol 2001; 19:2165–2170.
58. Wierda W, O'Brien SM, Faderl S, et al. Improved survival in patients with relapsed- refractory chronic lymphocytic leukemia (CLL) treated with fludarabine, cyclophosphamide, and rituximab (FCR) combination. Blood 2003; 102:110a.
59. Weiss M, Lamanna N, Jurcic J, et al. Pentostatin, cyclophosphamide, and rituximab (PCR therapy): a new active regimen for previously treated patients with chronic lymphocytic leukemia (CLL). Blood 2003; 102:673a.
60. Hale G, Dyer MJ, Clark MR, et al. Remission induction in non-Hodgkin lymphoma with reshaped human monoclonal antibody CAMPATH-1H. Lancet 1988; 2:1394–1399.
61. Keating MJ, Flinn I, Jain V, et al. Therapeutic role of alemtuzumab (Campath-1H) in patients who have failed fludarabine: results of a large international study. Blood 2002; 99:3554–3561.
62. Lundin J, Kimby E, Bjorkholm M, et al. Phase II trial of subcutaneous anti-CD52 monoclonal antibody alemtuzumab (Campath-1H) as first-line treatment for patients with B-cell chronic lymphocytic leukemia (B-CLL). Blood 2002; 100:768–773.

63. Wierda W, Faderl S, O'Brien S, et al. Combined cyclophosphamide, fludarabine, alemtuzumab, and rituximab (CFAR) is active for relapsed and refractory patients with CLL. Blood 2004; 104:101a.
64. Keating MJ, Cazin B, Coutre S, et al. Campath-1H treatment of T-cell prolymphocytic leukemia in patients for whom at least one prior chemotherapy regimen has failed. J Clin Oncol 2002; 20:205–213.
65. Dearden CE, Matutes E, Cazin B, et al. High remission rate in T-cell prolymphocytic leukemia with CAMPATH-1H. Blood 2001; 98:1721–1726.
66. Morris E, Thomson K, Craddock C, et al. Outcomes after alemtuzumab-containing reduced-intensity allogeneic transplantation regimen for relapsed and refractory non-Hodgkin lymphoma. Blood 2004; 104:3865–3871.
67. Chakrabarti S, MacDonald D, Hale G, et al. T-cell depletion with Campath-1H 'in the bag' for matched related allogeneic peripheral blood stem cell transplantation is associated with reduced graft-versus-host disease, rapid immune constitution and improved survival. Br J Haemat 2003; 121:109–118.
68. Nahta R, Esteva FJ. HER-2-targeted therapy: lessons learned and future directions. Clin Cancer Res 2003; 9:5078–5084.
69. Baselga J, Tripathy D, Mendelsohn J, et al. Phase II study of weekly intravenous recombinant humanized anti-p185HER2 monoclonal antibody in patients with HER2/neu-overexpressing metastatic breast cancer. J Clin Oncol 1996; 14:737–744.
70. Cobleigh MA, Vogel CL, Tripathy D, et al. Multinational study of the efficacy and safety of humanized anti-HER2 monoclonal antibody in women who have HER2-overexpressing metastatic breast cancer that has progressed after chemotherapy for metastatic disease. J Clin Oncol 1999; 17:2639–2648.
71. Slamon DJ, Leyland-Jones B, Shak S, et al. Use of chemotherapy plus a monoclonal antibody against HER2 for metastatic breast cancer that overexpresses HER2. N Engl J Med 2001; 344:783–792.
72. Esteva FJ, Valero V, Booser D, et al. Phase II study of weekly docetaxel and trastuzumab for patients with HER-2-overexpressing metastatic breast cancer. J Clin Oncol 2002; 20:1800–1808.
73. Hurwitz H, Fehrenbacher L, Novotny W, et al. Bevacizumab plus irinotecan, fluorouracil, and leucovorin for metastatic colorectal cancer. N Engl J Med 2004; 350:2335–2342.
74. Yang JC, Haworth L, Sherry RM, et al. A randomized trial of bevacizumab, an anti-vascular endothelial growth factor antibody, for metastatic renal cancer. N Engl J Med 2003; 349:427–434.
75. Cunningham D, Humblet Y, Siena S, et al. Cetuximab monotherapy and cetuximab plus irinotecan in irinotecan-refractory metastatic colorectal cancer. N Engl J Med 2004; 351:337–345.
76. Saltz LB, Meropol NJ, Loehrer PJ Sr, et al. Phase II trial of cetuximab in patients with refractory colorectal cancer that expresses the epidermal growth factor receptor. J Clin Oncol 2004; 22:1201–1208.
77. Baselga J, Trigo J, Bouthis J. Cetuximab (C225) plus cisplatin/carboplatin is active in patients with recurrent/metastatic squamous-cell carcinoma of the head and neck progressing on a same dose and schedule platinum-based regimen. Proc Am Soc Clin Oncol 2002; 21:226a.
78. Burtness BA, Li Y, Flood W, et al. Phase III trial comparing cisplatin (C) + placebo to C + anti-epidermal growth factor antibody (EGF-R) C225 in patients with metastatic/recurrent head & neck cancer (HNC). Proc Am Soc Clin Oncol 2002; 21:226a.
79. Sievers EL, Appelbaum FR, Spielberger RT, et al. Selective ablation of acute myeloid leukemia using antibody-targeted chemotherapy: a phase I study of an anti-CD33 calicheamicin immunoconjugate. Blood 1999; 93:3678–3684.
80. Sievers EL, Larson RA, Staudtmauer EA, et al. Efficacy and safety of gemtuzumab ozogamicin in patients with CD33-positive acute myeloid leukemia in first relapse. J Clin Oncol 2001; 19:3244–3254.
81. Adadori S, Suciu Willemze R, et al. Sequential administration of gemtuzumab ozogamcin and convential chemotherapy as first line therapy in elderly patients with acute myeloid leukemia: a phase II study (AML-15) of the EORTC and GIMEMA leukemia groups. Hematologica 2004; 89:950–956.

82. Sievers E, Larson R, Estey E, et al. Final report of prolonged disease-free survival in patients with acute myeloid leukemia in first relapse treated with gemtuzumab ozogamicin followed by hematpoietic stem cell transplantation. Blood 2002; 100:89a.
83. Rajvanshi P, Schulman H, Sievers E, et al. Hepatic sinusoidal obstruction after gemtuzumab ozogamicin (Mylotarg) therapy. Blood 2002; 99:10–14.
84. Giles FJ, Kantarjian HM, Kornblau SM, et al. Mylotarg (gemtuzumab ozogamicin) therapy is associated with hepatic venoocclusive disease in patients who have not received stem cell transplantation. Cancer 2001; 92:406–413.
85. Kell WJ, Burnett AK, Chopra R, et al. A feasibility study of simultaneous administration of gemtuzumab ozogamicin with intensive chemotherapy in induction and consolidation in younger patients with acute myeloid leukemia. Blood 2003; 102:4277–4283.
86. Estey E, Giles FJ, Beran M, et al. Experience with gemtuzumab ozogamicin ("Mylotarg") and all-*trans* retinoic acid in untreated acute promyelocytic leukemia. Blood 2002; 99:4222–4224.
87. Schwartz MA, Lovett DR, Redner A, et al. Dose-escalation trial of M195 labeled with iodine 131 for cytoreduction and marrow ablation in relapsed or refractory myeloid leukemias. J Clin Oncol 11:294–303.
88. Burke JM, Caron PC, Papadopoulos EB, et al. Cytoreduction with iodine-131-anti-CD33 antibodies before bone marrow transplantation for advance myeloid leukemias. Bone Marrow Transplant 2003; 32:549–556.
89. Matthews DC, Appelbaum FR, Eary JF, et al. Phase I study of (131)I-anti-CD45 antibody plus cyclophosphamide and total body irradiation for advanced acute leukemia and myelodysplastic syndrome. Blood 1999; 94:1237–1247.
90. Pagel JM, Appelbaum FR, Eary JF, et al. ^{131}I-anti-CD45 antibody plus busulfan/cyclophosphamide in matched related transplants for acute myeloid leukemia in first remission. Blood 2004; 104:232a.
91. Bunjes D. ^{188}Re-labeled anti-CD66 monoclonal antibody in stem cell transplantation for patients with high-risk acute myeloid leukemia. Leuk Lymph 2002; 43:2125–2131.
92. Kaminski MS, Zelenetz AD, Press OW, et al. Pivotal study of iodine I 131 tositumomab for chemotherapy-refractory low-grade or transformed low-grade B-cell non-Hodgkin's lymphomas. J Clin Oncol 2001; 19:3918–3928.
93. Kaminski MS, Tuck M,m Estes J, et al. ^{131}I tositumomab therapy as initial treatment for follicular lymphoma. N Engl J Med 2005; 352:441–449.
94. Press OW, Unger JM, Braziel RM, et al. A phase 2 trial of CHOP chemotherapy followed by tositumomab/iodine I 131 tositomomab for previously untreated follicular non-Hodgkin's lymphoma: Southwest Oncology Group protocol S9911.
95. Liu SY, Eary JF, Petersdorf SH, et al. Follow-up of relapsed B-cell lymphoma patients treated with iodine-131-labeled anti-CD20 antibody and autologous stem-cell rescue. J Clin Oncol 1998; 16:3270–3278.
96. Press OW, Eary JF, Gooley T, et al. A phase I/II trial of iodine-131-tositumomab (anti-CD20), etoposide, cyclophosphamide, and autologous stem cell transplantation for relapsed B-cell lymphomas. Blood 2000; 96:2934–2942.
97. Gopal AK, Rajendran JG, Petersdorf SH, et al. High-dose chemo-radioimmunotherapy with autologous stem cell support for relapsed mantle cell lymphoma. Blood 2002; 99:3158–3162.
98. Gordon LI, Molina A, Witzig T, et al. Durable responses after ibritumomab tiuxetan radioimmunotherapy for CD20+ B-cell lymphoma: long-term follow-up of a phase 1/2 study. Blood 2004; 103:4429–4431.
99. Witzig TE, Gordon LI, Cabanillas F, et al. Randomized controlled trial of yttrium-90-labeled ibritumomab tiuxetan radioimmunotherapy versus rituximab immunotherapy for patients with relapsed or refractory low-grade, follicular, or transformed B-cell non-Hodgkin's lymphoma. J Clin Oncol 2002; 20:2453–2463.

CHAPTER 15

ADOPTIVE CELLULAR THERAPY FOR THE TREATMENT OF CANCER

CASSIAN YEE

Program in Immunology Clinical Research Division Fred Hutchinson Cancer Research Center University of Washington Seattle, WA

INTRODUCTION

Over the last decade, advances in the field of tumor immunobiology have led to a renaissance in the use of adoptively transferred T cells for the treatment of patients with cancer. These advances include the identification of T cell-defined tumor-associated antigens, a greater understanding of the underlying molecular principles governing T cell activation, differentiation and expansion, and the development of novel strategies to elicit and characterize T cell responses both in vitro, and in vivo. In this chapter, the 'principles and practice' of adoptive cellular therapy are discussed in the context of translational studies arising from basic immunologic discoveries.

BIOLOGICAL BASIS FOR ADOPTIVE CELLULAR THERAPY

Adoptive cellular therapy involves the ex vivo expansion of immune cells for infusion with the goal of increasing the anti-tumor immune response in vivo. The scientific foundation that adoptive therapy could be directed in an antigen-specific fashion was established in the 1970's using mouse models. These studies, using tumor-bearing mice, led to several important principles that are still relevant today in developing clinical trials of adoptive cellular therapy.

For several immunogenic tumors, it was observed that the anti-tumor response could be transferred from previously immunized mice to syngeneic tumor-bearing

H.L. Kaufman and J.D. Wolchok (eds.), General Principles of Tumor Immunotherapy, 343–361.

recipients. Although CD8+ cytotoxic T lymphocytes (CTL) were identified as being the dominant effector cells responsible for the anti-tumor response [1–3], both CD4+ and CD8+ T cells were found to be essential for optimal efficacy, and in some cases, CD4+ T cells alone were found to sufficient [4,5] [6,7]. The Friend murine leukemia virus (FMuLV) tumor model was instructive in this regard. CD8+ CTL and CD4+ T cells recognizing, respectively, the *env* and *gag* proteins of the leukemia virus were found to be highly specific and effective in eradicating the FMuLV tumor, FBL from mice with micrometastatic disease. Co-administered CD4+ T helper cells or a source of helper function (e.g. co-administered IL-2) was required when antigen-specific CTL were used [8–10], whereas CD4+ T cells did not require exogenous help and were also found to be effective. Furthermore, the FBL tumor is Class I+, Class II- suggesting that, while CTL can exert a direct anti-tumor effect by engaging Class I-restricted epitopes, adoptively transferred CD4 T cells recruit non-specific effectors to mediate tumor killing.

Be they CD4+ or CD8+ T cells, effector cells of high avidity [11, 12] and sufficient magnitude [13] were required to induce durable remissions. When suboptimal doses, or T cells of low avidity were used, a limited non-curative effect was observed. In addition, successful therapy was observed only when recipients received a pre-infusion conditioning regimen. Tumor-bearing mice that were not conditioned with cyclophosphamide or irradiation prior to adoptive therapy, failed to be cured [13–15]. When this observation was made several decades ago, it was proposed that pre-infusion conditioning provided host immune suppression to foster an environment that favored the in vivo persistence of adoptively transferred T cells. With greater understanding of the role of regulatory T cells and homeostatic lymphoid regulation in tumor immunity, it has since been confirmed that these early hypotheses were largely accurate and that recipient conditioning may in fact be a means of suppressing regulatory obstacles to and upregulating homeostatic signals that lead to the enhanced anti-tumor effect of adoptively transferred T cells.

One important caveat of these early studies of adoptive therapy is that these models used ‘immunogenic’ tumors and could be eradicated only at a time when the tumor burden was relatively low – at the micrometastatic or microscopic level. An *immunogenic* tumor is one that is capable of immunizing and eliciting a specific anti-tumor response that could be adoptively transferred to non-immunized recipients and reject tumors in such mice. Often, immunogenic tumors express costimulatory ligands to enhance in vivo immunization and genetically modifying non-immunogenic tumors to enhance immunity using, for example, retroviral vectors encoding B7 or GM-CSF was sufficient to render a non-immunogenic tumor, immunogenic [16,17]. To more faithfully recapitulate the human condition, more rigorous models of adoptive therapy have since been evaluated using non-immunogenic tumors, such as B16 melanoma, in the setting of established disease. In such cases, a combination of pre-infusion immunodepletion (e.g. total body irradiation) followed by adoptive transfer and vaccination was required to eradicate established B16 melanoma tumors [18].

ADOPTIVE CELLULAR THERAPY- STRATEGIES FOR EX VIVO EXPANSION

Translating the murine studies to clinical trials has not been straightforward. However some of the principles established in these animal studies have served as guidelines towards developing more effective treatment. As described above, one of the major goals is to augment the number of tumor-reactive effectors for adoptive transfer. This can be achieved by ex vivo expansion - the degree of enrichment for antigen-specific effectors being dependent on the sophistication of methods and resources available. On this basis, the spectrum of adoptive therapy strategies can be divided pragmatically into two camps:

1. Non-specific expansion
2. Antigen-specific enrichment.

Non-specific expansion includes the use of donor lymphocyte infusions (DLI) in the allogeneic stem cell transplant setting, tumor-infiltrating lymphocytes culled from tumor sites and expanded ex vivo and the non-specific activation of effector cells in the peripheral blood using antibodies to the TCR-CD3 complex. Antigen-specific enrichment involves in vitro manipulation that preferentially expands or selects for T cells expressing a TCR of given specificity (endogenous receptor) or genetic modification that endows a population of lymphocytes with desired target specificity. In the latter case, this specificity can be the result of a transferred TCR or antibody recognition fragment. Although antigen-specific enrichment often represents a more labor and resource-intensive process, it may lead to more effective therapy. It can also provide a unique means of delineating the reasons for success or failure of a given approach and so, can contribute to a greater understanding in the development of improved strategies.

NON-SPECIFIC EXPANSION OF CELLULAR EFFECTORS

Donor Lymphocyte Infusions

The first evidence that T cells play a role in mediating anti-tumor responses in humans was observed in patients receiving T cell replete or T cell-depleted marrow for allogeneic stem cell transplantation almost 30 years ago [19, 20]. Patients receiving syngeneic (identical twin) and T-cell depleted marrow cells experienced rates of leukemia relapse after transplant that were more than twice as high as patients receiving unmanipulated (T cell replete) marrow from allogeneic donors. Furthermore, patients developing GVHD were even more likely to experience leukemia-free remission than those who did not develop GVHD. Taken together, these results suggest that the allogeneic effect of donor lymphocytes plays an important role in eradicating residual leukemia. The directed use of donor lymphocytes for infusion (DLI) for the treatment of leukemic relapse after transplant represents an extension of these findings and has been most successfully implemented in patients who relapse following transplantation for chronic myeloid leukemia [21, 22]. In general, donor lymphocyte infusions are considered for treatment of post-transplant relapse when patients have been tapered off immunosuppression without evidence of severe GVHD. DLI is administered at target doses of 10^6 to 10^8 CD3+ cells/kg. Severe GVHD and myelosuppression can result but these effects may be ameliorated by using a low initial cell dose and selective depletion of CD8+ T cells while preserving the CD4+ T cell population [23]. Efforts have also been made to introduce a suicide gene into donor lymphocytes, so that higher T cell doses to eradicate leukemic cells can be used while reserving the ability to later eliminate donor lymphocytes in vivo should GVHD be observed [24]. For example, lymphocytes transduced with the HSV thymidine kinase suicide gene, undergo cell death as the HSV-TK preferentially converts low-dose ganciclovir (which can be safely administered to patients), into a toxic intracellular metabolite.

While the use of DLI has been most effective for CML relapse (durable CR 60–75%), it is largely experimental therapy for patients with AML, ALL, myeloma and lymphoma where responses have been significantly weaker (< 30%) [25]. In an effort to boost these responses, investigators have turned to the use of donor lymphocytes that have undergone in vitro activation. In one form of this approach, microbeads coated with antibodies to the TCR-CDR3 complex (anti-CD3) and a T cell costimulatory molecule (anti-CD28) were used to activate and expand pheresis PBMCs collected from donors for infusion. In a Phase I study, this strategy proved to be particularly effective for patients relapsing post-transplant with ALL, AML and NHL without excessive GVHD [26].

Tumor-infiltrating Lymphocytes

Tumor-infiltrating lymphocytes are those mononuclear cells harvested from a tumor excisional biopsy and propagated in vitro, usually with high doses of IL-2 (6000 U/ml). These effectors were shown initially in murine models to be superior to 'LAK' cells or lymphokine activated killer cells which were generated by exposing peripheral mononuclear cells to high-dose IL-2. The Rosenberg lab at the NCI developed the use of TIL for eventual use in clinical trials and demonstrated an antitumor response in patients with metastatic melanoma ranging from 22–35% of patients when given together with high dose IL-2 which was required for TIL survival [27]. Although these results were promising, it was not apparent that TIL alone contributed to the response beyond what would be observed with high-dose IL-2 alone. The modest efficacy observed with TIL may be attributed to the limited numbers of tumor-reactive effectors in a largely heterogeneous population and the continued dependence of high doses of IL-2 in vivo.

Efforts to facilitate the expansion of tumor-reactive effectors have also been made by vaccinating patients and then harvesting TIL from tumor-vaccine draining lymph nodes followed by anti-CD3-mediated expansion in vitro [28]. Such approaches have met with modest success. More recently, using methods developed and optimized by Riddell and others for expanding T cell clones [29,30], the NCI group devised an improved strategy for expanding TIL effectors in vitro by a 'Rapid Expansion Protocol' involving the use of irradiated feeder cells, anti-CD3 antibody and IL-2. TIL expanded in this manner were subsequently used in the treatment of patients following nonmyeloablative conditioning and found to yield significant objective clinical responses (see below) [31].

ANTIGEN-SPECIFIC ENRICHMENT OF CELLULAR EFFECTORS

This section introduces two areas – T cell therapy targeting EBV-associated malignancies and the broader topic of T cell therapy targeting tumor-associated antigens. EBV-specific T cell therapy, as one of the most successful applications of antigen-specific adoptive cellular therapy for cancer, presents a powerful example of the clinical benefit that can be achieved.

EBV-specific T Cell Therapy

Patients receiving highly immunosuppressive therapy following stem cell or organ transplantation are at high risk for EBV-associated post-transplant lymphoproliferative disease (PTLD). In immunocompetent individuals EBV-infected B cells are constrained from developing into a lymphoproliferative disorder by the endogenous EBV-specific CTL population. However, immunosuppressive therapy can lead to unchecked proliferation of EBV-infected B cells. In the post-stem cell transplant setting, donor lymphocyte infusions can lead to reconstitution of EBV-specific CTL response and induce clinical remissions in patients developing PTLD [32]; however, DLI can often lead to GVHD and myelosuppression – both of which could be eliminated through the use of more specific effectors such as EBV-specific lymphocytes. Using autologous EBV-transformed lymphpblastoid cell lines (LCLs), Rooney and others were able generate high numbers of EBV reactive CTL ($>10^7$ cells/m^2) sufficient for repeated cycles of adoptive transfer and demonstrated that infusions of EBV-CTL could be used to effectively treat PTLD and prevent PTLD when given to patients with rising EBV DNA titers post-transplant [33–35]

The use of EBV-transformed B cells as stimulator cells to enrich for the population of EBV-specific CTL was ideally suited for the treatment of PTLD since the highly immunogenic immunodominant EBV nuclear antigens-EBNA 3A, B and C were well-expressed by the proliferating B cells. Treatment of other EBV-associated malignancies, however, would not be so straightforward

Nasopharyngeal cancer (NPC) and Hodgkin's Disease (HD) do not express the immunodominant EBV antigens; instead, less immunogenic antigens are expressed: EBNA1 in all NPCs and LMP1 and 2 in HD and 50% of NPCs. A recent study of patients with advanced NPC demonstrated complete and partial responses in patients receiving EBV-specific CTL [36]. CTL administered to patients with relapsed EBV+ HD persisted and expanded in vivo and led to significant tumor regression and long-term responses [37]. To enhance the efficacy of adoptive EBV-specific T cell therapy, methods being developed by this group include optimizing in vitro culture methods to elicit desired responses to subdominant cancer-associated viral antigens and genetic modification of T cells to render them TGF-beta resistant [38].

Tumor-associated Antigens for T Cell Therapy

A major obstacle to antigen-specific immunotherapy had been the identification of T cell-defined antigens for vaccine or adoptive therapy strategies. In 1991, the first human tumor-associated antigen recognized by T cells was discovered. This antigen, MAGE-1 (for Melanoma Antigen-1), was identified by first generating a tumor-reactive T cell clone and then using it to screen target cells transfected with a cosmid library generated using tumor DNA [39]. The transfected sequence from target cells that were lysed by the T cell clone were recovered and sequenced. Since this publication, similar strategies has been used to identify several T cell-defined tumor-associated antigens for both Class I and Class II-restricted targets.

Other approaches to the identification of tumor antigens for cellular immunotherapy include the use of serological methods to identify autoantibodies to tumor antigens. This approach, Serological Recombinant Expression cloning (SEREX) screens potential autoantibodies in patient serum against an expressed phage cDNA library derived from tumor cells and displayed on nitrocellulose filters [40]. cDNA from Phage plaques corresponding to the Immunoreactive plaques on the screening filters could then be recovered and sequenced. In this approach, the assumption is made that tumor antigens that can elicit an IgG autoantibody response are also those antigens that are likely to elicit a cellular (T cell) immune response. Although T cell reactivity to all of the over 2000 SEREX-defined tumor-associated autoantigens have yet to be confirmed, several T cell-defined antigens have been identified in this manner. Most notably, many of the cancer-testis antigens (see below) which represent tumor proteins expressed in both tumor cells and normal germinal tissues in the testis and fetal ovary [41].

A third approach uses gene expression profiling such as SAGE (Serial Analysis of Gene Expression), to identify overexpressed genes among tumor cells compared with benign cells [42]. The identification of such genes does not necessarily imply that they are immunogenic; Application of algorithms that predict for preferential binding to a given MHC allele or the use of a library of peptides that overlap the entire gene sequence may yield putative immunogenic epitopes that can then be used in efforts to elicit T cell responses. Such epitope or peptides identified in this manner, may in itself, not be sufficient to confirm that these responses are relevant until it can be shown that the T cells that are elicited will also recognize naturally processed peptides by screening against antigen-expressing tumor cells or transfectants.

Finally, a more resource intensive process of eluting peptides from the surface of tumor cells, (optionally identifying pools that are T cell-reactive) and then sequencing individual peptides by tandem mass spectrometric analysis, an enormous undertaking, is now becoming a more refined and feasible strategy for identifying directly those peptides presented by tumor cells and recognized by T cells [43–45]. Several tumor-associated antigens and their immunogenic epitopes have been identified in this manner with the added advantage that the posttranslational modification, and even peptide splicing and rearrangement observed with some epitopes that would foil other antigen-identification strategies, would not be an obstacle to the direct analysis of MHC-displayed peptide by mass spectrometry. The identification of T cell targets and, in some cases, the immunogenic epitope, afforded immunotherapists the opportunity to develop rational approaches to the generation and expansion of tumor-associated antigen-specific T cells for adoptive therapy.

STRATEGIES FOR THE IN VITRO GENERATION OF TUMOR ANTIGEN-SPECIFIC T CELLS

There are two broad approaches to generating tumor antigen-specific T cells for adoptive therapy. The first, is through the use of methods to cultivate from the peripheral blood or tumor-infiltrating site those T cells whose endogenous T cell receptors engage the target of interest. This is usually accomplished through iterative cycles of in vitro stimulation to further enrich for tumor antigen-specific T cells. The second, is through the transfer of a T cell receptor or antibody fragment that recognizes a tumor-derived epitope (in the context of MHC or as a surface protein, respectively) to lymphocytes to endow a population of T cells with antigen-specific properties. In recent studies, transfer of antigen-specific receptors has also been accomplished with other immune effector cells such as NK cells, eosinophils and even hematopoietic progenitor cells. In the latter case, it is hoped that a nascent population of potentially highly proliferative memory T cells will eventually develop in vivo from marrow-engrafted stem cells.

The first approach relies heavily on culture conditions and selection methods to identify T cells with the appropriate endogenous TCR and is constrained by the existent repertoire of T cells in any individual. The second approach, once the desired TCR or antibody fragment has been sequenced and cloned, relies on the efficiency and fidelity of gene transfer technologies and the appropriate display of the desired receptor on the cell surface to engage its ligand.

Enrichment of T Cells Expressing Endogenous T Cell Receptor for Tumor Antigens

The classical approach for eliciting antigen-specific responses in vitro has been through the use of tumor cell lines that are co-cultivated with autologous T cells. Due to limitations in generating autologous tumor cell lines of sufficient magnitude or longevity required for iterative restimulations, tumor-derived immunosuppressive factors and the generally poor costimulatory property of tumor cells, investigators have turned to the use of 'professional' antigen presenting cells such as dendritic cells [46, 47], monocytes and activated B cells for use as stimulators in vitro. For the most part, these APCs upregulate expression of costimulatory molecules and MHC upon activation or maturation and can be generated reliably, at least short term, from peripheral blood mononuclear cells. Activated B cells, i.e., those B cells which have been activated through their CD40 receptor, can be propagated to large numbers over several weeks to months under the proper conditions [48].

Dendritic cells, due to its innate capacity in its immature form, collect and/or phagocytose tumor membrane, apoptotic bodies and necrotic material, and are well suited to 'cross-present' tumor antigens. Lysed tumor cells have been used as a substrate for DC cross-presentation. However, more effective strategies that take advantage of specific inherent mechanisms that facilitate antigen uptake can be employed by exposing tumor cells to UV irradiation, apoptotic inducing agents (chemotherapy, butyrate), gamma-irradiation and opsonization by antibodies specific for tumor surface proteins (e.g. MICA [49] and syndecan [50]). These approaches have been used successfully to generate tumor-reactive CD8+ and CD4+ T cells. Professional APCs (DCs, activated B cells, LCLs) can also be engineered to express a target antigen of interest, in this way to generate T cells of desired specificity. Introducing genes encoding the target antigen can be achieved using a variety of viral vectors. Although retroviral transduction is feasible, genomic integration is not required, and infection with other viral vectors (adenoviral, fowlpox, canarypox and vaccinia virus) may be more efficient for immunization or in vitro stimulation. Non-viral delivery methods include electroporation, cationic lipid or polymer-mediated transfection, ballistic or hydrodynamic insertion and RNA transfection. RNA transfection represents one of the more readily available and potent technologies for engineering Class I and Class II presentation of antigen in dendritic cells. It has been used successfully to generate antigen-specific T cell responses against individual novel antigens; transfection of in vitro transcribed RNA representing the entire tumor cDNA library has also been used to elicit responses both in vivo and in vitro [51–53].

Generating responses against those antigens for which the immunogenic peptide epitope and restricting allele have been defined, is a more straightforward process. APCs pulsed with peptides corresponding to such epitopes have been commonly used to generate peptide-reactive T cells. However, not all peptide-specific T cells will engage their targets with sufficient affinity to be able to recognize tumor cells expressing endogenous antigen whose epitope is displayed at much lower concentrations than exogenously pulsed peptides. The ability to generate high affinity T cells in vitro is dependent on a number of factors including the T cell repertoire, peptide concentration, and the modulatory effect of cytokines and accessory signals in the culture from cells or costimulatory molecules and the peptide sequence itself. Alterations to the wild-type peptide sequence to identify superagonist peptide ligands have been variably successful in generating enhanced T cell responses against self antigens [54, 55].

In an effort to standardize optimal conditions for T cell stimulation, investigators have turned to 'artificial' antigen presenting cells (aAPC). Since these APCs are devoid of potentially allogeneic MHC they may be mass-produced and commercialized for use obviating the requirement for individually generating APCs from each patient. Beads coated with anti-CD3 and anti-CD28 and NK cell lines modified to accommodate antibodies, i.e. through Fc receptors for example, provide docking sites for anti-CD28 and 4-1BB for example have been used for non-specific lymphocyte expansion. Antigen specific stimulation using Insect cells (drosophila)

[56, 57], mouse fibroblast cells [58, 59] and NK cell lines (K562) [60] have been engineered to express the MHC of interest, and co-stimulatory molecules to enhance T cell activation e.g. B7.1 (CD80), ICAM-1 (CD54), , 4-1BBL (CD137) and LFA-3 (CD58) proteins. Since most epitopes are restricted to the A2 allele and its expression is prevalent among the Caucasian population, HLA-A*0201 MHC is more often co-expressed, however CD4+ T cell responses can also be elicited using surfaces coated with recombinant Class II peptide-MHC complexes [61]. Further, to provide a platform for presenting different antigens and epitopes, the MHC itself may be designed to easily accommodate peptide substitutions [62] or transfection strategies may be incorporated into a cell-based aAPC system [63]. Cell-based systems also provide of means of supplying cytokine such as IL-15, and have the further advantage of being propagated relatively easily in vitro, although regulatory constraints may be greater than that of synthetic or bead-based systems.

To date, about a half-dozen clinical trials using T cells generated against specific tumor-associated antigens have been reported, in all cases, for the treatment of patients with metastatic melanoma. A survey of these studies reveals that the method of T cell generation, the source of T cells, whether patients were pre-conditioned or not (see below) as well as the use of exogenous growth factors can all impact the in vivo persistence of the transferred T cells, the clinical responses observed and the severity of adverse events [64]. In one of the first reported studies using insect cells as APC for in vitro stimulation, adoptively transferred antigen-specific T cells failed to persist in vivo and only minor responses were observed, likely due to the absence of any co-administered IL-2 and the relatively low cell dose (10^8 cells) that was used [65]. The NCI reported two studies using antigen-specific T cell clones obtained from previously vaccinated patients failing peptide vaccine therapy and expanded in vitro with the identical peptide in the presence of high-dose IL-2 [66, 67]. These T cells failed to persist for any appreciable duration in vivo and no clinical responses were observed even when patients were pre-conditioned with a lymphodepleting regimen [67]. In these cases, it is postulated that the shortened period of in vivo T cell persistence (< 48 hr) was due to the requirement for supraphysiologic does of IL-2 help in vivo and a starting population of T cells that may have been exhausted by prior in vivo vaccination. By contrast, clinical studies using antigen-specific T cell clones generated from the peripheral blood of non-vaccinated patients using autologous dendritic cells, when administered at doses of up to 3.3×10^9 cells/m^2, led to enhanced in vivo survival, multiple tumor regressions and extended patient survival to more than 2 years in some cases [30]. These results have been confirmed in other studies using a similar protocol [68, 69]; the duration of in vivo persistence and the appearance of antigen-loss variants were also consistently observed among these studies suggesting that a uniform strategy can lead to reproducible results. Among the most dramatic clinical responses however, were those reported by the NCI using TIL cells expanded in vitro and infused following patient conditioning with a nonmyeloablative regimen in which half of all patients experienced partial or near complete responses [31].

Transfer of T Cell Receptor or Immunoglobulin Fragment Recognizing Target Epitope

The antigen specificity of effector cells may be redirected to a target antigen or epitope by introducing genes encoding the T cell receptor or Ig known to recognize the desired target. In the case of TCR transfer, antigens (intracellular or surface in origin) can be targeted so long as they are processed and presented in the context of its restricting MHC allele on the surface. For Ig receptors, the antigens must be displayed on the surface. The attractiveness of this strategy arises from the ability to: 1) rapidly generate large numbers of antigen-specific effectors by transferring vectors encoding TCR or Ig genes directly into the PBMC population without the requirement to individually isolate and expand for T cells expressing the endogenous receptor; 2) target surface antigens in MHC unrestricted fashion using Ig receptors; 3), select for high affinity receptors (previously isolated or genetically enhanced); since most tumor-associated antigens identified to date are represented by self antigens, high affinity endogenous T cell receptors may be difficult to isolate and introducing mutations to the binding site may enhance affinity over wild-type receptors; 4), redirect specificity of both helper CD4+ and cytotoxic CD8+ T cells [70]; 5) redirect specificity of non-T cell effectors, for example, NK cells, eosinophils, etc thus providing alternative modes of tumor killing; and 6) recruitment of memory or early precursor lymphocytes to directed killing thus providing a potentially highly proliferative effector pool [71].

TCR transfer

Genes encoding the alpha and beta chains of a T cell receptor can be isolated from tumor-reactive clones and introduced into lymphocytes using an expression vector (usually lentiviral or retroviral). For tumor-associated antigens, TCR transfer leading to productive recognition of the redirected target has been successfully performed for several melanoma antigens (MART-1, gp100, tyrosinase) [72,73], the prostate cancer antigen, PSMA [74] , NY-ESO-1 [75], MAGE-3 [76,77], CAMEL and several more universally expressed targets such as WT-1 [70,78], MDM2 [79]. One drawback has been the pairing of exogenously transferred alpha and beta TCR chains with endogenous TCR chains leading to non-productive T cell receptors and dilution of the desired TCR density on the surface. Chimeric TCR genes generated by fusing the signaling domain of the CD3 zeta chain to the exogenous TCR has limited pairing with endogenous TCR chains [76]. Other strategies to exclude endogenous pairing involve the use of mouse constant regions in the TCR alpha and beta chains and inclusion of unique cysteines to facilitate inter-chain disulfide bonding [78]. The latter approach has the added advantage of avoiding any immunogenicity that may arise from mutant or cross-species constructs. TCR-gene modified T cells have been used in a handful of studies to date [80]. Adoptive transfer of lymphocytes expressing TCR for the melanoma antigens demonstrated evidence of in vivo persistence and in some cases significant, measurable responses in patients with metastatic disease.

Chimeric antibody receptor transfer

Chimeric antibody or immunoglobulin receptors are comprised of the heavy and light chain variable regions of an antibody joined to the cytoplasmic signaling component of the lymphocyte signaling molecule (often CD3zeta). This enables activation of T cell effector function (lysis, cytokine release, proliferation) when antigen binds with the chimeric antibody receptor. Theoretically, any antibody that can be reconstituted in transfected T cells can be used; chimeric antibody receptors have been used to target CEA [81], Her-2/neu, Folate receptor [80], melanoma antigens, CD33 [82] and B cell antigens. In the case of B cell malignancies, CD19- and CD20-directed therapies have been developed by several groups which are now performing clinical trials. In an effort to augment the survival of T cells in vivo, the signaling domain of CD28, a costimulatory molecule associated with IL-2 production and induction of anti-apoptotic proteins, has been fused to the chimeric CD3zeta-antibody construct. Engagement of the target ligand led to IL-2 production and improved T cell persistence in animal studies [82, 83].

HOST CONDITIONING TO ENHANCE THE EFFECTIVENESS OF ADOPTIVE CELLULAR THERAPY

The effectiveness of adoptively transferred T cells may be enhanced in an in vivo environment that has been pre-conditioned by chemotherapy or irradiation. Tumor-sensitized T cells, when administered to tumor-bearing mice, are capable of eradicating disseminated cancer and providing long-term protection but only when recipient mice were pre-treated with cyclophosphamide; cyclophosphamide alone or T cell therapy alone in these mice failed to protect [13, 14, 84–87]. This was observed for both prophylactic and challenge tumor models (i.e. mice with 'large' tumor burdens) and has repeatedly been observed in a number of model systems. The immune-enhancing effects were believed to be dose-dependent and attributed to cyclophosphamide mediated elimination of 'suppressor' or 'regulatory' T cells [88], a 'bystander' effect leading to induction of homeostatic cytokines that support the growth of transferred T cells [87], or immunologic 'skewing' to a more favorable Th1 profile [89], with upregulation of type I interferon and augmentation in number of memory T cells in vivo [90]. This suggests that homeostatic regulation contributes to the favorable effects of recipient conditioning.

The effectiveness of immunotherapy may be enhanced when combined with conventional cytotoxic agents (cyclophosphamide, doxorubicin, paclitaxel) [89], and among these, cyclophosphamide (CY) has been the most extensively studied. Since the original observation almost 40 years ago that cyclophosphamide could augment immune responses [91], this effect has been evaluated in experimental animals and clinical studies at doses ranging from 40 to > 6000 mg/m2 [85, 87, 90, 92, 93]. In murine models, some studies report CY immunopotentiation only at high (175 mg/kg or > 6 g /m^2) but not low doses (12.5 mg/kg or 40 mg/m^2) claiming only a 'bystander effect, while others demonstrate benefit at low doses (30 mg/kg) attributable to decreases in Treg numbers and/or function [88, 92]. In adoptive therapy studies, transferred memory T cells from tumor-sensitized mice are capable of eradicating disseminated cancer and providing long-term protection but only when mice were pre-treated with cyclophosphamide (cyclophosphamide alone in these mice failed to protect) [13, 14, 84–87]; this was observed for both prophylactic and challenge tumor models (i.e. mice with 'large' tumor burdens). The immune-enhancing effects were believed to be dose-dependent and attributed to cyclophosphamide-mediated elimination of 'suppressor' or 'regulatory' T cells [88], a 'bystander' effect leading to induction of homeostatic cytokines that support the growth of transferred T cells [87], or immunologic 'skewing' to a more favorable Th1 profile [89], with upregulation of type I interferon and augmentation in number of memory T cells in vivo [90]. As early as the mid 1980s, Berd and Mastrangelo first demonstrated in humans cyclophosphamide potentiation of DTH responses to a vaccine in patients with metastatic cancer at doses of 1000 mg/m^2 [94]. They later reported that lower doses (300 mg/m^2) were also adequate, as a result of a reduction in suppressor function based on in vitro functional studies [95–97]. Other investigators have suggested that lower does of CY (200-400 mg/m^2) can selectively deplete suppressor activity (CD8) while higher doses may have a 'bystander' homeostatic effect [87, 96] although at the time, regulatory T cell phenotypes had not been defined. Other investigators have suggested the use of low-dose metronomic dosing (50 mg doses) for vaccine-elicited responses. However, these studies were undertaken to identify a dose and schedule that would on balance, be sufficient to deplete regulatory T cells while preserving in vivo response to vaccines. Adoptive therapy involving the ex vivo manipulation of effector cells would not be not subject to similar constraints.

It is now believed that a number of mechanisms may be involved in augmenting or resuscitating the function of tumor-specific T cells, including depletion of regulatory T cells and homeostatic upregulation of gamma chain-receptor cytokines such as IL-7 and IL-15 [98–101]. Clinical trials of adoptive therapy have exploited lymphodepletion as a means of improving T cell survival and function. Most notably, patients with metastatic melanoma treated with a nonmyeloablative regimen comprised of fludarabine, cyclophosphamide and low-dose irradiation experienced prolonged survival and robust engraftment of adoptively transferred TIL (up to 90% of reconstituted T cells) when coadministered with high-dose IL-2. Significant regressions were observed and about 50% of patients experienced measurable clinical responses although not all responses were durable and some cases were accompanied by serious autoimmune and infectious toxicities. A less potent lymphodepleting regimen comprised of fludarabine alone led to upregulation of IL-7 and IL-15 levels, increase in T cell persistence in vivo, minimal toxicities but a more modest clinical response. Although these studies are promising, the optimal regimen for lymphodepletion and patient conditioning (perhaps more selective regulatory T cell depletion) have yet to be defined in clinical trials.

CONCLUSION AND FUTURE PROSPECTS

Adoptive cellular therapy of cancer has progressed at a steady pace over the last decade as more and more benchtop discoveries culminate in clinical trials. Methods to isolate, modify and expand human tumor-specific T cells have been successfully developed, and the opportunity to refine and streamline some of these approaches will foster its evolution into a feasible and more broadly applicable treatment modality. Combination strategies that incorporate the use of irradiation, chemotherapy, vaccination and other targeted therapies have been shown to augment the immune response. Tumor immune escape mechanisms are becoming an increasingly apparent obstacle and reagents designed to reverse immune suppression (through depletion of regulatory cells [101, 102], counter-inhibitory antibodies [103, 104], cytokine immunomodulation [100] or downregulation of negative signaling pathways [105]) may be partnered with adoptive immunotherapy to mediate more effective and durable responses. As a non-cross-resistant therapy with the potential for minimal toxicity, high specificity and long-term immunoprotection, it is hoped that the advent of these technologies to the clinic will lead to the development of adoptive therapy as a treatment modality for patients with cancer.

REFERENCES

1. Overwijk, W.W., A. Tsung, K.R. Irvine, M.R. Parkhurst, T.J. Goletz, K. Tsung, M.W. Carroll, C. Liu, B. Moss, S.A. Rosenberg, and N.P. Restifo. 1998. gp100/pmel 17 is a murine tumor rejection antigen: induction of "self"-reactive, tumoricidal T cells using high-affinity, altered peptide ligand. *J Exp Med* 188:277–286.
2. Sakai, K., A.E. Chang, and S.Y. Shu. 1990. Phenotype analyses and cellular mechanisms of the pre-effector T-lymphocyte response to a progressive syngeneic murine sarcoma. *Cancer Res* 50:4371–4376.
3. Greenberg, P.D. 1986. Therapy of murine leukemia with cyclophosphamide and immune Lyt-2+ cells: cytolytic T cells can mediate eradication of disseminated leukemia. *Journal of Immunology* 136:1917–1922.
4. Ossendorp, F., E. Mengede, M. Camps, R. Filius, and C.J. Melief. 1998. Specific T helper cell requirement for optimal induction of cytotoxic T lymphocytes against major histocompatibility complex class II negative tumors. *J Exp Med* 187:693–702.
5. Surman, D.R., M.E. Dudley, W.W. Overwijk, and N.P. Restifo. 2000. Cutting edge: CD4+ T cell control of CD8+ T cell reactivity to a model tumor antigen. *J Immunol* 164:562–565.
6. Greenberg, P.D., D.E. Kern, and M.A. Cheever. 1985. Therapy of disseminated murine leukemia with cyclophosphamide and immune Lyt-1+,2- T cells. Tumor eradication does not require participation of cytotoxic T cells. *Journal of Experimental Medicine* 161:1122–1134.
7. Frey, A.B., and S. Cestari. 1997. Killing of rat adenocarcinoma 13762 in situ by adoptive transfer of CD4+ anti-tumor T cells requires tumor expression of cell surface MHC class II molecules. *Cell Immunol* 178:79–90.
8. Cameron, R.B., P.J. Spiess, and S.A. Rosenberg. 1990. Synergistic antitumor activity of tumor-infiltrating lymphocytes, interleukin 2, and local tumor irradiation. Studies on the mechanism of action. *J Exp Med* 171:249–263.
9. Cheever, M.A., J.A. Thompson, D.E. Kern, and P.D. Greenberg. 1985. Interleukin 2 (IL 2) administered in vivo: influence of IL 2 route and timing on T cell growth. *Journal of Immunology* 134:3895–3900.

10. Cheever, M.A., P.D. Greenberg, A. Fefer, and S. Gillis. 1982. Augmentation of the anti-tumor therapeutic efficacy of long-term cultured T lymphocytes by in vivo administration of purified interleukin 2. *J Exp Med* 155:968–980.
11. Zeh, H.J., D. Perry-Lalley, M.E. Dudley, S.A. Rosenberg, and J.C. Yang. 1999. High avidity CTLs for two self-antigens demonstrate superior in vitro and in vivo antitumor efficacy. *Journal of Immunology* 162:989–994.
12. Alexander-Miller, M.A., G.R. Leggatt, and J.A. Berzofsky. 1996. Selective expansion of high- or low-avidity cytotoxic T lymphocytes and efficacy for adoptive immunotherapy. *Proceedings of the National Academy of Sciences of the United States of America* 93:4102–4107.
13. Greenberg, P.D. 1991. Adoptive T cell therapy of tumors: mechanisms operative in the recognition and elimination of tumor cells. *Adv Immunol* 49:281–355.
14. Awwad, M., and R.J. North. 1989. Cyclophosphamide-induced immunologically mediated regression of a cyclophosphamide-resistant murine tumor: a consequence of eliminating precursor L3T4+ suppressor T-cells. *Cancer Res* 49:1649–1654.
15. North, R.J., and M. Awwad. 1987. T cell suppression as an obstacle to immunologically-mediated tumor regression: elimination of suppression results in regression. *Prog Clin Biol Res* 244:345–358.
16. Townsend, S.E., and J.P. Allison. 1993. Tumor rejection after direct costimulation of CD8+ T cells by B7-transfected melanoma cells [see comments]. *Science* 259:368–370.
17. Dranoff, G., E. Jaffee, A. Lazenby, P. Golumbek, H. Levitsky, K. Brose, V. Jackson, H. Hamada, D. Pardoll, and R.C. Mulligan. 1993. Vaccination with irradiated tumor cells engineered to secrete murine granulocyte-macrophage colony-stimulating factor stimulates potent, specific, and long-lasting anti-tumor immunity. *Proceedings of the National Academy of Sciences of the United States of America* 90:3539–3543.
18. Overwijk, W.W., M.R. Theoret, S.E. Finkelstein, D.R. Surman, L.A. de Jong, F.A. Vyth-Dreese, T.A. Dellemijn, P.A. Antony, P.J. Spiess, D.C. Palmer, D.M. Heimann, C.A. Klebanoff, Z. Yu, L.N. Hwang, L. Feigenbaum, A.M. Kruisbeek, S.A. Rosenberg, and N.P. Restifo. 2003. Tumor regression and autoimmunity after reversal of a functionally tolerant state of self-reactive CD8+ T cells. *J Exp Med* 198:569–580.
19. Weiden, P.L., K.M. Sullivan, N. Flournoy, R. Storb, and E.D. Thomas. 1981. Antileukemic effect of chronic graft-versus-host disease: contribution to improved survival after allogeneic marrow transplantation. *N Engl J Med* 304:1529–1533.
20. Porter, D.L., M.S. Roth, C. McGarigle, J.L. Ferrara, and J.H. Antin. 1994. Induction of graft-versus-host disease as immunotherapy for relapsed chronic myeloid leukemia. *N Engl J Med* 330:100–106.
21. Kolb, H.J., J. Mittermuller, C. Clemm, E. Holler, G. Ledderose, G. Brehm, M. Heim, and W. Wilmanns. 1990. Donor leukocyte transfusions for treatment of recurrent chronic myelogenous leukemia in marrow transplant patients. *Blood* 76:2462–2465.
22. Dazzi, F., R.M. Szydlo, N.C. Cross, C. Craddock, J. Kaeda, E. Kanfer, K. Cwynarski, E. Olavarria, A. Yong, J.F. Apperley, and J.M. Goldman. 2000. Durability of responses following donor lymphocyte infusions for patients who relapse after allogeneic stem cell transplantation for chronic myeloid leukemia. *Blood* 96:2712–2716.
23. Soiffer, R.J., E.P. Alyea, E. Hochberg, C. Wu, C. Canning, B. Parikh, D. Zahrieh, I. Webb, J. Antin, and J. Ritz. 2002. Randomized trial of CD8+ T-cell depletion in the prevention of graft-versus-host disease associated with donor lymphocyte infusion. *Biol Blood Marrow Transplant* 8:625–632.
24. Bonini, C., G. Ferrari, S. Verzeletti, P. Servida, E. Zappone, L. Ruggieri, M. Ponzoni, S. Rossini, F. Mavilio, C. Traversari, and C. Bordignon. 1997. HSV-TK gene transfer into donor lymphocytes for control of allogeneic graft-versus-leukemia [see comments]. *Science* 276:1719–1724.
25. Kolb, H.J., A. Schattenberg, J.M. Goldman, B. Hertenstein, N. Jacobsen, W. Arcese, P. Ljungman, A. Ferrant, L. Verdonck, D. Niederwieser, F. van Rhee, J. Mittermueller, T. de Witte, E. Holler, and H. Ansari. 1995. Graft-versus-leukemia effect of donor lymphocyte transfusions in marrow grafted patients. *Blood* 86:2041–2050.
26. Porter, D.L., B.L. Levine, N. Bunin, E.A. Stadtmauer, S.M. Luger, S. Goldstein, A. Loren, J. Phillips, S. Nasta, A. Perl, S. Schuster, D. Tsai, A. Sohal, E. Veloso, S. Emerson, and C.H. June.

2006. A phase 1 trial of donor lymphocyte infusions expanded and activated ex vivo via CD3/CD28 costimulation. *Blood* 107:1325–1331.
27. Rosenberg, S.A., J.R. Yannelli, J.C. Yang, S.L. Topalian, D.J. Schwartzentruber, J.S. Weber, D.R. Parkinson, C.A. Seipp, J.H. Einhorn, and D.E. White. 1994. Treatment of patients with metastatic melanoma with autologous tumor-infiltrating lymphocytes and interleukin 2 [see comments]. *Journal of the National Cancer Institute* 86:1159–1166.
28. Chang, A.E., A. Aruga, M.J. Cameron, V.K. Sondak, D.P. Normolle, B.A. Fox, and S. Shu. 1997. Adoptive immunotherapy with vaccine-primed lymph node cells secondarily activated with anti-CD3 and interleukin-2. *Journal of Clinical Oncology* 15:796–807.
29. Riddell, S.R., and P.D. Greenberg. 1990. The use of anti-CD3 and anti-CD28 monoclonal antibodies to clone and expand human antigen-specific T cells. *Journal of Immunological Methods* 128:189–201.
30. Yee, C., J.A. Thompson, D. Byrd, S.R. Riddell, P. Roche, E. Celis, and P.D. Greenberg. 2002. Adoptive T cell therapy using antigen-specific CD8+ T cell clones for the treatment of patients with metastatic melanoma: In vivo persistence, migration, and antitumor effect of transferred T cells. *Proc Natl Acad Sci U S A* 99:16168–16173.
31. Dudley, M.E., J.R. Wunderlich, P.F. Robbins, J.C. Yang, P. Hwu, D.J. Schwartzentruber, S.L. Topalian, R. Sherry, N.P. Restifo, A.M. Hubicki, M.R. Robinson, M. Raffeld, P. Duray, C.A. Seipp, L. Rogers-Freezer, K.E. Morton, S.A. Mavroukakis, D.E. White, and S.A. Rosenberg. 2002. Cancer regression and autoimmunity in patients after clonal repopulation with antitumor lymphocytes. *Science* 298:850–854.
32. Heslop, H.E., M.K. Brenner, and C.M. Rooney. 1994. Donor T cells to treat EBV-associated lymphoma. *N Engl J Med* 331:679–680.
33. Rooney, C.M., C.A. Smith, C.Y. Ng, S.K. Loftin, J.W. Sixbey, Y. Gan, D.K. Srivastava, L.C. Bowman, R.A. Krance, M.K. Brenner, and H.E. Heslop. 1998. Infusion of cytotoxic T cells for the prevention and treatment of Epstein-Barr virus-induced lymphoma in allogeneic transplant recipients. *Blood* 92:1549–1555.
34. Savoldo, B., J.A. Goss, M.M. Hammer, L. Zhang, T. Lopez, A.P. Gee, Y.F. Lin, R.E. Quiros-Tejeira, P. Reinke, S. Schubert, S. Gottschalk, M.J. Finegold, M.K. Brenner, C.M. Rooney, and H.E. Heslop. 2006. Treatment of solid organ transplant recipients with autologous Epstein Barr virus-specific cytotoxic T lymphocytes (CTL). *Blood*
35. Gustafsson, A., V. Levitsky, J.Z. Zou, T. Frisan, T. Dalianis, P. Ljungman, O. Ringden, J. Winiarski, I. Ernberg, and M.G. Masucci. 2000. Epstein-Barr virus (EBV) load in bone marrow transplant recipients at risk to develop posttransplant lymphoproliferative disease: prophylactic infusion of EBV-specific cytotoxic T cells. *Blood* 95:807–814.
36. Straathof, K.C., C.M. Bollard, U. Popat, M.H. Huls, T. Lopez, M.C. Morriss, M.V. Gresik, A.P. Gee, H.V. Russell, M.K. Brenner, C.M. Rooney, and H.E. Heslop. 2005. Treatment of nasopharyngeal carcinoma with Epstein-Barr virus–specific T lymphocytes. *Blood* 105:1898–1904.
37. Bollard, C.M., L. Aguilar, K.C. Straathof, B. Gahn, M.H. Huls, A. Rousseau, J. Sixbey, M.V. Gresik, G. Carrum, M. Hudson, D. Dilloo, A. Gee, M.K. Brenner, C.M. Rooney, and H.E. Heslop. 2004. Cytotoxic T Lymphocyte Therapy for Epstein-Barr Virus+ Hodgkin's Disease. *J Exp Med* 200:1623–1633.
38. Bollard, C.M., C. Rossig, M.J. Calonge, M.H. Huls, H.J. Wagner, J. Massague, M.K. Brenner, H.E. Heslop, and C.M. Rooney. 2002. Adapting a transforming growth factor beta-related tumor protection strategy to enhance antitumor immunity. *Blood* 99:3179–3187.
39. van der Bruggen, P., C. Traversari, P. Chomez, C. Lurquin, E. De Plaen, B. Van den Eynde, A. Knuth, and T. Boon. 1991. A gene encoding an antigen recognized by cytolytic T lymphocytes on a human melanoma. *Science* 254:1643–1647.
40. Sahin, U., O. Tureci, and M. Pfreundschuh. 1997. Serological identification of human tumor antigens. *Current Opinion in Immunology* 9:709–716.
41. Scanlan, M.J., A.O. Gure, A.A. Jungbluth, L.J. Old, and Y.T. Chen. 2002. Cancer/testis antigens: an expanding family of targets for cancer immunotherapy. *Immunol Rev* 188:22–32.
42. Hermeking, H. 2003. Serial analysis of gene expression and cancer. *Curr Opin Oncol* 15:44–49.

43. Cox, A.L., J. Skipper, Y. Chen, R.A. Henderson, T.L. Darrow, J. Shabanowitz, V.H. Engelhard, D.F. Hunt, and C.L. Slingluff, Jr. 1994. Identification of a peptide recognized by five melanoma-specific human cytotoxic T cell lines. *Science* 264:716–719.
44. Henderson, R.A., A.L. Cox, K. Sakaguchi, E. Appella, J. Shabanowitz, D.F. Hunt, and V.H. Engelhard. 1993. Direct identification of an endogenous peptide recognized by multiple HLA-A2.1-specific cytotoxic T cells. *Proc Natl Acad Sci U S A* 90:10275–10279.
45. Hunt, D.F., R.A. Henderson, J. Shabanowitz, K. Sakaguchi, H. Michel, N. Sevilir, A.L. Cox, E. Appella, and V.H. Engelhard. 1992. Characterization of peptides bound to the class I MHC molecule HLA-A2.1 by mass spectrometry. *Science* 255:1261–1263.
46. Van Voorhis, W.C., L.S. Hair, R.M. Steinman, and G. Kaplan. 1982. Human dendritic cells. Enrichment and characterization from peripheral blood. *J Exp Med* 155:1172–1187.
47. Steinman, R.M., and M.D. Witmer. 1978. Lymphoid dendritic cells are potent stimulators of the primary mixed leukocyte reaction in mice. *Proc Natl Acad Sci U S A* 75:5132–5136.
48. Schultze, J.L., S. Michalak, M.J. Seamon, G. Dranoff, K. Jung, J. Daley, J.C. Delgado, J.G. Gribben, and L.M. Nadler. 1997. CD40-activated human B cells: an alternative source of highly efficient antigen presenting cells to generate autologous antigen-specific T cells for adoptive immunotherapy. *J Clin Invest* 100:2757–2765.
49. Groh, V., Y.Q. Li, D. Cioca, N.N. Hunder, W. Wang, S.R. Riddell, C. Yee, and T. Spies. 2005. Efficient cross-priming of tumor antigen-specific T cells by dendritic cells sensitized with diverse anti-MICA opsonized tumor cells. *Proc Natl Acad Sci U S A* 102:6461–6466.
50. Dhodapkar, K.M., J. Krasovsky, B. Williamson, and M.V. Dhodapkar. 2002. Antitumor monoclonal antibodies enhance cross-presentation ofcCellular antigens and the generation of myeloma-specific killer T cells by dendritic cells. *J Exp Med* 195:125–133.
51. Liao, X., Y. Li, C. Bonini, S. Nair, E. Gilboa, P.D. Greenberg, and C. Yee. 2004. Transfection of RNA encoding tumor antigens following maturation of dendritic cells leads to prolonged presentation of antigen and the generation of high-affinity tumor-reactive cytotoxic T lymphocytes. *Mol Ther* 9:757–764.
52. Boczkowski, D., S.K. Nair, J.H. Nam, H.K. Lyerly, and E. Gilboa, editors. 2000. Induction of tumor immunity and cytotoxic T lymphocyte responses using dendritic cells transfected with messenger RNA amplified from tumor cells. 1028–1034 pp.
53. Boczkowski, D., S.K. Nair, D. Snyder, and E. Gilboa. 1996. Dendritic cells pulsed with RNA are potent antigen-presenting cells in vitro and in vivo. *Journal of Experimental Medicine* 184:465–472.
54. Zaremba, S., E. Barzaga, M. Zhu, N. Soares, K.Y. Tsang, and J. Schlom. 1997. Identification of an enhancer agonist cytotoxic T lymphocyte peptide from human carcinoembryonic antigen. *Cancer Research* 57:4570–4577.
55. Parkhurst, M.R., M.L. Salgaller, S. Southwood, P.F. Robbins, A. Sette, S.A. Rosenberg, and Y. Kawakami. 1996. Improved induction of melanoma-reactive CTL with peptides from the melanoma antigen gp100 modified at HLA-A*0201-binding residues. *Journal of Immunology* 157:2539–2548.
56. Jackson, M.R., E.S. Song, Y. Yang, and P.A. Peterson. 1992. Empty and peptide-containing conformers of class I major histocompatibility complex molecules expressed in Drosophila melanogaster cells. *Proc Natl Acad Sci U S A* 89:12117–12121.
57. Cai, Z., A. Brunmark, M.R. Jackson, D. Loh, P.A. Peterson, and J. Sprent. 1996. Transfected Drosophila cells as a probe for defining the minimal requirements for stimulating unprimed CD8+ T cells. *Proc Natl Acad Sci U S A* 93:14736–14741.
58. Latouche, J.B., and M. Sadelain. 2000. Induction of human cytotoxic T lymphocytes by artificial antigen-presenting cells. *Nat Biotechnol* 18:405–409.
59. Dupont, J., J.B. Latouche, C. Ma, and M. Sadelain. 2005. Artificial antigen-presenting cells transduced with telomerase efficiently expand epitope-specific, human leukocyte antigen-restricted cytotoxic T cells. *Cancer Res* 65:5417–5427.
60. Maus, M.V., A.K. Thomas, D.G. Leonard, D. Allman, K. Addya, K. Schlienger, J.L. Riley, and C.H. June. 2002. Ex vivo expansion of polyclonal and antigen-specific cytotoxic T lymphocytes

by artificial APCs expressing ligands for the T-cell receptor, CD28 and 4–1BB. *Nat Biotechnol* 20:143–148.
61. Maus, M.V., J.L. Riley, W.W. Kwok, G.T. Nepom, and C.H. June. 2003. HLA tetramer-based artificial antigen-presenting cells for stimulation of CD4+ T cells. *Clin Immunol* 106:16–22.
62. Oelke, M., M.V. Maus, D. Didiano, C.H. June, A. Mackensen, and J.P. Schneck. 2003. Ex vivo induction and expansion of antigen-specific cytotoxic T cells by HLA-Ig-coated artificial antigen-presenting cells. *Nat Med* 9:619–624.
63. Hirano, N., M.O. Butler, Z. Xia, A. Berezovskaya, A.P. Murray, S. Ansen, and L.M. Nadler. 2006. Efficient presentation of naturally processed HLA class I peptides by artificial antigen-presenting cells for the generation of effective antitumor responses. *Clin Cancer Res* 12:2967–2975.
64. Yee, C. 2005. Adoptive T cell therapy: Addressing challenges in cancer immunotherapy. *J Transl Med* 3:17.
65. Mitchell, M.S. 2002. Phase I trial of adoptive immunotherapy with cytolytic T lymphocytes immunized against a tyrosinase epitope. *Journal of Clinical Oncology* 20:1075–1086.
66. Dudley, M.E. 2001. Adoptive transfer of cloned melanoma-reactive T lymphocytes for the treatment of patients with metastatic melanoma. *Journal of Immunotherapy* 24:363–373.
67. Dudley, M.E., J.R. Wunderlich, J.C. Yang, P. Hwu, D.J. Schwartzentruber, S.L. Topalian, R.M. Sherry, F.M. Marincola, S.F. Leitman, C.A. Seipp, L. Rogers-Freezer, K.E. Morton, A. Nahvi, S.A. Mavroukakis, D.E. White, and S.A. Rosenberg. 2002. A phase I study of nonmyeloablative chemotherapy and adoptive transfer of autologous tumor antigen-specific T lymphocytes in patients with metastatic melanoma. *Journal of Immunotherapy* 25:243–251.
68. Meidenbauer, N., J. Marienhagen, M. Laumer, S. Vogl, J. Heymann, R. Andreesen, and A. Mackensen. 2003. Survival and tumor localization of adoptively transferred Melan-A-specific T cells in melanoma patients. *J Immunol* 170:2161–2169.
69. Mackensen, A., N. Meidenbauer, S. Vogl, M. Laumer, J. Berger, and R. Andreesen. 2006. Phase I study of adoptive T-cell therapy using antigen-specific CD8+ T cells for the treatment of patients with metastatic melanoma. *J Clin Oncol* 24:5060–5069.
70. Tsuji, T., M. Yasukawa, J. Matsuzaki, T. Ohkuri, K. Chamoto, D. Wakita, T. Azuma, H. Niiya, H. Miyoshi, K. Kuzushima, Y. Oka, H. Sugiyama, H. Ikeda, and T. Nishimura. 2005. Generation of tumor-specific, HLA class I-restricted human Th1 and Tc1 cells by cell engineering with tumor peptide-specific T-cell receptor genes. *Blood* 106:470–476.
71. Clay, T.M., M.C. Custer, P.J. Spiess, and M.I. Nishimura. 1999. Potential use of T cell receptor genes to modify hematopoietic stem cells for the gene therapy of cancer. *Pathol Oncol Res* 5:3–15.
72. Clay, T.M., M.C. Custer, J. Sachs, P. Hwu, S.A. Rosenberg, and M.I. Nishimura. 1999. Efficient transfer of a tumor antigen-reactive TCR to human peripheral blood lymphocytes confers anti-tumor reactivity. *J Immunol* 163:507–513.
73. Morgan, R.A., M.E. Dudley, Y.Y. Yu, Z. Zheng, P.F. Robbins, M.R. Theoret, J.R. Wunderlich, M.S. Hughes, N.P. Restifo, and S.A. Rosenberg. 2003. High efficiency TCR gene transfer into primary human lymphocytes affords avid recognition of melanoma tumor antigen glycoprotein 100 and does not alter the recognition of autologous melanoma antigens. *J Immunol* 171:3287–3295.
74. Gade, T.P., W. Hassen, E. Santos, G. Gunset, A. Saudemont, M.C. Gong, R. Brentjens, X.S. Zhong, M. Stephan, J. Stefanski, C. Lyddane, J.R. Osborne, I.M. Buchanan, S.J. Hall, W.D. Heston, I. Riviere, S.M. Larson, J.A. Koutcher, and M. Sadelain. 2005. Targeted elimination of prostate cancer by genetically directed human T lymphocytes. *Cancer Res* 65:9080–9088.
75. Zhao, Y., Z. Zheng, P.F. Robbins, H.T. Khong, S.A. Rosenberg, and R.A. Morgan. 2005. Primary human lymphocytes transduced with NY-ESO-1 antigen-specific TCR genes recognize and kill diverse human tumor cell lines. *J Immunol* 174:4415–4423.
76. Willemsen, R.A., M.E. Weijtens, C. Ronteltap, Z. Eshhar, J.W. Gratama, P. Chames, and R.L. Bolhuis. 2000. Grafting primary human T lymphocytes with cancer-specific chimeric single chain and two chain TCR. *Gene Ther* 7:1369–1377.
77. Calogero, A., G.A. Hospers, K.M. Kruse, P.I. Schrier, N.H. Mulder, E. Hooijberg, and L.F. de Leij. 2000. Retargeting of a T cell line by anti MAGE-3/HLA-A2 alpha beta TCR gene transfer. *Anticancer Res* 20:1793–1799.

78. Kuball, J., M.L. Dossett, M. Wolfl, W.Y. Ho, R.H. Voss, C. Fowler, and P.D. Greenberg. 2006. Facilitating matched pairing and expression of TCR-chains introduced into human T-cells. *Blood*
79. Stanislawski, T., R.H. Voss, C. Lotz, E. Sadovnikova, R.A. Willemsen, J. Kuball, T. Ruppert, R.L. Bolhuis, C.J. Melief, C. Huber, H.J. Stauss, and M. Theobald. 2001. Circumventing tolerance to a human MDM2-derived tumor antigen by TCR gene transfer. *Nat Immunol* 2:962–970.
80. Kershaw, M.H., J.A. Westwood, L.L. Parker, G. Wang, Z. Eshhar, S.A. Mavroukakis, D.E. White, J.R. Wunderlich, S. Canevari, L. Rogers-Freezer, C.C. Chen, J.C. Yang, S.A. Rosenberg, and P. Hwu. 2006. A phase I study on adoptive immunotherapy using gene-modified T cells for ovarian cancer. *Clin Cancer Res* 12:6106–6115.
81. Gyobu, H., T. Tsuji, Y. Suzuki, T. Ohkuri, K. Chamoto, M. Kuroki, H. Miyoshi, Y. Kawarada, H. Katoh, T. Takeshima, and T. Nishimura. 2004. Generation and targeting of human tumor-specific Tc1 and Th1 cells transduced with a lentivirus containing a chimeric immunoglobulin T-cell receptor. *Cancer Res* 64:1490–1495.
82. Finney, H.M., A.D. Lawson, C.R. Bebbington, and A.N. Weir. 1998. Chimeric receptors providing both primary and costimulatory signaling in T cells from a single gene product. *J Immunol* 161:2791–2797.
83. Kowolik, C.M., M.S. Topp, S. Gonzalez, T. Pfeiffer, S. Olivares, N. Gonzalez, D.D. Smith, S.J. Forman, M.C. Jensen, and L.J. Cooper. 2006. CD28 costimulation provided through a CD19-specific chimeric antigen receptor enhances in vivo persistence and antitumor efficacy of adoptively transferred T cells. *Cancer Res* 66:10995–11004.
84. North, R.J. 1982. Cyclophosphamide-facilitated adoptive immunotherapy of an established tumor depends on elimination of tumor-induced suppressor T cells. *J Exp Med* 155:1063–1074.
85. Greenberg, P.D., M.A. Cheever, and A. Fefer. 1981. Eradication of disseminated murine leukemia by chemoimmunotherapy with cyclophosphamide and adoptively transferred immune syngeneic Lyt-1+2- lymphocytes. *Journal of Experimental Medicine* 154:952–963.
86. Vierboom, M.P., G.M. Bos, M. Ooms, R. Offringa, and C.J. Melief. 2000. Cyclophosphamide enhances anti-tumor effect of wild-type p53-specific CTL. *Int J Cancer* 87:253–260.
87. Proietti, E., G. Greco, B. Garrone, S. Baccarini, C. Mauri, M. Venditti, D. Carlei, and F. Belardelli. 1998. Importance of cyclophosphamide-induced bystander effect on T cells for a successful tumor eradication in response to adoptive immunotherapy in mice. *J Clin Invest* 101:429–441.
88. Ghiringhelli, F., N. Larmonier, E. Schmitt, A. Parcellier, D. Cathelin, C. Garrido, B. Chauffert, E. Solary, B. Bonnotte, and F. Martin. 2004. CD4+CD25+ regulatory T cells suppress tumor immunity but are sensitive to cyclophosphamide which allows immunotherapy of established tumors to be curative. *Eur J Immunol* 34:336–344.
89. Machiels, J.P., R.T. Reilly, L.A. Emens, A.M. Ercolini, R.Y. Lei, D. Weintraub, F.I. Okoye, and E.M. Jaffee. 2001. Cyclophosphamide, doxorubicin, and paclitaxel enhance the antitumor immune response of granulocyte/macrophage-colony stimulating factor-secreting whole-cell vaccines in HER-2/neu tolerized mice. *Cancer Res* 61:3689–3697.
90. Schiavoni, G., F. Mattei, T. Di Pucchio, S.M. Santini, L. Bracci, F. Belardelli, and E. Proietti. 2000. Cyclophosphamide induces type I interferon and augments the number of CD44(hi) T lymphocytes in mice: implications for strategies of chemoimmunotherapy of cancer. *Blood* 95:2024–2030.
91. Maguire, H.C., Jr., and V.L. Ettore. 1967. Enhancement of dinitrochlorobenzene (DNCB) contact sensitization by cyclophosphamide in the guinea pig. *J Invest Dermatol* 48:39–43.
92. Lutsiak, M.E., R.T. Semnani, R. De Pascalis, S.V. Kashmiri, J. Schlom, and H. Sabzevari. 2005. Inhibition of CD4(+)25+ T regulatory cell function implicated in enhanced immune response by low-dose cyclophosphamide. *Blood* 105:2862–2868.
93. Vierboom, M.P.M., H.W. Nijman, R. Offringa, E.I.H. Vandervoort, T. Vanhall, L. Vandenbroek, G.J. Fleuren, P. Kenemans, W.M. Kast, and C.J.M. Melief. 1997. Tumor Eradication By Wild-Type P53-Specific Cytotoxic T Lymphocytes. *Journal of Experimental Medicine* 186:695–704.
94. Berd, D., M.J. Mastrangelo, P.F. Engstrom, A. Paul, and H. Maguire. 1982. Augmentation of the human immune response by cyclophosphamide. *Cancer Res* 42:4862–4866.

95. Berd, D., and M.J. Mastrangelo. 1987. Effect of low dose cyclophosphamide on the immune system of cancer patients: reduction of T-suppressor function without depletion of the CD8+ subset. *Cancer Res* 47:3317–3321.
96. Bast, R.C., Jr., E.L. Reinherz, C. Maver, P. Lavin, and S.F. Schlossman. 1983. Contrasting effects of cyclophosphamide and prednisolone on the phenotype of human peripheral blood leukocytes. *Clin Immunol Immunopathol* 28:101–114.
97. Berd, D., H.C. Maguire, Jr., and M.J. Mastrangelo. 1984. Potentiation of human cell-mediated and humoral immunity by low-dose cyclophosphamide. *Cancer Res* 44:5439–5443.
98. Goldrath, A.W., P.V. Sivakumar, M. Glaccum, M.K. Kennedy, M.J. Bevan, C. Benoist, D. Mathis, and E.A. Butz. 2002. Cytokine requirements for acute and Basal homeostatic proliferation of naive and memory CD8+ T cells. *J Exp Med* 195:1515–1522.
99. Brown, I.E., C. Blank, J. Kline, A.K. Kacha, and T.F. Gajewski. 2006. Homeostatic proliferation as an isolated variable reverses CD8+ T cell anergy and promotes tumor rejection. *J Immunol* 177:4521–4529.
100. Teague, R.M., B.D. Sather, J.A. Sacks, M.Z. Huang, M.L. Dossett, J. Morimoto, X. Tan, S.E. Sutton, M.P. Cooke, C. Ohlen, and P.D. Greenberg. 2006. Interleukin-15 rescues tolerant CD8+ T cells for use in adoptive immunotherapy of established tumors. *Nat Med* 12:335–341.
101. Wang, L.X., R. Li, G. Yang, M. Lim, A. O'Hara, Y. Chu, B.A. Fox, N.P. Restifo, W.J. Urba, and H.M. Hu. 2005. Interleukin-7-dependent expansion and persistence of melanoma-specific T cells in lymphodepleted mice lead to tumor regression and editing. *Cancer Res* 65:10569–10577.
102. Cesana, G.C., G. DeRaffele, S. Cohen, D. Moroziewicz, J. Mitcham, J. Stoutenburg, K. Cheung, C. Hesdorffer, S. Kim-Schulze, and H.L. Kaufman. 2006. Characterization of CD4+CD25+ regulatory T cells in patients treated with high-dose interleukin-2 for metastatic melanoma or renal cell carcinoma. *J Clin Oncol* 24:1169–1177.
103. Phan, G.Q., J.C. Yang, R.M. Sherry, P. Hwu, S.L. Topalian, D.J. Schwartzentruber, N.P. Restifo, L.R. Haworth, C.A. Seipp, L.J. Freezer, K.E. Morton, S.A. Mavroukakis, P.H. Duray, S.M. Steinberg, J.P. Allison, T.A. Davis, and S.A. Rosenberg. 2003. Cancer regression and autoimmunity induced by cytotoxic T lymphocyte-associated antigen 4 blockade in patients with metastatic melanoma. *Proc Natl Acad Sci U S A* 100:8372–8377.
104. Hodi, F.S., M.C. Mihm, R.J. Soiffer, F.G. Haluska, M. Butler, M.V. Seiden, T. Davis, R. Henry-Spires, S. MacRae, A. Willman, R. Padera, M.T. Jaklitsch, S. Shankar, T.C. Chen, A. Korman, J.P. Allison, and G. Dranoff. 2003. Biologic activity of cytotoxic T lymphocyte-associated antigen 4 antibody blockade in previously vaccinated metastatic melanoma and ovarian carcinoma patients. *Proc Natl Acad Sci U S A* 100:4712–4717.
105. Kortylewski, M., M. Kujawski, T. Wang, S. Wei, S. Zhang, S. Pilon-Thomas, G. Niu, H. Kay, J. Mule, W.G. Kerr, R. Jove, D. Pardoll, and H. Yu. 2005. Inhibiting Stat3 signaling in the hematopoietic system elicits multicomponent antitumor immunity. *Nat Med* 11:1314–1321.

CHAPTER 16

CHECKPOINT BLOCKADE AND COMBINATORIAL IMMUNOTHERAPIES

KARL S. PEGGS[1], SERGIO A. QUEZADA[2], AND JAMES P. ALLISON[3]

Howard Hughes Medical Institute, Department of Immunology, Memorial Sloan-Kettering Cancer Center, 1275 York Avenue, New York, NY, 10021, USA.

IMMUNOLOGICAL CHECKPOINTS

The mammalian adaptive immune system is capable of rapid targeted destruction of a multitude of pathogens. Specificity is endowed by the somatic generation of an extensive repertoire of T cell receptors (TCRs) and B cell antibodies/receptors, each exhibiting relatively small segments of highly variable sequence. However, a degree of cross-reactivity or promiscuity is perhaps a necessary feature of a system that must respond quickly to such a vast number of environmental antigenic challenges. Indeed, the clone size of peripheral CD8 T cells appears to be correlated with TCR promiscuity [1]. This feature broadens response capacity and theoretically increases the tempo of primary responses, but simultaneously heightens the risk of autoimmunity. The thymic positive selection model predicts that sub-threshold recognition of self antigens is an essential requirement for the generation and survival of both naïve and memory T cells, ultimately generating a system that is permissive to the persistence of autoreactive T cells of relatively low affinity following central tolerance induction. Inappropriate activation or targeting of the immune system would at the very least represent a biologically expensive waste of resource, but can also result in destruction of host tissues resulting in an array of autoimmune disorders. Hence it is no surprise that the promotion of protective immunity against pathogenic organisms or neoplastic cell growth and prevention of the emergence of autoreactive clonal populations are highly regulated processes.

H.L. Kaufman and J.D. Wolchok (eds.), General Principles of Tumor Immunotherapy, 363–390.

This regulation occurs at multiple levels throughout the processes of activation and termination of immune responses, and involves both mechanisms that are intrinsic to the activated cell population and mechanisms that are extrinsic to these cells and mediated via other populations such as regulatory T cells, dendritic cells (DCs) or macrophages. The molecular basis for the cell intrinsic control of T cell activation and tolerance resides within groups of activating and inhibitory receptors. Signalling through these receptors is integrated within a framework of overlapping or identical downstream signalling pathways. Together these pathways act as a rheostat for initial T cell activation. The apparent dependency of a productive immune response on a qualitative second 'co-stimulatory' signal mediated via CD28:B7 signalling provides an initial immunological checkpoint. In addition, co-stimulation can provide extra signals to promote cell division, augment cell survival, or induce effector functions such as cytokine secretion or cytotoxicity. Negative or 'co-inhibitory' signals may be more important both for the prevention of the initiation of inappropriately directed responses and for limiting the size, duration or premature focusing of immune responses once initiated. As a group the molecules controlling these signals therefore allow fine-tuning of the response to TCR ligation by cognate antigen.

Two major groups of co-stimulatory receptors have been described: the immunoglobulin superfamily, including CD28 and inducible T-cell co-stimulator (ICOS), and the tumour-necrosis factor receptor (TNFR) superfamily, including OX40, CD27, 4-1BB, CD30, GITR (glucocorticoid-induced TNFR family related gene) and HVEM (herpes-virus entry mediator). Members of the immunoglobulin superfamily share features in both sequence and structure, and the majority bind members of the B7 ligand family. Negative regulatory elements are likely a prerequisite of a system that is permissive to a degree of promiscuity in TCR recognition. The most well-established inhibitory members of the immunoglobulin 'co-stimulatory' family include cytotoxic T-lymphocyte-associated-antigen 4 (CTLA-4) and programmed cell death 1 (PD1). B and T lymphocyte attenuator (BTLA) is the most recently described member of the immunoglobulin superfamily and also appears to mediate inhibitory effects on T cell activation [2]. The identities of the receptors for the newer members of the B7 ligand family (B7-H3 and B7x/B7-H4) remain elusive, but these receptors may also mediate significant inhibitory activity, perhaps more so in the periphery given the tissue distribution of these more recently identified ligands.

ENDOGENOUS ANTI-TUMOR RESPONSES – ENHANCING ANTIGEN PRESENTATION AND IMMUNOGENICITY

Correlative studies in a number of human cancers demonstrating prolonged survival and/or reduced metastases in patients who have greater levels of tumor infiltrating T cells provide evidence suggesting the existence of tumor-reactive T cells *in vivo* and supporting their role in limiting tumor growth [3–7]. Clearly the presence of these cells is insufficient to prevent eventual tumor progression in these cases.

Defects in differentiation and cytotoxic pathways of intra-tumoral $CD8^+$ T cells have been demonstrated in human melanoma [8]. Numerous immunotherapeutic strategies aimed at increasing the frequency or activity of these populations have been postulated or enacted. One group of approaches aims at active immunization against relevant tumor targets. It is well recognised that tumor-induced defects in DC differentiation and function, which result in the accumulation of immature DCs and immature myeloid cells (iMCs) capable of direct suppression of antigen-specific T cell responses, are an important component of the inability of the immune system to respond adequately to tumor challenge [9]. Attempts to enhance antigen presentation, including those aimed at enhancing maturation (or, more precisely, immunogenicity) of immature precursors, may therefore be essential components of effective immunotherapies [10]. Prophylactic vaccination has proven an effective strategy in the combat of infectious pathogens and has also demonstrated considerable success at preventing tumor engraftment in a number of murine models of cancer using a variety of vaccination approaches (peptides, peptide- or tumor lysate-pulsed dendritic cells, GM-CSF secreting autologous or allogeneic tumor vaccines)[11–13]. However, just as vaccination approaches have proven far less effective in established infections in humans, such as those with chronic hepatitis or tuberculosis, recent clinical trials incorporating vaccination using the same approaches in human cancers have not produced compelling evidence of therapeutic benefit. Whilst T cell responses directed towards the antigens used for immunization can be detected, they have proven too weak and transient to eradicate tumors and the generation of prolonged, objectively quantifiable and clinically meaningful responses in patients has proven more difficult than initially envisaged [13, 14]. Tumor-reactive T cells may be expanded quite impressively, but the presence of active peripheral tolerance mechanisms may restrict responding clones to those of low avidity or impaired functionality [15,16]. Although part of the difficulty may relate to a tumor milieu characterised by significant populations of immunosuppressive iMCs within a background of readily available tumor antigen in tumor-bearing hosts [9], an additional obstacle to success arises from the fact that the tumors are host-derived and express mostly the same array of self antigens as the cell types from which they arise. Many of the molecules identified as potentially therapeutic targets in human cancers are self or 'altered self' antigens, either aberrantly expressed or over-expressed on malignant cells. Therapeutic interventions aimed at enhancement of tumor antigen presentation may be insufficient to overcome established immunological inhibitory checkpoints and might even result in a counter-balancing increase in inhibitory signaling [17,18]. Indeed, up-regulation of the ligands for the inhibitory receptors by tumor cells has become recognised as mechanism by which tumors might evade immunological destruction [19,20]. Overcoming multiple mechanisms of peripheral tolerance to these tumor-associated targets may therefore prove crucial for effective recruitment of the immune effectors required for successful immune-based therapies. Therapeutic manipulation of activation thresholds might recruit tumor-reactive cells, or enhance their functional capabilities sufficiently to effect meaningful anti-tumor activity.

THERAPEUTIC INHIBITION OF T CELL INTRINSIC CHECKPOINTS: CTLA-4 BLOCKADE

CD28 and CTLA-4 – the Archetypal T Cell Intrinsic Immune Regulators

CD28 is constitutively expressed by most mouse T cells, 90% of human $CD4^+$ T cells and 50% of human $CD8^+$ T cells. Expression of its two structurally-homologous ligands B7-1(CD80) and B7-2 (CD86) is restricted to lymphoid and antigen-presenting cells (such as DCs, macrophages and activated B and T cells). B7-2 is expressed at a low level in non-activated DCs and can be rapidly up-regulated by a variety of activating stimuli (infection, tissue injury, inflammatory cytokines, and interaction of DCs with activated T cells). B7-1 is virtually absent from non-activated DCs, is up-regulated by similar stimuli, but is expressed on the cell surface later than the peak of B7-2 expression. This compartmentalization of expression may direct early events in T cell activation to maintain peripheral tolerance by restricting T cell activation to areas of inflammation or injury.

The interaction between CD28 and B7-1 or B7-2 provides critical co-stimulatory activity that can rescue T cell clones from TCR-mediated anergy [21–23]. The importance of the pathway in the induction of immune responses is further highlighted by studies in which receptor-ligand binding is blocked with monoclonal antibodies or CTLA-Ig fusion protein. This results in diminution or elimination of T cell responses to a variety of *in vitro* and *in vivo* stimuli [24], although interpretation of the mechanism of inhibition has been complicated by the suggestion that the ligation of B7-1/B7-2 results in 'outside-in' signalling causing indoleamine 2,3-dioxygenase (IDO) induction, tryptophan depletion, production of pro-apoptotic metabolites, and reduced antigen-presenting function of DCs [25]. In addition, $CD28^{-/-}$ knockout mice show severe diminution of most T cell responses [26] and B7-1/B7-2 double knockout mice exhibit a virtual absence of T cell responses [27]. Isolated CD28 ligation results in transient expression of a restricted number of the same genes induced by TCR ligation with no discernable dedicated signalling element, but engagement in concert with TCR ligation strongly amplifies weak TCR signals and modifies the gene regulation induced by TCR stimulation [28,29]. Thus ligation of CD28 decreases the number of ligated TCRs that are required for a given biological response [30], resulting in an apparent dependency on a qualitative second signal when TCR occupancy is low.

CTLA-4 shares the B7-1 and B7-2 ligands with CD28 and acts as a counterbalancing inhibitory receptor. Their inter-dependence, coupled with the tight control of the temporal and spatial kinetics of their expression, allows fine tuning of the early events in T cell activation and may confer subtle influences over the shaping of the immune repertoire. The importance of the co-dependence of its activity on CD28-mediated signalling is emphasized by gene expression analyses demonstrating that CTLA-4 engagement selectively blocks augmentation of gene regulation by CD28-mediated co-stimulation, but does not ablate gene regulation induced by TCR triggering alone [29]. The function of CTLA-4 as a negative regulator of CD28-dependent T cell responses is perhaps most strikingly demonstrated by the phenotype of CTLA-4 knock-out mice, which succumb to a rapidly lethal polyclonal CD4-dependent lympho-proliferation within 3–4 weeks of birth [31–33]. CTLA-4 expression is difficult to detect on most resting T cells even though it influences some of the earliest events in T cell activation [34, 35]. It is mobilised from intracellular vesicles to the immunological synapse rapidly after TCR engagement [36]. Strong TCR agonists induce greater translocation of CTLA-4 suggesting that TCR signal strength itself may inversely influence subsequent signalling elements. In contrast to CD28, CTLA-4 has a short cell-surface half-life in activated T cells, and surface expression is thus tightly linked to gene transcription and/or translation. In the unphosphorylated state, an intracellular localization motif mediates rapid binding to AP-2, endocytosis and lysosomal targeting [37].

The structure of co-crystals of CTLA-4 and B7-1 suggests that these molecules may form extended lattice-like networks, enabled by the distal positioning of CTLA-4 binding sites from the B7-1 dimer interface [38, 39]. Together with its 500–2500 fold higher affinities for both B7 ligands than those of CD28 [40], this provides one possible physical mechanism of action for CTLA-4 as a negative regulator of CD28 signalling, i.e. exclusion of CD28 from the immunological synapse and out-competition for shared ligands [41, 42]. Expression of a mutant CTLA-4 molecule without a functional intracellular domain partially or completely blocks the massive lethal proliferation that characterizes CTLA-$4^{-/-}$ mice depending on the surface expression level [43–45], presumably as a consequence either of competition with CD28 for B7 ligation or of IDO induction [25]. Such competition may be most influential when B7 levels are limiting, as direct signalling through the tail appears to be necessary if B7 levels are high [42]. In addition, an alternatively spliced ligand independent form of CTLA-4 (liCTLA-4) lacking the B7-1/B7-2 ligand-binding domain has been reported to be expressed on resting T cells and to inhibit both T cell proliferation and cytokine production [46]. It has been speculated that this isoform controls survival and/or homeostasis of naive T cell subsets, althought his has not been confirmed. Taken together, the results suggest that inhibitory signals are affected via both ligand-independent and B7 ligation-dependent mechanisms.

Studies of TCR transgenic T cells from CTLA-4-deficient mice indicate that the inhibitory effect of CTLA-4 is more pronounced during secondary rather than primary responses *in vitro*, and indicate a role in both $CD4^+$ and $CD8^+$ T cell responses [47–49]. Together the data are consistent with a model in which chronic T cell stimulation results in persistently higher levels of CTLA-4 expression. Adoptive transfer experiments demonstrate that CTLA-4-deficient T cells show enhanced responsiveness to antigenic stimulation compared to wild type cells, confirming the importance of a cell-autonomous mechanism of CTLA-4-mediated inhibition [50]. Thus CTLA-4 blockade offers a potential mechanism by which to try to enhance the anti-tumor responses of pre-existent chronically stimulated tumor-reactive T cells by a combination of reducing the threshold for activation of weakly reacting clones and removal of the attenuation of subsequent T cell proliferation, the effect of which might be accentuated by prior up-regulation of CTLA-4 in the higher affinity population. Indeed, blockade might result in the promotion of higher affinity clones that would otherwise be more restricted by CTLA-4 signalling. In addition, the induction of $CD8^+$ T cell tolerance by non-immunogenic DCs requires engagement of the co-inhibitory molecules CTLA-4 and PD-1 [51]. Blockade could prevent the induction of tolerance in these cells and may be particularly suited to combination with vaccination strategies whose efficacy is limited by such inhibitory mechanisms.

Preclinical Models of CTLA-4 Targeted Checkpoint Blockade

Blockade of CTLA-4/B7 interactions with an anti-CTLA-4 monoclonal antibody is able to induce rejection of several types of established transplantable tumors in mice when used as a monotherapy. These include colon carcinoma, fibrosarcoma, prostatic carcinoma, lymphoma and renal carcinoma [52–56]. Anti-tumor activity appears dependent on inherent tumor immunogenicity and anti-CTLA-4 monotherapy fails to induce tumor eradication in the less immunogenic tumors (for example, B16 melanoma, SM1 mammary carcinoma). Irradiated tumor vaccines that are engineered to produce GM-CSF are highly effective prophylactics in tumor challenge experiments but poorly effective in treatment models. Combination with CTLA-4 blockade in treatment models results in synergism of activity, which can cause tumor rejection even of B16 melanoma [57] or SM1 mammary carcinoma [58]. In addition, this combination therapy significantly reduces the incidence of primary prostate tumors in transgenic (TRAMP) mice [59]. Analogous synergism is observed with DNA vaccines in prophylaxis models [60]. Tumor rejection following combination therapy in the B16 melanoma model is accompanied by depigmentation, reminiscent of the vitiligo seen in patients with melanoma who respond to immunotherapy, and suggesting that the immune targets for these responses may be normally expressed differentiation antigens. Depigmentation is uncommon following vaccination alone, suggesting that CTLA-4 blockade is important in breaking peripheral tolerance in this system, but importantly is also not seen with anti-CTLA-4 monotherapy. Vaccination of wild type mice with a GM-CSF secreting prostate carcinoma cell line together with anti-CTLA-4 similarly results in marked prostatitis accompanied by destruction of epithelium, suggesting that the immune response in the TRAMP model is directed, at least in part, against normal prostate antigens.

Combination of CTLA-4 blockade with a number of other therapeutic modalities has confirmed the enhanced efficacy of combinatorial immunotherapeutics. Multiple mechanisms may account for this effect including reduced tumor burden, increased availability of tumor antigen, upregulation of co-stimulatory molecules, or effects on regulatory T cell or APC function. Radiotherapy and chemotherapy are both important components of modern anti-tumor therapies, and both may synergise with CTLA-4 blockade. Survival in the poorly immunogenic metastatic mouse mammary carcinoma 4T1 model is not improved by either CTLA-4 blockade or radiotherapy when used as monotherapies [61], but mice treated with combined modality therapy demonstrate a statistically significant survival advantage, correlating with an inhibition of the formation of metastatic lesions within the lung.

Anti-CTLA-4 is also ineffective in retarding tumor growth in the murine MOPC-315 tumor system, but demonstrates significant therapeutic benefits when combined with a subtherapeutic dose of the chemotherapeutic agent melphalan [62]. Combination of anti-CTLA-4 with both peptide vaccination and CpG, which activates innate immunity via Toll like receptor (TLR)-9 signalling, enhances anti-tumor immunity in the B16 melanoma model [63]. Synergism of therapeutic activity between CTLA-4 blockade and an agonistic anti-GITR antibody occurs in the murine Meth A fibrosarcoma model, enabling rejection of larger tumors treated at later time points following engraftment than with either agent alone [64]. Finally, depletion of $CD4^+CD25^+$ regulatory T cells improves the therapeutic efficacy of a GM-CSF secreting cellular vaccine plus anti-CTLA-4 in the B16 melanoma model. Depletion prior to combination therapy results in induction of increased numbers of TRP-$2_{180-188}$-specific T cells (correlating with efficacy) and an enhanced ability to reject larger tumor burdens [65]. These data highlight the relevance of regulatory T cell populations as non cell-autonomous inhibitory checkpoints of immune responses in anti-tumor immunotherapeutics.

REGULATORY T CELLS AS A BARRIER TO SUCCESSFUL IMMUNOTHERAPY

Not all tumor-infiltrating lymphocytes are associated with a favorable prognostic impact on tumor outcomes. In particular, the functionality of tumor-specific $CD4^+$ populations can either help or hinder anti-tumor responses according to the precise cell type [66–70]. This phenomenon is at least partially explained by regulatory $CD4^+$ T cell subsets. A number of $CD4^+$ T cell subtypes with regulatory or suppressive activity are now recognized. They fall broadly into one of two categories: those which are produced by the thymus, express CD4, CD25, GITR and CTLA-4, and appear crucially dependent on the expression of the X-linked forkhead/winged helix transcription factor, Foxp3, for their development (so-called 'naturally occurring' regulatory T (T_R) cells); and those which arise from naïve $CD4^+$ T cells as a result of 'tolerogenic' encounters in the periphery. The latter 'inducible' or 'adaptive' regulatory T cells include interleukin (IL)-10-producing, Foxp3-negative Tr1 cells [71,72], transforming growth factor-β (TGFβ)-producing Th3 cells [73], and extra-thymically generated $CD4^+CD25^+Foxp3^+$ T cells [74–78]. In addition, $CD4^+CD25^-Foxp3^+$T cells with regulatory capabilities have been recognized [79]. To add further to this complexity, CD8+ T cells with suppressor activity have also been described [80–83]. The dominant inhibitory potential of regulatory T cell populations in murine models of malignancy is well established [84], and more recently their potential role in human malignancies has been demonstrated [69]. However, the level of tumor infiltration by regulatory T cells alone may not be the best predictor of outcome. Hodgkin's lymphoma tumors contain significant populations of both IL-10-secreting Tr1 and $CD4^+CD25^+$ regulatory T cells which induce a profoundly immunosuppressive environment [85]. However, the level of infiltration by $Foxp3^+$ cells may not be as good as predictor of outcome as combined assessment of both cells expressing Foxp3 and cells expressing TIA-1 (cytotoxic granule-associated RNA binding protein)[86] highlighting the potential importance of assessing the relative prevalence of multiple infiltrating populations. Indeed, identification of specific immunological signatures (based on flow cytometry, PCR or microarray analyses [87] that predict outcomes, or guide the institution or monitoring of therapies would be useful adjuncts to modern clinical practice. For example, it is plausible that tumors that contain few TIL, including T_R, will respond well to treatments that aim to enhance cytotoxic T cell numbers, function or migration, whilst those that contain significant numbers of T_R would benefit from therapies aimed at reducing T_R number or function. In addition, T_R represent another regulatory mechanism that may be enhanced in response to, and hence limit the efficacy of, current immunotherapeutic interventions. For example, IL-2 has entered clinical trials for a number of human cancers such as melanoma, renal cell carcinoma, rhabdomyosarcoma and ovarian cancer. Its initial use was based on the idea that it may directly enhance effector function of both innate and adaptive immune systems. However, IL-2 is recognised as crucial for the homeostasis and function of $CD4^+CD25^+$ regulatory T cells *in vivo* [88–90], and administration to patients with cancer results in increases in the numbers of peripheral T_R cells and stimulation of expression of CXC-chemokine receptor 4 (CXCR4) and CCR4 on T_R cells promoting their migration towards CXCL12 and CCL2 within the tumor microenvironment [91–93]. In addition, since the targets of many cancer vaccination strategies are self antigens, it is perhaps no surprise that 'therapeutic' cancer vaccines can induce amplification of tumor-specific regulatory T cells [94]. The 'immunogenicity' or 'tolerogenicity' of DCs also becomes an increasingly important consideration in vaccination programs since even conventionally 'mature' DCs can activate and expand autoantigen-specific T_R cells [95]. Overall, current evidence therefore suggests that regulatory T cells are potentially useful targets for immunotherapeutic interventions.

The mechanism(s) by which regulatory T cells induce suppression, however, remain controversial. $CD4^+CD25^+Foxp3^+$T cells suppress by contact-dependent mechanisms *in vitro* independently of TGF-β or IL-10 secretion [96–98], whereas suppression *in vivo* is cytokine-dependent. In addition, the mechanism(s) of action *in vivo* appear to be model dependent as certain forms of autoimmunity such as colitis can be suppressed by $CD4^+CD25^+$T cells in an IL-10 dependent manner [99,100], whereas others such as gastritis can be suppressed independently of IL-10 [100]. TGF-β has been implicated in the mechanism of T_R mediated suppression in some studies of autoimmune colitis [101–103] but not others [97]. A possible role for CTLA-4 in mediating suppression by $CD4^+CD25^-Foxp3^+$T cells has also been proposed. Again, this function has been implied by some but not all studies, including both *in vitro* and in vivo model systems of CTLA-4 blockade [104,105]. One tentative mechanism for this effect has been provided by the data suggesting that CTLA-4 can induce backward or "outside-in" signalling following ligation of B7-1/B7-2 on DCs, resulting in IDO generation [25]. Definitive experimental proof of the significance of CTLA-4 blockade in abrogating T_R function is currently lacking, in large part because of the confounding effects that CTLA-4 blockade has directly on effector T cells within the same systems. For example, normal mice treated with high doses of anti-CTLA-4 or a mixture of anti-CTLA-4 and anti-CD25 develop autoimmune gastritis, and the administration of anti-CTLA-4 reverses the T_R-mediated inhibition of $CD25^-$ T cell induced colitis *in vivo* [104]. However, exclusion of the possibility of a T cell intrinsic cell-autonomous mechanism of action of anti-CTLA-4 in these studies by a direct blockade of inhibitory signalling via CTLA-4 on effector populations is difficult. The demonstration that bone marrow chimeras generated from CTLA-$4^{-/-}$ and wild type CTLA-$4^{+/+}$ donors are protected from the lethal lymphoproliferative disorder that characterises the CTLA-$4^{-/-}$ mice [106] has also been used to suggest an important non cell-autonomous role for CTLA-4 in negative regulation of T cell responses. Wild type CTLA-4 expressing regulatory T cells are clearly intellectually viable candidate populations to mediate these effects. CTLA-4 could either be required for the normal development or maintenance of a regulatory population, or could be essential to the normal inhibitory function of these cells. However, CTLA-4 expression does not appear to be critical for the development of $CD4^+CD25^+$ T cells within the thymus of CTLA-$4^{-/-}$ mice [107], and $CD4^+CD25^+CD62L^+$ T cells from CTLA-4-deficient mice bearing a CTLA-4Ig transgene express levels of Foxp3 that are similarly high to those of wild type T_R by Western blot analysis, suggesting that they represent the same lineage [108]. Both of these CTLA-$4^{-/-}$ T_R populations exhibit regulatory function in suppressor assays that is equivalent to that of wild type T_R cells, although the mechanism of suppression may differ as they suppress in a partially TGF-β-dependent fashion in these assays, unlike their wild type counterparts [108]. In addition, anti-CTLA-4 does not successfully reverse *in vitro* suppression in all studies, which suggest that CTLA-4 blockade has only a moderate or no effect on the suppressive function of $CD4^+CD25^+$ regulatory T cells [109–112]. Thus current data suggest that the role of CTLA-4 in both the development and function of $CD4^+CD25^+$ T_R is, at least, partially redundant.

An interesting extension of the work suggesting that B7 molecules might be able to transduce inhibitory signals back into the cells on which they are expressed is provided by studies of B7 deficient T cells. B7-2 is constitutively expressed on some resting T cells, and both B7-1 and B7-2 can be up-regulated on activated T cells. $CD4^+CD25^-$ effector T cells from B7-1/B7-$2^{-/-}$ mice are resistant to suppression by $CD4^+CD25^+$ T_R compared to wild type $CD4^+CD25^-$ effector T cells *in vitro*, and these cells provoke a lethal wasting disease in lymphopenic mice despite the presence of regulatory T cells [113]. Restoration of the susceptibility of B7-1/B7-2-deficient cells to suppression is achievable by lentiviral-based expression of full-length B7-1 or B7-2, but not of truncated molecules lacking the transmembrane/cytoplasmic domain, despite restoration of CD28-dependent co-stimulatory activity by these truncation mutants. In addition, T cells that constitutively over-express B7-2 exhibit reduced alloreactivity and graft-versus-host disease mortality in murine transplantation models [114]. Conversely, T cells from B7-1/B7-$2^{-/-}$

mice effect accelerated alloresponses and increased graft-versus-host disease-related mortality. The down-regulation of responsiveness mediated via B7-1/B7-2 appears to be dependent on interaction with T cell-associated CTLA-4. Collectively these data suggest that bi-directional signalling may also be important in T-cell regulation by B7-1/B7-2 -CTLA-4 interactions.

Upregulation of particular molecules on regulatory T cell populations does not necessarily imply a role in suppressive function. An alternative explanation for the high levels of CTLA-4 is that its role in $CD4^+CD25^+$ T_R is the same as its proposed role in effector T cells i.e. it works in a cell-autonomous fashion to restrict proliferation of a population of T cells with higher affinities for self than those of non-regulatory populations, and that the higher levels of CTLA-4 are a manifestation of chronic stimulation by self antigen *in vivo*. A parallel may be drawn with CD25 expression. The IL-2 receptor consists of a heterotrimeric complex consisting of CD25 (α chain), CD122 (β chain) and CD132 (γ chain). This complex has a 100-fold higher affinity for IL-2 than the dimeric form (CD122 and CD132). Expression of high levels of this heterotrimeric receptor complex on T_R cells led to the suggestion that competition between T_R and effector/helper T cells for IL-2 might be a further mechanism of suppression [115]. The demonstration that $CD4^+CD25^+$ T_R can suppress autoimmunity in IL-2 receptor deficient mice excludes the possibility that competition for IL-2 is an essential mechanism of suppression *in vivo* [116].

TARGETING REGULATORY T CELLS

Monoclonal antibodies that result in depletion of regulatory T cell populations (e.g. anti-CD25 PC61 clone) have demonstrated the therapeutic potential of targeting regulatory T cells in murine models of cancer. *In vivo* administration suppresses growth of a number of murine tumors [84, 117], and combinatorial therapies show possible additive or synergistic activity [65,118–120]. Importantly, it was recognised early in these studies that T_R depletion was effective as a prophylactic or if given within 1 day of tumor inoculation, but failed to affect such anti-tumor responses if given at later time points [117]. Since CD25 is also upregulated on activated $CD4^+$and $CD8^+$ T cells, it is possible that the failure of delayed therapy relates to concomitant depletion of both regulatory and effector populations. This clearly has implications for attempts to clinically harness this approach in humans. Denileukin diftitox (ONTAK) is a fusion protein designed to direct the cytocidal action of diphtheria toxin to cells that overexpress the IL-2 receptor. *Ex vivo* studies indicate that it interacts with the high- and intermediate-affinity IL-2 receptor on the cell surface and undergoes internalization. Subsequent cleavage in the endosome releases the diphtheria toxin into the cytosol, which then inhibits cellular protein synthesis, resulting in rapid cell death. It is characterized by a relatively short half life (60 minutes) compared with monoclonal antibodies. Preliminary studies in ovarian and renal cell carcinoma demonstrate an early reduction in circulating T_R cells following denileukin diftitox therapy with preservation of the $CD4^+CD25^{int}$ memory T cell pool [121], but possible depletion of $CD25^+$ effector cells with prolonged/repeated administration [122]. Administration prior to tumor RNA-transfected DC vaccines enhanced tumor immunity as measured by subsequent *in vitro* analyses of cytokine production in recall responses to the DC vaccine [121].

Depletion of T_R from adoptively transferred lymphocyte populations provides an alternative therapeutic avenue by which to enhance anti-tumor activity. In a murine model of B16 melanoma therapy $CD4^+CD25^-$ T cells helped to break tolerance to a persisting self-antigen, induce depigmentation and treat established tumors through an IL-2-dependent mechanism, but this activity required simultaneous absence of naturally occurring $CD4^+CD25^+$ T cells to be effective [123]. These findings have obvious relevance for clinical studies utilising the adoptive transfer of expanded populations of tumor infiltrating lymphocytes following lymphodepleting chemoradiotherapy in humans [124].

The mechanism of action of other monoclonal antibodies that target molecules considered as activation markers, which are present on both regulatory and effector populations, is less clear. As previously stated, much of the difficulty arises from the confounding influences of effects on both populations. Examples include blocking antibodies to CTLA-4, and the agonistic antibodies to the TNFR family members GITR and OX40. All are recognised to enhance effector function, and all have anti-tumor activity in murine models of malignancy [64, 125–127]. More recent data suggest that signalling via GITR or OX40 on regulatory T cells may block their inhibitory activity [128, 129]. However, in a situation somewhat akin to that with CTLA-4 blockade, others have questioned the interpretation of some of the data from these studies. In particular, $GITR^{-/-}$ $CD4^+CD25^+$ T cells suppress to the same extent as wild type $CD4^+CD25^+$ T cells in suppressor assays [130]. In addition, experiments using $GITR^{-/-}$ $CD4^+CD25^-$ T cells suggest that GITR-L provides an important signal for $CD25^-$ T cells, rendering them resistant to $CD4^+CD25^+$-mediated regulation at the initiation of the immune response, and that engagement of GITR on $CD4^+CD25^+$ T cells plays no role in abrogation of the suppressive activity of $CD4^+CD25^+$ T cells *in vitro* [130]. Whilst debates about mechanism do not detract from the possible therapeutic efficacy of these approaches, a mechanistic understanding has relevance for the informed development of combinatorial approaches, and this becomes increasingly important in the midst of a proliferation of possible immunotherapeutic manipulations.

TOWARDS AN UNDERSTANDING OF THE MECHANISM OF COMBINATORIAL IMMUNOTHERAPIES: CTLA-4 BLOCKADE AND GM-CSF SECRETING CELLULAR VACCINES

GM-CSF secreting cellular vaccines have shown promise as anti-cancer immunotherapeutics in murine models and early clinical studies, inducing infiltrates of DCs, macrophages, eosinophils and lymphocytes at vaccination sites, and enhancing tumor infiltration by $CD4^+$ and $CD8^+$ lymphocytes [131]. In poorly immunogenic murine tumors such as B16BL6 melanoma vaccination alone is insufficient to cure pre-established tumors, whilst combination with CTLA-4 blockade results in tumor elimination [57]. Chronic anti-CTLA-4 therapy *in vivo* induces the accumulation of intra-nodal T_R, suggesting a direct cell-autonomous effect of blockade of CTLA-4-mediated inhibitory signalling on the T_R [112]. Growth of B16 tumor also induces the accumulation of T_R in the lymph nodes, which is further enhanced by anti-CTLA-4 monotherapy [112]. However, anti-CTLA-4 monotherapy does not result in increased intra-tumoral T cell infiltration. GM-CSF-expressing B16 cellular vaccine enhances tumor infiltration by $CD8^+$ T cells, but intra-tumoral proliferation is still presumably under the restraints imposed by CTLA-4 mediated signalling and tumor growth is not prevented. Combination with CTLA-4 blockade results in maximal effects on non-regulatory T cell numbers by allowing unrestrained proliferation driven by tumor antigens, resulting in the inversion of the ratio of effectors to regulators [112]. These data suggest that the priming induced by the cellular vaccine results in a massive increase in the effector compartment within the tumor and once the inhibitory cellular restraints imposed by CTLA-4 signalling are removed the inhibitory activities of the T_R are overwhelmed, resulting in tumor rejection. In the absence of the cellular vaccine, insufficient effector T cells infiltrate the tumor and the outcome of CTLA-4 blockade still favors T_R over the effector populations resulting in continued tumor growth. Hence, the overall outcome will depend on the priming history of the T cell populations and the local antigenic milieu. We believe that these results favor a T cell intrinsic cell-autonomous mode of action of anti-CTLA-4 on both the effector and regulatory compartments, although it remains difficult to completely exclude an additional non cell-autonomous effect mediated via inhibition of T_R function. If additional effects on T_R are absent or relatively modest then these cells may be good targets for further combinatorial therapies. The synergistic effect of T_R depletion and CTLA-4 blockade have already been demonstrated in murine models [65].

CLINICAL TRIALS OF CTLA-4 BLOCKADE

Early clinical trials incorporating human anti-CTLA-4 antibodies (MDX-010 or CP-675,206) developed using transgenic mouse technologies have predominantly focused on patients with metastatic melanoma or renal carcinoma, although smaller studies have also included patients with prostatic, ovarian, breast or colonic carcinomas [132–137]. A number of preliminary observations can be made from these phase 1 and early phase 2 protocols. When used as a monotherapy anti-CTLA-4 is capable of inducing objective tumor response rates of 7-15% in heavily pre-treated patients with melanoma or renal carcinoma and responses have involved multiple visceral sites including the lung and brain [138]. Evidence of immunological activity can be demonstrated in a larger number of patients who do not reach conventional objective response criteria. This includes the generation of immune cell infiltrates into the tumors and tumor necrosis [133]. Softer indices of benefit including disease stabilization and symptomatic improvements have also been noted in many studies [136]. Although not all responses have been maintained they have proven apparently durable in some cases, and most studies document ongoing responses at 18-35+ months. The dosing and scheduling of anti-CTLA-4 has varied between studies and the optimal approach remains unclear. Resolution of this issue would be considerably aided by the existence of a suitable biomarker for its activity other than response rate.

Data from preclinical models, in which monotherapy has proven insufficient in the more poorly immunogenic tumors and combinatorial therapies have shown synergistic activity, have pre-empted and informed the development of clinical trials combining CTLA-4 blockade with other therapeutic modalities. The majority of published studies to date have focused on co-administration of anti-CTLA-4 and melanoma peptides [132, 134, 135]. Both the rates and durations of responses appear similar to those in studies of anti-CTLA-4 monotherapy [134], as does the incidence, severity and pattern of adverse events. Interestingly, CTLA-4 blockade has not resulted in measurable increases in anti-peptide responses in peripheral blood over those demonstrated with peptide vaccine alone [134, 135]. One possible interpretation of this data is that anti-tumor responses with this combinatorial approach might be attributable to anti-CTLA-4 alone. However, these results could also reflect the sampling site (i.e. peripheral blood sampling may not reflect intra-tumoral populations) or, alternatively, vaccination with peptide vaccines may indirectly result in the activation of tumor specific T cells with specificity different from the tumor antigen immunogen [139]. A phase III trial will compare response rates among groups treated with vaccine alone, MDX-010 alone, and MDX-010 together with vaccine. Combination of CTLA-4 blockade with high dose bolus IL-2 is also being studied [140]. The latter is an approved treatment for metastatic melanoma and results in response rates of ~15% of which a high percentage can be durable [141, 142]. Preliminary results suggest that the combination may give additive therapeutic benefits [140]. Preliminary results from studies combining GM-CSF expressing cellular vaccines and CTLA-4 blockade have given similarly encouraging data in support of synergistic activity [131, 143].

ADVERSE IMMUNE MANIFESTATIONS OF CTLA-4 BLOCKADE IN PRE-CLINICAL MODELS AND CLINICAL TRIALS

Since immunological checkpoints have a vital physiological role in limiting the potential for damage inherent in harbouring an auto-reactive T cell repertoire, checkpoint blockade might theoretically result in uncontrolled auto-reactivity and significant toxicity. Anti-CTLA-4 can exacerbate autoimmunity in a variety of experimental models [144], although this has generally occurred when mice were vaccinated with self antigens in combination with CTLA-4 blockade (145, 146, 147, 148). Pre-clinical studies also illustrate the possibility of induction of autoimmunity. However, toxicities were essentially limited to predicted 'target' tissues sharing the same antigenic determinants as the cellular vaccines (depigmentation in the melanoma model [57], prostatitis in the prostate cancer model [59]. More serious systemic toxicities were not documented, perhaps in part due to the shorter duration of therapy, and shorter half life of the original hamster anti-mouse antibody (clone 9H10) used in these studies as compared to that of the fully human antibody used for subsequent clinical studies. Non-human primates treated with CTLA-4 blockade and a human melanoma whole cell vaccine showed enhanced development of antibodies to some self antigens, in particular to those present in lysates prepared from their melanocyte rich iris tissue [149]. Continued administration of anti-CTLA-4 in high doses for up to six months, however, did not result in any clinically or pathologically detectable end organ damage, even in those animals with detectable humoral anti-self responses.

In contrast to the limited autoreactive toxicities seen in preclinical models adverse immune events (AIE) have been a prominent feature of the early clinical studies with anti-CTLA-4. The commonest side effect in the initial study of MDX-010 was development of an asymptomatic, grade 1 reticular and erythematous rash on the trunk and extremities, particularly in the patients with melanoma [133]. Histological examination revealed perivascular lymphoid aggregates of both $CD4^+$ and $CD8^+$ T cells juxtaposed with dying melanocytes suggesting a loss of tolerance to melanocyte differentiation antigens. The generation of low titers of autoantibodies in a number of patients demonstrated that the therapy may at least partially compromise systemic tolerance, but no evidence for autoimmune disease was noted. Subsequent studies have confirmed that the most common AIE involve the skin and the gastrointestinal tract and that these adverse events are also due to inflammatory T cell infiltrates. Grade 3 and 4 adverse immune events, especially colitis, have been observed, with occasional cases of colonic perforation [137,150]. Immune mediated hypophysitis, uveitis, and hepatitis have also been documented [132,136,151,152]. Management of these adverse events includes cessation of drug and treatment with high dose steroids. The majority resolve with systemic immune suppression without long term sequelae, and anti-tumor responses do not appear to be compromised. Adverse events may also resolve without intervention [136] in keeping with the lack of progression of vitiligo in the murine melanoma model following cessation of therapy and antibody clearance, and suggesting a reversible effect on T cell function. In addition, the demonstration that $CD4^+CD25^+$ T cells isolated from mice following chronic CTLA-4 blockade *in vivo* are capable of suppressing normally in *ex vivo* assays mitigates against irreversible suppression of their function if they are involved in any way in the activity of CTLA-4 blockade [112].

Much has been written concerning the correlation of serious AIE (Grade 3 or 4) with anti-tumor responses [134] or freedom from relapse [135]. It has been suggested that this indicates either that TCR specificities are directed at antigens shared by tumor and normal cellular counterparts (as may be the case for melanoma differentiation antigens), or that the coincident development of separate populations mediating anti-tumor and anti-host activities is closely linked. It is, however, possible that non self-specific activation and subsequent infiltration of T cells propagates at least some of these AIE. The antigen specificity of T cell infiltrates in tissue where AIE are observed, as well as that of tumor-infiltrating T cells remains to be analyzed.

However, resolving the issue of whether such adverse events are an inherent part of effective checkpoint blockade, or whether they can be dissociated by manipulation of dose scheduling, or by targeting immunological rather than clinical endpoints as a primary objective is currently a vital imperative. Combinatorial approaches involving strategies that will enhance presentation of tumor-selective antigens to the immune system over-and-above those of normal tissues might help to improve the therapeutic index.

OTHER POTENTIAL CO-INHIBITORY TARGETS FOR CHECKPOINT BLOCKADE

Other members of the immunoglobulin superfamily that act as inhibitory checkpoints are also potential targets for therapeutic blockade. These include PD-1 and its ligands PD-L1 (B7-H1) and PD-L2 (B7-DC), and more speculatively B7-H3, B7x/B7-H4 and BTLA. PD-1 is more broadly expressed than CD28/CTLA-4. It is expressed on activated $CD4^+$ and $CD8^+$ T cells, B cells and monocytes, and at low levels on NK-T cells. PD-L1 is expressed on resting and upregulated on activated B, T, myeloid and dendritic cells, and on $CD4^+CD25^+$ T_R cells. It is also expressed on non-haematopoietic cells including microvascular endothelial cells and in non-lymphoid organs including heart, lung, pancreas, muscle and placenta. This distribution suggests that interactions of ligands and receptors may be important in regulating effector T cell responses in the peripheral tissues by antigen presenting cells such as DCs, macrophages and also endothelial cells. PD-L2 is induced by cytokines on macrophages and DCs.

PD-L1 is expressed on many human malignancies [19,20,153,154]. Its expression is associated with poor prognosis in renal and esophageal cancer [19, 155]. By contrast, PD-L2 is the best genomic discriminator between primary mediastinal B cell lymphoma and other less favourable diffuse large B cell lymphomas [156]. Transfection of murine tumors with PD-L1 renders them less susceptible to lysis by cytotoxic T cells *in vitro*, and markedly enhances tumor growth and invasiveness *in vivo* [157]. Both effects are reversed by blockade with anti-PD-L1 antibody [157, 158]. Murine myeloma cell lines naturally express PD-L1, and their growth *in vivo* is also inhibited significantly by the administration of anti-PD-L1 antibody. Their growth is suppressed completely in syngeneic PD-1-deficient mice [157]. In addition, PD-$1^{-/-}CD8^+$ TCR transgenic T cells cause tumor rejection in an adoptive transfer model in which wild type and CTLA-$4^{-/-}$ T cells fail to mediate rejection [20]. Activation of human T cells isolated from the ascites of patients with ovarian cancer, either in the presence or absence of PD-L1 blockade, followed by adoptive transfer into tumor-bearing NOD-SCID mice, also demonstrated enhanced anti-tumor activity of the cells that had been conditioned in the presence of anti-PD-L1 [159]. Overall, these results are consistent with a model in which CTLA-4 is more vital for regulation of $CD4^+$ T cell responses, particularly early at the APC interface, whereas PD-1 has a relatively minor role at this stage (when CD28 co-stimulation can overcome its inhibitory effects [160] but a more critical role in suppressing the execution of T cell effector function against cells that do not express CD80/86. Intriguingly, PD-L2 expression on J558 plasmacytoma cells actually enhances CD8-mediated immunity, tumor rejection and establishment of immunological memory to subsequent re-challenge [161]. The effect is evident for PD-1$^{-/-}$as well as wild type T cells, suggesting that it may be mediated by interaction with a receptor other than PD-1. A limited number of studies have examined the ability of anti-PD-1 antibodies to promote anti-tumor responses directly. Two metastatic models have been shown to be sensitive to PD-1 blockade [162]. Growth of the colonic carcinoma cell line CT26 was inhibited by 50% after treatment with anti-PD-1 antibody, and B16 melanoma metastasis to the liver after intrasplenic injection of tumor cells was also inhibited.

B7-H3 (B7-RP2) and B7x (B7-H4, B7-S1) are the most recently described B7 family members. Both currently remain orphan ligands and both appear to mediate inhibitory effects on immune responses [163–166]. They display greater similarity to each other than other family members and appear to bind to a receptor(s) expressed on activated but not naïve T cells, but the identity of the receptor(s) remains unclear. Expression of mRNA for either ligand is seen in both lymphoid and non-lymphoid tissues. The broad tissue distribution and inducible nature of both ligands has led to the suggestion that they down-regulate immune responses in the periphery and play a role in regulating T cell tolerance. B7x is expressed on several human tumors (e.g. ovarian and lung carcinoma) at higher levels than in the normal tissue counterparts [167–169] suggesting a possible role in immune evasion as suggested for PD-L1. The expression levels on antigen presenting cells are currently controversial. It has been suggested that human regulatory T cells may induce IL-10 production by APCs and an autocrine up-regulation of B7x, which is then inhibitory to subsequent T cell activation [170, 171]. If expression on either tumor cells or APCs mediates significant inhibition of tumor-reactive T cells, blockade may prove to be therapeutically beneficial.

Finally, BTLA is the most recently described member of the costimulatory immunoglobulin superfamily. It is expressed on activated T and B cells, shows high expression by resting B cells, is induced on anergic CD4^{+} T cells and has lower expression on macrophages, DCs and NK cells [2, 172, 173]. Its ligand has recently been identified as HVEM [174]. HVEM is constitutively expressed by naïve T cells, is down-regulated after activation, and then re-expressed as the T cell returns towards a resting (memory) state. BTLA exerts inhibitory effects on both B and T cells [2]. Both cell types show moderately enhanced responsiveness in BTLA$^{-/-}$ mice and blockade leads to inhibition of transplantation tolerance. Thus, the negative regulation induced by BTLA ligation on B cells and T cells can potently regulate the strength of the immune response and alter the balance governing immune tolerance. The consequences of immunological blockade in tumor models await further study.

CONCLUSIONS: ACCENTUATE THE POSITIVE, ELIMINATE THE NEGATIVE

The potential for therapeutic immunological checkpoint blockade has been amply demonstrated in pre-clinical murine models of a variety of cancers and in combination with a variety of other therapeutic interventions. Early clinical studies demonstrate an ability to elicit responses in a proportion of heavily pre-treated patients with advanced stage disease. The association of clinical responses with immune related adverse events is perhaps not surprising given the mode of action of these therapies. Whether such adverse events are an inherent part of effective checkpoint blockade, or whether they can be dissociated remains an area for future study. These reactions have been organ-specific and no clinical evidence of generalized systemic autoimmunity has been documented to date. The majority resolve with systemic immune suppression without long term sequelae, and anti-tumor responses do not appear to be compromised. Whilst CTLA-4 blockade remains the archetypal example of these approaches, other immunological checkpoints offer further targets for intervention.

Given the multitude of inhibitory checkpoints involved in the regulation of immune responses that can potentially impact negatively on interventions aimed at enhancing antigen presentation and augmenting T cell effector functions it is possible that the most effective immunotherapies will involve combinatorial approaches targeting multiple elements of the immune pathway. We are perhaps moving towards an era characterised by attempts to not only accentuate the positive but also simultaneously to eliminate the negative. Therapies aimed at enhancing tumor antigen presentation (dendritic cell vaccines, GM-CSF secreting cellular vaccines, CpG oligonucleotides, imiquimod), inhibiting cell-autonomous and non cell-autonomous negative immune regulation (e.g. CTLA-4 and PD-1/PD-L1 blockade, depletion or inhibition of T_R), and amplifying T cell effector functions (e.g. agonistic anti-GITR, anti-OX40, anti-4-1BB antibodies) have been shown to enhance immune responses directed towards tumors and should yield synergistic anti-cancer effects. Proof of principle for the idea of combinatorial therapeutics is available from murine models (e.g. CTLA-4 blockade with GM-CSF expressing cellular vaccines, anti-CD25 mediated regulatory T cell depletion, or agonistic anti-GITR antibody [57, 59, 64, 65], or cellular vaccines co-transfected with GM-CSF and OX-40L [175] and is currently being explored in the next phase of clinical studies [143]. Combined or sequential manipulation of multiple members of the co-stimulatory family may ultimately prove more effective in generation of sustained responses and immunological memory. It is hoped that combinatorial therapies may also offer the best balance of benefits and toxicities by directing the immune responses unleashed by blockade of inhibitory pathways towards relevant tumor targets. It is anticipated that the results from pre-clinical studies of combinatorial approaches will continue to inform the rational evolution of clinical strategies.

ACKNOWLEDGEMENTS:

Karl S Peggs is a Visiting Fellow funded by the Leukaemia Research Fund, London, United Kingdom; Sergio A Quezada is a Fellow of the Cancer Research Institute, USA. James P. Allison holds the David H. Koch Chair in Immunologic Studies at the Memorial Sloan-Kettering Cancer Center.

REFERENCES

1. Hao,Y., Legrand,N., & Freitas,A.A. (2006) The clone size of peripheral CD8 T cells is regulated by TCR promiscuity. *J.Exp.Med.*
2. Watanabe,N., Gavrieli,M., Sedy,J.R., Yang,J., Fallarino,F., Loftin,S.K., Hurchla,M.A., Zimmerman,N., Sim,J., Zang,X., Murphy,T.L., Russell,J.H., Allison,J.P., & Murphy,K.M. (2003) BTLA is a lymphocyte inhibitory receptor with similarities to CTLA-4 and PD-1. *Nat.Immunol.*, 4, 670–679.
3. Marrogi,A.J., Munshi,A., Merogi,A.J., Ohadike,Y., El Habashi,A., Marrogi,O.L., & Freeman,S.M. (1997) Study of tumor infiltrating lymphocytes and transforming growth factor-beta as prognostic factors in breast carcinoma. *Int.J.Cancer*, 74, 492–501.
4. Zhang,L., Conejo-Garcia,J.R., Katsaros,D., Gimotty,P.A., Massobrio,M., Regnani,G., Makrigiannakis,A., Gray,H., Schlienger,K., Liebman,M.N., Rubin,S.C., & Coukos,G. (2003) Intratumoral T cells, recurrence, and survival in epithelial ovarian cancer. *N.Engl.J.Med.*, 348, 203–213.
5. Nakano,O., Sato,M., Naito,Y., Suzuki,K., Orikasa,S., Aizawa,M., Suzuki,Y., Shintaku,I., Nagura,H., & Ohtani,H. (2001) Proliferative activity of intratumoral CD8(+) T-lymphocytes as a prognostic factor in human renal cell carcinoma: clinicopathologic demonstration of antitumor immunity. *Cancer Res.*, 61, 5132–5136.
6. Vesalainen,S., Lipponen,P., Talja,M., & Syrjanen,K. (1994) Histological grade, perineural infiltration, tumour-infiltrating lymphocytes and apoptosis as determinants of long-term prognosis in prostatic adenocarcinoma. *Eur.J.Cancer*, 30A, 1797–1803.
7. Naito,Y., Saito,K., Shiiba,K., Ohuchi,A., Saigenji,K., Nagura,H., & Ohtani,H. (1998) CD8+ T cells infiltrated within cancer cell nests as a prognostic factor in human colorectal cancer. *Cancer Res.*, 58, 3491–3494.
8. Mortarini,R., Piris,A., Maurichi,A., Molla,A., Bersani,I., Bono,A., Bartoli,C., Santinami,M., Lombardo,C., Ravagnani,F., Cascinelli,N., Parmiani,G., & Anichini,A. (2003) Lack of terminally differentiated tumor-specific CD8+ T cells at tumor site in spite of antitumor immunity to self-antigens in human metastatic melanoma. *Cancer Res.*, 63, 2535–2545.
9. Gabrilovich,D. (2004) Mechanisms and functional significance of tumour-induced dendritic-cell defects. *Nat.Rev.Immunol.*, 4, 941–952.
10. Furumoto,K., Soares,L., Engleman,E.G., & Merad,M. (2004) Induction of potent antitumor immunity by in situ targeting of intratumoral DCs. *J.Clin.Invest*, 113, 774–783.
11. Young,J.W. & Inaba,K. (1996) Dendritic cells as adjuvants for class I major histocompatibility complex-restricted antitumor immunity. *J.Exp.Med.*, 183, 7–11.
12. Dranoff,G., Jaffee,E., Lazenby,A., Golumbek,P., Levitsky,H., Brose,K., Jackson,V., Hamada,H., Pardoll,D., & Mulligan,R.C. (1993) Vaccination with irradiated tumor cells engineered to secrete murine granulocyte-macrophage colony-stimulating factor stimulates potent, specific, and long-lasting anti-tumor immunity. *Proc.Natl.Acad.Sci.U.S.A*, 90, 3539–3543.
13. Finn,O.J. (2003) Cancer vaccines: between the idea and the reality. *Nat.Rev.Immunol.*, 3, 630–641.
14. Rosenberg,S.A., Yang,J.C., & Restifo,N.P. (2004) Cancer immunotherapy: moving beyond current vaccines. *Nat.Med.*, 10, 909–915.
15. Rosenberg,S.A., Sherry,R.M., Morton,K.E., Scharfman,W.J., Yang,J.C., Topalian,S.L., Royal,R.E., Kammula,U., Restifo,N.P., Hughes,M.S., Schwartzentruber,D., Berman,D.M., Schwarz,S.L., Ngo,L.T., Mavroukakis,S.A., White,D.E., & Steinberg,S.M. (2005) Tumor progression can occur

despite the induction of very high levels of self/tumor antigen-specific CD8+ T cells in patients with melanoma. *J.Immunol.*, 175, 6169–6176.
16. Nishikawa,H., Qian,F., Tsuji,T., Ritter,G., Old,L.J., Gnjatic,S., & Odunsi,K. (2006) Influence of CD4+CD25+ regulatory T cells on low/high-avidity CD4+ T cells following peptide vaccination. *J.Immunol.*, 176, 6340–6346.
17. Dhodapkar,M.V., Steinman,R.M., Krasovsky,J., Munz,C., & Bhardwaj,N. (2001) Antigen-specific inhibition of effector T cell function in humans after injection of immature dendritic cells. *J.Exp.Med.*, 193, 233–238.
18. Chakraborty,N.G., Chattopadhyay,S., Mehrotra,S., Chhabra,A., & Mukherji,B. (2004) Regulatory T-cell response and tumor vaccine-induced cytotoxic T lymphocytes in human melanoma. *Hum.Immunol.*, 65, 794–802.
19. Thompson,R.H., Gillett,M.D., Cheville,J.C., Lohse,C.M., Dong,H., Webster,W.S., Krejci,K.G., Lobo,J.R., Sengupta,S., Chen,L., Zincke,H., Blute,M.L., Strome,S.E., Leibovich,B.C., & Kwon,E.D. (2004) Costimulatory B7-H1 in renal cell carcinoma patients: Indicator of tumor aggressiveness and potential therapeutic target. *Proc.Natl.Acad.Sci.U.S.A*, 101, 17174–17179.
20. Blank,C., Brown,I., Peterson,A.C., Spiotto,M., Iwai,Y., Honjo,T., & Gajewski,T.F. (2004) PD-L1/B7H-1 inhibits the effector phase of tumor rejection by T cell receptor (TCR) transgenic CD8+ T cells. *Cancer Res.*, 64, 1140–1145.
21. Harding,F.A., McArthur,J.G., Gross,J.A., Raulet,D.H., & Allison,J.P. (1992) CD28-mediated signalling co-stimulates murine T cells and prevents induction of anergy in T-cell clones. *Nature*, 356, 607–609.
22. Linsley,P.S., Brady,W., Grosmaire,L., Aruffo,A., Damle,N.K., & Ledbetter,J.A. (1991) Binding of the B cell activation antigen B7 to CD28 costimulates T cell proliferation and interleukin 2 mRNA accumulation. *J.Exp.Med.*, 173, 721–730.
23. Hathcock,K.S., Laszlo,G., Pucillo,C., Linsley,P., & Hodes,R.J. (1994) Comparative analysis of B7–1 and B7–2 costimulatory ligands: expression and function. *J.Exp.Med.*, 180, 631–640.
24. Lenschow,D.J. & Bluestone,J.A. (1993) T cell co-stimulation and in vivo tolerance. *Curr.Opin.Immunol.*, 5, 747–752.
25. Fallarino,F., Grohmann,U., Hwang,K.W., Orabona,C., Vacca,C., Bianchi,R., Belladonna,M.L., Fioretti,M.C., Alegre,M.L., & Puccetti,P. (2003) Modulation of tryptophan catabolism by regulatory T cells. *Nat.Immunol.*, 4, 1206–1212.
26. Shahinian,A., Pfeffer,K., Lee,K.P., Kundig,T.M., Kishihara,K., Wakeham,A., Kawai,K., Ohashi,P.S., Thompson,C.B., & Mak,T.W. (1993) Differential T cell costimulatory requirements in CD28-deficient mice. *Science*, 261, 609–612.
27. Borriello,F., Sethna,M.P., Boyd,S.D., Schweitzer,A.N., Tivol,E.A., Jacoby,D., Strom,T.B., Simpson,E.M., Freeman,G.J., & Sharpe,A.H. (1997) B7–1 and B7–2 have overlapping, critical roles in immunoglobulin class switching and germinal center formation. *Immunity.*, 6, 303–313.
28. Diehn,M., Alizadeh,A.A., Rando,O.J., Liu,C.L., Stankunas,K., Botstein,D., Crabtree,G.R., & Brown,P.O. (2002) Genomic expression programs and the integration of the CD28 costimulatory signal in T cell activation. *Proc.Natl.Acad.Sci.U.S.A*, 99, 11796–11801.
29. Riley,J.L., Mao,M., Kobayashi,S., Biery,M., Burchard,J., Cavet,G., Gregson,B.P., June,C.H., & Linsley,P.S. (2002) Modulation of TCR-induced transcriptional profiles by ligation of CD28, ICOS, and CTLA-4 receptors. *Proc.Natl.Acad.Sci.U.S.A*, 99, 11790–11795.
30. Viola,A. & Lanzavecchia,A. (1996) T cell activation determined by T cell receptor number and tunable thresholds. *Science*, 273, 104–106.
31. Waterhouse,P., Penninger,J.M., Timms,E., Wakeham,A., Shahinian,A., Lee,K.P., Thompson,C.B., Griesser,H., & Mak,T.W. (1995) Lymphoproliferative disorders with early lethality in mice deficient in Ctla-4. *Science*, 270, 985–988.
32. Tivol,E.A., Borriello,F., Schweitzer,A.N., Lynch,W.P., Bluestone,J.A., & Sharpe,A.H. (1995) Loss of CTLA-4 leads to massive lymphoproliferation and fatal multiorgan tissue destruction, revealing a critical negative regulatory role of CTLA-4. *Immunity.*, 3, 541–547.
33. Chambers,C.A., Sullivan,T.J., & Allison,J.P. (1997) Lymphoproliferation in CTLA-4-deficient mice is mediated by costimulation-dependent activation of CD4+ T cells. *Immunity.*, 7, 885–895.

34. Blair,P.J., Riley,J.L., Levine,B.L., Lee,K.P., Craighead,N., Francomano,T., Perfetto,S.J., Gray,G.S., Carreno,B.M., & June,C.H. (1998) CTLA-4 ligation delivers a unique signal to resting human CD4 T cells that inhibits interleukin-2 secretion but allows Bcl-X(L) induction. *J.Immunol.*, 160, 12–15.
35. Brunner,M.C., Chambers,C.A., Chan,F.K., Hanke,J., Winoto,A., & Allison,J.P. (1999) CTLA-4-Mediated inhibition of early events of T cell proliferation. *J.Immunol.*, 162, 5813–5820.
36. Egen,J.G. & Allison,J.P. (2002) Cytotoxic T lymphocyte antigen-4 accumulation in the immunological synapse is regulated by TCR signal strength. *Immunity.*, 16, 23–35.
37. Shiratori,T., Miyatake,S., Ohno,H., Nakaseko,C., Isono,K., Bonifacino,J.S., & Saito,T. (1997) Tyrosine phosphorylation controls internalization of CTLA-4 by regulating its interaction with clathrin-associated adaptor complex AP-2. *Immunity.*, 6, 583–589.
38. van der Merwe,P.A. & Davis,S.J. (2003) Molecular interactions mediating T cell antigen recognition. *Annu.Rev.Immunol.*, 21, 659–684.
39. Stamper,C.C., Zhang,Y., Tobin,J.F., Erbe,D.V., Ikemizu,S., Davis,S.J., Stahl,M.L., Seehra,J., Somers,W.S., & Mosyak,L. (2001) Crystal structure of the B7–1/CTLA-4 complex that inhibits human immune responses. *Nature*, 410, 608–611.
40. Greene,J.L., Leytze,G.M., Emswiler,J., Peach,R., Bajorath,J., Cosand,W., & Linsley,P.S. (1996) Covalent dimerization of CD28/CTLA-4 and oligomerization of CD80/CD86 regulate T cell costimulatory interactions. *J.Biol.Chem.*, 271, 26762–26771.
41. Nakaseko,C., Miyatake,S., Iida,T., Hara,S., Abe,R., Ohno,H., Saito,Y., & Saito,T. (1999) Cytotoxic T lymphocyte antigen 4 (CTLA-4) engagement delivers an inhibitory signal through the membrane-proximal region in the absence of the tyrosine motif in the cytoplasmic tail. *J.Exp.Med.*, 190, 765–774.
42. Carreno,B.M., Bennett,F., Chau,T.A., Ling,V., Luxenberg,D., Jussif,J., Baroja,M.L., & Madrenas,J. (2000) CTLA-4 (CD152) can inhibit T cell activation by two different mechanisms depending on its level of cell surface expression. *J.Immunol.*, 165, 1352–1356.
43. Masteller,E.L., Chuang,E., Mullen,A.C., Reiner,S.L., & Thompson,C.B. (2000) Structural analysis of CTLA-4 function in vivo. *J.Immunol.*, 164, 5319–5327.
44. Chikuma,S., Abbas,A.K., & Bluestone,J.A. (2005) B7-independent inhibition of T cells by CTLA-4. *J.Immunol.*, 175, 177–181.
45. Takahashi,S., Kataoka,H., Hara,S., Yokosuka,T., Takase,K., Yamasaki,S., Kobayashi,W., Saito,Y., & Saito,T. (2005) In vivo overexpression of CTLA-4 suppresses lymphoproliferative diseases and thymic negative selection. *Eur.J.Immunol.*, 35, 399–407.
46. Vijayakrishnan,L., Slavik,J.M., Illes,Z., Greenwald,R.J., Rainbow,D., Greve,B., Peterson,L.B., Hafler,D.A., Freeman,G.J., Sharpe,A.H., Wicker,L.S., & Kuchroo,V.K. (2004) An autoimmune disease-associated CTLA-4 splice variant lacking the B7 binding domain signals negatively in T cells. *Immunity.*, 20, 563–575.
47. Chambers,C.A., Sullivan,T.J., Truong,T., & Allison,J.P. (1998) Secondary but not primary T cell responses are enhanced in CTLA-4-deficient CD8+ T cells. *Eur.J.Immunol.*, 28, 3137–3143.
48. Chambers,C.A., Kuhns,M.S., & Allison,J.P. (1999) Cytotoxic T lymphocyte antigen-4 (CTLA-4) regulates primary and secondary peptide-specific CD4(+) T cell responses. *Proc.Natl.Acad.Sci.U.S.A*, 96, 8603–8608.
49. Luhder,F., Chambers,C., Allison,J.P., Benoist,C., & Mathis,D. (2000) Pinpointing when T cell costimulatory receptor CTLA-4 must be engaged to dampen diabetogenic T cells. *Proc.Natl.Acad.Sci.U.S.A*, 97, 12204–12209.
50. Greenwald,R.J., Boussiotis,V.A., Lorsbach,R.B., Abbas,A.K., & Sharpe,A.H. (2001) CTLA-4 regulates induction of anergy in vivo. *Immunity.*, 14, 145–155.
51. Probst,H.C., McCoy,K., Okazaki,T., Honjo,T., & van den,B.M. (2005) Resting dendritic cells induce peripheral CD8+ T cell tolerance through PD-1 and CTLA-4. *Nat.Immunol.*, 6, 280–286.
52. Leach,D.R., Krummel,M.F., & Allison,J.P. (1996) Enhancement of antitumor immunity by CTLA-4 blockade. *Science*, 271, 1734–1736.
53. Yang,Y.F., Zou,J.P., Mu,J., Wijesuriya,R., Ono,S., Walunas,T., Bluestone,J., Fujiwara,H., & Hamaoka,T. (1997) Enhanced induction of antitumor T-cell responses by cytotoxic T lymphocyte-

associated molecule-4 blockade: the effect is manifested only at the restricted tumor-bearing stages. *Cancer Res.*, 57, 4036–4041.

54. Kwon,E.D., Hurwitz,A.A., Foster,B.A., Madias,C., Feldhaus,A.L., Greenberg,N.M., Burg,M.B., & Allison,J.P. (1997) Manipulation of T cell costimulatory and inhibitory signals for immunotherapy of prostate cancer. *Proc.Natl.Acad.Sci.U.S.A*, 94, 8099–8103.
55. Shrikant,P., Khoruts,A., & Mescher,M.F. (1999) CTLA-4 blockade reverses CD8+ T cell tolerance to tumor by a CD4+ T cell- and IL-2-dependent mechanism. *Immunity.*, 11, 483–493.
56. Sotomayor,E.M., Borrello,I., Tubb,E., Allison,J.P., & Levitsky,H.I. (1999) In vivo blockade of CTLA-4 enhances the priming of responsive T cells but fails to prevent the induction of tumor antigen-specific tolerance. *Proc.Natl.Acad.Sci.U.S.A*, 96, 11476–11481.
57. van Elsas,A., Hurwitz,A.A., & Allison,J.P. (1999) Combination immunotherapy of B16 melanoma using anti-cytotoxic T lymphocyte-associated antigen 4 (CTLA-4) and granulocyte/macrophage colony-stimulating factor (GM-CSF)-producing vaccines induces rejection of subcutaneous and metastatic tumors accompanied by autoimmune depigmentation. *J.Exp.Med.*, 190, 355–366.
58. Hurwitz,A.A., Yu,T.F., Leach,D.R., & Allison,J.P. (1998) CTLA-4 blockade synergizes with tumor-derived granulocyte-macrophage colony-stimulating factor for treatment of an experimental mammary carcinoma. *Proc.Natl.Acad.Sci.U.S.A*, 95, 10067–10071.
59. Hurwitz,A.A., Foster,B.A., Kwon,E.D., Truong,T., Choi,E.M., Greenberg,N.M., Burg,M.B., & Allison,J.P. (2000) Combination immunotherapy of primary prostate cancer in a transgenic mouse model using CTLA-4 blockade. *Cancer Res.*, 60, 2444–2448.
60. Gregor,P.D., Wolchok,J.D., Ferrone,C.R., Buchinshky,H., Guevara-Patino,J.A., Perales,M.A., Mortazavi,F., Bacich,D., Heston,W., Latouche,J.B., Sadelain,M., Allison,J.P., Scher,H.I., & Houghton,A.N. (2004) CTLA-4 blockade in combination with xenogeneic DNA vaccines enhances T-cell responses, tumor immunity and autoimmunity to self antigens in animal and cellular model systems. *Vaccine*, 22, 1700–1708.
61. Demaria,S., Kawashima,N., Yang,A.M., Devitt,M.L., Babb,J.S., Allison,J.P., & Formenti,S.C. (2005) Immune-mediated inhibition of metastases after treatment with local radiation and CTLA-4 blockade in a mouse model of breast cancer. *Clin.Cancer Res.*, 11, 728–734.
62. Mokyr,M.B., Kalinichenko,T., Gorelik,L., & Bluestone,J.A. (1998) Realization of the therapeutic potential of CTLA-4 blockade in low-dose chemotherapy-treated tumor-bearing mice. *Cancer Res.*, 58, 5301–5304.
63. Davila,E., Kennedy,R., & Celis,E. (2003) Generation of antitumor immunity by cytotoxic T lymphocyte epitope peptide vaccination, CpG-oligodeoxynucleotide adjuvant, and CTLA-4 blockade. *Cancer Res.*, 63, 3281–3288.
64. Ko,K., Yamazaki,S., Nakamura,K., Nishioka,T., Hirota,K., Yamaguchi,T., Shimizu,J., Nomura,T., Chiba,T., & Sakaguchi,S. (2005) Treatment of advanced tumors with agonistic anti-GITR mAb and its effects on tumor-infiltrating Foxp3+CD25+CD4+ regulatory T cells. *J.Exp.Med.*, 202, 885–891.
65. Sutmuller,R.P., van Duivenvoorde,L.M., van Elsas,A., Schumacher,T.N., Wildenberg,M.E., Allison,J.P., Toes,R.E., Offringa,R., & Melief,C.J. (2001) Synergism of cytotoxic T lymphocyte-associated antigen 4 blockade and depletion of CD25(+) regulatory T cells in antitumor therapy reveals alternative pathways for suppression of autoreactive cytotoxic T lymphocyte responses. *J.Exp.Med.*, 194, 823–832.
66. Woo,E.Y., Chu,C.S., Goletz,T.J., Schlienger,K., Yeh,H., Coukos,G., Rubin,S.C., Kaiser,L.R., & June,C.H. (2001) Regulatory CD4(+)CD25(+) T cells in tumors from patients with early-stage non-small cell lung cancer and late-stage ovarian cancer. *Cancer Res.*, 61, 4766–4772.
67. Woo,E.Y., Yeh,H., Chu,C.S., Schlienger,K., Carroll,R.G., Riley,J.L., Kaiser,L.R., & June,C.H. (2002) Cutting edge: Regulatory T cells from lung cancer patients directly inhibit autologous T cell proliferation. *J.Immunol.*, 168, 4272–4276.
68. Liyanage,U.K., Moore,T.T., Joo,H.G., Tanaka,Y., Herrmann,V., Doherty,G., Drebin,J.A., Strasberg,S.M., Eberlein,T.J., Goedegebuure,P.S., & Linehan,D.C. (2002) Prevalence of regulatory T cells is increased in peripheral blood and tumor microenvironment of patients with pancreas or breast adenocarcinoma. *J.Immunol.*, 169, 2756–2761.

69. Curiel,T.J., Coukos,G., Zou,L., Alvarez,X., Cheng,P., Mottram,P., Evdemon-Hogan,M., Conejo-Garcia,J.R., Zhang,L., Burow,M., Zhu,Y., Wei,S., Kryczek,I., Daniel,B., Gordon,A., Myers,L., Lackner,A., Disis,M.L., Knutson,K.L., Chen,L., & Zou,W. (2004) Specific recruitment of regulatory T cells in ovarian carcinoma fosters immune privilege and predicts reduced survival. *Nat.Med.*, 10, 942–949.
70. Viguier,M., Lemaitre,F., Verola,O., Cho,M.S., Gorochov,G., Dubertret,L., Bachelez,H., Kourilsky,P., & Ferradini,L. (2004) Foxp3 expressing CD4+CD25(high) regulatory T cells are overrepresented in human metastatic melanoma lymph nodes and inhibit the function of infiltrating T cells. *J.Immunol.*, 173, 1444–1453.
71. Groux,H., O'Garra,A., Bigler,M., Rouleau,M., Antonenko,S., de Vries,J.E., & Roncarolo,M.G. (1997) A CD4+ T-cell subset inhibits antigen-specific T-cell responses and prevents colitis. *Nature*, 389, 737–742.
72. Levings,M.K., Sangregorio,R., Galbiati,F., Squadrone,S., de Waal,M.R., & Roncarolo,M.G. (2001a) IFN-alpha and IL-10 induce the differentiation of human type 1 T regulatory cells. *J.Immunol.*, 166, 5530–5539.
73. Weiner,H.L. (2001) Induction and mechanism of action of transforming growth factor-beta-secreting Th3 regulatory cells. *Immunol.Rev.*, 182, 207–214.
74. Walker,M.R., Kasprowicz,D.J., Gersuk,V.H., Benard,A., Van Landeghen,M., Buckner,J.H., & Ziegler,S.F. (2003) Induction of FoxP3 and acquisition of T regulatory activity by stimulated human CD4+. *J.Clin.Invest*, 112, 1437–1443.
75. Chen,W., Jin,W., Hardegen,N., Lei,K.J., Li,L., Marinos,N., McGrady,G., & Wahl,S.M. (2003) Conversion of peripheral CD4+CD25- naive T cells to CD4+CD25+ regulatory T cells by TGF-beta induction of transcription factor Foxp3. *J.Exp.Med.*, 198, 1875–1886.
76. Apostolou,I. & von Boehmer,H. (2004) In vivo instruction of suppressor commitment in naive T cells. *J.Exp.Med.*, 199, 1401–1408.
77. Kretschmer,K., Apostolou,I., Hawiger,D., Khazaie,K., Nussenzweig,M.C., & von Boehmer,H. (2005) Inducing and expanding regulatory T cell populations by foreign antigen. *Nat.Immunol.*, 6, 1219–1227.
78. Curotto de Lafaille,M.A., Lino,A.C., Kutchukhidze,N., & Lafaille,J.J. (2004) CD25- T cells generate CD25+Foxp3+ regulatory T cells by peripheral expansion. *J.Immunol.*, 173, 7259–7268.
79. Zhou,G., Drake,C.G., & Levitsky,H.I. (2005) Amplification of tumor-specific regulatory T cells following therapeutic cancer vaccines. *Blood.*
80. Gilliet,M. & Liu,Y.J. (2002) Generation of human CD8 T regulatory cells by CD40 ligand-activated plasmacytoid dendritic cells. *J.Exp.Med.*, 195, 695–704.
81. Zheng,S.G., Wang,J.H., Koss,M.N., Quismorio,F., Jr., Gray,J.D., & Horwitz,D.A. (2004) CD4+ and CD8+ regulatory T cells generated ex vivo with IL-2 and TGF-beta suppress a stimulatory graft-versus-host disease with a lupus-like syndrome. *J.Immunol.*, 172, 1531–1539.
82. Chang,C.C., Ciubotariu,R., Manavalan,J.S., Yuan,J., Colovai,A.I., Piazza,F., Lederman,S., Colonna,M., Cortesini,R., Dalla-Favera,R., & Suciu-Foca,N. (2002) Tolerization of dendritic cells by T(S) cells: the crucial role of inhibitory receptors ILT3 and ILT4. *Nat.Immunol.*, 3, 237–243.
83. Noble,A., Giorgini,A., & Leggat,J.A. (2006) Cytokine-induced IL-10-secreting CD8 T cells represent a phenotypically distinct suppressor T-cell lineage. *Blood*, 107, 4475–4483.
84. Shimizu,J., Yamazaki,S., & Sakaguchi,S. (1999) Induction of tumor immunity by removing CD25+CD4+ T cells: a common basis between tumor immunity and autoimmunity. *J.Immunol.*, 163, 5211–5218.
85. Marshall,N.A., Christie,L.E., Munro,L.R., Culligan,D.J., Johnston,P.W., Barker,R.N., & Vickers,M.A. (2004) Immunosuppressive regulatory T cells are abundant in the reactive lymphocytes of Hodgkin lymphoma. *Blood*, 103, 1755–1762.
86. Alvaro,T., Lejeune,M., Salvado,M.T., Bosch,R., Garcia,J.F., Jaen,J., Banham,A.H., Roncador,G., Montalban,C., & Piris,M.A. (2005) Outcome in Hodgkin's lymphoma can be predicted from the presence of accompanying cytotoxic and regulatory T cells. *Clin.Cancer Res.*, 11, 1467–1473.
87. Dave,S.S., Wright,G., Tan,B., Rosenwald,A., Gascoyne,R.D., Chan,W.C., Fisher,R.I., Braziel,R.M., Rimsza,L.M., Grogan,T.M., Miller,T.P., LeBlanc,M., Greiner,T.C., Weisenburger,D.D.,

Lynch,J.C., Vose,J., Armitage,J.O., Smeland,E.B., Kvaloy,S., Holte,H., Delabie,J., Connors,J.M., Lansdorp,P.M., Ouyang,Q., Lister,T.A., Davies,A.J., Norton,A.J., Muller-Hermelink,H.K., Ott,G., Campo,E., Montserrat,E., Wilson,W.H., Jaffe,E.S., Simon,R., Yang,L., Powell,J., Zhao,H., Goldschmidt,N., Chiorazzi,M., & Staudt,L.M. (2004) Prediction of survival in follicular lymphoma based on molecular features of tumor-infiltrating immune cells. *N.Engl.J.Med.*, 351, 2159–2169.

88. Furtado,G.C., Curotto de Lafaille,M.A., Kutchukhidze,N., & Lafaille,J.J. (2002) Interleukin 2 signaling is required for CD4(+) regulatory T cell function. *J.Exp.Med.*, 196, 851–857.
89. Almeida,A.R., Legrand,N., Papiernik,M., & Freitas,A.A. (2002) Homeostasis of peripheral CD4+ T cells: IL-2R alpha and IL-2 shape a population of regulatory cells that controls CD4+ T cell numbers. *J.Immunol.*, 169, 4850–4860.
90. Malek,T.R. & Bayer,A.L. (2004) Tolerance, not immunity, crucially depends on IL-2. *Nat.Rev.Immunol.*, 4, 665–674.
91. Zhang,H., Chua,K.S., Guimond,M., Kapoor,V., Brown,M.V., Fleisher,T.A., Long,L.M., Bernstein,D., Hill,B.J., Douek,D.C., Berzofsky,J.A., Carter,C.S., Read,E.J., Helman,L.J., & Mackall,C.L. (2005) Lymphopenia and interleukin-2 therapy alter homeostasis of CD4+CD25+ regulatory T cells. *Nat.Med.*, 11, 1238–1243.
92. Ahmadzadeh,M. & Rosenberg,S.A. (2006) IL-2 administration increases CD4+ CD25(hi) Foxp3+ regulatory T cells in cancer patients. *Blood*, 107, 2409–2414.
93. Zou,W. (2006) Regulatory T cells, tumour immunity and immunotherapy. *Nat.Rev.Immunol.*, 6, 295–307.
94. Zhou,G., Drake,C.G., & Levitsky,H.I. (2006) Amplification of tumor-specific regulatory T cells following therapeutic cancer vaccines. *Blood*, 107, 628–636.
95. Yamazaki,S., Iyoda,T., Tarbell,K., Olson,K., Velinzon,K., Inaba,K., & Steinman,R.M. (2003) Direct expansion of functional CD25+ CD4+ regulatory T cells by antigen-processing dendritic cells. *J.Exp.Med.*, 198, 235–247.
96. Thornton,A.M. & Shevach,E.M. (2000) Suppressor effector function of CD4+CD25+ immunoregulatory T cells is antigen nonspecific. *J.Immunol.*, 164, 183–190.
97. Piccirillo,C.A., Letterio,J.J., Thornton,A.M., McHugh,R.S., Mamura,M., Mizuhara,H., & Shevach,E.M. (2002) CD4(+)CD25(+) regulatory T cells can mediate suppressor function in the absence of transforming growth factor beta1 production and responsiveness. *J.Exp.Med.*, 196, 237–246.
98. Stephens,L.A., Mottet,C., Mason,D., & Powrie,F. (2001) Human CD4(+)CD25(+) thymocytes and peripheral T cells have immune suppressive activity in vitro. *Eur.J.Immunol.*, 31, 1247–1254.
99. Asseman,C., Mauze,S., Leach,M.W., Coffman,R.L., & Powrie,F. (1999) An essential role for interleukin 10 in the function of regulatory T cells that inhibit intestinal inflammation. *J.Exp.Med.*, 190, 995–1004.
100. Suri-Payer,E. & Cantor,H. (2001) Differential cytokine requirements for regulation of autoimmune gastritis and colitis by CD4(+)CD25(+) T cells. *J.Autoimmun.*, 16, 115–123.
101. Chen,M.L., Pittet,M.J., Gorelik,L., Flavell,R.A., Weissleder,R., von Boehmer,H., & Khazaie,K. (2005) Regulatory T cells suppress tumor-specific CD8 T cell cytotoxicity through TGF-beta signals in vivo. *Proc.Natl.Acad.Sci.U.S.A*, 102, 419–424.
102. Green,E.A., Gorelik,L., McGregor,C.M., Tran,E.H., & Flavell,R.A. (2003) CD4+CD25+ T regulatory cells control anti-islet CD8+ T cells through TGF-beta-TGF-beta receptor interactions in type 1 diabetes. *Proc.Natl.Acad.Sci.U.S.A*, 100, 10878–10883.
103. Fahlen,L., Read,S., Gorelik,L., Hurst,S.D., Coffman,R.L., Flavell,R.A., & Powrie,F. (2005) T cells that cannot respond to TGF-{beta} escape control by CD4+CD25+ regulatory T cells. *J.Exp.Med.*, 201, 737–746.
104. Read,S., Malmstrom,V., & Powrie,F. (2000) Cytotoxic T lymphocyte-associated antigen 4 plays an essential role in the function of CD25(+)CD4(+) regulatory cells that control intestinal inflammation. *J.Exp.Med.*, 192, 295–302.
105. Takahashi,T., Tagami,T., Yamazaki,S., Uede,T., Shimizu,J., Sakaguchi,N., Mak,T.W., & Sakaguchi,S. (2000) Immunologic self-tolerance maintained by CD25(+)CD4(+) regulatory T cells constitutively expressing cytotoxic T lymphocyte-associated antigen 4. *J.Exp.Med.*, 192, 303–310.

106. Bachmann,M.F., Kohler,G., Ecabert,B., Mak,T.W., & Kopf,M. (1999) Cutting edge: lymphoproliferative disease in the absence of CTLA-4 is not T cell autonomous. *J.Immunol.*, 163, 1128–1131.
107. Kataoka,H., Takahashi,S., Takase,K., Yamasaki,S., Yokosuka,T., Koike,T., & Saito,T. (2005) CD25(+)CD4(+) regulatory T cells exert in vitro suppressive activity independent of CTLA-4. *Int.Immunol.*, 17, 421–427.
108. Tang,Q., Boden,E.K., Henriksen,K.J., Bour-Jordan,H., Bi,M., & Bluestone,J.A. (2004) Distinct roles of CTLA-4 and TGF-beta in CD4+CD25+ regulatory T cell function. *Eur.J.Immunol.*, 34, 2996–3005.
109. Quezada,S.A., Peggs,K.S., Curran,M.A., & Allison,J.P. (2006) CTLA4 blockade and GM-CSF combination immunotherapy alters the intratumor balance of effector and regulatory T cells. *J.Clin.Invest*, 116, 1935–1945.
109. Thornton,A.M. & Shevach,E.M. (1998) CD4+CD25+ immunoregulatory T cells suppress polyclonal T cell activation in vitro by inhibiting interleukin 2 production. *J.Exp.Med.*, 188, 287–296.
110. Chai,J.G., Tsang,J.Y., Lechler,R., Simpson,E., Dyson,J., & Scott,D. (2002) CD4+CD25+ T cells as immunoregulatory T cells in vitro. *Eur.J.Immunol.*, 32, 2365–2375.
111. Levings,M.K., Sangregorio,R., & Roncarolo,M.G. (2001b) Human cd25(+)cd4(+) t regulatory cells suppress naive and memory T cell proliferation and can be expanded in vitro without loss of function. *J.Exp.Med.*, 193, 1295–1302.
112. Annunziato,F., Cosmi,L., Liotta,F., Lazzeri,E., Manetti,R., Vanini,V., Romagnani,P., Maggi,E., & Romagnani,S. (2002) Phenotype, localization, and mechanism of suppression of CD4(+)CD25(+) human thymocytes. *J.Exp.Med.*, 196, 379–387.
113. Paust,S., Lu,L., McCarty,N., & Cantor,H. (2004) Engagement of B7 on effector T cells by regulatory T cells prevents autoimmune disease. *Proc.Natl.Acad.Sci.U.S.A*, 101, 10398–10403.
114. Taylor,P.A., Lees,C.J., Fournier,S., Allison,J.P., Sharpe,A.H., & Blazar,B.R. (2004) B7 expression on T cells down-regulates immune responses through CTLA-4 ligation via T-T interactions [corrections]. *J.Immunol.*, 172, 34–39.
115. Shevach,E.M. (2002) CD4+ CD25+ suppressor T cells: more questions than answers. *Nat.Rev.Immunol.*, 2, 389–400.
116. Malek,T.R., Yu,A., Vincek,V., Scibelli,P., & Kong,L. (2002) CD4 regulatory T cells prevent lethal autoimmunity in IL-2Rbeta-deficient mice. Implications for the nonredundant function of IL-2. *Immunity.*, 17, 167–178.
117. Onizuka,S., Tawara,I., Shimizu,J., Sakaguchi,S., Fujita,T., & Nakayama,E. (1999) Tumor rejection by in vivo administration of anti-CD25 (interleukin-2 receptor alpha) monoclonal antibody. *Cancer Res.*, 59, 3128–3133.
118. Steitz,J., Bruck,J., Lenz,J., Knop,J., & Tuting,T. (2001) Depletion of CD25(+) CD4(+) T cells and treatment with tyrosinase-related protein 2-transduced dendritic cells enhance the interferon alpha-induced, CD8(+) T-cell-dependent immune defense of B16 melanoma. *Cancer Res.*, 61, 8643–8646.
119. Nagai,H., Horikawa,T., Hara,I., Fukunaga,A., Oniki,S., Oka,M., Nishigori,C., & Ichihashi,M. (2004) In vivo elimination of CD25+ regulatory T cells leads to tumor rejection of B16F10 melanoma, when combined with interleukin-12 gene transfer. *Exp.Dermatol.*, 13, 613–620.
120. Prasad,S.J., Farrand,K.J., Matthews,S.A., Chang,J.H., McHugh,R.S., & Ronchese,F. (2005) Dendritic cells loaded with stressed tumor cells elicit long-lasting protective tumor immunity in mice depleted of CD4+CD25+ regulatory T cells. *J.Immunol.*, 174, 90–98.
121. Dannull,J., Su,Z., Rizzieri,D., Yang,B.K., Coleman,D., Yancey,D., Zhang,A., Dahm,P., Chao,N., Gilboa,E., & Vieweg,J. (2005) Enhancement of vaccine-mediated antitumor immunity in cancer patients after depletion of regulatory T cells. *J.Clin.Invest*, 115, 3623–3633.
122. Barnett,B., Kryczek,I., Cheng,P., Zou,W., & Curiel,T.J. (2005) Regulatory T cells in ovarian cancer: biology and therapeutic potential. *Am.J.Reprod.Immunol.*, 54, 369–377.
123. Antony,P.A., Piccirillo,C.A., Akpinarli,A., Finkelstein,S.E., Speiss,P.J., Surman,D.R., Palmer,D.C., Chan,C.C., Klebanoff,C.A., Overwijk,W.W., Rosenberg,S.A., & Restifo,N.P. (2005) CD8+ T cell immunity against a tumor/self-antigen is augmented by CD4+ T helper cells and hindered by naturally occurring T regulatory cells. *J.Immunol.*, 174, 2591–2601.

124. Gattinoni,L., Powell,D.J., Jr., Rosenberg,S.A., & Restifo,N.P. (2006) Adoptive immunotherapy for cancer: building on success. *Nat.Rev.Immunol.*, 6, 383–393.
125. Turk,M.J., Guevara-Patino,J.A., Rizzuto,G.A., Engelhorn,M.E., Sakaguchi,S., & Houghton,A.N. (2004) Concomitant tumor immunity to a poorly immunogenic melanoma is prevented by regulatory T cells. *J.Exp.Med.*, 200, 771–782.
126. Cohen,A.D., Diab,A., Perales,M.A., Wolchok,J.D., Rizzuto,G., Merghoub,T., Huggins,D., Liu,C., Turk,M.J., Restifo,N.P., Sakaguchi,S., & Houghton,A.N. (2006) Agonist anti-GITR antibody enhances vaccine-induced CD8(+) T-cell responses and tumor immunity. *Cancer Res.*, 66, 4904–4912.
127. Sugamura,K., Ishii,N., & Weinberg,A.D. (2004) Therapeutic targeting of the effector T-cell co-stimulatory molecule OX40. *Nat.Rev.Immunol.*, 4, 420–431.
128. Shimizu,J., Yamazaki,S., Takahashi,T., Ishida,Y., & Sakaguchi,S. (2002) Stimulation of CD25(+)CD4(+) regulatory T cells through GITR breaks immunological self-tolerance. *Nat.Immunol.*, 3, 135–142.
129. Valzasina,B., Guiducci,C., Dislich,H., Killeen,N., Weinberg,A.D., & Colombo,M.P. (2005) Triggering of OX40 (CD134) on CD4(+)CD25+ T cells blocks their inhibitory activity: a novel regulatory role for OX40 and its comparison with GITR. *Blood*, 105, 2845–2851.
130. Stephens,G.L., McHugh,R.S., Whitters,M.J., Young,D.A., Luxenberg,D., Carreno,B.M., Collins,M., & Shevach,E.M. (2004) Engagement of glucocorticoid-induced TNFR family-related receptor on effector T cells by its ligand mediates resistance to suppression by CD4+CD25+ T cells. *J.Immunol.*, 173, 5008–5020.
131. Hodi,F.S. & Dranoff,G. (2006) Combinatorial cancer immunotherapy. *Adv.Immunol.*, 90, 341–368.
132. Phan,G.Q., Yang,J.C., Sherry,R.M., Hwu,P., Topalian,S.L., Schwartzentruber,D.J., Restifo,N.P., Haworth,L.R., Seipp,C.A., Freezer,L.J., Morton,K.E., Mavroukakis,S.A., Duray,P.H., Steinberg,S.M., Allison,J.P., Davis,T.A., & Rosenberg,S.A. (2003) Cancer regression and autoimmunity induced by cytotoxic T lymphocyte-associated antigen 4 blockade in patients with metastatic melanoma. *Proc.Natl.Acad.Sci.U.S.A*, 100, 8372–8377.
133. Hodi,F.S., Mihm,M.C., Soiffer,R.J., Haluska,F.G., Butler,M., Seiden,M.V., Davis,T., Henry-Spires,R., MacRae,S., Willman,A., Padera,R., Jaklitsch,M.T., Shankar,S., Chen,T.C., Korman,A., Allison,J.P., & Dranoff,G. (2003) Biologic activity of cytotoxic T lymphocyte-associated antigen 4 antibody blockade in previously vaccinated metastatic melanoma and ovarian carcinoma patients. *Proc.Natl.Acad.Sci.U.S.A*, 100, 4712–4717.
134. Attia,P., Phan,G.Q., Maker,A.V., Robinson,M.R., Quezado,M.M., Yang,J.C., Sherry,R.M., Topalian,S.L., Kammula,U.S., Royal,R.E., Restifo,N.P., Haworth,L.R., Levy,C., Mavroukakis,S.A., Nichol,G., Yellin,M.J., & Rosenberg,S.A. (2005) Autoimmunity correlates with tumor regression in patients with metastatic melanoma treated with anti-cytotoxic T-lymphocyte antigen-4. *J.Clin.Oncol.*, 23, 6043–6053.
135. Sanderson,K., Scotland,R., Lee,P., Liu,D., Groshen,S., Snively,J., Sian,S., Nichol,G., Davis,T., Keler,T., Yellin,M., & Weber,J. (2005) Autoimmunity in a phase I trial of a fully human anti-cytotoxic T-lymphocyte antigen-4 monoclonal antibody with multiple melanoma peptides and Montanide ISA 51 for patients with resected stages III and IV melanoma. *J.Clin.Oncol.*, 23, 741–750.
136. Ribas,A., Camacho,L.H., Lopez-Berestein,G., Pavlov,D., Bulanhagui,C.A., Millham,R., Comin-Anduix,B., Reuben,J.M., Seja,E., Parker,C.A., Sharma,A., Glaspy,J.A., & Gomez-Navarro,J. (2005) Antitumor activity in melanoma and anti-self responses in a phase I trial with the anti-cytotoxic T lymphocyte-associated antigen 4 monoclonal antibody CP-675,206. *J.Clin.Oncol.*, 23, 8968–8977.
137. Beck,K.E., Blansfield,J.A., Tran,K.Q., Feldman,A.L., Hughes,M.S., Royal,R.E., Kammula,U.S., Topalian,S.L., Sherry,R.M., Kleiner,D., Quezado,M., Lowy,I., Yellin,M., Rosenberg,S.A., & Yang,J.C. (2006) Enterocolitis in patients with cancer after antibody blockade of cytotoxic T-lymphocyte-associated antigen 4. *J.Clin.Oncol.*, 24, 2283–2289.
138. Peggs,K.S., Quezada,S.A., Korman,A.J., & Allison,J.P. (2006) Principles and use of anti-CTLA4 antibody in human cancer immunotherapy. *Curr.Opin.Immunol.*, 18, 206–213.

139. Lurquin,C., Lethe,B., De Plaen,E., Corbiere,V., Theate,I., van Baren,N., Coulie,P.G., & Boon,T. (2005) Contrasting frequencies of antitumor and anti-vaccine T cells in metastases of a melanoma patient vaccinated with a MAGE tumor antigen. *J.Exp.Med.*, 201, 249–257.
140. Maker,A.V., Phan,G.Q., Attia,P., Yang,J.C., Sherry,R.M., Topalian,S.L., Kammula,U.S., Royal,R.E., Haworth,L.R., Levy,C., Kleiner,D., Mavroukakis,S.A., Yellin,M., & Rosenberg,S.A. (2005) Tumor regression and autoimmunity in patients treated with cytotoxic T lymphocyte-associated antigen 4 blockade and interleukin 2: a phase I/II study. *Ann.Surg.Oncol.*, 12, 1005–1016.
141. . Atkins,M.B., Lotze,M.T., Dutcher,J.P., Fisher,R.I., Weiss,G., Margolin,K., Abrams,J., Sznol,M., Parkinson,D., Hawkins,M., Paradise,C., Kunkel,L., & Rosenberg,S.A. (1999) High-dose recombinant interleukin 2 therapy for patients with metastatic melanoma: analysis of 270 patients treated between 1985 and 1993. *J.Clin.Oncol.*, 17, 2105–2116.
142. Rosenberg,S.A. (2000) Interleukin-2 and the development of immunotherapy for the treatment of patients with cancer. *Cancer J.Sci.Am.*, 6 Suppl 1, S2-S7.
143. Fong,L., Kavanagh,B., Rini,B.I., Shaw,V., Weinberg,V., & Small,E.J. (2006) A phase I trial of combination immunotherapy with CTLA-4 blockade and GM-CSF in hormone-refractory prostate cancer. *Journal of Clinical Oncology, 2006 ASCO Annual Meeting Proceedings*, 24, 2508.
144. Hurwitz,A.A., Sullivan,T.J., Krummel,M.F., Sobel,R.A., & Allison,J.P. (1997) Specific blockade of CTLA-4/B7 interactions results in exacerbated clinical and histologic disease in an actively-induced model of experimental allergic encephalomyelitis. *J.Neuroimmunol.*, 73, 57–62.
145. Karandikar,N.J., Vanderlugt,C.L., Walunas,T.L., Miller,S.D., & Bluestone,J.A. (1996) CTLA-4: a negative regulator of autoimmune disease. *J.Exp.Med.*, 184, 783–788.
146. Perrin,P.J., Maldonado,J.H., Davis,T.A., June,C.H., & Racke,M.K. (1996) CTLA-4 blockade enhances clinical disease and cytokine production during experimental allergic encephalomyelitis. *J.Immunol.*, 157, 1333–1336.
147. Luhder,F., Hoglund,P., Allison,J.P., Benoist,C., & Mathis,D. (1998) Cytotoxic T lymphocyte-associated antigen 4 (CTLA-4) regulates the unfolding of autoimmune diabetes. *J.Exp.Med.*, 187, 427–432.
148. Wang,H.B., Shi,F.D., Li,H., Chambers,B.J., Link,H., & Ljunggren,H.G. (2001) Anti-CTLA-4 antibody treatment triggers determinant spreading and enhances murine myasthenia gravis. *J.Immunol.*, 166, 6430–6436.
149. Keler,T., Halk,E., Vitale,L., O'Neill,T., Blanset,D., Lee,S., Srinivasan,M., Graziano,R.F., Davis,T., Lonberg,N., & Korman,A. (2003) Activity and safety of CTLA-4 blockade combined with vaccines in cynomolgus macaques. *J.Immunol.*, 171, 6251–6259.
150. Korman,A., Yellin,M., & Keler,T. (2005) Tumor immunotherapy: preclinical and clinical activity of anti-CTLA4 antibodies. *Curr.Opin.Investig.Drugs*, 6, 582–591.
151. Robinson,M.R., Chan,C.C., Yang,J.C., Rubin,B.I., Gracia,G.J., Sen,H.N., Csaky,K.G., & Rosenberg,S.A. (2004) Cytotoxic T lymphocyte-associated antigen 4 blockade in patients with metastatic melanoma: a new cause of uveitis. *J.Immunother.*, 27, 478–479.
152. Blansfield,J.A., Beck,K.E., Tran,K., Yang,J.C., Hughes,M.S., Kammula,U.S., Royal,R.E., Topalian,S.L., Haworth,L.R., Levy,C., Rosenberg,S.A., & Sherry,R.M. (2005) Cytotoxic T-lymphocyte-associated antigen-4 blockage can induce autoimmune hypophysitis in patients with metastatic melanoma and renal cancer. *J.Immunother.*, 28, 593–598.
153. Dong,H., Strome,S.E., Salomao,D.R., Tamura,H., Hirano,F., Flies,D.B., Roche,P.C., Lu,J., Zhu,G., Tamada,K., Lennon,V.A., Celis,E., & Chen,L. (2002) Tumor-associated B7-H1 promotes T-cell apoptosis: a potential mechanism of immune evasion. *Nat.Med.*, 8, 793–800.
154. Brown,J.A., Dorfman,D.M., Ma,F.R., Sullivan,E.L., Munoz,O., Wood,C.R., Greenfield,E.A., & Freeman,G.J. (2003) Blockade of programmed death-1 ligands on dendritic cells enhances T cell activation and cytokine production. *J.Immunol.*, 170, 1257–1266.
155. Ohigashi,Y., Sho,M., Yamada,Y., Tsurui,Y., Hamada,K., Ikeda,N., Mizuno,T., Yoriki,R., Kashizuka,H., Yane,K., Tsushima,F., Otsuki,N., Yagita,H., Azuma,M., & Nakajima,Y. (2005) Clinical significance of programmed death-1 ligand-1 and programmed death-1 ligand-2 expression in human esophageal cancer. *Clin.Cancer Res.*, 11, 2947–2953.

156. Rosenwald,A., Wright,G., Leroy,K., Yu,X., Gaulard,P., Gascoyne,R.D., Chan,W.C., Zhao,T., Haioun,C., Greiner,T.C., Weisenburger,D.D., Lynch,J.C., Vose,J., Armitage,J.O., Smeland,E.B., Kvaloy,S., Holte,H., Delabie,J., Campo,E., Montserrat,E., Lopez-Guillermo,A., Ott,G., Muller-Hermelink,H.K., Connors,J.M., Braziel,R., Grogan,T.M., Fisher,R.I., Miller,T.P., LeBlanc,M., Chiorazzi,M., Zhao,H., Yang,L., Powell,J., Wilson,W.H., Jaffe,E.S., Simon,R., Klausner,R.D., & Staudt,L.M. (2003) Molecular diagnosis of primary mediastinal B cell lymphoma identifies a clinically favorable subgroup of diffuse large B cell lymphoma related to Hodgkin lymphoma. *J.Exp.Med.*, 198, 851–862.
157. Iwai,Y., Ishida,M., Tanaka,Y., Okazaki,T., Honjo,T., & Minato,N. (2002) Involvement of PD-L1 on tumor cells in the escape from host immune system and tumor immunotherapy by PD-L1 blockade. *Proc.Natl.Acad.Sci.U.S.A*, 99, 12293–12297.
158. Strome,S.E., Dong,H., Tamura,H., Voss,S.G., Flies,D.B., Tamada,K., Salomao,D., Cheville,J., Hirano,F., Lin,W., Kasperbauer,J.L., Ballman,K.V., & Chen,L. (2003) B7-H1 blockade augments adoptive T-cell immunotherapy for squamous cell carcinoma. *Cancer Res.*, 63, 6501–6505.
159. Curiel,T.J., Wei,S., Dong,H., Alvarez,X., Cheng,P., Mottram,P., Krzysiek,R., Knutson,K.L., Daniel,B., Zimmermann,M.C., David,O., Burow,M., Gordon,A., Dhurandhar,N., Myers,L., Berggren,R., Hemminki,A., Alvarez,R.D., Emilie,D., Curiel,D.T., Chen,L., & Zou,W. (2003) Blockade of B7-H1 improves myeloid dendritic cell-mediated antitumor immunity. *Nat.Med.*, 9, 562–567.
160. Carter,L., Fouser,L.A., Jussif,J., Fitz,L., Deng,B., Wood,C.R., Collins,M., Honjo,T., Freeman,G.J., & Carreno,B.M. (2002) PD-1:PD-L inhibitory pathway affects both CD4(+) and CD8(+) T cells and is overcome by IL-2. *Eur.J.Immunol.*, 32, 634–643.
161. Liu,X., Gao,J.X., Wen,J., Yin,L., Li,O., Zuo,T., Gajewski,T.F., Fu,Y.X., Zheng,P., & Liu,Y. (2003) B7DC/PDL2 promotes tumor immunity by a PD-1-independent mechanism. *J.Exp.Med.*, 197, 1721–1730.
162. Iwai,Y., Terawaki,S., & Honjo,T. (2005) PD-1 blockade inhibits hematogenous spread of poorly immunogenic tumor cells by enhanced recruitment of effector T cells. *Int.Immunol.*, 17, 133–144.
163. Suh,W.K., Gajewska,B.U., Okada,H., Gronski,M.A., Bertram,E.M., Dawicki,W., Duncan,G.S., Bukczynski,J., Plyte,S., Elia,A., Wakeham,A., Itie,A., Chung,S., Da Costa,J., Arya,S., Horan,T., Campbell,P., Gaida,K., Ohashi,P.S., Watts,T.H., Yoshinaga,S.K., Bray,M.R., Jordana,M., & Mak,T.W. (2003) The B7 family member B7-H3 preferentially down-regulates T helper type 1-mediated immune responses. *Nat.Immunol.*, 4, 899–906.
164. Zang,X., Loke,P., Kim,J., Murphy,K., Waitz,R., & Allison,J.P. (2003) B7x: a widely expressed B7 family member that inhibits T cell activation. *Proc.Natl.Acad.Sci.U.S.A*, 100, 10388–10392.
165. Prasad,D.V., Richards,S., Mai,X.M., & Dong,C. (2003) B7S1, a novel B7 family member that negatively regulates T cell activation. *Immunity.*, 18, 863–873.
166. Sica,G.L., Choi,I.H., Zhu,G., Tamada,K., Wang,S.D., Tamura,H., Chapoval,A.I., Flies,D.B., Bajorath,J., & Chen,L. (2003) B7-H4, a molecule of the B7 family, negatively regulates T cell immunity. *Immunity.*, 18, 849–861.
167. Choi,I.H., Zhu,G., Sica,G.L., Strome,S.E., Cheville,J.C., Lau,J.S., Zhu,Y., Flies,D.B., Tamada,K., & Chen,L. (2003) Genomic organization and expression analysis of B7-H4, an immune inhibitory molecule of the B7 family. *J.Immunol.*, 171, 4650–4654.
168. Salceda,S., Tang,T., Kmet,M., Munteanu,A., Ghosh,M., Macina,R., Liu,W., Pilkington,G., & Papkoff,J. (2005) The immunomodulatory protein B7-H4 is overexpressed in breast and ovarian cancers and promotes epithelial cell transformation. *Exp.Cell Res.*, 306, 128–141.
169. Tringler,B., Zhuo,S., Pilkington,G., Torkko,K.C., Singh,M., Lucia,M.S., Heinz,D.E., Papkoff,J., & Shroyer,K.R. (2005) B7-h4 is highly expressed in ductal and lobular breast cancer. *Clin.Cancer Res.*, 11, 1842–1848.
170. Kryczek,I., Wei,S., Zou,L., Zhu,G., Mottram,P., Xu,H., Chen,L., & Zou,W. (2006a) Cutting Edge: Induction of B7-H4 on APCs through IL-10: Novel Suppressive Mode for Regulatory T Cells. *J.Immunol.*, 177, 40–44.
171. Kryczek,I., Zou,L., Rodriguez,P., Zhu,G., Wei,S., Mottram,P., Brumlik,M., Cheng,P., Curiel,T., Myers,L., Lackner,A., Alvarez,X., Ochoa,A., Chen,L., & Zou,W. (2006b) B7-H4 expression

identifies a novel suppressive macrophage population in human ovarian carcinoma. *J.Exp.Med.*, 203, 871–881.

172. Han,P., Goularte,O.D., Rufner,K., Wilkinson,B., & Kaye,J. (2004) An inhibitory Ig superfamily protein expressed by lymphocytes and APCs is also an early marker of thymocyte positive selection. *J.Immunol.*, 172, 5931–5939.
173. Hurchla,M.A., Sedy,J.R., Gavrielli,M., Drake,C.G., Murphy,T.L., & Murphy,K.M. (2005) B and T lymphocyte attenuator exhibits structural and expression polymorphisms and is highly Induced in anergic CD4+ T cells. *J.Immunol.*, 174, 3377–3385.
174. Sedy,J.R., Gavrieli,M., Potter,K.G., Hurchla,M.A., Lindsley,R.C., Hildner,K., Scheu,S., Pfeffer,K., Ware,C.F., Murphy,T.L., & Murphy,K.M. (2005) B and T lymphocyte attenuator regulates T cell activation through interaction with herpesvirus entry mediator. *Nat.Immunol.*, 6, 90–98.
175. Gri,G., Gallo,E., Di Carlo,E., Musiani,P., & Colombo,M.P. (2003) OX40 ligand-transduced tumor cell vaccine synergizes with GM-CSF and requires CD40-Apc signaling to boost the host T cell antitumor response. *J.Immunol.*, 170, 99–106.

PART 4

CLINICAL TUMOR IMMUNOTHERAPY

CHAPTER 17

GENERAL APPROACHES TO MEASURING IMMUNE RESPONSES

MARY L. DISIS[1,*] AND KEITH L. KNUTSON[2]

[1]*Center for Translational Medicine in Women's Health, Tumor Vaccine Group, University of Washington;* [2]*Department of Immunology, Mayo Clinic*

INTRODUCTION

Our understanding of the T cell immune response directed against tumors has advanced significantly over the past several years. As a result, a host of immune-based strategies for treating and preventing cancer are being tested in the clinic. The development of reproducible and quantitative methods for monitoring tumor-specific immunity has also become better defined. Assays, such as ELISPOT and MHC tetramers, that a few years ago were used only by a very few investigators, have now become standard tools for tumor immunologists. Standard quantitative methods are undergoing a reevaluation as newer approaches are developed which focus on potential functions of the induced immune response. In the future, assessment of the tumor-specific immune response will entail a combination of assays directed against both measuring the direct effect of the immune manipulation as well as methods that assess the effect of such interventions on the immune microenvironment.

QUANTITATIVE ASSAYS FOR THE MEASUREMENT OF CELLULAR IMMUNITY

The ability to enumerate T cells specific for tumors has become standard and quite reproducible. The three methods most commonly used for the quantitative

*Center for Translational Medicine in Women's Health, Tumor Vaccine Group, 815 Mercer Street, 2nd Floor, University of Washington, Seattle WA 98109, e-mail: ndisis@u.washington.edu

H.L. Kaufman and J.D. Wolchok (eds.), General Principles of Tumor Immunotherapy, 393–404.

measurement of antigen-specific T cell responses include ELISPOT, intracellular cytokine staining by flow cytometry (CFC), and MHC tetramer analysis. ELISPOT and CFC measure parameters in T cells that are potentially related to antigen-induced function. Tetramer assays enumerate all potential antigen-specific T cells based on their peptide-MHC specificity.

The detection of cytokines secreted by antigen-specific T cells has driven the development of several assays to detect tumor antigen-specific responses. Common methods are to measure either cytokine production by an enzyme-linked immunosorbent assay (ELISA) or to enumerate individual cytokine-producing T cells by enzyme-linked immunospot assay (ELISPOT) [1]. The ELISA measures cytokine production from a bulk population of cells and therefore, it does not give information about individual cells and can not be used to enumerate antigen-specific T cells. An alternative to the ELISA is the ELISPOT assay, which can be used to directly determine the frequency of antigen-specific T cells within peripheral blood samples. The basic ELISPOT assay entails six sequential steps: (1) coating a 96-well nitrocellulose-backed microtiter plate with cytokine-specific antibody; (2) blocking the plate to prevent nonspecific binding of cellular proteins; (3) incubating the cytokine-secreting T cells with stimulator cells or antigens; (4) lysing and removing the cells from the plate; (5) adding a labeled second antibody; and (6) detecting the antibody-cytokine complex. The final detection step is typically an enzyme/substrate reaction that generates a colored spot, which represents a permanent mark that can be quantitated microscopically, visually, or electronically. Each spot presumably represents a single cytokine-secreting cell. The number of spots (i.e., cytokine-secreting cells), after subtraction of non-specific spots, is divided by the number of cells placed in each well which yields the antigen-specific T cell precursor frequency. ELISPOT can detect antigen-specific T cell precursors at levels as low as 1:100,000. The assay has also been shown to reliably detect the number of antigen-specific T cells in experiments in which known quantities of antigen-specific T cells were added to bulk PBMC preparations [2] and has been shown to correlate to the CD8+ T cell precursor frequency obtained by limiting dilution analysis [3]. Originally, the predominant use of ELISPOT was to measure the CD8 T cell immune responses to HLA class I peptides, but it has been applied to tumor cells, tumor cell lysates, HLA class II peptides, and protein antigens. The majority of ELISPOT assays are conducted to measure for IFN-gamma-secreting cells, but antibody pairs are being defined that permit measuring other cytokines such as TNF-alpha, IL-4, and IL-5.

A significant advantage of the ELISPOT, when compared to assays requiring flow cytometric readout, is that the limits of detection are typically low, ranging from 1:300,000 to 1:100,000. However, an *in vitro* stimulation step is often added and may introduce artifact. Two major formats for the ELISPOT are used to evaluate precursor frequencies, the 3-day and 10-day formats. The 3-day format is useful if the precursor frequencies are high, such as with the case of viral antigens [4]. In this assay, the effector cells are stimulated with antigen and antigen-presenting cells (APC) for 24 hours followed by an overnight incubation with the secondary detection antibody. Secreted cytokine bound to the nitrocellulose plate is then detected. In contrast, the longer 10-day ELISPOT developed by McCutcheon and colleagues requires an intermediate *in vitro* sensitization step [5]. The shorter assay format has been used successfully to monitor immunologic responses to viral vaccines. For example, Smith and colleagues used it to monitor the increase in varicella-zoster virus-specific immunity in elderly individuals following booster immunizations. The precursor frequencies of varicella zoster-specific T cells are typically measured in the range of 1:20,000 to 1:2,000 [4]. We have used the 10-day format to monitor low level CD8 T cell precursor frequencies that were specific for HLA-A2 motifs contained with the tumor antigen HER-2/neu. Patients with advanced stage breast and ovarian cancer received a vaccine that consisted of three helper peptides 14–18 amino acids in length, all of which encompassed HLA-A2 binding 9-mer peptides [6]. Prior to immunization, less than 10% of patients had preexistent immunity to either the full-length helper peptides or the HLA-A2 peptides. After immunization, the 10-day IFN-gamma ELISPOT demonstrated that CTL precursors specific for the encompassed HLA-A2 peptides could be detected in greater than 60% of subjects following vaccination. The assay was taken through validation steps prior to use in the clinical trial with IFN-gamma-coated beads which revealed that the assay had a detection limit of 1:100,000 and a detection efficiency of about 93%. Preliminary assays evaluating for CTL precursors specific for the HLA-A2 influenza matrix peptide using a range of PBMC concentrations showed that the assay was linear over a PBMC range of 1.0–3.5 x 10^5 cells.

ELISPOT, like most assays that measure T cell function, has a higher variability than assays that do not directly measure a functional response. The variability of ELISPOT has been reported [7]. Lathey studied the intra-assay, inter-assay, and biological variability of ELISPOT. He analyzed the background (i.e. no antigen, low) spots, response to Candida antigen (intermediate), and PHA (high). If the spot counts were below 20, the intra-assay coefficient of variation was >30. The variability, however, decreases with increasing numbers of spots until a plateau of 200 spots is achieved, at which time the CV is 7–8. The mean CV at baseline in the absence of antigen is high at 45–50%. Lathey also observed that the inter-assay variability CVs were approximately double of the intra-assay variability CVs, suggesting the assays be done in batch rather than sequentially. The inability of the assay to reproducibly detect response at lower precursor frequencies has led to the development of strategies to improve the signal without extending the time of *in vitro* stimulation by the inclusion of IL-7 and IL-15 [8]. The addition of the cytokines to the 3-day format improved detection of antigen-specific CD4 T cells up to 2.4-fold, and antigen-specific CD8 T cells up to 7.5-fold.

Although ELISPOT has become the "comparator" assay for immunologic monitoring, the sensitivity and limits of detection of the assay vary greatly from laboratory to laboratory. Obstacles to be overcome to translate ELISPOT from a laboratory tool to a clinical grade monitoring technique include maximizing assay parameters to avoid any *in vitro* expansion step, developing the assay for use in cryopreserved cells, determining optimal antigen preparations used in analysis, and defining the reliability of the assay to perform over time in multiple clinical samples.

Despite such obstacles, T cell immunity detected by ELISPOT assay has been correlated with survival in some studies. For example, Enk and colleagues reported that MAGE-specific T cell precursor frequencies detected by ELISPOT in patients who received IFN-alpha following melanoma resection correlated with improved survival [9]. In another study, Reynolds and colleagues immunized melanoma patients with a polyvalent vaccine and quantified the MAGE3 and Melan-A/MART-1 specific IFNγ secreting T cells. Those who had demonstrated antigen-specific T cell precursors had a longer recurrence-free survival (greater than 12 months) than non-responders (3–5 months) [10]. Thus, ELISPOT may be a useful tool in the readout of cancer-specific immunotherapy clinical trials.

CFC is another cytokine-based assay that has evolved into a method that can be applied directly to the monitoring of human clinical trials of immune-based therapies. CFC has the unique advantage of providing a rapid simultaneous determination of cytokine production as well as the identification of leukocyte subsets. In addition, quantitation of cytokine production is not compromised by the presence of variable concentrations of cellular or soluble receptors. The overall approach of the assay is to stimulate the T cells with antigen, leading to the production of cytokines which are then trapped in the cell with the use of chemicals that block intracellular transit and secretion. The cytokines are stained with fluorochrome-conjugated specific antibodies following permeabilization and fixation of the cells. Several cytokine-specific antibodies are now commercially available that are conjugated to a wide variety of fluorochromes. Co-staining is performed with antibodies that detect cell surface markers or other surface molecules that demonstrate phenotype (e.g. CD4, CD8, and CD45). The cells are analyzed using flow cytometry. With the technological improvements in flow cytometers allowing for the simultaneous detection of multiple colors, exquisite phenotypic detail of the cytokine-producing cells can be obtained. A typical CFC assay uses three- or four-color staining, for example, cytokine FITC, CD69 PE, and CD4 PerCP-Cy5.5. The fourth color is reserved for an additional phenotypic marker or for use as an "exclusion channel" to reduce non-specific background. CD69, an early activation antigen, is used to ensure that the cells registered as cytokine-positive have an activated phenotype, and to allow easier clustering of small populations of responsive cells. The cytokines most frequently analyzed, because they yield the highest frequency of positive cells, are TNF-alpha, IFN-gamma, and IL-2. Cells are gated on CD4 (or CD8), and the proportion of CD69+cytokine+ cells in a resting control sample is subtracted from that in an antigen-stimulated sample to report the percent of specifically responsive cells.

A significant advantage of CFC is that it has been adapted for measurement of cytokine-producing cells from whole blood without prior processing with agents such as ficoll [11]. The CFC assay has a limit of detection at greater than 1 antigen-specific T cells in 10,000 PBMC or other (e.g. CD3, CD4 T cells). Nonspecific background staining, which is likely attributable to many potential sources, is a major shortcoming of CFC, keeping its limit of detection/quantification relatively high at >1:10,000 (antigen-specific T cells per total cell count). One source of error that has been identified is cytokine production by platelets and monocytes. Nomura and colleagues developed an exclusion gating strategy to minimize the signal contributed by monocytes and platelets. Staining with either CD33- or CD62P-specific 4th-color antibodies allowed them to filter out activated monocytes and platelets, respectively [11]. Although CFC is advantageous because it has been adapted to measuring responses after only short periods (e.g. 6–8 hrs) of *in vitro* manipulation, this could pose a limitation on its ability to accurately measure all of the antigen-specific precursors since it would be expected that there would be a broad variability in the amount of time it takes to generate an immune response. Some studies indicate that different cytokines are elevated at different times during the recall response [12]. Furthermore, there are noted differences in the time required to activate a CD4 T cell as compared to a CD8 T cell [13]. The duration of exposure to toxic uncoupling agents such as Brefeldin or Monensin is one limitation to extended *in vitro* stimulation. Efforts have been made to enhance the response to antigen. Waldrop and colleagues showed enhanced activation of antigen-specific T cells by inclusion of monoclonal antibodies to the CD28 and CD49b costimulatory molecules [14]. Nomura and colleagues reported that the intra-assay CVs for IFN-gamma and TNF-alpha were 8.4 and 4.1, respectively [11]. However, the inter-assay variability was somewhat higher for both cytokines at 23.7% and 18.4%.

Tetramers represent a direct approach to the identification and visualization of antigen-specific T cells. Tetramers are composed of four MHC class I molecules, each bound to a specific peptide of interest. The MHC molecules are held together by biotinylating each monomer followed by binding to fluorochrome-conjugated avidin. As a tetramer, the MHC class I molecules bind with greater affinity to the TCR than they would as monomers [15–16]. Recently, MHC class II tetramers have been developed to identify CD4 T cells [17]. The limit of detection of the assay has been reported to be greater than 1 CD8+ T cell per 10,000 freshly prepared peripheral blood mononuclear cells, which is consistent with limitations of flow cytometry-based methods such as CFC [15–16]. Cells are typically co-stained with fluorochrome-conjugated anti-CD8 T cells in order to enumerate only those cells that co-express both CD8 and the antigen-specific TCR. When used alone with CD8 staining, tetramers provide only information about the TCR of the CD8 T cell but nothing related to the overall phenotype or function of the cell. Because tetramer staining of cells does not require activation of the T cells, the variability is similar to regular flow-cytometry with intra- and inter-assay variability typically less than 10%. A problem with this strategy is that activated T cells tend to down regulate surface expression of the TCR following activation. An alternative approach would be to run parallel samples, one stained with tetramers and the other taken through a CFC assay, ELISPOT, or CTL assay. Studies comparing tetramer assays to these other assays have, however, revealed that the tetramer assays consistently tend to show higher precursor frequencies [18–21]. Although the reason for these discrepancies is unclear, there are some potential mechanisms that may be implicated in the observation. First, as previously mentioned, if the cytokine-based assays to be used as comparators are not optimized to detect all of the responding cells, discrepancies may become apparent. Alternatively, it could be possible that not all of the tetramer binding antigen-specific T cells are functional as has been reported [22]. Whatever the mechanism for the discrepancy, one caveat to tetramer analysis is that it may overestimate functional immunity. There are other obstacles associated with the use of tetramers: the need for knowledge of biologically relevant MHC epitopes contained within tumor antigens, and the limited sources for obtaining tetramers. Tetramer analysis as a tool for immunologic monitoring is typically confined to clinical trials involving immunization with the peptides to which the tetramers are targeted. The bulk of the human clinical trials in which tetramers were used focused on melanoma where many biologically relevant tumor antigen-derived peptides have been identified, including Mart-1, gp-100, and tyrosinase [15–16].

Both benefits and pitfalls have been described for all three of these quantitative assays; however, each one is well adapted to use in clinical trials. A recent report demonstrated that the assays corresponded well with each other, suggesting any of the assays would be useful in the readout of immune interventions for cancer [29].

ANTIBODY IMMUNITY AS A MEASURE OF THE INDUCED RESPONSE

Antigen-specific antibodies are a surrogate measure of immunologic and clinical efficacy in infectious disease vaccine models. For some infectious diseases, especially those with relatively long incubation periods, induction of seroconversion by vaccines is paralleled by the induction of immunologic memory. It is the induction of a memory response that provides the mechanisms for long-term protection even if the antibody levels wane [30].

Antibody levels, in some instances, may even serve as a reflection of the T cell response generated. In many infectious disease models, the total levels of antigen-specific IgG or IgA has been shown to correlate with protection from disease in the clinical setting [31]. A classic example is that of diphtheria vaccine antigen (DT). The degree of protection against clinical disease has been shown to be correlated well to the level of serum antibody against the toxin [30]. The assays to measure antibodies are stringently standardized and, although a level of 0.01 IU anti-D/ml is accepted as a protective levels, >0.05 IU anti-D/ml is considered to indicate optimal protection [32]. Likewise, viral antigens systems also have developed immunologic correlates. The induction of >10 mIU anti-HBs/ml has become accepted as the correlate of efficacy for Hepatitis B vaccines. This level of antibody has been associated with the generation of T cell memory more than five years after primary immunization as validated by ELISPOT analysis and by the ability of a booster shot to elicit a rapid anti-HBs response [33]. Thus, the total quantitative level of antibody induced, particularly a class of antibody that indicates Ig class switch and cognate T cell help such as IgG or IgA, may serve as a surrogate for the development of a T cell response and memory. There is some suggestion, in these early phase studies, that the generation of antibody immunity to tumors may have a positive clinical effect [34,35].

Antigen-specific antibody isotype is a potential indicator of the T-helper phenotype elicited after immunization. Cytokines induced in the immune environment play a major role in selecting the isotypes of antibody that are produced in an immune response [36]. Two dominant cytokines influencing the generation of specific antibody responses are IL-4 and IFN-gamma. Studies have demonstrated that IL-4 can induce activated B cells to secrete IgE as well as IgG_1 and that IFN-gamma would inhibit that secretion [37]. In addition IFN-gamma has been shown to impact Ig isotype selection in both T cell dependent and T cell independent systems, stimulating IgG_{2a} production [37]. Most investigations evaluating the correlation between T helper subsets and IgG isotype have been performed in animal models. For example, one recent study immunized mice with Hepatitis antigens and evaluated both T helper cytokine secretion and IgG isotypic antibody response [38]. Results demonstrated a strong correlation between IFN-gamma production and IgG_{2a} and, between IL-4 production and IgG_1. Furthermore, both T cell cytokine production and the associated antibody responses could be modulated by *in vivo* cytokine treatment. Other investigators propose using the development of a specific IgG isotype response as a surrogate for the T cell helper subset stimulated during lipid vesicle immunization with ova [39]. In these studies, not only did IFN-gamma/IgG_{2a} and IL-4/IgG_1 correlate, but both responses could be manipulated by the delivery vehicle of the antigen. No clear parallel has been made in the human system to IL-4 and IFN-gamma control of IgG_1 and IgG_{2a} as it has in the mouse. Lack of established antigen systems with known correlations and difficulty in establishing quantitative isotype antibody analysis might contribute to the lack of data in human models. If tumor antigen-specific antibody immunity were a reflection of the development of T cell immunity, perhaps a simple serologic analysis could replace more complex T cell assays.

EXPERIMENTAL METHODS FOR THE ASSESSMENT OF CELLULAR IMMUNITY

The next generation of assays is, for the most part, based on increasing the sensitivity of detection of the immune response while maximizing the amount of information obtained concerning the character of the immune response. In addition, newer techniques are being developed that more closely simulate the terminal function of tumor antigen-specific effector cells such as proliferation and lysis.

The analysis of the cellular immune response by real time PCR (RT-PCR) can be quantitative and sensitive. The method can be used not only to assess changes in PBMC after active immunization, but also changes in the tumor itself. RT-PCR has been used to determine a comprehensive cytokine profile in stimulated PBMC after immunization. A benefit of RT-PCR in immunologic monitoring is that the method is sensitive and can detect approximately 1/20,000–1/50,000 antigen-specific T cells. Furthermore the assay does not require *in vitro* expansion and yields a great deal of information about the phenotype of the response [40]. Most notably, RT-PCR can be performed on very minimal amounts of material. In fact, using RT-PCR to analyze the cellular immune response occurring after vaccination against a tumor antigen in mice can be monitored serially in murine blood without euthanizing the animal [41]. The disadvantage of RT-PCR is that, while the assay can give comprehensive information concerning gene expression, the method does not provide any indication of actual protein expression and can not discriminate between various cell subsets [40]. Methods have been developed to detect secreted cytokines in small samples of peripheral blood [42]. Beads coupled with antibodies specific for a variety of cytokines can be used to capture secreted proteins found in blood after the activation of a specific immune response. Techniques have been developed to allow the simultaneous detection of 15 immune-related cytokines in a single blood sample. This type of analysis has demonstrated performance characteristics well within guidelines for a clinical assay [42]. The use of antibody-coated beads will allow adaptation to flow cytometric analysis where specific evaluation of cellular subsets can be performed readily. Development of highly reproducible assays that can determine multiple immune response-related parameters will allow exquisite characterization of the tumor antigen-specific immune response generated after vaccination. Both these newer methods give a broad based analysis of the tumor antigen-specific immune response evaluating multiple parameters simultaneously.

Newer methods of measuring cellular immunity focus on function, such as T cell proliferation and lysis and the development of immunologic memory. Techniques have been developed, such as the measurement of serial halving of the fluorescent intensity of the vital dye carboxyfluorescein diacetate succinimidyl ester (CFSE), that reflect a lifespan of proliferation in a highly quantitative fashion. CSFE diffuses through the cell membrane, and the protein has a very low turnover rate. One can assess the rate of proliferation by measuring the serial halving of the number of CFSE staining cells. Studies have demonstrated that this method of analysis can detect 8–10 cycles of cell division by flow cytometry [43]. Not only can CFSE analysis assess the proliferative potential of the immune response, the technique can also determine the kinetics of that response. Likewise, effective immunization results in the development of immunological memory which is antigen-specific. After immunization, T cells undergo quantitative and qualitative changes which result in the development of memory T cells. First, there is an increase in the frequency of antigen-reactive T cells, and this increased frequency can be maintained for long periods of time. Secondly, unlike naïve T cells, memory T cells express different cell surface markers and behave in functionally different ways [44, 45]. The characteristic surface phenotype of memory T cells includes upregulation of CD44 and integrins and downregulation of CD62L and high molecular weight CD45 isoforms [44]. Based on their proliferation *in vivo* and the expression of activation markers, memory T cells comprise two distinct subsets, "central memory" T cells (T_{CM}) and "effector memory" T cells (T_{EM}). T_{CM} express the lymph node homing receptors CD62L and CCR7 and lack immediate effector function. However, upon a secondary challenge, they can stimulate DCs and also differentiate into effector T cells. T_{EM} do not express CD62L or CCR7 but rather express receptors for migration to non-lymphoid peripheral tissues to mediate inflammatory reactions or cytotoxicity. The molecular definition of the changes that occur in a T cell to make it a memory cell have allowed the development of methods that can more specifically quantitate and phenotype memory cells, e.g. flow cytometric methods. Memory/effector subsets of CD4+ T cells are delineated by differential expression of CD45RO isoforms which can be easily characterized with flow cytometry. In addition, other surface markers, specifically CD62L and CCR7, can be evaluated to differentiate between effector memory T cells and central memory T cells. Thus, phenotyping the antigen-specific memory T cell can be performed by using flow cytometry evaluating surface markers or be coupled to a more functional assay such as CFC.

The lytic potential of an antigen-specific T cell has long been acknowledged as the functional measure of viral eradication. Likewise, the generation of cancer-specific CTL has been touted as the major goal of a tumor antigen-specific vaccine. Quantitative assays are being developed that measure specific lytic and apoptotic functions ascribed to antigen-specific CTL. The release of chromium from labeled target cells after they have been destroyed by cytolytic T cells has been the gold standard for the assessment of CTL activity. Unfortunately, chromium release (^{51}Cr) assays are fraught with technical problems that make them difficult to adapt to analysis of multiple specimens and even more difficult to standardize. Investigators have circumvented the need for ^{51}Cr by developing non-toxic methods of cell labeling. Snyder and colleagues describe a "Lysispot" assay as a measure of direct target cell killing [46]. In the Lysispot, target cells are transduced to express a foreign marker, in this case *Escherichia coli* β-galactosidase or β-gal. Simply, β-gal is introduced into a target cell via a viral vector such as herpes simplex. Maximal amounts of β-gal are produced in the target cell within three hours; thus, the lytic assay can be performed in a minimal period of time. If CTL specific for the target are present, the target cell will be lysed, β-gal will be released and imbedded on a nitrocellulose membrane impregnated with anti-β-gal antibodies. Complementary antibodies specific for β-gal can be used to develop the membrane, and then spots are counted that correspond to individual lyse target cells. Results demonstrate that the Lysispot compares favorably to both ELISPOT and chromium release assays. Further variations on the analysis of lytic activity actually focus on the measurement of enzymes. The measurement of granzyme B production and release by CTL has been adapted to a highly quantitative format [47]. The development of the assay is based on the basic biologic function of antigen-specific CTL that release granzyme B and perforin when they recognize antigen in the context of MHC. Similar to the Lysispot described above, nitrocellulose membranes are impregnated with antibodies specific for granzyme B. When the enzyme is released by activated T cells in the presence of their specific target, secreted granzyme is bound to antibody and presumably can be detected by an additional granzyme B-specific antibody. Individual spots on plates represent an activated T cell in the process of lysing its target [47]. Measurement of granzyme B release results in markedly decreased assay backgrounds as compared with the standard chromium release assay.

Abbreviations: APC: antigen-presenting cell
CFC: cytokine flow cytometry
CMV: cytomegalovirus
CTL: cytotoxic T cell
IFN: interferon
IL: interleukin
MHC: major histocompatibility complex
PBMC: peripheral blood mononuclear cells

CONCLUSION

Our ability to measure and characterize the tumor-specific cellular immune response has advanced rapidly in the last decade. Assays such as ELISPOT which were highly experimental years ago are now standard tools in most immunologic laboratories. Newer cell-based assays further define the potential therapeutic function of the induced immune response. Finally, simultaneous analysis of tumor-specific antibody and T cell immunity may indicate a simple serologic method which might predict a robust T cell response.

ACKNOWLEDGEMENTS

KLK is supported by a Department of Defense Breast Cancer Research Program Fellowship (DAMD 17-00-1-0492), a Department of Defense Concept Award (BC023177) and NCI grant (R01101190). MLD is supported by NCI grant U-54 CA 090818 and K24 CA85218. We would like to thank Mr. Robert Schroeder for assistance in manuscript preparation.

REFERENCES

1. Tanguay S, Killion JJ (1994) Direct comparison of ELISPOT and ELISA-based assays for detection of individual cytokine-secreting cells. Lymphokine Cytokine Res 13(4):259–63
2. Schmittel A, et al. (2000) Quantification of tumor-specific T lymphocytes with the ELISPOT assay. J Immunother 23(3):289–95
3. Miyahira Y, et al. (1995) Quantification of antigen specific CD8+ T cells using an ELISPOT assay. J Immunol Methods 181(1):45–54
4. Smith JG, et al. (2001) Development and validation of a gamma interferon elispot assay for quantitation of cellular immune responses to varicella-zoster virus. Clin Diagn Lab Immunol 8(5):871–9
5. McCutcheon M, et al. (1997) A sensitive ELISPOT assay to detect low-frequency human T lymphocytes. J Immunol Methods 210(2):149–66
6. Knutson KL, et al. (2001) Immunization with a HER-2/neu helper peptide vaccine generates HER-2/neu CD8 T-cell immunity in cancer patients. J Clin Invest 107(4):477–84
7. Lathey J (2003) Preliminary steps toward validating a clinical bioassay. BioPharm Int 18:42–50
8. Jennes W, et al. (2002) Enhanced ELISPOT detection of antigen-specific T cell responses from cryopreserved specimens with addition of both IL-7 and IL-15–the Amplispot assay. J Immunol Methods 270(1):99–108
9. Enk AH, et al. (1999) Decreased rate of progression and induction of tumor-specific immune response by adjuvant immunotherapy in stage IV melanoma. Hautarzt 50(2):103–8
10. Reynolds SR, et al. (1997) Stimulation of CD8+ T cell responses to MAGE-3 and Melan A/MART-1 by immunization to a polyvalent melanoma vaccine. Int J Cancer 72(6):972–6

11. Nomura LE, et al. (2000) Optimization of whole blood antigen-specific cytokine assays for CD4(+) T cells. Cytometry 40(1):60–8
12. McHugh S, et al. (1996) Kinetics and functional implications of Th1 and Th2 cytokine production following activation of peripheral blood mononuclear cells in primary culture. Eur J Immunol 26(6):1260–5
13. Seder RA, Ahmed R (2003) Similarities and differences in CD4(+) and CD8(+) effector and memory T cell generation. Nat Immunol 4(9):835–42
14. De Rosa SC, et al. (2001) 11-color, 13-parameter flow cytometry: identification of human naive T cells by phenotype, function, and T-cell receptor diversity. Nat Med 7(2):245–8
15. Pittet MJ, et al. (2001a) Expansion and functional maturation of human tumor antigen-specific CD8+ T cells after vaccination with antigenic peptide. Clin Cancer Res 7(3 Suppl):796s–803s
16. Pittet MJ, et al. (2001b) Ex vivo analysis of tumor antigen specific CD8+ T cell responses using MHC/peptide tetramers in cancer patients. Int Immunopharmacol 1(7):1235–47
17. Kwok WW, et al. (2002) Use of class II tetramers for identification of CD4+ T cells. J Immunol Methods 268(1):71–81
18. Dunbar PR, et al. (1998) Direct isolation, phenotyping and cloning of low-frequency antigen-specific cytotoxic T lymphocytes from peripheral blood. Curr Biol 8(7):413–6
19. He XS, et al. (1999) Quantitative analysis of hepatitis C virus-specific CD8(+) T cells in peripheral blood and liver using peptide-MHC tetramers. Proc Natl Acad Sci U S A 96(10):5692–7
20. Tan LC, et al. (1999) A re-evaluation of the frequency of CD8+ T cells specific for EBV in healthy virus carriers. J Immunol 162(3):1827–35
21. Xiong Y, et al. (2001) Simian immunodeficiency virus (SIV) infection of a rhesus macaque induces SIV-specific CD8(+) T cells with a defect in effector function that is reversible on extended interleukin-2 incubation. J Virol 75(6):3028–33
22. Engstrand M, et al. (2003) Cellular responses to cytomegalovirus in immunosuppressed patients: circulating CD8+ T cells recognizing CMVpp65 are present but display functional impairment. Clin Exp Immunol 132(1):96–104
23. Jager E, et al. (2002) Peptide-specific CD8+ T-cell evolution in vivo: response to peptide vaccination with Melan-A/MART-1. Int J Cancer 98(3):376–88
24. Lau R, et al. (2001) Phase I trial of intravenous peptide-pulsed dendritic cells in patients with metastatic melanoma. J Immunother 24(1):66–78
25. Lee KH, et al. (1999) Increased vaccine-specific T cell frequency after peptide-based vaccination correlates with increased susceptibility to in vitro stimulation but does not lead to tumor regression. J Immunol 163(11):6292–300
26. Lee P, et al. (2001) Effects of interleukin-12 on the immune response to a multipeptide vaccine for resected metastatic melanoma. J Clin Oncol 19(18):3836–47
27. Nielsen MB, Marincola FM (2000) Melanoma vaccines: the paradox of T cell activation without clinical response. Cancer Chemother Pharmacol 46 Suppl:S62–6
28. Oertli D, et al. (2002) Rapid induction of specific cytotoxic T lymphocytes against melanoma-associated antigens by a recombinant vaccinia virus vector expressing multiple immunodominant epitopes and costimulatory molecules in vivo. Hum Gene Ther 13(4):569–75
29. Maecker HT, et al. (2005) Impact of cryopreservation on tetramer, cytokine flow cytometry, and ELISPOT. BMC Immunol 6(1):17
30. Ellis RW (1999a) Immunological Correlates for Efficacy of Combination Vaccines. In: Ellis RW (ed) Combination Vaccines: Development, Clinical Research, and Approval. Humana Press, Totowa, pp 107–131
31. Ellis RW (1999b) Development of combination vaccines. Vaccine 17(13–14):1635–42
32. Volk V, et al. (1962) Antigenic responses to booster dose of diptheria and tetanus toxoids: Seven to thirteen years after primary inoculation of noninstitutionalized children. Public Health Rep 77:185
33. Van Hattum J, et al. (1991) In vitro anti-HBs production by indiviual B cells of responders to hepatitis B vaccine who subsequently lost antibody. In: Hollinger F, Lemon S, Margolis H (eds) Viral Hepatitis and Liver Disease. Williams and Wilkins, Baltimore, pp 774

34. Hsueh EC, et al. (1998) Correlation of specific immune responses with survival in melanoma patients with distant metastases receiving polyvalent melanoma cell vaccine. J Clin Oncol 16(9):2913–20
35. Quan WD, Jr., et al. (1997) Active specific immunotherapy of metastatic melanoma with an antiidiotype vaccine: a phase I/II trial of I-Mel-2 plus SAF-m. J Clin Oncol 15(5):2103–10
36. Finkelman FD, et al. (1990) Lymphokine control of in vivo immunoglobulin isotype selection. Annu Rev Immunol 8:303–33
37. Coffman RL, et al. (1986) B cell stimulatory factor-1 enhances the IgE response of lipopolysaccharide-activated B cells. J Immunol 136(12):4538–41
38. Milich DR, et al. (1997) The hepatitis B virus core and e antigens elicit different Th cell subsets: antigen structure can affect Th cell phenotype. J Virol 71(3):2192–201
39. Brewer JM, et al. (1998) Lipid vesicle size determines the Th1 or Th2 response to entrapped antigen. J Immunol 161(8):4000–7
40. Panelli MC, et al. (2002) The role of quantitative PCR for the immune monitoring of cancer patients. Expert Opin Biol Ther 2(5):557–64
41. Hempel DM, et al. (2002) Analysis of cellular immune responses in the peripheral blood of mice using real-time RT-PCR. J Immunol Methods 259(1–2):129–38
42. de Jager W, et al. (2003) Simultaneous detection of 15 human cytokines in a single sample of stimulated peripheral blood mononuclear cells. Clin Diagn Lab Immunol 10(1):133–9
43. Lyons AB (2000) Analysing cell division in vivo and in vitro using flow cytometric measurement of CFSE dye dilution. J Immunol Methods 243(1–2):147–54
44. Dutton RW, et al. (1998) T cell memory. Annu Rev Immunol 16:201–23
45. Zinkernagel RM, et al. (1996) On immunological memory. Annu Rev Immunol 14:333–67
46. Snyder JE, et al. (2003) Measuring the frequency of mouse and human cytotoxic T cells by the Lysispot assay: independent regulation of cytokine secretion and short-term killing. Nat Med 9(2):231–5
47. Rininsland FH, et al. (2000) Granzyme B ELISPOT assay for ex vivo measurements of T cell immunity. J Immunol Methods 240(1–2):143–55

CHAPTER 18

INTERFERON THERAPY

STERGIOS J. MOSCHOS AND JOHN M. KIRKWOOD

The University of Pittsburgh Cancer Institute Melanoma Center, Hillman Cancer Center, UPCI Research Pavilion, Suite 1.32 5117 Centre Avenue, Pittsburgh, PA 15213-2584

INTRODUCTION

In 1957, Issacs and Lindenmann discovered that cells previously infected with a virus are resistant to infection by another virus. This phenomenon, termed interference, was attributed to a substance, called interferon (IFN) [1]. Despite unsuccessful attempts to isolate the protein for more than 20 years it soon became known that IFN is not a single molecule but a family of structurally related molecules which have a broader than the originally discovered antiviral role with important cytostatic, direct antitumor and indirect immunomodulatory effects. The interaction of the type I IFN system with the phylogenetically more recently developed specialized immune system imply a role of type I IFNs in the integrity of the organism by allogeneic inhibition [2, 3]. Purification to heterogeneity and cloning of the first interferon gene [4] further advanced IFN research field and IFN was the first protein to become available for the clinical treatment of malignancies.

THE MOLECULES AND THEIR RECEPTORS

The Interferon Superfamily

IFNs are divided in two groups, based on structural, physicochemical, and biological properties. IFN-γ is the only type II and 8 type I IFNs families have been described in mammals, namely IFN-α, IFN-β, IFN-δ, IFN-ε, IFN-κ, IFN-λ, IFN-τ, IFN-ω. Among these families IFN-τ and IFN-δ are not produced in humans. In the human IFN system there are 21 functional non-allelic genes encoding for different IFN species; 13 subtypes for IFN-α, 3 for IFN-λ and single species of IFN-β, ω, ε, κ.

H.L. Kaufman and J.D. Wolchok (eds.), General Principles of Tumor Immunotherapy, 405–430.

Type I IFNs have likely diverged from a common ancestral gene through gene duplication and are evolutionary conserved, except for INF-λ, as reflected by their common intron-less structure and their clustering in the short arm of chromosome 9. It has therefore been suggested that type I IFNs may be divided in two subgroups, designated Ia (IFN-α, β, ω, ε, κ.) and Ib (IFN-λ) [5]. The physiologic significance of the large number of type I IFN subtypes (especially IFN-α) remains obscure but given that individual subtypes show quantitatively distinct patterns of antiviral, anti-proliferative and natural killer (NK) stimulatory activities, it is tempting to speculate that this redundancy of alternative defense pathways provides a survival advantage for protection.

Production of Endogenous IFNs

Recent progress on the pathways regulating IFN production has more firmly established that type I IFNs are an important link between innate and adaptive immunity and by their constitutive, low-level production they contribute to immunosurveillance against tumors and exogenous pathogens [2, 6]. Upon exposure to 'danger' stimuli type I IFNs are produced by almost all cells of the body "sounding the alarm". IFN gene induction is the end result from activation of signaling pathways originating from several pathogen recognition receptors, termed toll-like receptors (TLRs), expressed on the surface of antigen presenting cells (APCs). These receptors 'sense' specific pathogen-associated molecular, non-protein patterns normally not expressed by host tissues or endogenous molecules released from 'stressed' cells. TLRs are transmembrane proteins with a cytoplasmic domain that is conserved between the members of the interleukin-1 receptor (IL-1R) family (Toll/IL-1R or TIR domain). The TLR expression profile on APCs varies accounting for the induction of different sets of pro-inflammatory cytokines in response to the respective TLR ligands from invading pathogens. All TLRs use the adaptor MyD88 for signaling, but different TLRs also use different additional adaptors, such as the TIR domain-containing adaptor inducing IFN-β (TRIF or TICAM-1) or the tumor necrosis factor receptor-associated factor (TRAF) 6 resulting in activation of divergent signaling cascades, such as the MAPK and NF-κB [7]. The TLR adaptor complex interacts with several members of a growing family of transcription factors, termed interferon regulatory factors (IRFs), which bind to the regulatory sequences of IFN-α and IFN-β genes, termed virus-inducible enhancer-like response elements (VREs) and regulate their transcription. To date, IRF-3 [8], IRF-5 [9], and IRF-7 [10] positively regulate whereas IRF-2 is a negative regulator of IFN production [11]. Cross-talk with other signaling pathways is required for full activation of IRFs [12].

Type I IFN production has been most extensively studied in the model of viral infection. Although IRF-1 and IRF-2 are constitutively expressed at low levels intracellularly, the negative regulator IRF-2 accumulates due to its longer half life than IRF-1 and therefore allows only for low-level constitutive IFN production [6]. In the early phase of viral infection IRF-3, is activated and induces weak expression of IFN-α4 and IFN-β genes, as well as IRF-7 and IRF-1 gene expression. In the late phase of viral induction both IRF-3 and IRF-7 amplify the induction of IFN-β and certain other IFN-α genes. This autocrine-paracrine loop not only amplifies type I IFN production but also the production of other inflammatory cytokines via IFN or TLR-mediated signaling pathways which activate immune and other cells [13–16] and result in a more efficient activation of the immune system. In fact, defects in IFNα gene transcription related with inactivity of the IFN-α2 and α4 promoter have recently been associated with melanoma development [17].

Although all cells are capable of producing type I IFNs, a distinct subset of bone marrow-derived dendritic cells (DCs), termed plasmacytoid dendritic cells (pDCs), express large amounts (100-1,000 fold more than any other cell type) of type I IFNs in response to viral infection [18]. pDCs express lymphoid rather than myeloid surface markers, have a distinct pattern of TLR expression (TLR7, TLR9≫ TLR1, TLR6, TLR10, CD303/BDCA2) and are dependent on FLT3 ligand for their development. These differences between pDCs and $CD11c^+$ immature DCs suggest that they may have been developed through different evolutionary trails to preferentially recognize viruses and bacteria, respectively. The mechanism of rapid and robust transcription of type I IFNs by pDCs is probably related with the constitutive rather than inducible expression of IRF-7 in pDCs and therefore the independence of IFNα production on the positive feedback of IFNβ [19]. pDCs have recently shown to play an important role beyond viral immunity and preliminary data in several cancer types suggest that they are recruited in the tumor microenvironment [20], but they become dysfunctional [21, 22], remain immature [23] and in some cases have been associated with adverse overall survival [24].

The Interferon Receptors

All IFN receptors belong to the class II cytokine receptor family, which also contains receptors for signaling by IL-10 related proteins. Human IFNs utilize three different receptors. The type Ia cytokines bind to a common receptor, termed IFN-AR, whereas IFN-λ (type Ib) exploits a different receptor, termed IFN-LR, and IFN-γ (type II) binds to a distinct receptor, termed IFN-GR. Each receptor is comprised of two transmembrane polypeptide chains, termed R1 and R2, with distinct complementary functions, but, in general, one subunit has ligand-binding property and the other has a signal-transducing one. Of note, the R2 subunit for IFN-LR is shared with the IL-10 and the IL-22 receptor complexes, accounting for the close functional relationship between IL-10 and IFN-λ. The clinical importance of IFNAR expression is reflected by recent data showing that the expression level of IFNAR1 subunit and/or its downregulation with IFNα treatment has been correlated with response to treatment in various diseases [25, 26]. Moreover, free circulating IFNARs were found to be higher in patients with a variety of malignancies compared with normal individuals [27] and specific IFNAR haplotypes have been correlated with higher incidence of several nonmalignant diseases [28].

Type I Interferon Signaling

Delineation of the signal transduction pathways following IFN-R stimulation has significantly contributed in better understanding of the anti-tumor mechanisms of type I IFNs. Binding of type I IFNs to IFN-AR results in activation of the two Jak proteins, Jak1 and Tyk2, which are non-covalently pre-associated with each IFN-AR subunit. Jak activation induces tyrosine phosphorylation of both receptor subunits and activation of several STAT proteins, such as STAT-1 and STAT-2. STATs then form homo- and/or hetero-dimers and translocate to the nucleus regulating gene transcription [29]. Recent studies have shown that both IFN-AR subunits may directly affect gene transcription independent of other signal transduction pathways. More specifically, the R2 subunit of the IFN-AR undergoes regulated intramembrane proteolysis releasing the intracellular domain which translocates to the nucleus and modulates gene transcription [30] whereas the R1 subunit contains a nuclear localization sequence which mediates its translocation to the nucleus after type I IFN stimulation [31]. Moreover, intracellular type I IFNs were shown to equally activate Jak-STAT pathway compared with extracellular IFNs implying a more prompt effect of IFN on the IFN producing cells compared with the slower classic IFN-AR pathway triggered in an autocrine, paracrine or endocrine fashion [32].

Although the Jak-STAT pathway is the most extensively studied, other pathways are also important for type I IFN-mediated effects which collaborate with the Jak-STAT pathway (reviewed in [33]). Protein kinase delta (PKCδ) is also activated by IFN and further phosphorylates STAT-1, a necessary step for full STAT-1 activation. CrkL and CrkII, members of the Crk-family of adaptor proteins which link cytokine receptors to downstream signaling elements, act via STAT-dependent and independent effects. IFN activated CrkL regulates the transcriptional function of STAT-5 and by indirectly antagonizing the Ras pathway has tumor suppressor activity. IFN-AR also activates insulin receptor substrate (IRS) -1 and 2, members of the IRS family of docking proteins which associate with STAT-3 and further activate PI 3'-kinase. PI 3'-kinase regulates the 40S ribosomal S6 protein which plays an important role in the regulation of cell cycle progression, cell survival and mRNA translation and transduces signals through Akt activation which is involved in cell survival.

ACTIONS AND "RE"-ACTIONS OF TYPE I IFNS

The Role of Interferon in Intracellular Functions

IFNα has long been considered as a 'negative growth factor' which contributes to the eradication of pathogens or cancer-'allogeneic' cells by inducing cell cycle arrest or apoptosis [34]. This is predominantly mediated by modulating gene expression of number or key proteins involved in cell cycle, and apoptosis. More specifically, induction of p53 expression confers cells a more dynamic response to a variety of 'stress' signals [35]. Induction of the retinoblastoma protein pRBb [36] or cdk inhibitors [37] with concomitant downregulation of cyclins [38] results in prolongation of cell cycle and cell cycle arrest.

IFN-induced apoptosis has been well established in several physiologic processes [39,40] and is an important mechanism for elimination of pathogens and cancer cells [41]. Type I IFNs induce *direct* expression of pro-apoptotic genes, such as members of the tumor necrosis factor receptor family (Fas/CD95, TRAIL/Apo2L), caspases (caspase-4 and -8), the double strand-activated kinase PKR, the 2-5A oligoadenylate synthetase pathway, and others (reviewed in [42]). The clinical significance of apoptosis induction is reflected in a recent study of patients with multiple sclerosis which showed that IFN-β1a responders compared to non-responders had an increase in soluble TRAIL protein [43]. Type I IFNs may *indirectly* induce apoptosis either by endothelial cell apoptosis and therefore anti-angiogenesis or augmentation of cell mediated cytotoxicity against cancer cells or pathogens.

Escape Mechanisms to Antiproliferative or Apoptotic Effects of IFNα

The magnitude and duration of the transcriptional activation of IFN responsive genes should be *physiologically* controlled to minimize pathology. STAT signaling induces expression of genes encoding suppressors of cytokine signaling (SOCS)-1 and 3 which negatively regulate the Jak-STAT pathway by blocking access of STATs to the receptor sites. Constitutive SOCS expression has been correlated with impaired DC antigen presentation [44] and resistance to IFNα therapy in several malignancies including melanoma [45, 46]. Two cytoplasmic protein tyrosine phosphatases, termed Shp-1 and -2, provide additional negative feedback by dephosphorylating STATs and other IFNAR-associated kinases and have been associated with protection of cells from the cytotoxic effects of IFNα. A third physiologic mechanism of both type I and type II IFN signaling is the expression of the protein inhibitor of activated STATs (PIAS-1), which has been similarly associated with impairment of innate immunity against pathogens [47].

Apart from the physiologic feedback regulation of type I IFN signaling, a number of *pathologic* mechanisms confer resistance to endogenously or exogenously administered IFNs. Although the Jak/STAT pathway is important for IFNα's immunomodulatory [48, 49] and direct antiproliferative effects, STAT signaling is not sufficient to sustain antitumor effect in cell lines [50] and tumors [51]. Moreover, high throughput analysis in IFNα resistant and sensitive melanoma cell lines suggests that induction of IFNα stimulated genes is more complicated than previously thought [52]. Also, cancer cells may have acquired a survival benefit secondary to more widespread defects in their IFNα signaling [53] or apoptotic machinery [54] and therefore combination IFNα-based strategies to overcome IFNα resistance may be an important consideration for treatment of cancer (see *rational combinations of interferons with other agents*).

Immunoregulatory Mechanisms of IFNα Action

Effect on life, death, cell cycle, and activation

Type IFNs exert multiple direct and indirect effects on the innate and adaptive immune system. More specifically, IFNα prevents apoptosis of neutrophils [55], T lymphocytes [56], and B cells [57] and attenuated proliferation of NK cells at any developmental stage [58]. However, in lymphocytes the balance between proliferation and cell death is more complex [39]; their anti-proliferative effect in lymphocytes is dynamic [59] and may be partially overcome by mitogenic stimuli resulting in an overall shaping of immune response during activation and prevention of activation-induced cell death [60].

Intuitively, the negative effects of type I IFNs in cell proliferation and prevention of apoptosis may serve the purpose of differentiation, antigen presentation and overall activation. Type I IFNs are major inducers of major histocompatibility molecules (MHC, especially class HLA-I) [61] and by restoring their expression in cancer cells may become more amenable to cytotoxic induced cell death. This has been suggested as one of the mechanisms to explain the therapeutic benefit of adjuvant high dose interferon (HDI) in melanoma [62].

Induction of NK cell proliferation and cytotoxicity are the earliest described immunological effects of type I IFNs [63–65] and similar observations have now been extended to lymphocytes and macrophages [66]. More specifically, IFNα induces polyclonal activation of $CD8^+$ cells during viral infections [67], and antitumor cell-mediated cytotoxicity [68, 69] and increases perforin and granzyme A expression in NK cells of patients with melanoma [70]. IFNα also upregulates the B lymphocyte stimulator protein (BLyS) and the proliferation-inducing ligand (APRIL) both of which activate a CD40–like pathway thereby enhancing B cell survival and inducing isotype class switch DNA recombination in IgD^+ and/IgM^+ B cells [57]. The induction of humoral immune responses may partially explain the increased autoantibody production frequently associated with IFNα therapy.

Maturation-polarization

Exogenously administered type I IFNs enhance function of antigen presenting and effector cells via a variety of mechanisms. Thus, type I IFNs upregulate expression of several TLRs on macrophages optimizing their antigen presenting function [71] and may induce differentiation to myeloid DCs [72]. In patients with completely resected, high risk for relapse melanoma adjuvant IFNα treatment upregulates expression of transport proteins associated with antigen processing (TAP1 and TAP2) and proteasome activator 28 in peripheral blood mononuclear cells [73]. Activation of TLRs on antigen presenting cells (APCs) induces type I IFN production by DC subsets [74–76] and further production of more type I IFNs as well as other DC-derived cytokines, such as IL-15, which have a dual activation–survival effect on DCs [77–79]. Type I IFNs act as maturation factors for DCs by upregulating class I and class II MHC (HLA-A, -B, -C, -DR) and costimulatory molecules (CD80, CD 83 and CD86) [80,81]. IFNα stimulates DCs to promote differentiation of naïve CD4 cells, expands non-polarized antigen-primed IL-2 secreting T cells towards Th_1 response [82, 83], and cooperates with NK cells to prime anti-tumor CD8 cells [84]. The mechanism of promoting Th_1 cell response by type I IFNs is secondary to a combination of antagonism of the suppressive effect of IL-4, suppression of IL-5 production on IFN-γ secreting $CD4^+$ cells, and upregulation of the β_2 chain of IL-12 receptor in $CD4^+$ cells [85–87].

IFNα also contributes to the formation and maintenance of immunologic memory. Adenoviral–IFNα engineered DCs delivered into intracranial tumors in mice enhanced antitumor efficacy of prior vaccination with an ovalbumin-derived MHC class II-restricted epitope [88]. Administration of high-dose interferon α2b (HDI) following vaccination leads to immunologic recall of gp100-specific $CD8^+$ T cells [89]. This finding has important implications for the maintenance of memory T lymphocytes, and suggests that IFNα may potentially be useful in cancer vaccines to assist in overcoming immunologic tolerance to tumor antigens.

Migration

IFN induces chemokinesis of T cells at various stages of differentiation by upregulating integrins, such as LFA-1, VLA-4, and ICAM-1 [90] and induces different sets of chemokines with their corresponding receptors on APCs thereby affecting their maturation-trafficking pattern. More specifically, type I IFNs upregulate the anaphylatoxin C3a receptor, the chemokine receptor CCR7, its natural ligand, MIP-3β, the Th_1 chemokine, IP-10, the MCP-1/CCL2, and the interferon-induced protein 10 (IP10,CXCL10) on the maturing antigen-loaded pDCs facilitating their homing to draining lymph nodes to encounter CCR7-expressing specific T cells among others [91–93]. They also upregulate the expression of CCR1 and CCR3 chemokine receptors on monocyte-derived cell subsets [94]. Thus, locally produced IFN induces a large number of cytokines to recruit early NK cells and macrophages which may contribute to the influx of Th_1 rather than Th_2 lymphocytes expressing the corresponding chemokine receptor CXCR3 into tissue [95–97]. The clinical importance of the IFN-induced enhanced migration and enhanced cell survival is reflected by the correlation of increased the number of lymphocytes and/or monocytes/macrophages infiltrating the tumor in patients with melanoma receiving interferon [98, 99] .

Interferon and autoimmunity

Given the diverse effects of type I IFNs in the innate and adaptive immune responses, it is not surprising that these cytokines play a pivotal pathogenic role in the exacerbation of pre-existing or *de novo* induction of a wide variety of clinical autoimmune disorders (reviewed in [100]). Systemic lupus erythematosus (SLE) is the most prevalent autoimmune disease in which increased serum levels of IFNα have been correlated with induction [101] or disease exacerbations [102]. Treatment-related autoimmunity has been recently correlated with higher incidence of antitumor responses [103] and HDI has shown prolonged overall survival in patients with melanoma [104]. Therefore, understanding the mechanisms of IFNα-induced autoimmunity in cancer may help select patients most likely to respond to IFNα therapy.

In patients with SLE, high serum levels of IFNa have not been fully explained but both exogenous and endogenous inducers may be considered. Exogenous agents may consist of pathogens (viruses, bacteria) or ultraviolet light exposure whereas endogenous agents may be products of apoptotic-necrotic cells or immune complexes (anti-ribonucleoprotein, anti-DNA) which trigger IFNα production in pDCs. Peripheral blood pDCs are reduced presumably owing to their migration to tissues following acquisition of IFNα/β-induced chemokine receptors and normally quiescent monocytes are differentiated under the influence of circulating IFNα/β into DCs. These DCs may capture apoptotic cells and nucleosomes in the SLE patients' blood and subsequently presentautoantigens to $CD4^+$ T cells thereby initiating the expansion of autoreactive T cells,followed by differentiation of autoantibody-producing B cells [105]. In psoriasis, pDCs were abundantly present and activated in primary plaque lesions and were producing IFNa early during the disease [106]. Interestingly, TNF-α which frequently overexpressed in late stages of cancer antagonizes IFN α/β- by inhibiting generation of pDCs, or inhibiting IFN-α release from immature pDCs [107].

Risk for development of chronic autoimmunity is inherited as a complex polygenic trait and is partially associated with the MHC class II region, which *per se* is not sufficient for clinically significant manifestation of autoimmune disease. Development of chronic autoimmunity during IFNα treatment is favored in individuals who carry important genetic susceptibility genes frequently contained in the MHC class II region. Indeed, specific haplotypes [108] or single nucleotide polymorphisms of cytokines [109], immune suppressive molecules [110], or members of the interferon signaling pathway [111] have been correlated with therapeutic response to type I IFNs in a variety of human diseases. Moreover, a study on the peripheral blood lymphocyte immune response in patients with IFNα-induced autoimmune thyroiditis showed that Th_1 response was predominant only in patients who developed autoimmune dysfunction [112] suggesting that all the immunoregulatory properties of IFNα are also potentially relevant for autoimmunity.

INTERFERON IN THE TREATMENT OF HUMAN CANCERS

Introduction

IFNα has been the second biologic agent after insulin to be tested for treatment of human illnesses. It was originally considered only as a 'viral penicillin' for therapy of a variety of viral-related illnesses, and in fact, in medical practice, type I IFNs have now been approved for diseases such as viral hepatitis, multiple sclerosis, and condyloma accuminatum. The application of IFNs in the treatment of malignancies was led by a clinical observation that partially purified IFNα could regress a variety of tumors [113].

Toxicity and Pharmacokinetics of IFNs; Results of Phase I Trials

Administration of IFNs results in wide range side effects reflecting the multitude of organs it affects (reviewed in [114]). The incidence and severity of these side effects are dose-, route-, and duration-related and in most cases predictable and fully reversible upon treatment discontinuation. Acutely, nearly all patients experience flu-like symptoms, such as fever, chills, myalgia, headache, nausea, vomiting which are overall manageable and abate over time (tachyphylaxis). Over time, constitutional symptoms, such as fatigue, appetite loss, and weight loss accumulate which may significantly affect patient's quality of life and may call for dose reduction or even treatment discontinuation. At any time hematologic toxicities may occur as a result of a direct cytostatic effect of IFNs, with neutropenia being the most frequent. Other laboratory abnormalities, such as liver function tests or CPK elevations may occur which may or may not be associated with clinical rhabdomyolysis. Neurological effects may affect behavior, cognition, mood or personality with depression being most frequent.

In the pivotal HDI trial E1684, approximately 78% of patients experienced grade 3 toxicity, and 24% discontinued therapy because of toxicity and despite proper dose reduction and symptomatic management. The management and prevention of HDI-related toxicities is one of the greatest challenges in broadening and improving the efficacy of this regimen because low dose interferon regimens though less toxic are also less effective [115]. During the recent years understanding the mechanisms of IFN-induced toxicity and identifying the patient subgroups most likely to develop symptoms has contributed to treatment, prevention or palliation of several of these side effects. Exogenously administered IFNα-induced releases of cytokines, such as TNFα, IL-1, IL-2, IL-6, IFNγ, and alteration of several hypothalamo-pituitary endocrine axes, such as the thyroid and the adrenal account for most of the constitutional symptoms observed. IFNα-induced depression was associated with induction of indoleamine-2,3-dioxygenase (IDO), the enzyme for the rate-limiting step of tryptophan conversion to kynurenine. In other words, IFNα shuttles tryptophan metabolism away from conversion to serotonin, a important neurotransmitter for mood stability [116]. Proactive treatment with antidepressants may prevent or minimize mood disorders, a hypothesis currently being tested in a prospective fashion in patients with high risk for relapse melanoma who are actively treated with HDI (UPCI 01-163). The mechanism of fatigue is not clear but anti-inflammatory agents are inefficient whereas low grade exercise and methylphenidate may moderately increased functional ability of IFNα treated patients in a small size preliminary study [117]. IFNα mediated suppression of hematopoietic progenitor cell proliferation, increased autoimmune mediated destruction of erythroid precursor cells and renal dysfunction with resultant reduction of erythropoietin release are the most account for most of IFN's hematologic side effects [118].

In phase I trials of patients with solid tumors, IFNα was administered using variable schedules, and by different routes. The most intensely studied route of administration was intramuscular but it was associated with higher incidence of toxicities without clear benefit at higher doses (reviewed in [119]). A single phase

I study comparing intramuscular with intravenous administration of IFNα in solid tumors showed that the reason for the lower tolerance to intramuscular treatment was increasing serum IFNα levels whereas daily intravenous administration was more tolerable and achieved higher peak serum levels than the intramuscular route [120]. Moreover, IFNα treatment in this study was associated with a 17% response rate (4/23) in patients with melanoma which provided the basis for the adjuvant trials of high dose IFNα therapy in melanoma.

Early Successess of Type I IFNs in the Treatment of Hematologic Malignancies

Hairy cell leukemia (HCL), a rare B-cell neoplasm for which no treatment existed in 1982 except for splenectomy, was the first neoplasm to be successfully treated with IFNα based on the ability of type I IFNs to induce remission in some patients with well-differentiated B-cell tumors. IFNα showed 70-85% hematologic response, resolution of splenomegaly and recovery of immunologic function, although partial remission was rare, infiltration of bone marrow by hairy cells was persistent, and relapse rate or disease progression following its discontinuation was high [121]. The effect of IFNα in HCL may be more direct on hairy cells, inducing malignant cell differentiation toward a stage less responsive to growth stimulation and therefore cytostasis [122].

More impressive clinical benefit of IFNα was shown in *chronic myelogenous leukemia* (CML) which was initially investigated in single institution studies [123] and was subsequently confirmed in several international large prospective randomized trials comparing IFNα-based vs. standard chemotherapeutic agents, such as busulfan and hydroxyurea (Italian, French, UK-MRC, Benelux, German). A meta-analysis of these trials showed that IFNα treatment significantly improved overall survival [124]. IFNα may restore the differentiation program of CML cells by suppressing Bcr-abl expression and cell proliferation and by increasing adhesion of CML progenitors to the bone marrow stroma [125]. IFNα reduces the number of $CD34^+$ bone marrow stem cells, increases cytotoxicity of NK and $CD8^+$ T cells, stimulates generation of DCs that can present CML-specific antigens and polarizes T cells responses towards a Th_1 pro-inflammatory phenotype [126].

Effect of Interferon in the Treatment of Several Solid Tumors

Type I IFNs have been successfully used for treatment of several solid tumors. In *renal cell carcinoma* (RCC) single agent IFNα had up to 30% response rate in earlier phase II studies with a few durable responses which led to its evaluation in randomized controlled trials alone or in combination with other treatment modalities. The response rate from these IFNα-based combinations was low and survival benefit was noted in a few of them [127–129]. Interestingly, IFNα following nephrectomy prolongs overall survival in the metastatic but not the adjuvant setting [130]. Addition of other agents to IFNα for RCC was associated with increased toxicity and clinical benefit in only a few of the studies [131,132]. *Kaposi sarcoma* (KS), an angiogenic-inflammatory neoplasm and one of the most frequent oncologic manifestations of AIDS, was responsive to IFNα [133]. Response rates were superior with higher doses [134] and in patients with higher peripheral blood $CD4^+$ counts[135]. Combination with concurrent antiretroviral therapy was superior to IFNα alone irrespective of the HIV-related immune dysfunction [136]. Single agent IFNα given in patients with *neuroendocrine tumors* resulted in biochemical and objective tumor responses and improved OS in small underpowered studies [137] and were confirmed in larger studies comparing variable doses of IFNα vs. chemotherapy [138]. In *hepatocellular carcinoma* the greatest benefit was seen in treatment of chronic hepatitis C infection, an important etiologic factor for development HCC with rising incidence in the United States. IFNα treatment decreased incidence of HCC in patients with chronic hepatitis C in a large retrospective Japanese study [139] whereas a prospective randomized Japanese study showed that in patients with compensated HCV-related liver cirrhosis, low HCV RNA load, and completely resected HCC nodules, IFNα improved 5-year OS [140]. Similar to hepatocellular carcinoma, studies of IFNa in *head and neck cancer* (HNC) showed an overall survival benefit in chemoprevention. One-year of IFNα combined with oral isotretitoin and oral a-tocopherol in patients with advanced premalignant lesions of the upper aerodigestive tract resulted in a 30% response rate in 12 months of observation [141]. A similar regimen used as adjuvant therapy in patients previously treated for advanced stage III and IV HNC was associated with 91% 2-year survival rate which needs to be confirmed in a phase III randomized trial [142].

Adjuvant Applications of IFNα in the Treatment of Melanoma

The early pharmacokinetic analysis of IFNα given in daily or three-times-weekly schedules via intramuscular, subcutaneous or intravenous routes had consistently shown responses of up to 20% in patients with metastatic melanoma [120]. Because therapeutic benefit to IFNα was noted only in patients with metastatic disease but small tumor burden it was hypothesized that the highest benefit from IFNα therapy would be in the adjuvant setting. A large number of international and cooperative group trials utilizing IFNα at varying dosages and schedules were begun in the United States and Europe. (Table 1)

In the E1684 trial, adjuvant HDI (20 $MU/m^2/d$, intravenously 5 days a week for 4 weeks, followed by 10 MU/m2 subcutaneously, three times a week for 48 weeks) was compared to observation in patients with previously resected deep primary melanoma (AJCC, T4N0M0) or regional lymph node positive disease (AJCC, any TN1) [143]. The study accrued 287 patients and reported a significant 5-year relapse-free survival (RFS, 37% vs. 26%, p=0.0023) and 5-year overall survival rate (OS, 46% vs. 37%, p=0.0237) in patients who received IFNα vs. observation. HDI was associated with dosing delays or reductions in about 50% of patients whereas 2/3 of patients experienced severe (grade 3) toxicity during the year of treatment. The high incidence of adverse events along with the overall cost against the small but

Table 1. International and Cooperative Group Trials Utilizing IFNα

Study (ref)	Patient number	Stage	Treatment arm[1]	Outcome	
				DFS	OS
		High dose			
Eastern Cooperative Oncology Group (ECOG)-E1684 [143]	287	IIB III	IFNα-2b 20 MU/m^2 iv qd 5d/wk, x4 wks then 10 MU/m^2 sc tiw, x48 wks	S[2]	S
Eastern COG-E1690 [144]	642	IIB III	IFNα-2b 20 MU/m^2 iv qd 5d/wk, x4 wks then 10 MU/m^2 sc tiw, x48 wks vs. 3 MU tiw, x2 yrs	S	NS
Eastern COG-E1694 [145]	774	IIB III	IFNα-2b 20 MU/m^2 iv qd 5d/wk, x4 wks then 10 MU/m^2 sc tiw, x48 wks vs. GMK vaccine 1cc sc on d1, 8, 15, 22 q12 wks (wks 12 to 96)	NS	NS
North Central Cancer Treatment Group 83-7052 [146]	262	IIB III	IFNα-2a 20 MU/m^2 im qd, x3 m	NS	NS
		Intermediate dose			
European Organization for Research and Treatment of Cancer (EORTC)			IFNα-2b 10 MU sc 5d/wk, x4 wks then 10 MU sc tiw, x1 yr vs.	NS	NS
Melanoma Trial 18952	1418	IIB III	IFNα-2b 10 MU sc 5d/wk, x4 wks then 5 MU sc tiw, x2 yrs		
		Low dose			
Scottish Melanoma Cooperative Trial [147]	96	II III	IFNα-2b 3 MU sc tiw, x6 m	NS	NS
Austrian Melanoma Cooperative Trial [148]	311	II	IFNα-2a 3 MU sc qd x3 wks then 3 MU sc tiw, x1 yr	S	NS
French Melanoma Cooperative Trial [149]	499	II	IFNα-2a 3 MU sc tiw, x18 m	NSNS	NS
World Health Organization-Melanoma Trial-16 [150]	444	IIB III	IFNα-2a 3 MU sc tiw, x3 yrs	NSNS	NS
AIM HIGH (UKCCCR) [151]	654	IIB III	IFNα-2a 3 MU sc tiw, x2 yrs	NS	NS

EORTC 18871/DKG-80 [152]	830	IIB III	IFNα-2b 1 MU sc alternate days, x1 yr vs. IFNγ 0.2 mg sc alternate days, x1 yr vs. Iscador M®	NS	NS

Abbreviations: MRC, Medical Research Council; MPA, medroxyprogesterone acetate; po, orally; qd, every day; bid, twice a day; VLB, vinblastine; 5-FU, 5-fluouracil; civ, continuous intravenous infusion; DGCIN, German Cooperative Renal Carcinoma Chemoimmunotherapy Group [1]statistically significant unless reported otherwise

significant overall survival benefit raised serious societal questions regarding the overall benefit. A series of quality of life (QOL) analyses were performed based on the E1684 trial which showed that IFNα-treated patients had more QOL-adjusted survival time than the observation group [153] and overall costs per life-year of quality-adjusted life-years which are less compared to other accepted adjuvant therapies of breast and colorectal cancer [154]. However the severe toxicity profile and the non-uniform acceptance of HDI by the medical community led to testing of less intense IFNα schedules. The E1690 trial was designed to compare high dose and low dose IFNa (LDI). 642 patients with completely resected deep primary or regional lymph node involvement were randomized to receive either standard HDI, or LDI given for longer periods (IFNα2b, 3 MU s.c., tiw for two-years) or observation [144]. At a median follow up of 52 months, comparison of the hazard ratios of the treatment arms vs. observation for RFS showed statistical significance only for the HDI arm (1.28 vs. 1.19) whereas neither study arm showed any OS benefit. The paradoxical absence of any OS benefit in the E1690 compared to the E1684 trial, while the RFS benefit of HDI was the same was mainly attributed to the confounding effect of post-relapse 'crossover' to HDI treatment of patients who were assigned to the observation arm and relapsed, since the E1690 trial was conducted in part before, but in part after, the FDA approval of HDI. The Intergroup E1694 study attempted to resolve the discrepancy regarding the overall survival benefit or not by HDI of the previous 2 HDI trials. Furthermore, it compared the efficacy of a vaccine preparation designed against the most immunogenic ganglioside expressed on melanoma cells (ganglioside GM2, GMK vaccine, Progenics, Inc, Tarrytown NY), which had earlier shown in a single-institution phase III study to induce antibody response against GM2 that was correlated with improved RFS and OS in stage III melanoma patients [155]. 880 patients with stage IIB/III melanoma were assigned to either the GMK vaccine (for 96 weeks) or the standard HDI treatment [145]. The study was unblinded at a median follow up of 1.3 yrs at the decision of the external data safety and monitoring committee, when the interim analysis revealed the superiority of HDI in both DFS and OS.

The updated results (median follow up intervals of 2.1-12.6 years) of all major 3 trials showed that although the HDI-induced RFS benefit is consistent and durable compared with observation there is not OS benefit associated with HDI [156]. This may be because of development of HDI-related long term side effects that have not been studied beyond the time of follow up [157]. However, no other IFNα regimen in melanoma has ever shown consistent OS benefit in prospective randomized controlled studies except for inconsistent DFS benefit [148].

The molecular mechanism accounting for the clinical benefit of HDI in the adjuvant setting for melanoma was examined in a neoadjuvant study of 20 patients with palpable regional lymphadenopathy (AJCC Stage IIIB & C) who had initial pretreatment excisional biopsy followed by the standard induction-intravenous HDI. The intravenous phase was then followed by definitive lymph node dissection and subsequent completion of standard subcutaneous maintenance HDI. At 4 weeks of assessment standard intravenous HDI was associated with 55% response rate. Moreover, clinical responders compared to non-responders had a longer DFS and OS and more significant increase in the number $CD3^+$ and $CD11c^+$ mononuclear cells infiltrating the tumor detected by immunohistochemistry on tumor biopsies before and after 4 weeks of treatment. There were no significant changes in angiogenesis or expression of melanoma antigens, overall suggesting that the effect of HDI may be more indirect and immunomodulatory rather than direct and cytotoxic. Future studies need to address the issue of predictive markers of IFNα response in order to apply this treatment schedule to a more selective group of patients who would most likely respond to treatment.

The Past: Failed Combinations of IFN with other Agents

It was thought that the efficacy of IFNα treatment would increase if IFNα would be combined with other treatment modalities. Based on preclinical studies that type I IFNs were thought to exert a radiosensitizing effect on tumor cells *external beam radiation therapy* was combined with IFNs in non small cell lung cancer [158], melanoma [159] and rectal cancer [160] with uniform significantly increased toxicity without any overall benefit. The combination of IFNα with other conventional chemotherapeutic agents and biologic agents (*biochemotherapy*) significantly increased overall toxicity of the regimen although the results from several phase II studies were promising with high objective response rates [161]. However, no phase III randomized cooperative group controlled study in melanoma and other tumors ever showed improvement in overall survival [162, 163]. The reason(s) for this failure may be twofold: In the overall regimen administered the fractional dose of IFNα given was small, which we now know plays significant role based on the direct experience from the randomized prospective studies of adjuvant IFNα in melanoma and other indirect evidence [164]. Also, several of the chemotherapeutic agents added may antagonize the immunomodulatory role of IFNα and promote immunosuppression [165]. Although in preclinical studies retinoids may synergize with IFNs in promoting differentiation, combination of IFNα with retinoids has shown conflicting results in different malignancies [141, 142, 166]. Finally IFNα did not potentiate the anti-angiogenic effect of endostatin in patients with metastatic melanoma [167].

The Future: Rational Combinations of Interferons with other Agents.

The clinical benefit of HDI in stage III melanoma combined with its limited efficacy in stage IV disease implies that IFNα resistance may be potentially overcome by building other molecularly targeted therapies upon HDI (reviewed in [115]). *Melanoma vaccines* have been investigated for more than 40 years and most of the vaccine-induced immune responses have been transient and with no correlation with clinical outcomes. Only recently have melanoma vaccines became more well defined and evaluated in terms of intermediate immunological endpoints resulting in their testing by Cooperative Group evaluations, such as in the recent phase II trial E1696 and the ongoing E4697 in which preliminary analysis showed suggestion for overall survival benefit in patients who have been successfully vaccinated [168]. A number of murine [169, 170] as well as small clinical studies [171, 172] have suggested that type I IFNs may enhance immune response to vaccination or may recall immune response of previously vaccinated subjects resulting in objective tumor responses. Based on these results we have initiated a clinical study of HDI in patients with metastatic melanoma (UPCI 04-125) who were previously vaccinated with defined melanoma epitopes, but have clinically progressed at the time of study entry. The primary aim of the study is to assess whether HDI can recall previously recorded immunologic responses, defined by ELISPOT.

Gangliosides are complex membranous amphipathic structures specifically overexpressed in a variety of tumors including melanoma. G_{D3} is one of the most abundant gangliosides in melanoma cells [173] and has been shown to 'shed' into the tumor environment where it is passively incorporated by nearby immune cells causing immunosuppression and apoptosis [174]. Anti-G_{D3} murine monoclonal antibody (mAb) R_{24} therapy was used for treatment of metastatic melanoma with a modest (~10%) response rate [175, 176]. The latter was primarily attributed to the development of human anti-mouse antibodies (HAMA), which decreased serum levels of anti-G_{D3} mAb in serum. The more recently developed chimeric anti-G_{D3} mAb (KW2871) exhibits a superior cytotoxic, pharmacodynamic, and pharmacokinetic profile owing in large part to the absence of any detectable HAMA response, long serum half life and superior bioavailability [177]. However these superior properties were not translated into meaningful clinical antitumor response in a recent phase I study of KW2871 in patients with metastatic melanoma [178]. We hypothesize that the lack of antibody efficacy is secondary to tumor-induced immunosuppression which suppresses effector cells in mediating antibody-dependent cell cytotoxicity (ADCC), among other mechanisms. Preliminary results in our lab suggest that IFN at clinically relevant concentrations augments KW2871-mediated cytotoxicity against a G_{D3} expressing melanoma cell line. We therefore plan to investigate the effect of concurrent administration of HDI and KW2871 in response rate and time-to-progression in patients with metastatic melanoma (UPCI-193).

IFNα-mediated induction of apoptosis activates survival and proliferative pathways in tumor cells, such as the *epidermal growth factor receptor* (EGF-R) pathway [179, 180], which abrogates IFNα-induced apoptosis [181, 182]. This adaptive cellular response to IFNα treatment has been clinically exploited in lung cancer. Cancer cells exposed to IFNα became highly sensitive to specific signaling inhibitors ("target prioritization"), such as EGFR inhibitors (ZD1839 Iressa™) [182].

Research on the "two signal model" of T cell activation established that the engagement of CD28 on the T cell surface by the B7-1 and B7-2 on the APC provides the necessary costimulatory signal for T cell activation. The discovery of the *cytotoxic T lymphocyte antigen* (CTLA-4) [183] originally left more questions than answers about its function until the advent of monoclonal antibodies specific for CTLA-4 which suggested that it plays a negative costimulatory role by attenuating T cell activation and expansion (reviewed in [184]). The first clinical trials of CTLA-4 antibody therapy in patients with advanced metastatic melanoma have shown significant response rates, with several durable responses at the cost of significant autoimmune manifestations [103,185]. CTLA-4 blockade and IFNα have common, though complementary mechanisms of action. Their effect is immunomodulatory, promote Th_1 rather than Th_2 responses [186, 187], they affect tryptophan metabolism[188], and promote autoimmunity. Therefore, we plan to study the effect of combination IFNα with CTLA-4 in patients with metastatic melanoma.

REFERENCES

1. Isaacs A, Lindenmann J. Virus Interference, I: Interferon. *Proc Royal Soc Lond* 1957;147:258–67.
2. Gresser I, Belardelli F. Endogenous type I interferons as a defense against tumors. *Cytokine Growth Factor Rev* 2002;13(2):111–8.
3. Dunn GP, Bruce AT, Sheehan KC, et al. A critical function for type I interferons in cancer immunoediting. *Nat Immunol* 2005;6(7):722–9. Epub 2005 Jun 12.
4. Taniguchi T. Construction and Identification of a Bacterial Plasmid Containing the Human Fibroblast Interferon Gene Sequences. *Proc Japan Acad* 1979;55B(464–9).
5. Kontsek P, Karayianni-Vasconcelos G, Kontsekova E. The human interferon system: characterization and classification after discovery of novel members. *Acta Virol* 2003;47(4):201–15.
6. Taniguchi T, Takaoka A. A weak signal for strong responses: interferon-alpha/beta revisited. *Nat Rev Mol Cell Biol* 2001;2(5):378–86.
7. Gohda J, Matsumura T, Inoue J. Cutting edge: TNFR-associated factor (TRAF) 6 is essential for MyD88-dependent pathway but not toll/IL-1 receptor domain-containing adaptor-inducing IFN-beta (TRIF)-dependent pathway in TLR signaling. *J Immunol* 2004;173(5):2913–7.
8. Fitzgerald KA, McWhirter SM, Faia KL, et al. IKKepsilon and TBK1 are essential components of the IRF3 signaling pathway. *Nat Immunol* 2003;4(5):491–6.
9. Takaoka A, Yanai H, Kondo S, et al. Integral role of IRF-5 in the gene induction programme activated by Toll-like receptors. *Nature* 2005;434(7030):243–9.
10. Honda K, Yanai H, Negishi H, et al. IRF-7 is the master regulator of type-I interferon-dependent immune responses. *Nature* 2005;434(7034):772–7.
11. Harada H, Fujita T, Miyamoto M, et al. Structurally similar but functionally distinct factors, IRF-1 and IRF-2, bind to the same regulatory elements of IFN and IFN-inducible genes. *Cell* 1989;58(4):729–39.

12. Sarkar SN, Peters KL, Elco CP, Sakamoto S, Pal S, Sen GC. Novel roles of TLR3 tyrosine phosphorylation and PI3 kinase in double-stranded RNA signaling. *Nat Struct Mol Biol* 2004;11(11): 1060–7.
13. Siren J, Pirhonen J, Julkunen I, Matikainen S. IFN-alpha regulates TLR-dependent gene expression of IFN-alpha, IFN-beta, IL-28, and IL-29. *J Immunol* 2005;174(4):1932–7.
14. Tissari J, Siren J, Meri S, Julkunen I, Matikainen S. IFN-alpha enhances TLR3-mediated antiviral cytokine expression in human endothelial and epithelial cells by up-regulating TLR3 expression. *J Immunol* 2005;174(7):4289–94.
15. Kamath AT, Sheasby CE, Tough DF. Dendritic cells and NK cells stimulate bystander T cell activation in response to TLR agonists through secretion of IFN-alpha beta and IFN-gamma. *J Immunol* 2005;174(2):767–76.
16. Gautier G, Humbert M, Deauvieau F, et al. A type I interferon autocrine-paracrine loop is involved in Toll-like receptor-induced interleukin-12p70 secretion by dendritic cells. *J Exp Med* 2005;201(9):1435–46.
17. Price KL, Herlyn M, Dent CL, Gewert DR, Linge C. The prevalence of interferon-alpha transcription defects in malignant melanoma. *Melanoma Res* 2005;15(2):91–8.
18. Siegal FP, Kadowaki N, Shodell M, et al. The nature of the principal type 1 interferon-producing cells in human blood. *Science* 1999;284(5421):1835–7.
19. Liu YJ. IPC: professional type 1 interferon-producing cells and plasmacytoid dendritic cell precursors. *Annu Rev Immunol* 2005;23:275–306.
20. Zou W, Machelon V, Coulomb-L'Hermin A, et al. Stromal-derived factor-1 in human tumors recruits and alters the function of plasmacytoid precursor dendritic cells. *Nat Med* 2001;7(12):1339–46.
21. Wei S, Kryczek I, Zou L, et al. Plasmacytoid Dendritic Cells Induce CD8+ Regulatory T Cells In Human Ovarian Carcinoma. *Cancer Res* 2005;65(12):5020–6.
22. Hishizawa M, Imada K, Kitawaki T, Ueda M, Kadowaki N, Uchiyama T. Depletion and impaired interferon-alpha-producing capacity of blood plasmacytoid dendritic cells in human T-cell leukaemia virus type I-infected individuals. *Br J Haematol* 2004;125(5):568–75.
23. Vermi W, Bonecchi R, Facchetti F, et al. Recruitment of immature plasmacytoid dendritic cells (plasmacytoid monocytes) and myeloid dendritic cells in primary cutaneous melanomas. *J Pathol* 2003;200(2):255–68.
24. Treilleux I, Blay JY, Bendriss-Vermare N, et al. Dendritic cell infiltration and prognosis of early stage breast cancer. *Clin Cancer Res* 2004;10(22):7466–74.
25. Ito K, Tanaka H, Ito T, et al. Initial expression of interferon alpha receptor 2 (IFNAR2) on CD34-positive cells and its down-regulation correlate with clinical response to interferon therapy in chronic myelogenous leukemia. *Eur J Haematol* 2004;73(3):191–205.
26. Massirer KB, Hirata MH, Silva AE, Ferraz ML, Nguyen NY, Hirata RD. Interferon-alpha receptor 1 mRNA expression in peripheral blood mononuclear cells is associated with response to interferon-alpha therapy of patients with chronic hepatitis C. *Braz J Med Biol Res* 2004;37(5):643–7. Epub 2004 Apr 22.
27. Ambrus JL, Sr., Dembinski W, Ambrus JL, Jr., et al. Free interferon-alpha/beta receptors in the circulation of patients with adenocarcinoma. *Cancer* 2003;98(12):2730–3.
28. Leyva L, Fernandez O, Fedetz M, et al. IFNAR1 and IFNAR2 polymorphisms confer susceptibility to multiple sclerosis but not to interferon-beta treatment response. *J Neuroimmunol* 2005;163 (1–2):165–71.
29. Stark GR, Kerr IM, Williams BR, Silverman RH, Schreiber RD. How cells respond to interferons. *Annu Rev Biochem* 1998;67:227–64.
30. Saleh AZ, Fang AT, Arch AE, Neupane D, El Fiky A, Krolewski JJ. Regulated proteolysis of the IFNaR2 subunit of the interferon-alpha receptor. *Oncogene* 2004;23(42):7076–86.
31. Subramaniam PS, Johnson HM. The IFNAR1 subunit of the type I IFN receptor complex contains a functional nuclear localization sequence. *FEBS Lett* 2004;578(3):207–10.
32. Shin-Ya M, Hirai H, Satoh E, et al. Intracellular interferon triggers Jak/Stat signaling cascade and induces p53-dependent antiviral protection. *Biochem Biophys Res Commun* 2005;329(3):1139–46.

33. Platanias LC. Mechanisms of type-I- and type-II-interferon-mediated signalling. *Nat Rev Immunol* 2005;5(5):375–86.
34. Balkwill F, Taylor-Papadimitriou J. Interferon affects both G1 and S+G2 in cells stimulated from quiescence to growth. *Nature* 1978;274(5673):798–800.
35. Takaoka A, Hayakawa S, Yanai H, et al. Integration of interferon-alpha/beta signalling to p53 responses in tumour suppression and antiviral defence. *Nature* 2003;424(6948):516–23.
36. Kumar R, Atlas I. Interferon alpha induces the expression of retinoblastoma gene product in human Burkitt lymphoma Daudi cells: role in growth regulation. *Proc Natl Acad Sci U S A* 1992;89(14):6599–603.
37. Subramaniam PS, Cruz PE, Hobeika AC, Johnson HM. Type I interferon induction of the Cdk-inhibitor p21WAF1 is accompanied by ordered G1 arrest, differentiation and apoptosis of the Daudi B-cell line. *Oncogene* 1998;16(14):1885–90.
38. Tiefenbrun N, Melamed D, Levy N, et al. Alpha interferon suppresses the cyclin D3 and cdc25A genes, leading to a reversible G0-like arrest. *Mol Cell Biol* 1996;16(7):3934–44.
39. Dondi E, Roue G, Yuste VJ, Susin SA, Pellegrini S. A dual role of IFN-alpha in the balance between proliferation and death of human CD4+ T lymphocytes during primary response. *J Immunol* 2004;173(6):3740–7.
40. Ozaki T, Takahashi K, Kanasaki H, Iida K, Miyazaki K. Expression of the type I interferon receptor and the interferon-induced Mx protein in human endometrium during the menstrual cycle. *Fertil Steril* 2005;83(1):163–70.
41. Thyrell L, Erickson S, Zhivotovsky B, et al. Mechanisms of Interferon-alpha induced apoptosis in malignant cells. *Oncogene* 2002;21(8):1251–62.
42. Chawla-Sarkar M, Lindner DJ, Liu YF, et al. Apoptosis and interferons: role of interferon-stimulated genes as mediators of apoptosis. *Apoptosis* 2003;8(3):237–49.
43. Wandinger KP, Lunemann JD, Wengert O, et al. TNF-related apoptosis inducing ligand (TRAIL) as a potential response marker for interferon-beta treatment in multiple sclerosis. *Lancet* 2003;361(9374):2036–43.
44. Shen L, Evel-Kabler K, Strube R, Chen SY. Silencing of SOCS1 enhances antigen presentation by dendritic cells and antigen-specific anti-tumor immunity. *Nat Biotechnol* 2004;22(12):1546–53. Epub 2004 Nov 21.
45. Li Z, Metze D, Nashan D, et al. Expression of SOCS-1, suppressor of cytokine signalling-1, in human melanoma. *J Invest Dermatol* 2004;123(4):737–45.
46. Roman-Gomez J, Jimenez-Velasco A, Castillejo JA, et al. The suppressor of cytokine signaling-1 is constitutively expressed in chronic myeloid leukemia and correlates with poor cytogenetic response to interferon-alpha. *Haematologica* 2004;89(1):42–8.
47. Liu B, Mink S, Wong KA, et al. PIAS1 selectively inhibits interferon-inducible genes and is important in innate immunity. *Nat Immunol* 2004;5(9):891–8. Epub 2004 Aug 15.
48. Lesinski GB, Anghelina M, Zimmerer J, et al. The antitumor effects of IFN-alpha are abrogated in a STAT1-deficient mouse. *J Clin Invest* 2003;112(2):170–80.
49. Lesinski GB, Kondadasula SV, Crespin T, et al. Multiparametric flow cytometric analysis of inter-patient variation in STAT1 phosphorylation following interferon Alfa immunotherapy. *J Natl Cancer Inst* 2004;96(17):1331–42.
50. Jackson DP, Watling D, Rogers NC, et al. The JAK/STAT pathway is not sufficient to sustain the antiproliferative response in an interferon-resistant human melanoma cell line. *Melanoma Res* 2003;13(3):219–29.
51. Lesinski GB, Valentino D, Hade EM, et al. Expression of STAT1 and STAT2 in malignant melanoma does not correlate with response to interferon-alpha adjuvant therapy. *Cancer Immunol Immunother* 2005;25:25.
52. Certa U, Wilhelm-Seiler M, Foser S, Broger C, Neeb M. Expression modes of interferon-alpha inducible genes in sensitive and resistant human melanoma cells stimulated with regular and pegylated interferon-alpha. *Gene* 2003;315:79–86.
53. Wong LH, Krauer KG, Hatzinisiriou I, et al. Interferon-resistant human melanoma cells are deficient in ISGF3 components, STAT1, STAT2, and p48-ISGF3gamma. *J Biol Chem* 1997;272(45):28779–85.

54. Soengas MS, Lowe SW. Apoptosis and melanoma chemoresistance. *Oncogene* 2003;22(20): 3138–51.
55. Sakamoto E, Hato F, Kato T, et al. Type I and type II interferons delay human neutrophil apoptosis via activation of STAT3 and up-regulation of cellular inhibitor of apoptosis 2. *J Leukoc Biol* 2005;78(1):301–9. Epub 2005 Apr 21.
56. Marrack P, Kappler J, Mitchell T. Type I interferons keep activated T cells alive. *J Exp Med* 1999;189(3):521–30.
57. Litinskiy MB, Nardelli B, Hilbert DM, et al. DCs induce CD40-independent immunoglobulin class switching through BLyS and APRIL. *Nat Immunol* 2002;3(9):822–9.
58. Loza MJ, Perussia B. Differential regulation of NK cell proliferation by type I and type II IFN. *Int Immunol* 2004;16(1):23–32.
59. Petricoin EF, 3rd, Ito S, Williams BL, et al. Antiproliferative action of interferon-alpha requires components of T-cell-receptor signalling. *Nature* 1997;390(6660):629–32.
60. Dondi E, Rogge L, Lutfalla G, Uze G, Pellegrini S. Down-modulation of responses to type I IFN upon T cell activation. *J Immunol* 2003;170(2):749–56.
61. Imai K, Ng AK, Glassy MC, Ferrone S. Differential effect of interferon on the expression of tumor-associated antigens and histocompatibility antigens on human melanoma cells: relationship to susceptibility to immune lysis mediated by monoclonal antibodies. *J Immunol* 1981;127(2): 505–9.
62. Wagner SN, Rebmann V, Willers CP, Grosse-Wilde H, Goos M. Expression analysis of classic and non-classic HLA molecules before interferon alfa-2b treatment of melanoma. *Lancet* 2000;356(9225):220–1.
63. Ortaldo JR, Mason A, Rehberg E, et al. Effects of recombinant and hybrid recombinant human leukocyte interferons on cytotoxic activity of natural killer cells. *J Biol Chem* 1983;258(24): 15011–5.
64. Biron CA, Sonnenfeld G, Welsh RM. Interferon induces natural killer cell blastogenesis in vivo. *J Leukoc Biol* 1984;35(1):31–7.
65. Carballido JA, Molto LM, Manzano L, Olivier C, Salmeron OJ, Alvarez de Mon M. Interferon-alpha-2b enhances the natural killer activity of patients with transitional cell carcinoma of the bladder. *Cancer* 1993;72(5):1743–8.
66. Uchida A, Vanky F, Klein E. Natural cytotoxicity of human blood lymphocytes and monocytes and their cytotoxic factors: effect of interferon on target cell susceptibility. *J Natl Cancer Inst* 1985;75(5):849–57.
67. Tough DF, Borrow P, Sprent J. Induction of bystander T cell proliferation by viruses and type I interferon in vivo. *Science* 1996;272(5270):1947–50.
68. Palmer KJ, Harries M, Gore ME, Collins MK. Interferon-alpha (IFN-alpha) stimulates anti-melanoma cytotoxic T lymphocyte (CTL) generation in mixed lymphocyte tumour cultures (MLTC). *Clin Exp Immunol* 2000;119(3):412–8.
69. Steitz J, Bruck J, Lenz J, Knop J, Tuting T. Depletion of CD25(+) CD4(+) T cells and treatment with tyrosinase-related protein 2-transduced dendritic cells enhance the interferon alpha-induced, CD8(+) T-cell-dependent immune defense of B16 melanoma. *Cancer Res* 2001;61(24): 8643–6.
70. Guillot B, Portales P, Thanh AD, et al. The expression of cytotoxic mediators is altered in mononuclear cells of patients with melanoma and increased by interferon-alpha treatment. *Br J Dermatol* 2005;152(4):690–6.
71. Miettinen M, Sareneva T, Julkunen I, Matikainen S. IFNs activate toll-like receptor gene expression in viral infections. *Genes Immun* 2001;2(6):349–55.
72. Gabriele L, Borghi P, Rozera C, et al. IFN-alpha promotes the rapid differentiation of monocytes from patients with chronic myeloid leukemia into activated dendritic cells tuned to undergo full maturation after LPS treatment. *Blood* 2004;103(3):980–7. Epub 2003 Oct 2.
73. Abuzahra F, Heise R, Joussen S, et al. Adjuvant interferon alfa treatment for patients with malignant melanoma stimulates transporter proteins associated with antigen processing and proteasome activator 28. *Lancet Oncol* 2004;5(4):250.

74. Ito T, Amakawa R, Kaisho T, et al. Interferon-alpha and interleukin-12 are induced differentially by Toll-like receptor 7 ligands in human blood dendritic cell subsets. *J Exp Med* 2002;195(11):1507–12.
75. Diebold SS, Montoya M, Unger H, et al. Viral infection switches non-plasmacytoid dendritic cells into high interferon producers. *Nature* 2003;424(6946):324–8. Epub 2003 Jun 22.
76. Pollara G, Jones M, Handley ME, et al. Herpes simplex virus type-1-induced activation of myeloid dendritic cells: the roles of virus cell interaction and paracrine type I IFN secretion. *J Immunol* 2004;173(6):4108–19.
77. Montoya M, Schiavoni G, Mattei F, et al. Type I interferons produced by dendritic cells promote their phenotypic and functional activation. *Blood* 2002;99(9):3263–71.
78. Mattei F, Schiavoni G, Belardelli F, Tough DF. IL-15 is expressed by dendritic cells in response to type I IFN, double-stranded RNA, or lipopolysaccharide and promotes dendritic cell activation. *J Immunol* 2001;167(3):1179–87.
79. Tourkova IL, Yurkovetsky ZR, Gambotto A, et al. Increased function and survival of IL-15-transduced human dendritic cells are mediated by up-regulation of IL-15Ralpha and Bcl-2. *J Leukoc Biol* 2002;72(5):1037–45.
80. Luft T, Pang KC, Thomas E, et al. Type I IFNs enhance the terminal differentiation of dendritic cells. *J Immunol* 1998;161(4):1947–53.
81. Radvanyi LG, Banerjee A, Weir M, Messner H. Low levels of interferon-alpha induce CD86 (B7.2) expression and accelerates dendritic cell maturation from human peripheral blood mononuclear cells. *Scand J Immunol* 1999;50(5):499–509.
82. Carbonneil C, Saidi H, Donkova-Petrini V, Weiss L. Dendritic cells generated in the presence of interferon-alpha stimulate allogeneic CD4+ T-cell proliferation: modulation by autocrine IL-10, enhanced T-cell apoptosis and T regulatory type 1 cells. *Int Immunol* 2004;16(7):1037–52. Epub 2004 Jun 7.
83. Krug A, Veeraswamy R, Pekosz A, et al. Interferon-producing cells fail to induce proliferation of naive T cells but can promote expansion and T helper 1 differentiation of antigen-experienced unpolarized T cells. *J Exp Med* 2003;197(7):899–906.
84. Tosi D, Valenti R, Cova A, et al. Role of cross-talk between IFN-alpha-induced monocyte-derived dendritic cells and NK cells in priming CD8+ T cell responses against human tumor antigens. *J Immunol* 2004;172(9):5363–70.
85. Brinkmann V, Geiger T, Alkan S, Heusser CH. Interferon alpha increases the frequency of interferon gamma-producing human CD4+ T cells. *J Exp Med* 1993;178(5):1655–63.
86. Schandene L, Del Prete GF, Cogan E, et al. Recombinant interferon-alpha selectively inhibits the production of interleukin-5 by human CD4+ T cells. *J Clin Invest* 1996;97(2):309–15.
87. Rogge L, Barberis-Maino L, Biffi M, et al. Selective expression of an interleukin-12 receptor component by human T helper 1 cells. *J Exp Med* 1997;185(5):825–31.
88. Okada H, Tsugawa T, Sato H, et al. Delivery of interferon-alpha transfected dendritic cells into central nervous system tumors enhances the antitumor efficacy of peripheral peptide-based vaccines. *Cancer Res* 2004;64(16):5830–8.
89. Astsaturov I, Petrella T, Bagriacik EU, et al. Amplification of virus-induced antimelanoma T-cell reactivity by high-dose interferon-alpha2b: implications for cancer vaccines. *Clin Cancer Res* 2003;9(12):4347–55.
90. Foster GR, Masri SH, David R, et al. IFN-alpha subtypes differentially affect human T cell motility. *J Immunol* 2004;173(3):1663–70.
91. Gutzmer R, Lisewski M, Zwirner J, et al. Human monocyte-derived dendritic cells are chemoattracted to C3a after up-regulation of the C3a receptor with interferons. *Immunology* 2004;111(4): 435–43.
92. Stylianou E, Yndestad A, Sikkeland LI, et al. Effects of interferon-alpha on gene expression of chemokines and members of the tumour necrosis factor superfamily in HIV-infected patients. *Clin Exp Immunol* 2002;130(2):279–85.
93. Parlato S, Santini SM, Lapenta C, et al. Expression of CCR-7, MIP-3beta, and Th-1 chemokines in type I IFN-induced monocyte-derived dendritic cells: importance for the rapid acquisition of potent migratory and functional activities. *Blood* 2001;98(10):3022–9.

94. Zella D, Barabitskaja O, Casareto L, et al. Recombinant IFN-alpha (2b) increases the expression of apoptosis receptor CD95 and chemokine receptors CCR1 and CCR3 in monocytoid cells. *J Immunol* 1999;163(6):3169–75.
95. Hokeness KL, Kuziel WA, Biron CA, Salazar-Mather TP. Monocyte chemoattractant protein-1 and CCR2 interactions are required for IFN-alpha/beta-induced inflammatory responses and antiviral defense in liver. *J Immunol* 2005;174(3):1549–56.
96. Wenzel J, Uerlich M, Haller O, Bieber T, Tueting T. Enhanced type I interferon signaling and recruitment of chemokine receptor CXCR3-expressing lymphocytes into the skin following treatment with the TLR7-agonist imiquimod. *J Cutan Pathol* 2005;32(4):257–62.
97. Wenzel J, Worenkamper E, Freutel S, et al. Enhanced type I interferon signalling promotes Th1-biased inflammation in cutaneous lupus erythematosus. *J Pathol* 2005;205(4):435–42.
98. Hakansson A, Gustafsson B, Krysander L, Hakansson L. Tumour-infiltrating lymphocytes in metastatic malignant melanoma and response to interferon alpha treatment. *Br J Cancer* 1996;74(5):670–6.
99. Moschos SJ, Edington HD, Rao UN, et al. High dose Interferon- 2b (HDI): Toxicity, response, and predicitve markers in a neoadjuvant trial for regional lymph node metastatic melanoma. 2005. *Proc Am Soc Clin Oncol* 2005;23(16S):714s.
100. Gota C, Calabrese L. Induction of clinical autoimmune disease by therapeutic interferon-alpha. *Autoimmunity* 2003;36(8):511–8.
101. Hooks JJ, Moutsopoulos HM, Geis SA, Stahl NI, Decker JL, Notkins AL. Immune interferon in the circulation of patients with autoimmune disease. *N Engl J Med* 1979;301(1):5–8.
102. Bengtsson AA, Sturfelt G, Truedsson L, et al. Activation of type I interferon system in systemic lupus erythematosus correlates with disease activity but not with antiretroviral antibodies. *Lupus* 2000;9(9):664–71.
103. Sanderson K, Scotland R, Lee P, et al. Autoimmunity in a phase I trial of a fully human anti-cytotoxic T-lymphocyte antigen-4 monoclonal antibody with multiple melanoma peptides and Montanide ISA 51 for patients with resected stages III and IV melanoma. *J Clin Oncol* 2005;23(4):741–50. Epub 2004 Dec 21.
104. Tsoutsos D, Ioannovich J, Frangia K, et al. The prevalence and prognostic significance of autoantibodies detected in patients with high risk melanoma receiving adjuvant therapy with high-dose interferon (Abstr 7519). *Proc Am Soc Clin Oncol* 2005;25.
105. Blanco P, Palucka AK, Gill M, Pascual V, Banchereau J. Induction of dendritic cell differentiation by IFN-alpha in systemic lupus erythematosus. *Science* 2001;294(5546):1540–3.
106. Nestle FO, Conrad C, Tun-Kyi A, et al. Plasmacytoid predendritic cells initiate psoriasis through interferon-{alpha} production. *J Exp Med* 2005;202(1):135–43.
107. Palucka AK, Blanck JP, Bennett L, Pascual V, Banchereau J. Cross-regulation of TNF and IFN-alpha in autoimmune diseases. *Proc Natl Acad Sci U S A* 2005;102(9):3372–7. Epub 2005 Feb 22.
108. Zang GQ, Xi M, Feng ML, Ji Y, Yu YS, Tang ZH. Curative effects of interferon-alpha and HLA-DRB1 -DQA1 and -DQB1 alleles in chronic viral hepatitis B. *World J Gastroenterol* 2004;10(14):2116–8.
109. Wergeland S, Beiske A, Nyland H, et al. IL-10 promoter haplotype influence on interferon treatment response in multiple sclerosis. *Eur J Neurol* 2005;12(3):171–5.
110. Yee LJ, Perez KA, Tang J, van Leeuwen DJ, Kaslow RA. Association of CTLA4 polymorphisms with sustained response to interferon and ribavirin therapy for chronic hepatitis C virus infection. *J Infect Dis* 2003;187(8):1264–71. Epub 2003 Apr 2.
111. Takahashi M, Okada J, Ito K, et al. Electrochemical DNA array for simultaneous genotyping of single-nucleotide polymorphisms associated with the therapeutic effect of interferon. *Clin Chem* 2004;50(3):658–61.
112. Mazziotti G, Sorvillo F, Piscopo M, et al. Innate and Acquired Immune System in Patients Developing Interferon-{alpha}-Related Autoimmune Thyroiditis: A Prospective Study. *J Clin Endocrinol Metab* 2005;90(7):4138–44. Epub 2005 Apr 26.

113. Gutterman JU, Blumenschein GR, Alexanian R, et al. Leukocyte interferon-induced tumor regression in human metastatic breast cancer, multiple myeloma, and malignant lymphoma. *Ann Intern Med* 1980;93(3):399–406.
114. Kirkwood JM, Bender C, Agarwala S, et al. Mechanisms and management of toxicities associated with high-dose interferon alfa-2b therapy. *J Clin Oncol* 2002;20(17):3703–18.
115. Moschos SJ, Kirkwood JM, Konstantinopoulos PA. Present status and future prospects for adjuvant therapy of melanoma: time to build upon the foundation of high-dose interferon alfa-2b. *J Clin Oncol* 2004;22(1):11–4. Epub 2003 Dec 9.
116. Capuron L, Neurauter G, Musselman DL, et al. Interferon-alpha-induced changes in tryptophan metabolism. relationship to depression and paroxetine treatment. *Biol Psychiatry* 2003;54(9): 906–14.
117. Schwartz AL, Thompson JA, Masood N. Interferon-induced fatigue in patients with melanoma: a pilot study of exercise and methylphenidate. *Oncol Nurs Forum* 2002;29(7):E85–90.
118. Kowdley KV. Hematologic side effects of interferon and ribavirin therapy. *J Clin Gastroenterol* 2005;39(1 Suppl):S3–8.
119. Houglum JE. Interferon: mechanisms of action and clinical value. *Clin Pharm* 1983;2(1):20–8.
120. Kirkwood JM, Ernstoff MS, Davis CA, Reiss M, Ferraresi R, Rudnick SA. Comparison of intramuscular and intravenous recombinant alpha-2 interferon in melanoma and other cancers. *Ann Intern Med* 1985;103(1):32–6.
121. Quesada JR, Reuben J, Manning JT, Hersh EM, Gutterman JU. Alpha interferon for induction of remission in hairy-cell leukemia. *N Engl J Med* 1984;310(1):15–8.
122. Vedantham S, Gamliel H, Golomb HM. Mechanism of interferon action in hairy cell leukemia: a model of effective cancer biotherapy. *Cancer Res* 1992;52(5):1056–66.
123. Talpaz M, Kantarjian HM, McCredie K, Trujillo JM, Keating MJ, Gutterman JU. Hematologic remission and cytogenetic improvement induced by recombinant human interferon alpha A in chronic myelogenous leukemia. *N Engl J Med* 1986;314(17):1065–9.
124. Interferon alfa versus chemotherapy for chronic myeloid leukemia: a meta-analysis of seven randomized trials: Chronic Myeloid Leukemia Trialists' Collaborative Group. *J Natl Cancer Inst* 1997;89(21):1616–20.
125. Verma A, Platanias LC. Signaling via the interferon-alpha receptor in chronic myelogenous leukemia cells. *Leuk Lymphoma* 2002;43(4):703–9.
126. de Castro FA, Palma PV, Morais FR, et al. Immunological effects of interferon-alpha on chronic myelogenous leukemia. *Leuk Lymphoma* 2003;44(12):2061–7.
127. Interferon-alpha and survival in metastatic renal carcinoma: early results of a randomised controlled trial. Medical Research Council Renal Cancer Collaborators. *Lancet* 1999;353(9146):14–7.
128. Atzpodien J, Kirchner H, Illiger HJ, et al. IL-2 in combination with IFN- alpha and 5-FU versus tamoxifen in metastatic renal cell carcinoma: long-term results of a controlled randomized clinical trial. *Br J Cancer* 2001;85(8):1130–6.
129. Pyrhonen S, Salminen E, Ruutu M, et al. Prospective randomized trial of interferon alfa-2a plus vinblastine versus vinblastine alone in patients with advanced renal cell cancer. *J Clin Oncol* 1999;17(9):2859–67.
130. Flanigan RC, Salmon SE, Blumenstein BA, et al. Nephrectomy followed by interferon alfa-2b compared with interferon alfa-2b alone for metastatic renal-cell cancer. *N Engl J Med* 2001;345(23):1655–9.
131. Aass N, De Mulder PH, Mickisch GH, et al. Randomized phase II/III trial of interferon Alfa-2a with and without 13-cis-retinoic acid in patients with progressive metastatic renal cell Carcinoma: the European Organisation for Research and Treatment of Cancer Genito-Urinary Tract Cancer Group (EORTC 30951). *J Clin Oncol* 2005;23(18):4172–8.
132. Atzpodien J, Kirchner H, Jonas U, et al. Interleukin-2- and interferon alfa-2a-based immunochemotherapy in advanced renal cell carcinoma: a Prospectively Randomized Trial of the German Cooperative Renal Carcinoma Chemoimmunotherapy Group (DGCIN). *J Clin Oncol* 2004;22(7):1188–94. Epub 2004 Feb 23.

133. Groopman JE, Gottlieb MS, Goodman J, et al. Recombinant alpha-2 interferon therapy for Kaposi's sarcoma associated with the acquired immunodeficiency syndrome. *Ann Intern Med* 1984;100(5):671–6.
134. Real FX, Oettgen HF, Krown SE. Kaposi's sarcoma and the acquired immunodeficiency syndrome: treatment with high and low doses of recombinant leukocyte A interferon. *J Clin Oncol* 1986;4(4):544–51.
135. Evans LM, Itri LM, Campion M, et al. Interferon-alpha 2a in the treatment of acquired immunodeficiency syndrome-related Kaposi's sarcoma. *J Immunother* 1991;10(1):39–50.
136. Krown SE, Gold JW, Niedzwiecki D, et al. Interferon-alpha with zidovudine: safety, tolerance, and clinical and virologic effects in patients with Kaposi sarcoma associated with the acquired immunodeficiency syndrome (AIDS). *Ann Intern Med* 1990;112(11):812–21.
137. Eriksson B, Oberg K, Alm G, et al. Treatment of malignant endocrine pancreatic tumours with human leucocyte interferon. *Lancet* 1986;2(8519):1307–9.
138. Bajetta E, Zilembo N, Di Bartolomeo M, et al. Treatment of metastatic carcinoids and other neuroendocrine tumors with recombinant interferon-alpha-2a. A study by the Italian Trials in Medical Oncology Group. *Cancer* 1993;72(10):3099–105.
139. Yoshida H, Shiratori Y, Moriyama M, et al. Interferon therapy reduces the risk for hepatocellular carcinoma: national surveillance program of cirrhotic and noncirrhotic patients with chronic hepatitis C in Japan. IHIT Study Group. Inhibition of Hepatocarcinogenesis by Interferon Therapy. *Ann Intern Med* 1999;131(3):174–81.
140. Shiratori Y, Ito Y, Yokosuka O, et al. Antiviral therapy for cirrhotic hepatitis C: association with reduced hepatocellular carcinoma development and improved survival. *Ann Intern Med* 2005;142(2):105–14.
141. Shin DM, Khuri FR, Murphy B, et al. Combined interferon-alfa, 13-cis-retinoic acid, and alpha-tocopherol in locally advanced head and neck squamous cell carcinoma: novel bioadjuvant phase II trial. *J Clin Oncol* 2001;19(12):3010–7.
142. Shin DM, Glisson BS, Khuri FR, et al. Phase II and biologic study of interferon alfa, retinoic acid, and cisplatin in advanced squamous skin cancer. *J Clin Oncol* 2002;20(2):364–70.
143. Kirkwood JM, Strawderman MH, Ernstoff MS, Smith TJ, Borden EC, Blum RH. Interferon alfa-2b adjuvant therapy of high-risk resected cutaneous melanoma: the Eastern Cooperative Oncology Group Trial EST 1684. *J Clin Oncol* 1996;14(1):7–17.
144. Kirkwood JM, Ibrahim JG, Sondak VK, et al. High- and low-dose interferon alfa-2b in high-risk melanoma: first analysis of intergroup trial E1690/S9111/C9190. *J Clin Oncol* 2000;18(12):2444–58.
145. Kirkwood JM, Ibrahim JG, Sosman JA, et al. High-dose interferon alfa-2b significantly prolongs relapse-free and overall survival compared with the GM2-KLH/QS-21 vaccine in patients with resected stage IIB-III melanoma: results of intergroup trial E1694/S9512/C509801. *J Clin Oncol* 2001;19(9):2370–80.
146. Creagan ET, Dalton RJ, Ahmann DL, et al. Randomized, surgical adjuvant clinical trial of recombinant interferon alfa-2a in selected patients with malignant melanoma. *J Clin Oncol* 1995;13(11):2776–83.
147. Cameron DA, Cornbleet MC, Mackie RM, et al. Adjuvant interferon alpha 2b in high risk melanoma - the Scottish study. *Br J Cancer* 2001;84(9):1146–9.
148. Pehamberger H, Soyer HP, Steiner A, et al. Adjuvant interferon alfa-2a treatment in resected primary stage II cutaneous melanoma. Austrian Malignant Melanoma Cooperative Group. *J Clin Oncol* 1998;16(4):1425–9.
149. Grob JJ, Dreno B, de la Salmoniere P, et al. Randomised trial of interferon alpha-2a as adjuvant therapy in resected primary melanoma thicker than 1.5 mm without clinically detectable node metastases. French Cooperative Group on Melanoma. *Lancet* 1998;351(9120):1905–10.
150. Cascinelli N, Belli F, MacKie RM, Santinami M, Bufalino R, Morabito A. Effect of long-term adjuvant therapy with interferon alpha-2a in patients with regional node metastases from cutaneous melanoma: a randomised trial. *Lancet* 2001;358(9285):866–9.

151. Hancock BW, Wheatley K, Harris S, et al. Adjuvant interferon in high-risk melanoma: the AIM HIGH Study–United Kingdom Coordinating Committee on Cancer Research randomized study of adjuvant low-dose extended-duration interferon Alfa-2a in high-risk resected malignant melanoma. *J Clin Oncol* 2004;22(1):53–61. Epub 2003 Dec 9.
152. Kleeberg UR, Suciu S, Brocker EB, et al. Final results of the EORTC 18871/DKG 80–1 randomised phase III trial. rIFN-alpha2b versus rIFN-gamma versus ISCADOR M versus observation after surgery in melanoma patients with either high-risk primary (thickness >3 mm) or regional lymph node metastasis. *Eur J Cancer* 2004;40(3):390–402.
153. Cole BF, Gelber RD, Kirkwood JM, Goldhirsch A, Barylak E, Borden E. Quality-of-life-adjusted survival analysis of interferon alfa-2b adjuvant treatment of high-risk resected cutaneous melanoma: an Eastern Cooperative Oncology Group study. *J Clin Oncol* 1996;14(10):2666–73.
154. Hillner BE, Kirkwood JM, Atkins MB, Johnson ER, Smith TJ. Economic analysis of adjuvant interferon alfa-2b in high-risk melanoma based on projections from Eastern Cooperative Oncology Group 1684. *J Clin Oncol* 1997;15(6):2351–8.
155. Livingston PO, Wong GY, Adluri S, et al. Improved survival in stage III melanoma patients with GM2 antibodies: a randomized trial of adjuvant vaccination with GM2 ganglioside. *J Clin Oncol* 1994;12(5):1036–44.
156. Kirkwood JM, Manola J, Ibrahim J, Sondak V, Ernstoff MS, Rao U. A pooled analysis of eastern cooperative oncology group and intergroup trials of adjuvant high-dose interferon for melanoma. *Clin Cancer Res* 2004;10(5):1670–7.
157. Sonnenblick M, Rosin A. Cardiotoxicity of interferon. A review of 44 cases. *Chest* 1991;99(3): 557–61.
158. Bradley JD, Scott CB, Paris KJ, et al. A phase III comparison of radiation therapy with or without recombinant beta-interferon for poor-risk patients with locally advanced non-small-cell lung cancer (RTOG 93–04). *Int J Radiat Oncol Biol Phys* 2002;52(5):1173–9.
159. Gyorki DE, Ainslie J, Joon ML, Henderson MA, Millward M, McArthur GA. Concurrent adjuvant radiotherapy and interferon-alpha2b for resected high risk stage III melanoma – a retrospective single centre study. *Melanoma Res* 2004;14(3):223–30.
160. Perera F, Fisher B, Kocha W, Plewes E, Taylor M, Vincent M. A phase I pilot study of pelvic radiation and alpha-2A interferon in patients with locally advanced or recurrent rectal cancer. *Int J Radiat Oncol Biol Phys* 1997;37(2):297–303.
161. Legha SS, Ring S, Eton O, et al. Development of a biochemotherapy regimen with concurrent administration of cisplatin, vinblastine, dacarbazine, interferon alfa, and interleukin-2 for patients with metastatic melanoma. *J Clin Oncol* 1998;16(5):1752–9.
162. Falkson CI, Ibrahim J, Kirkwood JM, Coates AS, Atkins MB, Blum RH. Phase III trial of dacarbazine versus dacarbazine with interferon alpha-2b versus dacarbazine with tamoxifen versus dacarbazine with interferon alpha-2b and tamoxifen in patients with metastatic malignant melanoma: an Eastern Cooperative Oncology Group study. *J Clin Oncol* 1998;16(5):1743–51.
163. Atkins MB, Lee S, Flaherty EJ, Sosman JA, Sondak VK, Kirkwood JM. A prospective randomized phase III trial of concurrent biochemotherapy (BCT) with cisplatin, vinblastine, dacarbazine (CVD), IL-2 and interferon alpha-2b (IFN) versus CVD alone in patients with metastatic melanoma (E3695): An ECOG-coordinated intergroup trial (abstract 2847). *Proc Am Soc Clin Oncol* 2003.
164. Fluck M, Kamanabrou D, Lippold A, Reitz M, Atzpodien J. Dose-dependent treatment benefit in high-risk melanoma patients receiving adjuvant high-dose interferon alfa-2b. *Cancer Biother Radiopharm* 2005;20(3):280–9.
165. Su YB, Sohn S, Krown SE, et al. Selective CD4+ lymphopenia in melanoma patients treated with temozolomide: a toxicity with therapeutic implications. *J Clin Oncol* 2004;22(4):610–6. Epub 2004 Jan 15.
166. Motzer RJ, Murphy BA, Bacik J, et al. Phase III trial of interferon alfa-2a with or without 13-cis-retinoic acid for patients with advanced renal cell carcinoma. *J Clin Oncol* 2000;18(16):2972–80.
167. Moschos SJ, Odoux C, Land SR, et al. Endostatin plus Interferon-a2b therapy in patients with metastatic melanoma: a novel anti-angiogenic and immumodulatory cancer treatment. *submitted*.

168. Kirkwood JM, Lee S, Land S, et al. E1696: Final analysis of the clinical and immunological results of a multicenter ECOG phase II trial of multi-epitope peptide vaccination for stage IV melanoma with MART-1 (27–35), gp100 (209–210M), and tyrosinase (368–376, 370D) (MGT) +/- IFNa2b and GM-CSF (abstr 7502). Proc Am Soc Clin Oncol, 2004.
169. Okada H, Tsugawa T, Sato H, et al. Delivery of interferon-alpha transfected dendritic cells into central nervous system tumors enhances the antitumor efficacy of peripheral peptide-based vaccines. *Cancer Res* 2004;64(16):5830–8.
170. Arico E, Robertson K, Allen D, Ferrantini M, Belardelli F, Nash AA. Humoral immune response and protection from viral infection in mice vaccinated with inactivated MHV-68: effects of type I interferon. *J Interferon Cytokine Res* 2002;22(11):1081–8.
171. Gehring S, Gregory SH, Kuzushita N, Wands JR. Type 1 interferon augments DNA-based vaccination against hepatitis C virus core protein. *J Med Virol* 2005;75(2):249–57.
172. Astsaturov I, Petrella T, Bagriacik EU, et al. Amplification of virus-induced antimelanoma T-cell reactivity by high-dose interferon-alpha2b: implications for cancer vaccines. *Clin Cancer Res* 2003;9(12):4347–55.
173. Dippold WG, Dienes HP, Knuth A, Meyer zum Buschenfelde KH. Immunohistochemical localization of ganglioside GD3 in human malignant melanoma, epithelial tumors, and normal tissues. *Cancer Res* 1985;45(8):3699–705.
174. Caldwell S, Heitger A, Shen W, Liu Y, Taylor B, Ladisch S. Mechanisms of ganglioside inhibition of APC function. *J Immunol* 2003;171(4):1676–83.
175. Vadhan-Raj S, Cordon-Cardo C, Carswell E, et al. Phase I trial of a mouse monoclonal antibody against GD3 ganglioside in patients with melanoma: induction of inflammatory responses at tumor sites. *J Clin Oncol* 1988;6(10):1636–48.
176. Kirkwood JM, Mascari RA, Edington HD, et al. Analysis of therapeutic and immunologic effects of R(24) anti-GD3 monoclonal antibody in 37 patients with metastatic melanoma. *Cancer* 2000;88(12):2693–702.
177. Lee FT, Rigopoulos A, Hall C, et al. Specific localization, gamma camera imaging, and intracellular trafficking of radiolabelled chimeric anti-G(D3) ganglioside monoclonal antibody KM871 in SK-MEL-28 melanoma xenografts. *Cancer Res* 2001;61(11):4474–82.
178. Scott AM, Lee FT, Hopkins W, et al. Specific targeting, biodistribution, and lack of immunogenicity of chimeric anti-GD3 monoclonal antibody KM871 in patients with metastatic melanoma: results of a phase I trial. *J Clin Oncol* 2001;19(19):3976–87.
179. Qu XJ, Yang JL, Russell PJ, Goldstein D. Changes in epidermal growth factor receptor expression in human bladder cancer cell lines following interferon-alpha treatment. *J Urol* 2004;172(2): 733–8.
180. Budillon A, Tagliaferri P, Caraglia M, et al. Upregulation of epidermal growth factor receptor induced by alpha-interferon in human epidermoid cancer cells. *Cancer Res* 1991;51(4): 1294–9.
181. Boccellino M, Giuberti G, Quagliuolo L, et al. Apoptosis induced by interferon-alpha and antagonized by EGF is regulated by caspase-3-mediated cleavage of gelsolin in human epidermoid cancer cells. *J Cell Physiol* 2004;201(1):71–83.
182. Tagliaferri P, Caraglia M, Budillon A, et al. New pharmacokinetic and pharmacodynamic tools for interferon-alpha (IFN-alpha) treatment of human cancer. *Cancer Immunol Immunother* 2005;54(1):1–10.
183. Brunet JF, Denizot F, Luciani MF, et al. A new member of the immunoglobulin superfamily–CTLA-4. *Nature* 1987;328(6127):267–70.
184. Egen JG, Kuhns MS, Allison JP. CTLA-4: new insights into its biological function and use in tumor immunotherapy. *Nat Immunol* 2002;3(7):611–8.
185. Phan GQ, Yang JC, Sherry RM, et al. Cancer regression and autoimmunity induced by cytotoxic T lymphocyte-associated antigen 4 blockade in patients with metastatic melanoma. *Proc Natl Acad Sci U S A* 2003;100(14):8372–7. Epub 2003 Jun 25.
186. Ubaldi V, Gatta L, Pace L, Doria G, Pioli C. CTLA-4 engagement inhibits Th2 but not Th1 cell polarisation. *Clin Dev Immunol* 2003;10(1):13–7.

187. Reuben JM, Lee BN, Shen DY, et al. Therapy with human monoclonal anti-CTLA-4 antibody, CP-675,206, reduces regulatory T cells and IL-10 production in patients with advanced malignant melanoma (MM). 2005.
188. Boasso A, Herbeuval JP, Hardy AW, Winkler C, Shearer GM. Regulation of indoleamine 2,3-dioxygenase and tryptophanyl-tRNA-synthetase by CTLA-4-Fc in human CD4+ T cells. *Blood* 2005;105(4):1574–81. Epub 2004 Oct 5.

CHAPTER 19

HIGH DOSE INTERLEUKIN-2 THERAPY

CHRISTIAN A. PETRULIO, GAIL DERAFFELE,
AND HOWARD L. KAUFMAN*

The Tumor Immunology Laboratory, Division of Surgical Oncology, Columbia University, New York, NY USA

Keywords: Immunotherapy, Interleukin-2, Melanoma, Renal Cell Carcinoma, Treatment

INTRODUCTION

Interleukin-2 (IL-2) is a cytokine that is produced predominantly by activated T lymphocytes and acts in an autocrine manner to promote the proliferation and effector function of T cells. The recognition that T cells depended on IL-2 for growth and differentiation revolutionized the field of T cell biology since exposure of T cells to IL-2 in vitro provided a mechanism for prolonging T cell survival and manipulating T cell responses under experimental conditions. Following the availability of recombinant IL-2 in the late 1970's, studies documented the ability of IL-2 to support the development of lymphocyte activated killer (LAK) cells from peripheral blood and later tumor-infiltrating lymphocytes (TIL) from established tumors. In early clinical studies pioneered by Steven A. Rosenberg patients with cancer were treated with adoptively transferred LAK or TIL cells and survival of these cells in vivo was maintained by adjuvant IL-2. Careful analysis of these early clinical trials suggested that metastatic melanoma and renal cell carcinoma were the most responsive tumors to this form of immunotherapy. Further analysis also revealed that IL-2 alone was responsible for much of the therapeutic activity of the regimen, and this was subsequently confirmed in several animal models.

*Chief, Division of Surgical Oncology, Columbia University Medical Center, 177 Fort Washington Avenue, MHB-7SK, New York, NY USA E-mail: hlk2003@columbia.edu

H.L. Kaufman and J.D. Wolchok (eds.), General Principles of Tumor Immunotherapy, 431–452.

The effects of high-dose IL-2 was later confirmed in clinical trials conducted by the Cytokine Working Group. In general, high-dose, bolus IL-2 administration results in a defined objective clinical response in 15–20% of melanoma and renal cell carcinoma patients with durable complete responses in 5–10% of patients. These data resulted in FDA approval of high-dose IL-2 for metastatic renal cell carcinoma in 1992 and for metastatic melanoma in 1998.

While high-dose IL-2 resulted in durable clinical responses, treatment was often associated with significant toxicity. In early studies a mortality rate of approximately 2% was reported with high-dose IL-2 administration. The deaths reported in early IL-2 studies was largely related to bacterial sepsis as it was not recognized that patients receiving high-dose IL-2 are susceptible to infection due to a limited period of neutrophil dysfunction. In 1990 the use of gram positive antibiotic coverage became routine and the number of deaths from IL-2 in experienced centers decreased dramatically. Furthermore, the induction of a capillary leak syndrome by IL-2 characterized by hypotension, decreased vascular tone and third space fluid sequestration has allowed a more rationale management plan for preventing and/or treating the adverse effects of IL-2. Despite our understanding of IL-2 pharmacology and toxicology, high-dose IL-2 is still best administered at centers with expertise and facilities designed for managing patients undergoing intensive therapy with immunologic agents. The availability of physicians and nurses with such expertise and patient access to such centers currently limit the number of patients receiving IL-2.

In 2006, an estimated 59,580 new cases of metastatic melanoma and 31,160 new cases of renal cell carcinoma will be diagnosed in the United States [1]. Together, they will account for more than 20,000 deaths. Melanoma and renal cell carcinoma have both been highly resistant to chemotherapy although recent evidence does support the role of tyrosine kinase inhibitors as potential therapeutic agents, especially in renal cell carcinoma. There has not, however, been consistent evidence that these agents result in survival benefit. Thus, high-dose IL-2 remains the treatment of choice for patients with metastatic melanoma or renal cell carcinoma who can tolerate treatment. Additional investigation combining IL-2 with molecular pathway inhibitors will be a furtive area of research. Ideally, a biomarker that can identify patients likely to respond to IL-2 prior to treatment would significantly improve our management of these patients.

Although IL-2 was introduced to clinical trials over 20 years ago and has been approved since 1992 the mechanism responsible for tumor regression in IL-2 treated patients is not entirely defined. Preliminary data strongly supported a role for activated T cells or natural killer (NK) cells in IL-2 mediated tumor rejection. There is now, however, data suggesting that IL-2 may actually promote the activity of a naturally occurring regulatory T cell population that suppresses anti-tumor T cell responses. These new insights into the biology of IL-2 need to be reconciled with the clinical observations of therapeutic benefit in selected patients [2]. Clearly, a better understanding of the biology of IL-2 is needed to select appropriate patients for treatment with IL-2 and to increase the likelihood of beneficial responses for those patients receiving IL-2 therapy. This chapter will focus on the clinical management of patients treated with high-dose IL-2, particularly those with metastatic melanoma or renal cell carcinoma. The chapter will emphasize our current understanding of IL-2 biology, the clinical evidence supporting high-dose IL-2, the indications for IL-2, selection of patients for treatment and management of IL-2 related toxicity.

BIOLOGY OF INTERLEUKIN-2

Interleukin-2 is a four bundle α-helical cytokine produced mainly by activated T lymphocytes. It binds to the high-affinity IL-2 receptor (IL-2R), which consists of three subunits—the α-chain (CD25), the β-chain (CD122), and the common cytokine receptor γc-chain (CD132), of which only the latter two are required for signal transduction. Janus activated kinase (JAK) 1 and 3 are associated with the IL-2Rβ and γc chains, respectively, and phosphorylate tyrosine kinase residues in the cytoplasmic tail of the IL-2R after trimerization of the receptor complex. These events amplify downstream pathways of the mitogen-activated protein kinase (MAPK) and signal transducers and activators of transcription (STAT) pathways initiating T-cell proliferation and cytokine release [3]. Activated T cells and regulatory T cells express high levels of IL-2Rα, whereas, IL-2Rβ and γc are shared by other cytokine receptors. For example, the IL-2Rβ is a component of the IL-15 receptor and is also expressed on NK cells, NKT cells and $CD8^+$ memory T cells. The γc chain is expressed on most hemoatopoietic cells and is a subunit of the receptors for IL-4, IL-7, IL-9, IL-15, and IL-21 [4,5].

IL-2 was first described and studied as a growth factor and promoter of T-cell immunity. The ability of IL-2 to provide a stimulus for T cell survival led to its use *in vivo* as an agent for supporting the survival of adoptively transferred lymphokine-activated killer (LAK) and tumor-infiltrating lymphocyte (TIL) cells [6]. Subsequent studies demonstrated that single agent IL-2 had anti-tumor activity in murine tumor models and in patients with metastatic renal cell carcinoma and melanoma. The mechanism of this effect was thought to be related to the T-cell growth promoting effects of IL-2 on naturally occurring tumor-specific T cells. This was supported by the frequent finding of infiltrating T cells at sites of tumor regression following treatment with IL-2 [7]. This mechanism was questioned when IL-2 and IL-2R knockout mice showed unexpected lymphoproliferation followed by lethal autoimmunity [8–10] suggesting that IL-2 played a critical role in regulating T-cell homeostasis and may be even more important for maintenance of tolerance. Thus, it was hypothesized that lymphoproliferation in IL-2 deficient mice was due to failure of IL-2 to sensitize autoreactive T cells to undergo apoptosis. Further studies, however, implicated the role of IL-2 in maintaining $CD4^+CD25^+$ regulatory T (Treg) cells, a population that inhibits autoreactive and tumor-reactive T cells. There is increasing evidence that IL-2/IL-2R signaling plays a major role in the development and activation of Tregs. In fact, the number of Tregs is markedly reduced in mice that are deficient in IL-2, IL-2R, or STAT5, and administration of IL-2 or re-introduction of IL-2-producing cells to IL-2-deficient mice restores the production of Tregs and lymphoid homeostasis [11–14]. Adoptive transfer of wild-type Treg cells to IL-2Rβ or STAT5-deficient mice prevents lymphoproliferation and lethal autoimmunity [12–18]. Thymic expression of IL-2Rβ in *IL-2R*β knockout mice reconstitutes the production of Tregs and prevents lymphoproliferation and lethal autoimmunity [11, 12].

There is also data to support the role of IL-2 in regulating Treg function. CD62L is a Treg-cell ligand necessary for lymphocyte homing to lymph nodes. It has been shown that IL-2 is necessary for optimal CD62L expression on these cells, and its lack of expression in IL-2- and IL-2R-deficient animals might lead to improper trafficking of Tregs accounting for their low numbers [13].

In contrast to the effects of IL-2 on Tregs, IL-2 also plays a role in promoting effector T cells functions and thus induction of T cell immunity. This is supported by three significant observations from *in vitro* studies. First, IL-2 has potent T cell growth-factor activity as documented by the effects of exogenous IL-2 on recently activated $CD4^+$ and $CD8^+$ T cells, which undergo clonal expansion in the presence of IL-2. Second, T cell proliferation and function can be inhibited by monoclonal antibodies specific for IL-2 or the IL-2R [14, 15] with blockade of the IL-2/IL-2R interaction abrogating T-cell proliferation. Finally, IL-2 sensitizes activated T cells to undergo apoptosis or activation-induced cell death (AICD) by fas- and TNF-dependent pathways, which was postulated to account for the lymphoproliferation and autoimmunity associated with IL-2- and IL-2R-deficiency [16].

These findings, however, were not borne out in *in vivo* studies, where IL-2 has been shown to be dispensable for T-cell immunity. *IL-2* knockout mice developed protective immunity and recall responses after infection with various immune-stimulating agents [17, 20]. In many of these studies, both antigen-specific clonal expansion and contraction were observed, suggesting that IL-2 is not mandatory for either function *in vivo*, despite earlier *in vitro* findings. Studies have shown that IL-2 may be required for optimal late stage effector responses, however, and the absence of signaling induced by IL-2 leads to an almost normal increase in the number of antigen-specific T cells in secondary lymphoid tissues but lower levels of effector-cell responses and fewer antigen-specific T cells in non-lymphoid tissues [18, 19]. Malek and colleagues postulated a model in which TCR and co-stimulatory molecules induce limited clonal expansion of T cells, but that their extensive amplification and differentiation into effector cells requires signaling through the IL-2R *in vitro* but not *in vivo* - likely due to sufficient redundancy obviating the need for IL-2 [13]. Thus, the emerging data suggests that IL-2 has a mandatory role in Treg expansion and functional regulation, but a non-essential role in T cell proliferation and activation. Further research is needed to better understand how IL-2 mediates T cell homeostasis *in vivo* and this information can be used to better apply IL-2 as a therapeutic agent alone or in combination with other immunotherapeutic and non-immunotherapeutic drugs.

CLINICAL TRIALS SUPPORTING HIGH DOSE INTERLEUKIN-2 FOR METASTATIC MELANOMA

Recombinant IL-2 became available in 1976 and Rosenberg and colleagues injected mice with IL-2 stimulated lymphocytes, demonstrating regression of pulmonary metastases derived from sarcoma and melanoma cell lines [21, 22]. They went on to show that directly administered high-dose IL-2 generated LAK cell-mediated regression of metastases with a strong-dose response relationship [22]. A phase I clinical study conducted by Rosenberg and colleagues confirmed the safety of administering IL-2 and LAK cells in 1985 [23]. In this study, they treated 25 patients with a variety of refractory tumors, including seven with melanoma. Eleven of the 25 patients had a partial response, with 7 of the 11 responding patients being melanoma patients, and these responses seemed to be durable. Lotze and colleagues treated ten patients with high-dose IL-2 alone, six of whom had melanoma [24]. They found that three of the six melanoma patients showed disease regression, whereas the remaining patients, with colorectal or ovarian cancer, showed no response. Biopsy material from regressing lesions showed marked lymphocytic infiltrate. Following this, 157 patients were treated with either high-dose IL-2 alone or with autologous transfer of LAK cells [25]. Of the 106 patients treated with combination therapy, 21.6% had an objective response with 7.5% having a complete response. Of the 46 patients treated with IL-2 alone, 13% had an objective response with a complete response seen in only one patient (2.1%). The complete responses were durable in both arms of the study.

Between 1985 and 1993, clinical trials investigated the efficacy of single-agent high-dose IL-2. These studies included a total of 270 patients with metastatic melanoma. IL-2 was administered at doses ranging from 360,000 to 720,000 IU/kg given intravenously over 15 minutes every 8 hours for up to 14 doses over five days as tolerated. IL-2 was administered in settings with maximal supportive care, including pressor support for hypotension. The first cycle was followed by a second cycle after six to nine days of recovery. The two cycles comprised one course of IL-2 treatment, and further courses were given every six to twelve weeks as tolerated. Atkins and colleagues followed the patients through 1996 with a follow-up interval ranging from three to eleven years [26]. The overall objective response rate was 16%, including 17 complete responders (6%). Median duration of response was six months for partial responders and had not been reached by the time of analysis for the complete responders. By a median follow-up of five years, nearly half of the responders were still alive with 15 having survived more than five years. The median survival for the entire group was 11.4 months. Toxicities included hypotension (64%), grade four hypotension (1%), mental status changes, tachyarrhythmias, and respiratory events (<4%). Nausea, vomiting, and diarrhea were common but not life threatening. While serum creatinine and bilirubin frequently rose, there was no evidence for chronic renal or hepatic dysfunction. The infection rate was 15% with *Staphylococcus aureas* sepsis leading to six deaths. These deaths all occurred before 1990, when antibiotic prophylaxis became standard practice during therapy.

Rosenberg and colleagues further studied high-dose IL-2 (720,000 IU/kg every eight hours, up to 14 doses over five days) in 409 patients with melanoma or renal cell carcinoma between 1985 and 1996 [27]. Of the 11.7% of melanoma patients who had a complete response, 83.3% remained in remission by the time of publication with a range of duration from 70 to 148 months. On the basis of these findings, the FDA approved high-dose bolus IL-2 for the treatment of metastatic melanoma in 1998.

Other clinical trials have focused on combining high-dose IL-2 with other cytokines and chemotherapeutic agents (biochemotherapy) in order to improve response rates or lessen toxicity (by using lower doses of IL-2). A phase III study of high-dose IL-2 with or without interferon-(IFN)-alpha was conducted with 85 patients with advanced metastatic melanoma [28] and showed an overall partial response rate of only 7.1% for the whole study population, without a significant difference between two groups. There were no complete responders, and the median duration of response was 11.5 months. Therefore, co-administration of these two cytokines remains investigational.

Several small, single-institution trials reporting high response rates with biochemotherapy have led to at least five randomized trials evaluating various doses and schedules of IL-2, IFN-alpha, and chemotherapy agents such as dacarbazine, cisplatin, and vinblastine. The group at M.D Anderson randomized

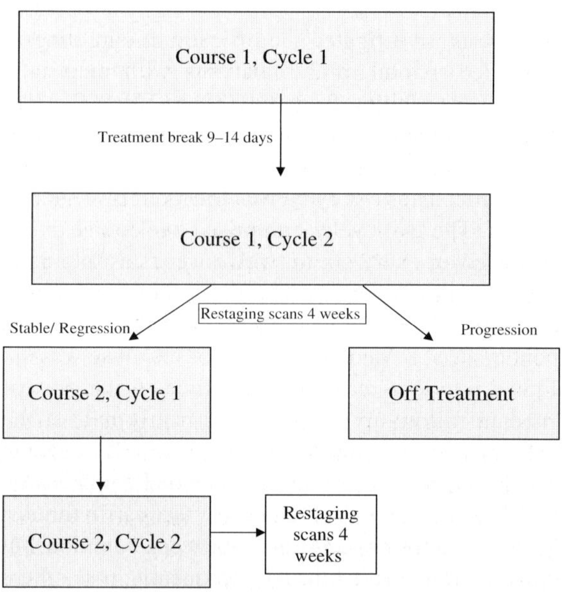

Figure 1. The standard treatment regimen for high-dose IL-2 (600,000 or 720,000 I.U./kg) is given by 15 minute I.V. bolus administration every 8 hours to a maximum of 14 doses or irreversible Grade 3 toxicity. The cycle is repeated in 9–14 days to complete one course of therapy. Courses are repeated if patients exhibit objective responses or stable disease on re-staging scans

patients to treatment with chemotherapy comprising cisplatin, vinblastine, and dacarbazine, or the same regimen combined with high-dose continuous infusion IL-2 and subcutaneous IFN-alpha [28]. The biochemotherapy arm boasted statistically significant improvements in response rate, time to progression, and median survival. However, hemodynamic, constitutional, and myelosuppressive toxicity was significantly worse in this arm. Four other studies, including a large intergroup trial, however, have not confirmed these results [29–33]. Therefore, biochemotherapy remains an experimental option for highly selected patients with symptomatic or rapidly progressive disease in whom tumor response might palliate specific symptoms or allow further immunotherapy or other clinical trial involvement.

A large number of trials exploring low doses of intravenous or subcutaneous IL-2 have shown no therapeutic benefit compare to high-dose IL-2. Similarly, alternative infusion regimens, including continuous dosing schedules, have not been effective in patients with melanoma. Thus, the standard of care continues to be high-dose bolus IL-2 (see Figure 1).

CLINICAL TRIALS SUPPORTING HIGH DOSE INTERLEUKIN-2 FOR RENAL CELL CARCINOMA

As with melanoma, partial responses were noted in patients with metastatic renal cell carcinoma in the initial studies using autologous LAK cells and IL-2 [23]. In the follow-up report of 157 patients treated with LAK cells and IL-2, the highest response rates were seen in 36 patients with metastatic renal cell carcinoma, with 33% having a complete or partial response [25]. A separate phase II trial of IL-2 with LAK cells in 32 patients with metastatic renal cell carcinoma found an overall response rate of 16% with disease-free survival of 4 to 16+ months [34]. In 1995, Fyfe and colleagues initially reported the results of seven independent phase II studies evaluating single agent bolus high-dose IL-2 conducted at 21 institutions [35]. Long term follow-up became available in 2000 [35]. In these trials, 255 patients were treated with the same high-dose bolus regimens used for metastatic melanoma. Five to nine days after completion of the first cycle of therapy a second cycle of was administered. Complete and partial responses were noted in 17 (7%) and 20 (8%) patients, respectively. Grade three and four toxicity rates were similar to those noted in the melanoma studies. Toxicities included hypotension (74%), oliguria/anuria (46%), mental status changes (28%), nausea and vomiting (25%), fever/chills (24%), diarrhea (22%), elevated bilirubin (21%), thrombocytopenia (21%), anemia (18%), dyspnea (17%), elevated BUN/creatinine (14%), and elevated transaminase levels (10%). Coma was noted in 2% and sepsis in 6%. These toxicities were generally reversed with discontinuation of therapy. Mortality, however, was 4% in these seven phase II studies. The median survival for the entire population was 16.3 months, and the median duration of response was 20 months for partial responders and 54 months for all responders, and had yet to be reached for complete responders by 131 months. The FDA approved high-dose bolus IL-2 for the treatment of metastatic renal cell carcinoma in 1992 based on these seven studies. Subsequent studies have confirmed the response rates and durability of response for high-dose bolus IL-2 [36,37].

In contrast to melanoma, renal cell carcinoma patients treated with low doses of IL-2 appear to have clinical benefit, although the response rates are lower than that observed for high-dose IL-2. Yang, et al. conducted a three arm randomized clinical trial comparing high-dose bolus IL-2 (720,000 I.U./kg i.v.), low-dose bolus IL-2 (72,000 I.U./kg i.v.) and subcutaneous IL-2 (250,000 I.U./kg s.c. first week, then 125,000 I.U./Kg sc for 5 weeks) [38]. Overall there was a statistically significant benefit favoring the high-dose Il–2 treated group but meaningful responses were also reported in the other two groups. The authors concluded that high-dose IL-2 should remain the standard of care for patients with metastatic renal cell carcinoma who can tolerate therapy. The data, however, also supports the use of lower doses of IL-2 in patients with renal cell carcinoma who might not be able to tolerate high-dose regimens.

A particular challenge in renal cell carcinoma has been the management of patients who present with metastatic disease and a synchronous primary tumor. The clinical benefit of nephrectomy for metastatic renal cell carcinoma has long been debated. Arguments against pre-treatment nephrectomy cite the high morbidity and mortality associated with surgery and the potential delay of systemic therapy. Arguments for pre-treatment nephrectomy cite evidence of spontaneous regression in some tumors and better responses to immunotherapy in situations of lower tumor burden. In 1989, the Southwest Oncology Group (SWOG) initiated a study to determine whether nephrectomy affects survival in metastatic renal-cell cancer [39]. They compared the outcomes of 120 metastatic renal cell carcinoma patients randomized to receive IFN-alpha 2b alone or following nephrectomy with endpoints being survival and tumor regression. The nephrectomy arm of the study had a significant survival advantage (11.1 months vs. 8.1 months). The authors found no delays in systemic therapy and only one surgery-related death, and concluded that nephrectomy should remain the standard of care before immunotherapy in patients with a primary tumor. The UCLA group has also reported a survival benefit of 16.5 months for patients treated with IL-2 following nephrectomy, confirming the conclusion that survival is improved when immunotherapy is given after nephrectomy [40].

BIOMARKERS PREDICTIVE OF RESPONSE TO IL-2 THERAPY

A variety of factors likely modulates the response to IL-2 and could be potentially useful as markers to predict response rates to IL-2 therapy. Although there are no prospectively validated markers to date, several putative biomarkers have been proposed. This includes such factors as HLA type since induction of HLA-DR has been associated with response to high-dose IL-2 therapy [41,42]. Other parameters being investigated in melanoma patients include lactate dehydrogenase (LDH), 5-S-cysteinyldopa, melanoma-inhibiting activity (MIA), S100-beta, and the presence of circulating melanoma cells, as well as molecular profiling of metastatic lesions, but none has yet been proven clinically relevant in patient selection [43–48].

Patient characteristics before, during, and after high-dose IL-2 therapy have also been evaluated to identify correlates of treatment response. Heretofore, no factors have been identified that consistently predict response to therapy. Atkins and colleagues found that prior systemic therapy and baseline performance status (PS) were the only factors predictive of response to high-dose IL-2 therapy in patient with metastatic melanoma [26]. Fifteen of the 17 complete responses were in treatment-naïve patients, and the response rate in patients with an ECOG PS of 0 was twice that of those with a PS of 1. Factors found not to be associated with response were visceral involvement, number of involved organs, and dose intensity of IL-2. Rosenberg and colleagues reported that prior immunotherapy was the only factor negatively correlated with complete response in both melanoma and renal cell carcinoma patients [23]. These investigators also reported that the total cumulative dose of IL-2 and a high rebound lymphocytosis after treatment were associated with complete tumor regression. A follow-up study at the National Cancer Institute revealed several factors associated with response to IL-2 in melanoma patients: the presence of subcutaneous or cutaneous only metastases, increased number of doses received during the first course, rebound lymphocytosis, abnormal thyroid function, and the development of autoimmune vitiligo [44].

Analysis performed on the data from trials of high-dose IL-2 in patients with renal cell carcinoma have similarly found variable associations between response rates and pretreatment or treatment related factors. Pretreatment factors that have been associated with higher response rates for renal cell carcinoma to high-dose IL-2 include performance status, prior nephrectomy, erythropoietin production, treatment-related thrombocytopenia, no thyroid dysfunction, rebound lymphocytosis, post-treatment elevations of blood TNF-a and IL-1 levels, no prior immunotherapy, fewer sites of disease, retention of the primary tumor in place, and bone or liver metastases [25, 34, 35, 45, 46]. Study of Atkins et al. reviewing pathology slides of 163 RCC patients from seven separate clinical trials revealed that patients with clear cell carcinomas having alveolar features and the absence of papillary and granular features correlated to response to IL-2, while patients with non-clear cell cancers did not respond well to IL-2 [47].

A novel renal cell carcinoma marker, carbonic anydrase IX (CA IX) has been investigated as a prognostic factor. In non-metastatic RCC patients, low CA IX predicted a worse outcome similar to patients with metastatic disease. Overall CA IX expression was found to decrease with the development of metastases [48]. CA IX is expressed in 94% of clear cell RCC specimens, and early studies at UCLA revealed that all patients who had a complete response to IL-2 had high CA IX expression [48]. The biological role of CA IX in tumor progression or response to IL-2 is not defined. However, CA IX-specific cytotoxic T cells have been generated, and this may provide a target for vaccine development and explain why CA IX expression may predict a better response to IL-2 therapy [50].

SELECTION OF PATIENTS FOR IL-2 THERAPY

Il–2 is indicated for the treatment of patients with metastatic melanoma and renal cell carcinoma. The safe administration of IL-2 depends on careful patient selection, constant management of clinical toxicity and treatment in experienced centers. In considering IL-2 therapy the overall clinical condition of the patient, including performance status, comorbid conditions, location of metastatic disease and wishes of the patient need to be carefully considered. Table 1 lists the contraindications to high-dose IL-2 therapy. In general, a poor performance status or presence of significant underlying cardiac, pulmonary or autoimmune disease is a contraindication to IL-2 therapy. Patients with significant cardiac disease, especially those with reversible ischemic damage or heart failure, are also not candidates for IL-2 because they will not tolerate the hypotension and fluid shifts that typically occur during treatment. Patients with supraventricular dysrhythmias, however, can often be safely treated but require careful evaluation and cardiology consultation. Similarly, significant pulmonary disease may result in rapid onset shortness of breath and early pulmonary edema. Patients with underlying pulmonary disease or a history of smoking should undergo pre-treatment pulmonary function studies to assess their eligibility for treatment and to provide a baseline level of pulmonary status in case of change induced during IL-2 therapy [1].

Patients with unsuspected brain metastases may be at risk for seizure, coma and death if treated with high-dose IL-2. Thus, pre-treatment brain MRI is mandatory before starting therapy. In selected cases of brain metastasis, IL-2 may be safely administered following craniotomy and surgical resection or local radiation therapy

Table 1. Contraindications to IL-2 Therapy

Contraindication	Comment
Poor performance status (< ECOG 1)	Need to assess before each cycle
Untreated brain metastasis	Can consider IL-2 if treated and minimal residual edema is present
Concurrent infection	Can result in uncontrolled sepsis and death
Chronic beta blocker use	Can potentiate hypotension during treatment
Congestive heart failure	Cannot tolerate fluid shifts
Ischemic heart disease	Can precipitate MI during hypotension
Significant pulmonary disease	Can result in pulmonary edema and need for mechanical ventilation
Ulcerative colitis	Can result in bowel perforation
Autoimmune disease	Can worsen with IL-2
Chronic steroid medication	Counteracts the effects of IL-2

provided there is no residual edema and patients do not require steroids [52]. There is also a significantly increased risk of complications if patients have underlying infections at the time of IL-2 administration. This can usually be avoided by careful history and physical examination in concert with a pre-treatment chest X-ray, urinalysis and complete blood count. Patients should also avoid steroid medications, which can counteract the effects of IL-2, and beta blockers, which can potentiate hypotension during therapy.

The initial pre-treatment screening for patients being considered for high-dose IL-2 therapy are shown in Table 2. In addition to a careful history and physical examination, routine blood work (including thyroid function studies), brain MRI, staging CT scans, EKG, urinalysis and chest X-rays are obtained on all patients. Patients with a history of cardiac disease or over the age of 50 should also have a stress test to document the lack of reversible ischemic disease. Pulmonary function studies are also useful in patients with underlying chronic lung disease. Although major organ dysfunction and autoimmunity are relative contraindications to IL-2 treatment, each case may need to be evaluated independently and in consultation with an expert. For example, while IL-2 can be safely given to patients with well controlled diabetes mellitus, those patients with brittle diabetes may experience an exacerbation of their disease upon exposure to IL-2. The risk-benefit ratio may need to be carefully considered in those with known mild autoimmune disease or borderline performance status.

Table 2. IL-2 Screening

Screening Test	Indication
Brain MRI	All patients
Cardiac stress test	All patients over 50 years old or any patient with a history of cardiac disease
Pulmonary function studies	Any patient with extensive lung disease or history of heavy smoking
EKG	All patients for baseline
Chest X-ray	All patients to rule out infection, verify central line placement
Urinalysis	All patients to rule out urinary tract infection
Complete blood count, electrolytes, blood urea nitrogen, creatinine, liver function studies	All patients to rule out infection or other organ dysfunction
Thyroid function studies	All patients to rule out autoimmunity and have a baseline level
CT scans of chest, abdomen and pelvis	All patients for staging and response evaluation
History and physical examination	All patients to document unsuspected infection or steroid use, confirm performance status

The management of patients being treated with high-dose IL-2 usually requires intensive nursing care and close clinical monitoring. Although many centers utilize an intensive care unit or step-down setting, patients can be managed safely on a hospital unit with skilled nurses and telemetry monitoring. Frequent vital signs with attention to daily weight, pulse, blood pressure, urine output and oxygen saturation are required. In contrast to many drug regimens, patients must be clinically evaluated before each dose of IL-2 and decisions to give the dose must consider the physiologic status of the patient, presence of underlying toxicity, mental status and psychological state of the patient and availability of physician and nurse support in the event of toxicity. Daily weights and lab studies are needed to identify shifts in fluid status and organ dysfunction. Most IL-2 side effects are reversible and it is possible to hold a dose for grade 3 or greater toxicity and resume treatment if the effect resolved within 12-24 hours.

The guidelines for management of IL-2 patients are shown in Table 3. Patients are monitored by continuous cardiac telemetry with daily weights and vital signs, urine output and oxygen saturation tested as needed during therapy. Routine medications administered prior to IL-2 include acetaminophen and indomethacin to prevent fever/chills, famotidine to avoid gastric irritation, anti-emetics and gram positive antibiotic prophylaxis. Patients are evaluated before each dose and if parameters are favorable the dose is given. If grade 3 or greater toxicity is observed the dose may be held until the side effect resolves. Failure to resolve within 24 hours, however, is usually an indication to halt further IL-2 treatment during the cycle. Patients will return in 9-14 days for a second cycle and the length of this interval depends

Table 3. Management of IL-2 Patients During Therapy

Pre-treatment labs	CBC with diff, electrolytes, blood urea nitrogen, creatinine, liver function studies, prothrombin and partial thromboplastin times, LDH (melanoma patients) and thyroid panel
Pre-treatment tests	Electrocardiogram Chest X-ray Brain MRI Cardiac stress test for age>50 Pulmonary function studies for patients with chronic lung disease
Pre-treatment medications	Acetaminophen 650 mg po q 6 hours Indomethacin 50 mg po q 8 hours Famotidine 20 mg po/IV q 12 hours Granisetron 1 mg po or 0.7 mg IV q day Oxacillin 2 grams IV q 6 hours Vancomycin 1 gram IV q 12 hours (If allergic to penicillin) Discontinue antihypertensives
During treatment	Continuous cardiac telemetry Periodic vital signs, Strict urine output and oxygen saturation Daily weight Daily blood work (cbc, electrolytes, creatinine and liver function studies) 1 dose may be held for grade III or IV toxicity; If toxicity not improved or resolved within 24 hours IL-2 therapy should be stopped.

on resolution of symptoms and organ dysfunction induced by the first cycle of IL-2. Re-staging scans are typically performed four or more weeks after the second cycle of treatment since IL-2 often takes a longer time to induce regression when compared to cytotoxic chemotherapy agents. This is an important point and often stable disease on re-staging may imply an early objective response to IL-2 and generally warrants further treatment if the patient is able to tolerate further therapy.

MANAGEMENT OF HIGH DOSE INTERLEUKIN-2 TOXICITY

The management of IL-2-related side effects is well established, and most patients can be treated with minimal morbidity. Safe administration of IL-2 begins with vigilant patient selection. As mentioned, only patients with adequate cardiac, pulmonary, renal, and hepatic function should be offered therapy. As previously stated, performance status has been shown to be a predictor of response, and patients with ECOG performance status of 2 or higher should be excluded. Patients over age 50 should undergo stress testing. Respiratory complaints, smoking history, heavy tumor burden, or known pulmonary disease (FEV1 and FVC < 65% predicted) mandate pulmonary function testing. Untreated cerebral metastases predispose to altered mental status and other neurological complications due to IL-2, so all patients should undergo pre-treatment brain MRI screening. Many of the adverse effects of IL-2 can be prevented or treated with proper fluid and pharmacologic management, and nearly all adverse effects are reversible upon cessation of therapy. Guidelines for safe administration of high-dose IL-2 have been previously published [51]. A list of common IL-2-related side effects and their management are listed in Table 4.

Cardiac and Hemodynamic Side Effects. IL-2 induces a capillary leak syndrome that leads to hypotension, decreased systemic vascular resistance, tachycardia, increased cardiac index, and third space fluid sequestration. The pathophysiology of this effect is not well described. Significant hypotension is common, occurring in 85% of IL-2 treated patients. Initial management includes fluid challenge and most patients will respond to this, although careful attention should be paid to the pulmonary status since excess fluid can result in pulmonary edema and respiratory compromise. Those patients who do not respond to fluid or who cannot tolerate excessive fluid may be treated with vasopressors such as dopamine or phenylephrine. Hypotension tends to occur gradually and will often manifest several hours after IL-2 dosing. Most patients will tolerate further IL-2 dosing once the hypotensive episode has been properly treated or corrected with fluid or vasopressors. While tachycardia is common, overt arrhythmias are not. Atrial arrhythmias associated with hypotension occur in about 10% of patients and usually respond to supportive management.

The capillary leak syndrome also results in significant third space sequestration of fluid during therapy. This typically manifests as peripheral edema although fluid may accumulate in any organ, including the lungs where pulmonary edema is possible. Patients often gain 10–20 kg during a single cycle of IL-2 and the

Table 4. Management of IL-2 Related Toxicity

Hypotension	If systolic BP < 80–90 mmHg hold dose 250cc NS fluid bolus; repeat as necessary up to 1.5 L per day Phenlyephrine or dopamine drip
Pulmonary edema	If unresolved in 8 hours chest X-ray Persistence, then hold dose Lasix
Arrhythmias	Cardiac monitor Obtain 12 lead EKG Stop IL-2 treatment Check cardiac enzymes Replace electrolytes Supportive care
Altered mental status	Observe Anti-anxiolytics If severe, stop treatment If persistent, obtain brain MRI
Elevated creatinine	If > 4.0 mg/dl, hold dose If > 8.0 mg/dl stop therapy Replace electrolytes, correct acidosis Careful fluid management
Elevated bilirubin	If > 3.7 mg/dl consider holding dose If > 7.5 mg/dl consider stopping therapy
Nausea and vomiting	Anti-emetics
Mucositis	Magic mouthwash
Diarrhea	Lomotil Tincture of opium
Pruritus	Eucerin cream Diphenhydramine 50 mg po q 6 hrs Hydroxyzine 50 mg po q 8 hrs Oatmeal baths
Anemia	Observe after fluid sequestration Check for rectal bleeding Consider transfusion if persistent and symptomatic
Electrolyte imbalances	Replete Mg^{2+}, Ca^{2+}, Phosphorus daily
Thrombocytopenia	If < 75 k/ul and > 50 k/ul hold dose If < 50 k/ul consider stopping therapy

weight is a sensitive indicator of the fluid status in these patients. Most patients with normal cardiac reserve will mobilize this fluid once the capillary leak stops. In some cases, however, this can be hastened by administration of diuretics. This must be done cautiously and only after the capillary leak has resolved.

Based on these hemodynamic changes, adequate cardiac reserve is essential. Thus, IL-2 administration should be considered on an individual basis for patients over 50 and these patients should have a normal cardiac stress test. Patients over the age of 70 have difficulty tolerating IL-2 and should be considered on an individual basis and only at experienced centers. Children have been given IL-2 and the hemodynamic changes appear to be similar to those observed in the adult population but are often better tolerated. Furthermore, due to the high potential for cardiovascular side effects, all patients require on-going monitoring during therapy. Although rare, myocardial infarction has been reported after IL-2 treatment and patients with acute rhythm changes, chest pain, shortness of breath or other signs of acute infarction should discontinue IL-2 and have regular EKG and cardiac enzymes tested.

IL-2 rarely induces an acute cardiomyopathy characterized by a lymphocytic infiltrate in the myocardium. Symptoms are often non-specific and may include chest pain, shortness of breath, fever, and malaise. The diagnosis is usually made when cardiac enzymes are elevated in the face of a normal EKG. The diagnosis can be confirmed by myocardial biopsy but this is usually not necessary. Treatment is usually symptomatic and includes the use of non-steroidal anti-inflammatory agents. The condition is typically self-limited and resolved within a few weeks.

Pulmonary Side Effects

The capillary leak syndrome commonly results in pulmonary fluid sequestration. This can result in shortness of breath, dyspnea, and, less commonly, pleural effusion. Because of this, patients with serious underlying pulmonary disease or tumor-related effusions should not be offered IL-2. Pre-treatment pulmonary function studies may be helpful to define those patients who may be at risk for developing complications and establishing a baseline for pulmonary performance should changes occur during therapy. Regular pulse oximetry may identify impending pulmonary compromise and allow early cessation of treatment. Most pulmonary side effects are mild and easily treated with diuretics and supplemental oxygen via nasal cannula. More serious pulmonary issues may require mechanical ventilation or thoracentesis with cessation of treatment.

Renal Side Effects

Oliguria is the most common renal side effect of IL-2 treatment. This is often seen within 48 hours of starting treatment and is associated with an increased creatinine, azotemia, low fractional excretion of sodium, and fluid retention. Electrolyte derangements are also common and include hypocalcemia, hypomagnesemia, hypophosphatemia, and metabolic acidosis. These effects are usually transient and respond to fluid challenge and repletion of the deficient electrolytes. While renal function normally recovers upon cessation of IL-2, treatment is usually halted once serum creatinine levels reach 4.0 mg/dl. Diuretics encourage quick recovery and may be administered once hypotension has resolved. The renal manifestations of IL-2 may be more significant in the renal cell carcinoma population since many of these patients have only one kidney. Hemodialysis is rarely, if ever, indicated in these patients although careful attention to renal status is important during therapy with high-dose IL-2.

Gastrointestinal Side Effects

IL-2 therapy often causes nausea, vomiting, mucositis and diarrhea. Many patients also experience hypoalbuminemia and elevation of hepatic enzymes and bilirubin. Prophylactic anti-emetics are the standard of care but may need to be adjusted throughout the course of treatment depending on the severity of the patient's reaction. Secretory diarrhea occurs in about 10% of patients and usually responds to symptomatic management (see Table 4). IL-2 is contraindicated in patients with active colitis due to rare reports of colonic perforation seen especially in those with inflammatory bowel disease. Abdominal pain is uncommon, so if it does occur it should be evaluated carefully. Signs and symptoms of bowel perforation may be masked as these patients are on standing non-steroidal anti-inflammatory agents. An inflammatory hepatitis may cause right upper quadrant pain and a reversible cholestasis is common. These entities normally resolve without treatment. Mucositis is typically self limited but may be relieved with symptomatic management. Anorexia may occur during therapy and avoidance of food will usually lessen the incidence of nausea and vomiting in this situation. The appetite returns within a few days if related to IL-2 treatment.

Hematological Effects

IL-2 can affect nearly all cells of the hematopoeitic system and requires careful monitoring during treatment. Anemia, thrombocytopenia, lymphopenia, and eosinophilia have all been reported. While neutrophil counts are normal, the function of these cells may be impaired by IL-2, and this can lead to an increased risk of infectious complications. It is standard practice to place all patients on broad-spectrum antibiotics during IL-2 treatment. It is mandatory to monitor blood counts at least daily during active treatment, and blood transfusions should be considered for symptomatic patients. Although bleeding is rare during IL-2 administration, treatment should be stopped if the platelet count falls below 20,000–30,000 /m^3. There is often a rebound lymphocytosis that occurs within 3–10 days of stopping IL-2 therapy. This is important to note since the white blood count may not be reliable for diagnosing infection in the post-IL-2 setting.

Neurological Side Effects

The neuropsychiatric effects of IL-2 are often the most disturbing to patients and family. Typical effects include lethargy, confusion, visual hallucinations, and rarely coma. While significant neurological sequelae are rare, mental status and the neurological exam should be monitored closely during IL-2 treatment. Changes in mental status are often preceded by impaired memory, vague or incoherent responses, irritability, lack of attention, and vivid dreams. IL-2 should be held or discontinued if there is evidence of mental status changes, and patients should be monitored closely or restrained to prevent trauma from falling during periods of disorientation. The use of anti-anxiolytics and anti-psychotics may be useful for IL-2 induced mental status changes and irritability. If symptoms do not improve promptly, other causes should be sought including new brain metastases.

Cutaneous Side Effects

Peripheral vasodilation as part of the capillary leak syndrome will often manifest as facial and cutaneous flushing. Less commonly, patients may experience significant dessication and dequamation of the skin with associated pruritis. This can be managed with emollients and systemic pharmacologic treatments including diphenhydramine and hydroxyzine (see Table 4)

Immunological Side Effects

IL-2 induces significant fever and chills following administration. This can be effectively prevented by premedicating patients with acetaminophen and indomethacin. Long-term immunologic side effects have included vitiligo and autoimmune thyroiditis. Therefore, thyroid function should be monitored before, during, and after IL-2 therapy. There has been a correlation between the development of autoimmune phenomenon and therapeutic anti-tumor activity with IL-2.

NOVEL METHODS FOR REDUCING IL-2 RELATED TOXICITY

High-dose IL-2 toxicity can be reduced pharmacologically. Dexamethasone prevents induction of tumor necrosis factor (TNF) alpha by IL-2 and reduces treatment-related toxicity resulting in a threefold increase in the maximum tolerated dose [52]. Potential interference with IL-2 anti-tumor efficacy, however, limits the utility of this approach in the routine clinical setting. Co-administration of IL-2 with soluble TNF receptors has shown promise in animal models, inhibiting some of the adverse effects associated with high-dose IL-2 without interfering with the anti-tumor effects of IL-2. Unfortunately, these agents did not significantly block IL-2-related toxicity in humans [54]. A strategy to reduce IL-2-associated vasodilation by inhibiting synthesis of nitric oxide with NG-monomethyl-L-arginine was tested in a phase I study of renal cell carcinoma patients who developed hypotension secondary to IL-2 infusion. In this trial, hypotension was completely or partially reversed in all patients. This was accompanied by increased pulmonary vascular resistance and reversal of IL-2-induced hyperdynamic cardiac output [55].

IL-2 induces release of superoxide, a potent mediator of hemodynamic instability and organ dysfunction during septic shock. In an animal model, IL-2-associated hypotension was ameliorated by combining IL-2 with the superoxide dismutase mimetic, M40403, with improvement of anti-tumor efficacy (56). Continuous intravenous infusion of IL-2 has been compared to the standard bolus regimen, but clinical efficacy was not superior and toxicities were excessive [57,58].

Another approach to reduce IL-2 toxicity is to avoid systemic administration and to localize IL-2 to the tumor microenvironment. Liu and Rosenberg evaluated the transduction of tumor infiltrating lymphocytes with the IL-2 gene using a retroviral vector [59]. In this model, tumor cell antigens stimulate production of IL-2 resulting in T-cell proliferation without requiring exogenous IL-2, thereby circumventing systemic toxicity. Radny and colleagues studied injecting IL-2 directly into tumors and confirmed its safety and tolerability [60]. Toxicity was mild, and 85% of treated lesions completely regressed leading to an extraordinarily high systemic complete response rate of 62.5% with the longest ongoing remission lasting more than 38 months. Furthermore, based on data suggesting that Tregs may be increased by IL-2 and since Tregs may inhibit effective anti-tumor immunity, studies are underway to inhibit Tregs in combination with IL-2 or other forms of immunotherapy [61, 62]. The results from such studies need to be carefully evaluated to determine the potential for increasing therapeutic responses while limiting toxicity associated with IL-2 treatment.

CONCLUSIONS

The prognosis for patients with metastatic melanoma remains poor and few treatment options are available. Patients with metastatic renal cell carcinoma seem to benefit from tyrosine kinase inhibitors although the survival benefit with these agents is limited. Thus, the limited survival benefit with currently available agents and the inherent immunogenicity of melanomas and renal cell carcinomas suggests that high-dose IL-2 should be considered for all patients who are able to tolerate treatment. IL-2 has been well studied as a single agent in metastatic melanoma and durable responses can be expected in 15–20% of patients with many achieving long term survival. A better understanding of the biology of IL-2 and its receptor, as well as the identification of a regulatory T cell subset has yielded new clues to how IL-2 mediates therapeutic effects in cancer patients. Further research is required to define the mechanism of tumor regression and may provide new targets for immune manipulation. Vigilant screening of patients prior to IL-2 treatment and adherence to practical guidelines for the management of toxicity allows safe administration of IL-2 in most patients. There have been considerable efforts aimed at reducing the frequency and severity of IL-2 side effects, and these will require further clinical investigation before they can be recommended. Potential biomarkers, such as CA IX in renal cell carcinoma, may play a role in selecting patients who are more likely to respond to IL-2 therapy but this requires prospective validation. Patients with metastatic melanoma or renal cell carcinoma should be evaluated for IL-2 and treatment can be safely administered to most eligible patients especially at experienced high-dose IL-2 centers.

REFERENCES

1. Jemal, A., Murray, T., Ward, E., Samuels, A., Tiwari, R.C., Ghafoor, A., Feuer, E.J. and Thun, M.J: Cancer statistics *CA Cancer J Clin* 55:10–30, 2005.
2. Nelson, BH: Regulatory T-cells and Tolerance. *J. Immunol.* 172:3983–3988, 2004.
3. Gaffen, S.L.: Signaling domains of the interleukin 2 receptor. *Cytokine* 14:63–77, 2001.
4. He, Y.W. and Malek T.R: The structure and function of γc-dependent cytokines and receptors: regulation of T lymphocytes development and homeostasis. *Crit. Rev. Immunol* 18, 503–524, 1998.
5. Parrish-Novak, J., Foster, D.C., Holly, R.D. and Clegg, C.H: Interleukin-21 and the IL-21 receptor; novel effectors of NK and T cell responses. *J. Leukoc. Biol* 72, 856–863, 2002.

6. Rosenberg, S., Lotze, M., Muul, L., Leitman, S., Chang, A., Ettinghausen, S., Matory, Y., Skibber, J., Shiloni, E., Vetto, J., et al: Observations on the systemic administration of autologous lymphokine-activated killer cells and recombinant interleukin-2 to patients with metastatic cancer. *N Eng J Med* 313:1485–1492, 1985.
7. Lotze, M., Chang, A., Seipp, C., Simpson, C., Vetto, J., and Rosenberg, S: High-dose recombinant interleukin-2 in the treatment of patients with disseminated cancer. *JAMA* 256:3117–3124, 1986.
8. Sadlack, B. et al: Ulcerative colitis-like disease in mice with a disrupted interleukin-gene.*Cell* 75, 253–261 1993.
9. Sadlack, B. et al: Generalized autoimmune disease in interleukin-2-deficient mice is triggered by an uncontrolled activation and proliferation of CD4+ T cells. *Eur. J. Immunol* 25, 3053–3059,1995.
10. Sadlack, B., Kuhn, R., Schorle, H., Muller, W. & Horak, I: Development and proliferation of lymphocytes in mice deficient for both interleukins-2 and -4. *Eur. J. Immunol.* 24, 281–284, 1994.
11. Malek, T. R., Yu, A., Vincek, V., Scibelli, P. & Kong, L: CD4 regulatory T cells prevent lethal autoimmunity in IL-2R-deficient mice. Implications for the nonredundant function of IL-2. *Immunity* 17, 167–178, 2002.
12. Malek, T. R., Porter, B. O., Codias, E. K., Scibelli, P. & Yu, A: Normal lymphoid homeostasis and lack of lethal autoimmunity in mice containing mature T cells with severely impaired IL-2 receptors. *J. Immunol* 164, 2905–2914, 2004.
13. Malek TR, Bayer AL. Tolerance, not immunity, crucially depends on IL-2. Nature Rev Immunol 4:665–674, 2004.
14. Depper, J. M., Leonard, W. J., Robb, R. J., Waldmann, T. A. & Greene, W. C: Blockade of the interleukin-2 receptor by anti-Tac antibody: inhibition of human lymphocyte activation. *J. Immunol* 131, 690–696, 1983.
15. Gillis, S., Gillis, A. E. & Henney, C. S: Monoclonal antibody directed against interleukin 2 : Inhibition of T lymphocyte mitogenesis and the *in vitro* differentiation of alloreactive cytolytic T cells. *J. Exp. Med.* 154, 983–988, 1981.
16. Van Parijs, L. et al: Functional responses and apoptosis of CD25 (IL-2Rα)-deficient T cells expressing a transgenic antigen receptor.*J. Immunol.* 158, 3738–3745,1997.
17. Kundig, T. M. et al. Immune responses in interleukin-2-deficient mice. Science 262, 1059–1061, 1993.
18. D'Souza, W. N. & Lefrancois, L: IL-2 is not required for the initiation of CD8 T cell cycling but sustains expansion. *J. Immunol* 171, 5727–5735, 2003.
19. Leung, D. T., Morefield, S. & Willerford, D. M: Regulation of lymphoid homeostasis by IL-2 receptor signals in vivo. *J. Immunol* 164, 3527–3534, 2000.
20. Lotze, M., Grimm, E., Mazumder, A., Strausser, J., and Rosenberg, S: In vitro growth of cytotoxic human lymphocytes. Lysis of fresh and cultured autologous tumor by lymphocytes cultured in T cell growth factor (TCGF). *Cancer Res* 41:4420, 1981.
21. Mazumder, A., and Rosenberg, S: Successful immunotherapy of natural killer-resistant established pulmonary metastases by the intravenous adoptive transfer of syngeneic lymphocytes activated in vitro by interleukin-2. *J Exp Med* 159:495, 1984.
22. Rosenberg, S., Mule, J., Spiess, P., Reichert, C., and Schwarz, S: Regression of Established Pulmonary Metastases and Subcutaneous Tumor Mediated by the Systemic Administration of High-Dose Recombinant Interleukin 2. *J Exp Med* 161:1169–1188, 1985.
23. Rosenberg, S., Lotze, M., Muul, L., Leitman, S., Chang, A., Ettinghausen, S., Matory, Y., Skibber, J., Shiloni, E., Vetto, J., et al: Observations on the systemic administration of autologous lymphokine-activated killer cells and recombinant interleukin-2 to patients with metastatic cancer. *N Eng J Med* 313:1485–1492.
24. Lotze, M., Chang, A., Seipp, C., Simpson, C., Vetto, J., and Rosenberg, S. 1986. High-dose recombinant interleukin-2 in the treatment of patients with disseminated cancer. *JAMA* 256: 3117–3124, 1985.
25. Rosenberg, S., Lotze, M., Muul, L., Chang, A., Avis, F., Leitman, S., Linehan, W., Robertson, C., Lee, R., Rubin, J., et al: A progress report on the treatment of 157 patients with advanced cancer

using lymphokine-activated killer cells and interleukin-2 or high-dose interleukin-2 alone. *N Eng J Med* 316:889–897, 1987.

26. Atkins, M., Lotze, M., Dutcher, J., Fisher, R., Weiss, G., Margolin, K., Abrams, J., Sznol, M., Parkinson, D., Hawkins, M., et al: High-dose recombinant interleukin-2 therapy for patients with metastatic melanoma: analysis of 270 patients treated between 1985 and 1993. *J Clin Oncol* 17:2105–2116, 1999.
27. Rosenberg, S., Yang, J., White, D., and Steinberg, S: Durability of complete responses in patients with metastatic cancer treated with high-dose interleukin-2: identification of the antigens mediating response. *Ann Surg*. 228:307–319, 1998.
28. Sparano, J., Fisher, R., Sunderland, M., Margolin, K., Ernest, M., Sznol, M., Atkins, M., Dutcher, J., Micetich, K., Weiss, G., et al: Randomized phase III trial of treatment with high-dose interleukin-2 either alone or in combination with interferon alpha-2a in patients with advanced melanoma. *J Clin Oncol* 11:1969–1977, 1993.
29. Eton, O., Legha, S., Bedikian, A., Lee, J., Buzaid, A., Hodges, C., Ring, S., Papadopoulos, N., Plager, C., East, M., et al: Sequential biochemotherapy versus chemotherapy for metastatic melanoma: results from a phase III randomized trial. *J Clin Oncol* 20:2045–2052, 2002.
30. Keilholz, U., Goey, S., Punt, C., Proebstle, T., Salzmann, R., Scheibenbogen, C., Schadendorf, D., Liendard, D., Enk, A., Dummer, R., et al: Interferon-alfa-2a and interleukin-2 with or without cisplatin in metastatic melanoma: a randomized trial of the European Organization for the Research and Treatment of Cancer Melanoma Cooperative Group. *J Clin Oncol* 15:2579–2588, 1997.
31. Rosenberg, S., Yang, J., Schwartzentruber, D., Hwu, P., Marincola, F., Topalian, S., Seipp, C., Einhorn, J., White, D., and Steinberg, S: Prospective randomized trial of the treatment of patients with metastatic melanoma using chemotherapy with cisplatin, dacarbazine, and tamoxifen alone, or in combination with interleukin-2 and interferon-alfa-2b. *J Clin Oncol* 17:968–975, 1999.
32. Keilholz, U., Punt, C., Gore, M., Suciu, S., Kruit, W., Patel, P., Lienard, D., Thomas, J., Lehmann, F., and Eggermont, A: Dacarbazine, cisplatin and IFN-a2b with or without IL-2 in advanced melanoma: Final analysis of EORTC randomized phase III trial 18951. In *ASCO*. Chicago. 708 (abst 2848), 2003.
33. Atkins, M., Lee, S., Flaherty, L., Sosman, J., Sondak, V., and Kirkwood, J: A prospective randomized phase III trial of concurrent biochemotherapy (BCT) with cisplatin, vinblastine, dacarbazine (CVD), IL-2 and interferon alpha-2b (IFN) versus CVD alone in patients with metastatic melanoma (E3695): An ECOG-coordinated intergroup trial. In *ASCO*. Chicago. 708 (abstr 2847), 2003.
34. Fisher, R.I., Coltman, C.A., Jr., Doroshow, J.H., Rayner, A.A., Hawkins, M.J., Mier, J.W., Wiernik, P., McMannis, J.D., Weiss, G.R., Margolin, K.A., et al: Metastatic renal cancer treated with interleukin-2 and lymphokine-activated killer cells. A phase II clinical trial. *Ann Intern Med* 108:518–523, 1988.
35. Fyfe, G., Fisher, R.I., Rosenberg, S.A., Sznol, M., Parkinson, D.R., and Louie, A.C: Results of treatment of 255 patients with metastatic renal cell carcinoma who received high-dose recombinant interleukin-2 therapy. *J Clin Oncol* 13:688–696, 1995.
36. Fisher, R.I., Rosenberg, S.A., and Fyfe, G: Long-term survival update for high-dose recombinant interleukin-2 in patients with renal cell carcinoma. *Cancer J Sci Am* 6 Suppl 1:S55–57, 2000.
37. Bukowski, R.M: Natural history and therapy of metastatic renal cell carcinoma: the role of interleukin-2. *Cancer* 80:1198–1220, 1997.
38. Yang, JC, Sherry, RM, Steinberg, SM, Topalian, SL, Schwartzentruber, DJ, Hwu, P, Seipp, CA, Rogers-Freezer, L, Morton, KE, White, DE, Liewehr, DJ, Merino, MJ, Rosenberg, SA: Randomized Study of High-Dose and Low Dose Interleukin-2 in patients with Metastatic Renal Cancer. *J Clin Oncol* Aug 15;21 (16):3127–32, 2003.
39. Flanigan RC, Salmon SE, Blumenstein BA, Bearman SI, Roy V, McGrath PC, Caton JR Jr, Munshi N, Crawford ED: Nephrectomy followed by interferon alfa-2b compared with interferon alfa-2b alone for metastatic renal-cell cancer *N Eng J Med* 345(23): 1655–59, 2001.
40. Pantuck AJ, Belldegrun AS, Figlin RA: Nephrectomy and interleukin-2 for metastatic renal-cell carcinoma. *N Engl J Med* 345(23) 1711–1712, 2001.
41. Marincola, F., Venzon, D., White, D., Rubin, J., Lotze, M., Simonis, T., Balkissoon, J., Rosenberg, S., and Parkinson, D: HLA association with response and toxicity in melanoma patients treated with interleukin 2-based immunotherapy. *Cancer Res* 52:6561–6566, 1992.

42. Rubin, J., Elwood, L., Rosenberg, S., and Lotze, M: Immunohistochemical correlates of response to recombinant interleukin-2-based immunotherapy in humans. *Cancer Res* 49:7086–7092, 1986.
43. Horikoshi, T., Ito, S., Wakamatsu, K., Onodera, H., and Eguchi, H: Evaluation of melanin-related metabolites as markers of melanoma progression. *Cancer* 73:629–636, 1994.
44. Phan, G., Attia, P., Steinberg, S., White, D., and Rosenberg, S: Factors associated with response to high-dose interleukin-2 in patients with metastatic melanoma. *J Clin Oncol.* 19:3477–3482, 2001.
45. Jonasch E, George D, Atkins MB: Renal neoplasia. In: Brenner B, ed. Brenner & Rector's The Kidney, 7th ed. Philadelphia: Saunders; 1895–1923, 2004.
46. Royal RE, Steinberg SM, Krouse RS, et al: Correlates of response to IL-2 therapy in patients treated for metastatic renal cancer and melanoma. *Cancer J Sci Am* 2:91, 1996.
47. Upton MP, Parker RA, Youmans A, McDermott DF, Atkins MB: Histologic predictors of renal cell carcinoma response to interleukin-2-based therapy. *J Immunol* 28: 488–95, 2005.
48. Said J: Biomarker discover in urogenital cancer. *Biomarkers* Nov;10 Suppl 1:S83–6, 2005.
49. Bui MH, Seligson D, Han KR, et al: Carbonic anhydrase IX is an independent predictor of survival in advanced renal cell carcinoma: implications for pronosis and therapy. Clin Cancer Res 9:802–811, 2003.
50. Mukouyama H, Janzen NK, Hernandez JM, et al: Generation of kidney cancer-specific antitumor immune responses using peripheral blood moncytes transduced with a recombinant adenovirus encoding carbonic anhydrase 9. *Clin Cancer Res* 10:1421–1429, 2004.
51. Schwartzentruber, D: Guidelines for the Safe Administration of High-Dose Interleukin-2. *J Immunother* 24:287–293, 2001.
52. Guirguis, LM, Yang, JC, White, DE, Steinberg SM, Liewehr, DJ, Rosenberg ,SA, Schwartzentruber, DJ: Safety and efficacy of high-dose Interleukin-2 therapy in patients with brain metastases. J Immunother Jan-Feb; 25(1):82–7, 2002.
53. Mier, J., Vachino, G., Klempner, M., Aaronson, F., Noring, R., Smith, S., Brandon, E., Laird, W., and Atkins, M: Inhibition of interleukin-2-induced tumor necrosis factor release by dexamethasone: prevention of an acquired neutrophil chemotaxis defect and differential suppression of interleukin-2-associated side effects. *Blood* 76:1933–1940, 1990.
54. Du Bois, J., Trehu, E., Mier, J., Shapiro, L., Epstein, M., Klempner, M., Dinarello, C., Kappler, K., Ronayne, L., Rand, W., et al: Randomized placebo-controlled clinical trial of high-dose interleukin-2 in combination with a soluble p75 tumor necrosis factor receptor immunoglobulin G chimera in patients with advanced melanoma and renal cell carcinoma. *J Clin Oncol* 15:1052–1062, 1997.
55. Kilbourn, R., Fonseca, G., Trissel, L., and Griffith, O: Strategies to reduce side effects of interleukin-2: evaluation of the antihypotensive agent NG-monomethyl-L-arginine. *Cancer J Sci Am* 6:S21–30, 2000.
56. Samlowski, W., Petersen, R., Cuzzocrea, S., Macarthur, H., Burton, D., McGregor, J., and Salvemimi, D: A nonpeptidyl mimic of superoxide dismutase, M40403, inhibits dose-limiting hypotension associated with interleukin-2 and increases its antitumor effects. *Nat Med* 9:750–755, 2003.
57. Dillman, R., O'Connor, A., Simpson, L., Barth, N., VanderMolen, L., and Vanderplas, P: Does Continuous-Infusion Interleukin-2 Increase Survival in Metastatic Melanoma? *Am J Clin Oncol* 26:141–145, 2003.
58. Thompson, J., Lee, D., Lindgren, C., Benz, L., Collins, C., Levitt, D., and Fefer, A: Influence of dose and duration of infusion of interleukin-2 on toxicity and immunomodulation. *J Clin Oncol* 6:669–678, 1988.
59. Liu, K., and Rosenberg, S: Interleukin-2-independent proliferation of human melanoma-reactive T lymphocytes transduced with an exogenous IL-2 gene is stimulation dependent. *J Immunother* 26:190–201, 2003.
60. Radny, P., Caroli, U., Bauer, J., Paul, T., Schlegel, C., Eigentler, T., Weide, B., Schwarz, M., and Garbe, C: Phase II trial of intralesional therapy with interleukin-2 in soft-tissue melanoma metastases. *Br J Cancer* 89:1620–1626, 2003.

61. Mahnke, K., Qian, Y., Knop, J., and Enk, A: Induction of CD4+/CD25+ regulatory T cells by targeting of antigens to immature dendritic cells. *Blood* 101:4862–4869, 2003.
62. Shimizu, J., Yamazaki, S., and Sakaguchi, S: Induction of tumor immunity by removing CD25+CD4+ T cells: a common basis between tumor immunity and autoimmunity. *J Immunol.* 163:5211–5218, 1999.

CHAPTER 20

MONOCLONAL ANTIBODIES IN CANCER THERAPY

CHRISTOPH RADER AND MICHAEL R. BISHOP
Experimental Transplantation and Immunology Branch, Center for Cancer Research, National Cancer Institute, National Institutes of Health, Bethesda, MD, USA

INTRODUCTION

In concert with their clinical acceptance, monoclonal antibodies (mAbs) have become an exemplary biotechnology drug with revenues from global sales in 2003 amounting to more than $7 billion. A major indication of biotechnology drugs in general and mAbs in particular has been cancer therapy. In fact, out of 270 biotechnology drugs that were in clinical trials in 2003, 101 were investigated in the field of cancer therapy, and of these, 47 were mAbs [1], targeting both "blockbuster" and "nichebuster" markets. Since the approval of rituximab for the treatment of non-Hodgkin's lymphoma (NHL) in 1997, seven additional mAbs were approved by the Food and Drug Administration (FDA) for cancer therapy (Figure 1) and many more are in clinical trials [2]. The mounting success of the antibody molecule as therapeutic agent is based on at least three properties; (*i*) a Fab moiety that permits antigen binding with high specificity and affinity, (*ii*) a Fc moiety that mediates effector functions, such as antibody-dependent cellular cytotoxicity (ADCC) and complement-dependent cytotoxicity (CDC), (*iii*) a molecular mass of approximately 150 kDa that, in concert with Ig recycling through the neonatal Fc receptor, allows a circulatory half-life of up to 21 days. In addition, mAbs have been conjugated to radioisotopes, chemotherapeutic agents, bacterial toxins, cytokines, and enzymes in order to enhance their effector functions [3].

H.L. Kaufman and J.D. Wolchok (eds.), General Principles of Tumor Immunotherapy, 453–484.

Antibody name	Company	Antibody type	Conjugation/ combination	Antigen target	Tumor target	Approval date
Rituximab (Rituxan™)	Biogen Idec/ Genentech	chimeric mouse/human IgG1	none/ chemotherapy	CD20	NHL	1997
Ibritumomab tiuxetan (Zevalin™)	Biogen Idec	mouse IgG1	^{90}yttrium/ none	CD20	NHL	2002
Tositumomab (Bexxar™)	Corixa/ GlaxoSmithKline	mouse IgG2a	^{131}iodine/ none	CD20	NHL	2003
Gemtuzumab ozogamicin (Mylotarg™)	Wyeth	humanized IgG4	calicheamicin/ none	CD33	AML	2000
Alemtuzumab (Campath™)	Millenium/ ILEX	humanized IgG1	none/ none	CD52	CLL	2001
Trastuzumab (Herceptin™)	Genentech	humanized IgG1	none/ chemotherapy	c-erbB-2 (HER2)	breast cancer	1998
Cetuximab (Erbitux™)	ImcloneSystems/ Bristol-Myers Squibb	chimeric mouse/human IgG1	none/ chemotherapy	c-erbB-1 (HER1)	colorectal cancer	2004
Bevacizumab (Avastin™)	Genentech	humanized IgG1	none/ chemotherapy	VEGF	colorectal cancer	2004

Figure 1. Monoclonal antibodies approved for cancer therapy by the Food and Drug Administration. Since 1997, eight mAbs have been approved for the treatment of a variety of cancers. Until 2004, hematologic malignancies dominated cancers targeted by approved mAbs. With the availibility of trastuzumab, cetuximab, and bevacizumab, mAb treatment has also become an option for patients with metastatic breast and colorectal cancer. Bevacizumab, which was approved most recently, is a unique drug in several ways. First, it is the only approved treatment that intentionally targets tumor angiogenesis and, second, the only approved mAb for cancer therapy that targets a soluble rather than a cell surface antigen. Bevacizumab is currently in clinical trials for the treatment of a variety of cancers that depend on tumor angiogenesis

MOLECULAR FEATURES OF MONOCLONAL ANTIBODIES IN CANCER THERAPY

Structure and Formats

The antibody, or immunoglobulin (Ig), molecule consists of a defined covalent assembly of Ig domains (Figure 2). Probably due to its conformational stability and resistance to proteases, the Ig module is found in a variety of extracellular proteins referred to as the Ig superfamily. It is thought that the evolutionary success of the Ig module was driven by the Metazoan evolution with its demand for stable protein modules mediating recognition and adhesion at the cell surface [4]. Though most cell adhesion molecules of the Ig superfamily are single chain molecules, they form homophilic and heterophilic intermolecular interactions that resemble the chain associations found in the antibody molecule (Figure 2). It has therefore been suggested that the antibody molecule evolved from cell adhesion molecules [4]. With its new phenotype, the hypervariable antigen binding site, whose diversity in humans is based on the random combination of approximately 160 functional variable (V), diversity (D), and joining (J) gene segments and somatic mutation, evolved rapidly

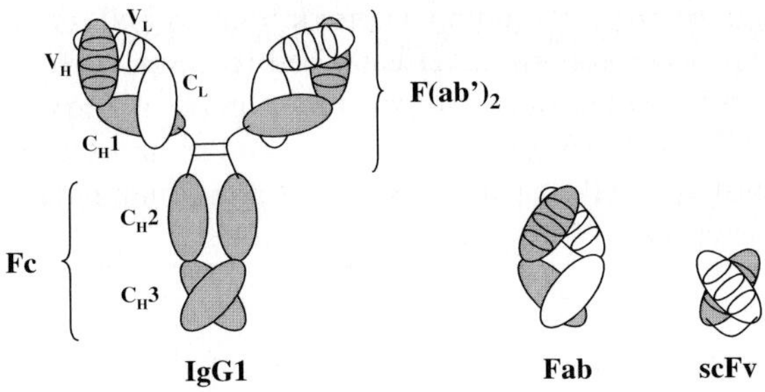

Figure 2. Formats of monoclonal antibodies. The 150-kDa IgG1 molecule (**left**) contains two identical light chains and two identical heavy chains. The light chain consists of one N-terminal variable Ig domain (V_L) followed by one constant Ig domain (C_L). The heavy chain consists of one N-terminal variable Ig domain (V_H) followed by three constant Ig domains (C_H1, C_H2, and C_H3). C_H1 and C_H2 are linked through a flexible hinge region that anchors four interchain disulfide bridges of the IgG1 molecule, one for each of the two light and heavy chain pairs (not shown) and two for the heavy chain pair (shown). The antibody combining site results from the convergence of six hypervariable peptide loops or complementarity determining regions (CDRs), three provided by each V_L and V_H. Each of the twelve Ig domains of the IgG1 molecule consists of approximately 100 amino acids which form a sandwich of two opposing antiparallel beta-sheets that surround a hydrophobic core and are linked by a disulfide bridge. Thus, in addition to its four interchain disulfide bridges the IgG1 molecule is comprised of twelve intrachain disulfide bridges. The 50-kDa monovalent Fab fragment (**center**) contains a single light chain associated with a heavy chain fragment lacking the C-terminal hinge region and constant Ig domains C_H2 and C_H3. Two heterophilic (V_L/V_H and C_L/C_H1) domain interactions and one interchain disulfide bridge between C_L and C_H1 contribute to the stability of the Fab fragment. The 25-kD single chain Fv (scFv) molecule (**right**) consists of variable domains V_L and V_H covalently linked by a polypeptide linker

to become a central protein module of the immune system. The antigen binding site results from the convergence of six hypervariable peptide loops or complementarity determining regions (CDRs), three provided by each light and heavy chain variable domain. The six CDRs are clustered at one end of the antibody molecule (Figure 2). It is primarily the variation in amino acid sequence in the CDRs that produces mAbs of differing antigen specificities. CDR1 and CDR2 of light and heavy chain are encoded within the V gene segments. The most hypervariable CDRs, CDR3 of light and heavy chain are generated by the recombination of V and J gene segments or V, D, and J gene segments, respectively [5]. Intriguingly, the same features that led to the evolutionary success of the Ig domain, namely its stability and versatility, also underlie the success of antibody engineering by rational design and directed evolution. In fact, the ability to functionally express and display Ig domains as antibody fragments by phage, bacteria, and yeast is the *sine qua non* of antibody engineering. Two formats of the antibody molecule that have been predominately used in antibody engineering (Figure 2) are the 50-kD Fab fragment the 25-kD single chain Fv (scFv) fragment [6]. The modular nature of the antibody molecule permits a variety of additional multivalent formats [7]. Of particular interest are multivalent antibody constructs with specificity for two different antigens, which are referred to as bispecific antibodies [8]. For the most part, bispecific antibodies have been engineered for recruiting cytotoxic T cells or NK cells to the tumor site through combining specificity for an effector cell receptor, such as CD3 or FcγRIIIa (CD16), with specificity for a tumor antigen. For example, a recently described bispecific antibody, which combines an anti-CD3 scFv and an anti-CD19 scFv, was shown to redirect cytotoxic T cells for the efficient killing of malignant B-cells at subpicomolar concentrations [9].

Molecular Targets

The use of mAb therapy for cancer depends on the identification of molecular targets, *i.e.*, antigens that are specifically expressed on the cell surface of tumor cells or tumor supporting cells. In addition, growth factors that are specifically expressed by tumor or tumor supporting cells can serve as molecular targets for mAb therapy. By binding to these extracellular antigens, mAbs mediate the selective destruction of tumor cells. In contrast to conventional treatments, mAb therapy does not harm healthy cells that do not express these antigens and, consequently, will cause fewer side effects. As candidates for mAb therapy, antigens should be expressed at high levels on the cell surface of tumor cells or tumor supporting cells and should be absent from critical tissue, including bone marrow, heart, central and peripheral nervous system. Although the ideal molecular target is expressed in the context of the tumor only, few truly tumor-specific antigens have been identified [10]. However, a number of molecular targets with broader expression have proven to be useful for antibody therapy as long as their expression is restricted to less critical tissues. Antigens CD20, CD33, and CD54, which are targeted by five out of eight approved mAbs (Figure 1), are broadly expressed on hematopoietic cells; EGF receptor (ErbB1 or HER1), which is targeted by approved mAb cetuximab, as well as EGF receptor family protein ErbB2 or HER2, which is targeted by approved mAb trastuzumab (Figure 1), are overexpressed in some carcinomas but are also expressed at lower levels in normal epithelial cells [11]; similarly, the target of approved mAb bevacizumab, vascular endothelial growth factor (VEGF), is overexpressed in tumor compared to healthy tissue [12]. Nevertheless, a number of preclinical and clinical mAbs target antigens with a more restricted expression pattern. For example, mAb L19, which, like bevacizumab, targets tumor angiogenesis, binds to the extra-domain B of fibronectin, which is inserted into the fibronectin molecule by alternative splicing during angiogenesis and tissue remodeling but is virtually undetectable in healthy adult tissues [13]. A truly tumor-specific antigen is the B-cell receptor, the idiotype, expressed by malignant B-cells. Custom-made mAbs against individual idiotypes were among the first mAbs that entered the clinic in the early 1980s [14].

Mechanisms of Activity

How does the interaction of mAb and antigen mediate tumor cell killing? Various mechanisms of activity[15] are summarized in Figure 3. By binding to its antigen,

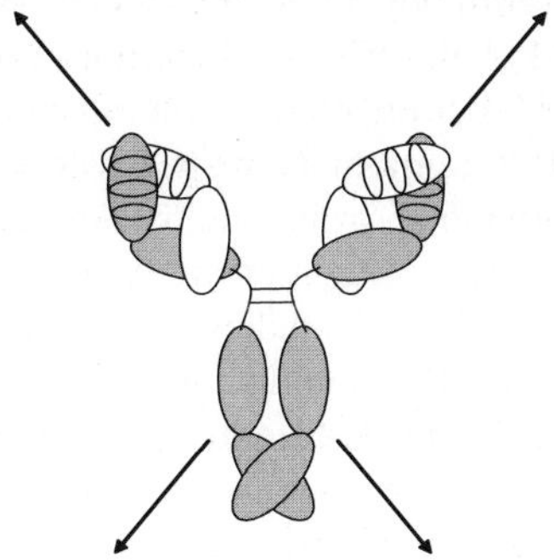

Figure 3. Mechanisms of activity by which monoclonal antibodies mediate tumor cell killing. MAbs can block receptor/ligand interactions that are crucial for cell survival by binding to either receptor or ligand. Receptor cross-linking triggering tumor cell apoptosis is another mechanism of activity that is mediated by the bivalent Fab moiety of the antibody molecule. Immunologic effector functions include antibody-dependent cellular cytotoxicity (ADCC) and complement-dependent cytotoxicity (CDC), both of which are mediated by the Fc moiety of the antibody molecule. To enhance the limited immunologic effector functions of the naked antibody molecule, mAbs have been conjugated to radioisotopes, chemotherapeutic agents, bacterial toxins, cytokines, and enzymes

which could be a receptor or ligand, the mAb can block receptor/ligand interactions that are crucial for cell survival. For example, by binding to VEGF secreted by tumor cells, bevacizumab blocks its interaction with VEGF receptor 2 on endothelial cells that line tumor-infiltrating blood vessels. VEGF receptor 2 blockade leads to endothelial cell apoptosis that precedes tumor cell apoptosis [12]. MAb cetuximab has a similar mechanisms of activity that targets tumor cells directly by blocking the EGF receptor [16]. In addition to the blockade of receptor/ligand interactions, receptor cross-linking is another mechanism of activity that is mediated by the bivalent Fab moiety of the antibody molecule. For example, cross-linking of the B-cell receptor by anti-idiotype mAbs has been shown to induce tumor cell apoptosis [17]. However, the perhaps dominating mechanisms of activity of mAbs are the effector functions mediated by the Fc moiety, *i.e.*, ADCC and CDC. In ADCC, the Fc moiety of IgG1 complexed on the tumor cell surface activates FcγRIIIa (CD16) on natural killer (NK) cells, triggering a cytolytic response. ADCC is thought to be a key mechanism of activity of the approved mAbs rituximab and trastuzumab [18]. In fact, polymorphisms in the sequence of the FcγRIIIa (CD16) receptor, known to modulate human IgG1 binding and ADCC, also influence responses to rituximab [19]. In CDC, on the other hand, the Fc moiety of IgG1 complexed on the tumor cell surface binds to complement protein C1q, triggering a cytolytic response through activation of the complement cascade. CDC is thought to contribute to the activity of rituximab [20]. In addition to these natural mechanisms of activity of the naked antibody molecule, which constitutes five out of eight approved mAbs (Figure 1), the effector functions of the three remaining approved mAbs were enhanced by conjugation to β-emitting radioisotopes ^{90}Y and ^{131}I (ibritumomab tiuxetan and tositumomab, respectively) and the chemotherapeutic agent calicheamicin (gemtuzumab ozagamicin). Another strategy to enhance the effector function of mAbs is by conjugation to cytokines. For example, mAb EMD 273063, which has entered clinical studies for the treatment of metastatic melanoma [21], consists of an anti-GD2 ganglioside IgG1 molecule recombinantly fused to a molecule of interleukin-2 at the C-terminus of each heavy chain. Immunotoxins are chemical conjugations or recombinant fusions of antibody fragments to truncated bacterial or plant toxins, foremost *Pseudomonas* exotoxin A, diphtheria toxin, and ricin toxin [22]. Immunotoxin BL22, which consist of an anti-CD22 scFv recombinantly fused to a truncated form of *Pseudomonas* exotoxin A, has entered clinical studies for the treatment of hairy cell leukemia [23]. Yet another strategy that has entered clinical studies is the conjugation of mAbs to enzymes for the selective activation of prodrugs at the tumor site [24].

Generating Monoclonal Antibodies

Today, mAbs are generated by either hybridoma technology or phage display [25]. All eight mAbs approved for cancer therapy today are derived from mAbs that were generated by hybridoma technology conceived thirty years ago [26]. The hallmark of hybridoma technology is the ability to produce unlimited amounts of defined antibodies. Recently, the approval of adalimumab (Humira™)[27], an anti-TNF-α antibody for the treatment of rheumatoid arthritis, marks the first approval of a mAb generated by phage display. The generation of mAbs through hybridoma technology and phage display is compared in Figure 4. While phage display [28] has a broad range of applications, its utilization for the generation of mAbs has been particularly successful [29,30]. More recently, display technologies other than phage display have been applied to the generation of mAbs, including yeast and ribosome display [31, 32]. What are the advantages of display technologies over hybridoma technology for the generation of mAbs? The physical connection of antibody phenotype (protein) and genotype (cDNA) effectively allows selection rather than screening of mAbs. Selectable phenotypes include stability, affinity, and specificity among other features. In contrast to hybridoma technology, which was practically confined to rodents until recently [33], display technologies permit the generation of mAbs from virtually any species whose Ig genes are known [34]. In particular, the generation of human mAbs has been greatly facilitated by the accessibility of large naïve and synthetic human antibody libraries through display technologies [35–37]. A striking advantage of naïve and synthetic repertoires is their antigen independence, *i.e.*, one library can be used for the selection of mAbs against any antigen. In addition, immune antibody repertoires from humans, rabbits, chickens as well as other species are attractive alternatives to the mouse antibody

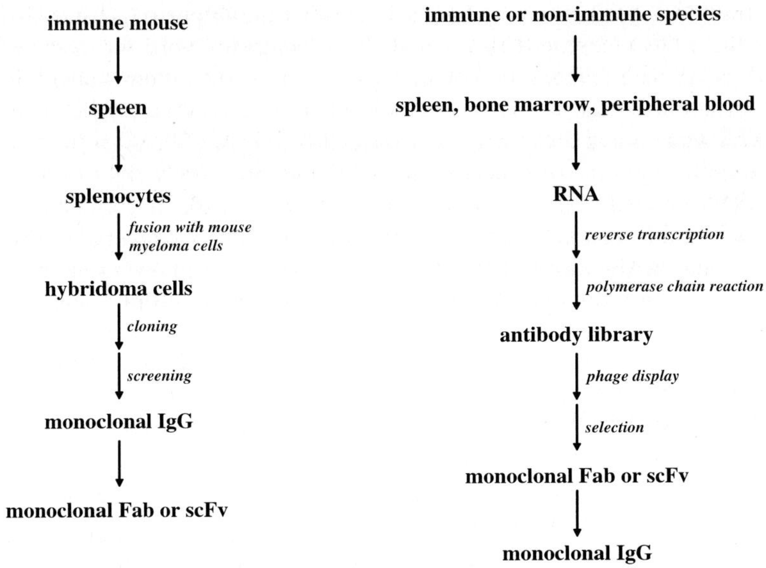

Figure 4. Generation of monoclonal antibodies through hybridoma technology or phage display. This simplified flow chart highlights the differences between the two main routes to mAbs. Whereas the key element of hybridoma technology is the fusion of primary splenocytes with immortal myeloma cells to hybridoma cells, phage display is entirely based on recombinant technology, utilizing retro-transcribed cDNA for the amplification and subsequent combinatorial assembly of light chain and heavy chain encoding sequences. The resulting library of randomly combined antibody light and heavy chains are displayed on the surface of a filamentous phage particle. The displayed protein is encoded on a plasmid, also called phagemid, harbored by the filamentous phage particle. Thus, protein phenotype and DNA genotype are physically linked, allowing their reamplification and enrichment over several rounds of selection for binding to the antigen of interest. Hybridoma technology, on the other hand, preserves the original light chain and heavy chain pairs; hybridoma cells expressing a mAb that binds to the antigen of interest are identified by screening rather than selection

repertoire for the generation of mAbs to human antigens. As was demonstrated more recently, rabbit and chicken mAbs can be humanized while retaining both high specificity and affinity to the human antigen [38,39]. Rabbit and chicken mAbs are of particular interest for the development of therapeutic antibodies that are evaluated in mouse models of human cancer where antibodies are required to recognize both the human antigen in the xenografted tissue and its mouse homologue in the host tissue.

Despite the rapid progress of mAb generation through display technologies, hybridoma technology has maintained a competitive position through further advancements, such as the development of transgenic [40] or transplanted [41] mice expressing human antibodies and the development of transgenic mice with conditionally immortal splenocytes [42]. In particular, the generation of fully human mAbs from transgenic mice promises to become a major contributor to the growing list of mAbs approved for cancer therapy by the FDA. One of the most advanced human mAbs from transgenic mice in clinical studies is panitumumab (ABX-EGF) which targets the EGF receptor (ErbB1) and, thus, competes with the recently approved mAb cetuximab (Figure 1). Another fully human mAb from transgenic mice is MDX-010, which targets CTLA-4, a molecule on T cells that is believed to be responsible for suppressing the immune response. Blocking of CTLA-4 is thought to enable the immune systems of cancer patients to more effectively fight tumors. In 2004, the FDA granted fast track designation for MDX-010, in combination with a melanoma peptide vaccine, for the treatment of metastatic melanoma. A new generation of human mAbs directed to CD20, which might be more potent than rituximab when used as a single agent, have also been generated from transgenic mice [43].

Tailoring Monoclonal Antibodies: From Rational Design to Directed Evolution

The ability to humanize antibodies revolutionized the utilization of mAbs for cancer therapy [44]. Mouse mAbs generated through hybridoma technology are highly immunogenic in humans, triggering a human anti-mouse antibody (HAMA) response, which severely limits their clinical applications and makes antibody humanization mandatory if repeated administration is required for therapy. Among the eight approved mAbs for cancer therapy (Figure 1), four are fully humanized mAbs, two are chimeric mAbs, and only two, which are conjugated to radioisotopes and administered as a single dose, are not humanized.

The first generation of engineered mAbs with human sequences (Figure 5) were chimeric, *i.e.*, they consisted of mouse variable domains V_L and V_H recombinantly fused to human constant domains [45]. Due to their remaining mouse sequences, chimeric antibodies can still trigger a human anti-chimera antibody (HACA) response. To overcome this limitation, the next generation of engineered mAbs was further humanized by grafting the six CDRs that comprise the antigen binding site of the mouse or rat mAb into corresponding human framework regions [46]. This rational design strategy takes advantage of the conserved structure of the variable Ig domain, with the framework regions forming a rigid, yet adjustable [47] β-sheet scaffold that displays the CDRs loops. In addition to residues in the CDRs, framework residues contribute to antigen binding, either indirectly, by supporting the conformation of the CDR loops, or directly, by contacting the antigen [48,49]. Therefore, to maintain antigen binding, usually it is necessary to replace residues of the human framework in addition to CDR grafting. This fine tuning step, which until recently required computer modeling and iterative optimization by site directed mutagenesis, can also be subjected to directed evolution by phage display [38,50,51]. Using directed evolution by phage display, even CDR sequences can be humanized so that the resulting humanized antibody is fully human[52], as in the case of adalimumab[53], or just preserves the most hypervariable sequences, the CDR3 sequences, of the mouse mAb [54]. However, humanized [55] and perhaps even human antibodies can still trigger a human anti-human antibody (HAHA)

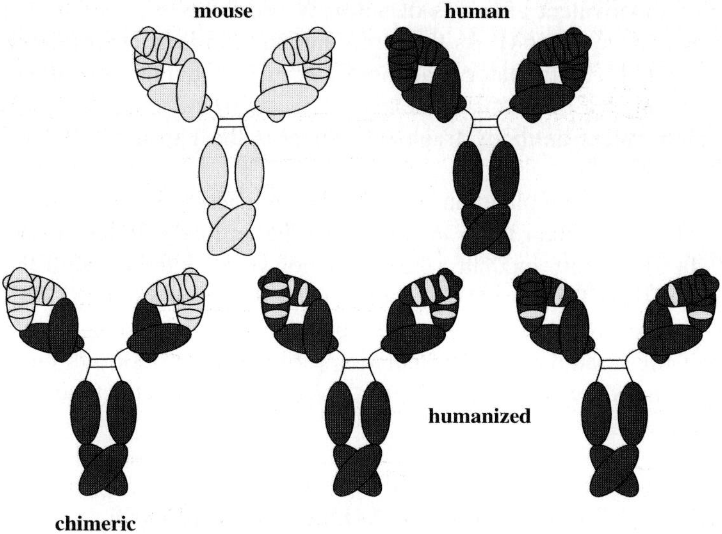

Figure 5. Mouse, chimeric, humanized, and human monoclonal antibodies. Mouse sequences are shown in yellow, human sequences in blue. Mouse or, less commonly, rat mAbs (top left) are generated by hybridoma technology and can be humanized to various degrees. Chimeric mAbs (bottom left), such as the approved mAbs rituximab and cetuximab, preserve the entire rodent variable domains V_L and V_H recombinantly fused to human constant domains. Humanized mAbs (bottom center), which already constitute the largest group among approved mAbs, are generated by grafting all six CDRs from the rodent variable domains V_L and V_H into a human framework. Using phage display, the number of preserved CDRs can be further reduced as shown here for a humanized mAb that retains only the two CDR3 sequences of the rodent mAb (bottom right). Human mAbs (top right) are generated from large naïve and synthetic or, less commonly, immune human antibody libraries by phage display or from transgenic mice by hybridoma technology

response, suggesting that antibody immunogenicity in humans is influenced by additional factors, including the nature of the antigen [56].

In addition to humanization, affinity maturation *in vitro* is a highly relevant step in engineering mAbs for cancer therapy. By increasing the affinity to its target antigen, the therapeutic dose of a mAb is reduced whereas its therapeutic duration is increased [57]. The affinity maturation of mAbs using phage display recapitulates the process of its natural counterpart, which is based on sequence diversification followed by selection [58]. Sequence diversification *in vitro* is accomplished by dispersed or focused mutagenesis strategies. For therapeutic applications, a focused mutagenesis strategy known as CDR walking [59] stands out as a the most general approach for affinity maturation of antibodies. A refined strategy targets mutations to CDR sequences naturally prone to hypermutations [60,61]. CDR walking involves the sequential or parallel optimization of CDRs by sequence randomization and subsequent selection by phage display. The CDRs are an obvious choice for focused mutagenesis because they comprise the antigen binding site and they are naturally diverse, suggesting that mutations in these regions are less likely to be immunogenic.

Using CDR walking, monovalent affinities of antibody fragments were improved into the subnanomolar range [62–64]. As the tumor-targeting properties of a mAb are determined by its size (*i.e.*, circulatory half-life), avidity (*i.e.*, number of antigen binding sites), and affinity, affinity maturation *in vitro* is particularly relevant in the generation of monovalent antibody fragments, such as the Fab and scFv[65] (Figure 2).

Perhaps the most interesting application of antibody engineering in recent years has focused on the Fc rather than the Fab moiety of the antibody molecule. As mentioned above, the Fc moiety mediates the interaction of an antibody with the NK cell receptor FcγRIIIa (CD16) in ADCC and C1q complement protein in CDC. The Fc moiety also interacts with the neonatal receptor FcRn, which is responsible for the extended half-life of antibodies in circulation [66]. Fc optimization through rational design and directed evolution has allowed the tuning of effector functions as well as circulatory half-life of mAbs [67].

CLINICAL INVESTIGATION OF MONOCLONAL ANTIBODIES IN HEMATOLOGIC MALIGNANCIES

Rituximab (Rituxan^{TM})

The CD20 antigen is expressed by more than 95% of B-cell lymphoma cells, but it is not expressed on early lymphocyte progenitor cells[68]. Rituximab is a chimeric mAb produced by combining the variable regions from the anti-CD20 murine mAb ibritumomab with human IgG1 constant regions [69]. Rituximab induces CDC and ADCC, as well as inhibiting proliferation, inducing apoptosis and sensitizing lymphoma cells to the effects of chemotherapy through binding of CD20 [69–71]. The most common toxicities associated with rituximab administration are infusion-related including fevers, chills, chest pain, back pain, bronchospasm and hypotension.

Rituximab monotherapy. The safety and efficacy of rituximab as monotherapy was established in a trial of 166 patients with low-grade non-Hodgkin's lymphoma (NHL) that had progressed after prior chemotherapy (Table 1) [72–74]. Rituximab was administered at 375mg/m[2] weekly for four doses resulting in an overall response rate of approximately 48% with 6% complete remissions (CR); the median duration of response was 13.0 months. When the International Workshop for standardization of response criteria in NHL were applied to this study, the overall and complete response rates were 62% and 32%, respectively [75]. It was observed that serum levels of rituximab correlated with response [76]. The safety and efficacy of re-treatment with rituximab was reported in a trial of 60 NHL patients who had relapsed at least 6 months following prior rituximab therapy [77]. An additional four week course of rituximab resulted in an overall response rate of 40%. The median time to progression in responders and median duration of response were 17.8 months and 16.3 months, respectively, which were longer than the patients' median durations of response achieved from their prior course of

Table 1. Selected trials of monoclonal antibody therapy for hematologic malignancies

Monoclonal Antibody	Indication	Trial Design	Patient Number	Response	Response Duration	Overall Survival	Reference Number
Rituximab	Relapsed "low-grade" NHL	Single-arm, phase II; rituximab 375mg/m^2 weekly x 4 doses	166	ORR = 48%, CR = 6%	TTP = 13.0 months	95% at median follow-up of 13.8 months	74
Rituximab	Untreated stage II-IV "low-grade" NHL	Single-arm; rituximab 375mg/m^2 weekly x 4 doses; responders received additional courses every 6 months	62 (60 assessable)	ORR = 73%, CR = 37%	PFS = 34 months at median follow-up of 30 months	82% at median follow-up of 30 months	78
Rituximab	Previously untreated or treated follicular NHL	Rituximab 375mg/m^2 weekly x 4 doses; patients with responding or stable disease randomized to maintenance rituximab or observation	202 (182 evaluable)	All patients: ORR = 52%, CR = 8%Observation arm (n = 78): ORR = 77%, CR = 31%;Maintenance arm (n = 73): ORR= 75%, CR = 38%	Observation arm: EFS = 11.8 monthsMaintenance arm:EFS = 23.2 months	Not reported.	80

(*Continued*)

Table 1. (Continued)

Monoclonal Antibody	Indication	Trial Design	Patient Number	Response	Response Duration	Overall Survival	Reference Number
Rituximab	Newly diagnosed or relapsed/refractory "low-grade" NHL	Single-arm; rituximab 375mg/m^2 plus CHOP x 6 cycles	40	ORR = 95%, CR = 52%	PFS = 74% at median follow-up of 29 months	Not reported.	81
Rituximab	Newly diagnosed, stage II- IV, diffuse large B-cell NHL in patients 60 - 80 years old	Randomized, phase III trial of rituximab 375mg/m^2 plus CHOP (R-CHOP) x 6 cycles vs. CHOP alone	398	R-CHOP arm (n = 202): ORR = 82%, CR/CRu = 75% vs.CHOP arm (n = 196): ORR = 69%, CR/CRu = 63%	R-CHOP arm: EFS = 57% at 2 years vs.CHOP arm: EFS = 38% at 2 years	R-CHOP arm = 70% at 2 years vs.CHOP arm = 57% at 2 years	85
Ibritumomab tiuxe-tanvs.rituximab	Relapsed or refractory "low-grade" NHL	Randomized, phase III trial of ibritumomab tiuxetan 0.4 mCi/kg vs. rituximab 375 mg/m^2 weekly x 4 doses	143	Ibritumomab tiuxetan arm (n = 73): ORR = 80%, CR/CRu = 34% vs.rituximab arm (n = 70): ORR = 56%, CR/CRu = 20%	Ibritumomab tiuxetan arm: TTP = 11.2 months vs.rituximab: EFS = 10.1 months	Ibritumomab tiuxetan arm: 84% at 2 years vs.rituximab arm: 86% at 2 years	98

Tositumomab	Untreated, stage III-IV, follicular NHL	Single arm, phase II trial of single course of tositumomab	76	ORR = 95%, CR = 75%	PFS = 59% at 5 years	67% at 5 years	101
Gemtuzumab ozogamicin	CD33-positive AML in first relapse	Three multi-center phase II trials of gemtuzumab ozogamicin at 9 mg/m^2 at 2-week intervals x 2 doses	142	CR/CRp = 29%	RFS = 6.8 months	OAS = 31% at 1 year	108
Alemtuzumab	Relapsed or refractory B-cell CLL	Phase II trial of Alemtuzumab at a target dose of 30 mg, 3 times weekly x a maximum of 12 weeks	93	ORR = 33%, CR = 25	TTP = 9.5 months	OAS = 35% at median follow-up of 29 months	119

NHL = non-Hodgkin's lymphoma; ORR = overall response rate; CR = complete response; TTP = time to progression; EFS = event-free survival; CHOP = cyclophosphamide, adriamycin, vincristine, and prednisone; CRu = complete response undetermined; PFS = progression-free survival; AML = acute myelogenous leukemia; CRp = complete remission with platelet recovery; CLL = chronic lymphocytic leukemia

rituximab. Rituximab monotherapy has been investigated as initial therapy in newly-diagnosed low-grade NHL [78–80]. Rituximab monotherapy was used as initial treatment in 62 previously untreated stage II-IV low-grade NHL patients resulting in an overall response rate of 71% [78]. The median progression free survival had still not been reached at a median follow-up of 15 months. The Swiss Group for Clinical Cancer Research trial studied the extended use of single-agent rituximab as maintenance therapy in 202 patients with untreated or previously treated follicular NHL [80]. Patients initially received standard rituximab for four weeks, and patients with responding or stable disease at 12 weeks after the start of therapy were then randomized to either observation or to receive additional single-agent rituximab every 2 months for 4 doses. The rituximab maintenance arm was observed to have a higher event-free survival (23 months vs. 12 months) than in the observation arm (p =.0.02).

Rituximab in combination with chemotherapy. Rituximab is capable of sensitizing lymphoma cells to chemotherapy. Czuczman and colleagues treated 40 patients with low-grade NHL with CHOP (cyclophosphamide, vincristine, doxorubicin and prednisone) plus rituximab (R-CHOP) combination [81]. The R-CHOP combination produced an overall response rate of 95%, including 55% CR. The median progression-free survival had not yet been reached at a median follow-up of 5.5 years. Similar high response rates have been observed in low-grade NHL patients after treatment with rituximab plus single agent (*e.g.*, fludarabine) and multi-agent chemotherapy [82, 83].

Rituximab has been studied in other B-cell malignancies expressing CD20 (*e.g.*, diffuse large B-cell NHL and chronic lymphocytic leukemia) [84–88]. A phase III study, LNH98-5, by Groupe d'Etude Des Lymphomes de L'Adulte (GELA) compared the efficacy and tolerability of R-CHOP with those of CHOP alone in 399 elderly (age 60–80 years) patients with previously untreated diffuse large B-cell NHL [85]. The rate of complete response was significantly higher in the group that received R-CHOP than in the group that received CHOP alone (76 percent vs. 63 percent, p = 0.005). An update of these results demonstrated that event-free, progression-free, disease-free, and overall survival all remain statistically significant in favor of the combination of R-CHOP [86].

Hainsworth and colleagues assessed the efficacy and toxicity of first-line single-agent rituximab, followed by re-treatment with rituximab at 6-month intervals, in 44 previously untreated patients with chronic lymphocytic leukemia (CLL) or small lymphocytic lymphoma [88]. Patients with objective response or stable disease continued to receive identical 4-week rituximab courses at 6-month intervals, for a total of four courses. The objective response rate after the first course of rituximab was 51% with 4% complete responses. Twenty-eight patients received one or more additional courses of rituximab. At the time of this report the overall response rate was 58%, with a median progression-free survival time of 18.6 months. In a multi-center phase II trial 31 patients with fludarabine- and anthracycline-naive B-CLL received a regimen containing rituximab and fludarabine [89]. The overall response rate was 87%; 10 patients achieved a CR. The median duration of response was 75 weeks. The effects of adding rituximab to fludarabine therapy in CLL patients were retrospectively assessed by comparing the treatment outcomes of patients enrolled on two multi-center clinical trials performed by the Cancer and Leukemia Group B (CALGB) that used fludarabine alone (CALGB 9011, n = 178) or fludarabine combined with rituximab (CALGB 9712, n = 104) [90]. In multivariate analyses, the patients receiving fludarabine and rituximab had a significantly better progression-free and overall survival than patients receiving fludarabine therapy.

Ibritumomab Tiuxetan (Zevalin™)

As previously described, radio-immunoconjugates are produced by directly conjugating a radioisotope to an antigen-specific mAb permitting the targeted radiation of tumor cells while minimizing the toxicity to normal tissue. The choice of radioisotopes, yttrium 90 (^{90}Y), a β-emitter, or iodine 131 (^{131}I), a β- and γ-emitter, varies depending on the clinical situation [91]. Ibritumomab tiuxetan is composed of ibritumomab (Y2B8), an anti-CD20 IgG1 mAb, conjugated to the linker-chelator tiuxetan (MX-DTPA), which forms a strong covalent bond with stable retention of ^{90}Y [92].Wiseman and colleagues performed a phase I/II study to determine the optimal distribution, the maximum tolerated dose, and the absorbed radiation dose to normal organs and bone marrow following ibritumomab tiuxetan administration [93]. The maximum tolerated dose of ibritumomab tiuxetan was 0.4 mCi/kg in patients with normal platelet counts and 0.3 mCi/kg in patients with mild thrombocytopenia. The primary toxicity of ibritumomab tiuxetan is reversible, delayed myelosuppression; the nadir occurring seven to nine weeks following therapy [94]. Hematological toxicity does not correlate with dosimetric measurements of ibritumomab tiuxetan, but it appears to be related to a patient's bone marrow reserve and history of prior chemotherapy. The reported incidence of HAMA formation is approximately 2%. Another significant concern is the risk for treatment-related myelodysplasia and acute myelogenous leukemia (AML), which has been identified in 1–2% of patients treated with ibritumomab tiuxetan [94].

In an initial phase I/II trial of ibritumomab tiuxetan, the overall and complete response rates in 32 patients with low-grade NHL were 82% and 26%, respectively [95]. Among 14 patients with intermediate-grade NHL the overall and complete response rate were 43% and 29%, respectively. The median response duration was 12.9 months. Long-term follow-up of 51 patients for relapsed or refractory B-cell NHL treated with ibritumomab tiuxetan demonstrated an overall response rate of 73% [96]. The median time to progression was 12.6 months; however, in the patients who achieved CR the time to progression was 28.3 months.

Witzig and colleagues studied whether NHL patients refractory to rituximab could subsequently respond to ibritumomab tiuxetan [97]. Treatment of 54 patients with rituximab-refractory follicular NHL with ibritumomab tiuxetan resulted in an overall response rate of 74%. In a phase III study, 143 patients with relapsed or refractory low grade or transformed B-cell NHL were randomized to receive either ibritumomab tiuxetan or rituximab [98]. Ibritumomab tiuxetan resulted in higher overall (80% vs. 56%; p = 0.002) and complete (30% vs. 16%; p = 0.04) response rates. However, there was no significant difference in time to disease progression (11.2 vs. 10.1 months; p = 0.173) or in overall survival.

Tositumomab (Bexxar™)

Tositumomab is a murine IgG2a anti-CD20 mAb linked to ^{131}I. The use of ^{131}I increases the whole body dose and requires shielding of hospital personnel and contact with pregnant women or children is not permissible [91]. Free ^{131}I in the blood may be taken up by the thyroid, therefore patients are treated with potassium iodine solution (SSKI) before and during therapy to prevent thyroid damage. The dose-limiting toxicity of tositumomab administration is reversible hematological toxicity with nadirs occurring at weeks 4 to 6 after treatment [99]. As a consequence, most clinical trials with tositumomab require less than 25% bone marrow involvement by lymphoma. Other toxicities include mild infusion reactions. The development of HAMA after of tositumomab administration appears to be less than 20%.

In a phase I/II single-center study, 59 patients with chemotherapy-relapsed or refractory NHL were treated with tositumomab [99]. Unlabeled mAb was given prior to labeled dosimetric and therapeutic doses to improve bio-distribution. The overall and complete response rates were 71% and 34%, respectively. A multi-center study investigated the efficacy, dosimetry, and safety of tositumomab in 47 patients with relapsed or refractory low-grade and transformed B-cell NHL [100]. The overall response rate was 57% with a median duration of response of 9.9 months.

Tositumomab was used as initial therapy in 76 patients with advanced-stage, follicular NHL [101]. Tositumab resulted in overall and complete response rates of 95% and 75%, respectively. Molecular remissions were observed in 80% of assessable patients who had a clinical complete response. At a median follow-up of 5.1 years, the actuarial 5-year progression-free survival for all patients was 59%. Similar to results with ibritumomab tiuxetan, tositumab has also been demonstrated to have efficacy in patients who have received prior rituximab [102].

Radio-immunoconjugates targeting CD20 have been used in combination with autologous hematopoietic stem cell transplantation (HSCT). Researchers at the Fred Hutchinson Cancer Research Center performed a multivariable comparison of 125 consecutive patients with follicular NHL treated with either high-dose radio-immunotherapy using ^{131}I-anti-CD20 (n = 27) or conventional high-dose therapy (n = 98) and autologous HSCT [103]. The 100-day treatment-related mortality was 3.7% in the high-dose radio-immunotherapy group and 11% in the conventional high-dose therapy group. Patients treated with high-dose radio-immunotherapy experienced improved 5-year progression-free (48% vs. 29%) and overall survival (67% vs. 53%), as compared to patients who received conventional high-dose therapy.

Gemtuzumab Ozogamicin (Mylotarg™)

The CD33 antigen is expressed on the majority of blasts in AML, but it is not widely expressed by cells outside the hematopoietic system [104]. Gemtuzumab ozogamicin is a humanized murine anti-CD33 mAb that is chemically linked to calicheamicin, an enediyne anti-tumor antibiotic that results in DNA cleavage and apoptosis [105]. Gemtuzumab ozogamicin is rapidly internalized by AML cells and results in G_2 arrest followed by apoptosis [106, 107]. Minor infusion related reactions have been documented with gemtuzumab ozogamicin administration. The most significant toxicities associated with gemtuzumab ozogamicin administration include myelosuppression and hepatotoxicity. In an analysis of 142 patients neutropenia and thrombocytopenia occurred in 99% and 97% respectively [108]. Hepatoxicity occurs in 30–40% of patients treated with gemtuzumab ozogamicin which is transient in the majority of cases; however, life-threatening veno-occlusive disease (VOD) has been noted in a small minority of patients. Prior exposure to gemtuzumab ozogamicin is an independent risk factor for the development of VOD in AML patients undergoing HSCT [109].

In a phase I dose escalation study 41 patients with refractory or relapsed CD33-positive AML were treated with single agent gemtuzumab ozogamicin in doses ranging from 0.25–9.0 mg/m^2 [110]. Eight patients (20%) had a reduction in peripheral blood and/or bone marrow blast counts to less than 5%. There was a cohort of patients who had apparent blast clearance but persistent thrombocytopenia (<100 x 10^9/L) that lead to a new response category termed complete remission without platelet recovery (CRp). Based on a recommended dose of 9.0mg/m^{2}for 2 doses with a 14-day interval, three open label, multi-center phase II trials were initiated that included a total of 142 patients [108]. All patients received the first dose, 77% received a second, and only 3% received a third dose. The complete remission rate, including CRp, was 29% with a median time to remission of 60 days.

Gemtuzumab ozogamicin is currently being evaluated in combination with conventional chemotherapy and HSCT protocols. A pilot study of gemtuzumab ozogamicin, idarubicin and cytarabine combination induced 3 complete remissions and 3 CRp in 14 patients with primary refractory or relapsed AML[111]. Another study treated 17 AML patients with a combination of cytarabine and topotecan with gemtuzumab ozogamicin resulting in complete remissions in 2 patients; the median survival was 8.2 weeks [112]. Gemtuzumab ozogamicin has also been used with all-trans retinoic acid to treat 19 patients with acute promyelocytic leukemia resulting in 16 complete remissions (84%) including 14 molecular remissions [113].

Alemtuzumab (Campath™)

Alemtuzumab is a humanized mAb (IgG1) directed against CD52, which is expressed on the majority of B-cell lineage neoplasms express the CD52 antigen, particularly on B-cell chronic lymphocytic leukemia (B-CLL) and T- cell prolymphocytic leukemia (T-PLL) [114]. CD52 is expressed on mature B and T lymphocytes, monocytes, and spermatozoa; it is not expressed on hematopoietic stem cells, erythrocytes or platelets. *In vitro* data demonstrated that cross-linking CD52 with the humanized mAb induces growth inhibition and apoptosis; however, the effector mechanisms of alemtuzumab are not completely understood [115].

The most common toxicities associated with alemtuzumab administration are infusion related. Hematological toxicity is common with severe lymphopenia occurring in almost all patients and grade 4 neutropenia occurring in approximately 20% of patients by 4 weeks after treatment [116]. The profound lymphopenia and reduced cell-mediated immunity leads to increased risk of opportunistic infections particularly latent viral infection such as cytomegalovirus [116–118].

Rai et al. reported the results of their phase II study on the safety and efficacy of intravenous alemtuzumab in 24 CLL patients [118]. The overall response rate was 33%, median duration of response was 15.4 months, and the median survival was 35.8 months. A multi-institutional, phase II study examined the safety and clinical efficacy of intravenous alemtuzumab in 93 patients with relapsed or refractory B-CLL who had received alkylating agents and had failed fludarabine therapy [119]. The overall response and complete response rates were 33% and 2%, respectively; the median time to progression was 9.5 months for responding patients. Osterborg and colleagues reported that the use of alemtuzumab as initial therapy of B-cell CLL resulted in an overall response rate of 89% and a CR of 33% [120].

Alemtuzumab was used to treat 76 patients with refractory and recurrent T-PLL resulting in an overall response rate of 51% with a 39.5% complete responses [121]. The median duration of CR was 8.7 months, and the median time to progression was 4.5 months. Uppenkamp and colleagues investigated alemtuzumab in patients with relapsed low- and high-grade NHL; however, responses were only observed in patients with low-grade NHL [122].

The combination of alemtuzumab and rituximab was reported in 48 patients with relapsed and refractory lymphoid malignancies; however, responses were only noted in the CLL or T-PLL subgroups [123]. Responses were observed in 20 of 32 CLL patients, while there were 4 responses in 9 patients with T-PLL. The combination of alemtuzumab and fludarabine has been shown to induce responses in CLL patients previously refractory to either treatment [124]. Alemtuzumab is also being studied as part of conditioning regimens to deplete host lymphocytes prior to allogeneic HSCT and to control graft-versus-host disease both *in vivo* and *ex vivo* [125].

Other Monoclonal Antibodies Under Investigation for the Treatment of Hematologic Malignancies

RFB4(dsFv)-PE38 (BL22) is a recombinant immunotoxin, in which a disulfide-linked Fv fragment of a mAb targeting CD22 is fused to truncated *Pseudomonas* exotoxin A [23]. BL22 was administered to 16 patients with purine analog-refractory hairy cell leukemia resulting in 11 complete remissions and 2 partial remissions. Numerous additional mAbs are under investigation to treat hematologic malignancies including epratuzumab (anti-CD22), apolizumab (anti-1D10), and SGN-30 (anti-CD30).

CLINICAL INVESTIGATION OF MONOCLONAL ANTIBODIES IN SOLID MALIGNANCIES

Trastuzumab (Herceptin™)

Human epidermal growth factor receptor-2 (ErbB2; HER2; HER2/neu) is a tyrosine kinase membrane receptor which is expressed on approximately 30% of breast cancer cells; its expression is associated with a poor prognosis in breast cancer patients [126, 127]. Laboratory studies demonstrated that antibodies directed against HER2 can inhibit growth of tumors and of transformed cells that express high levels of this receptor [128, 129]. Trastuzumab is relatively well tolerated with the most common side effects being infusion-related symptoms occurring in approximately 40% of patients. The most significant adverse event is cardiac dysfunction, which has been most commonly observed in patients receiving trastuzumab concomitantly with adriamycin.

Trastuzumab monotherapy is capable of providing prolonged disease stability in a significant number of patients with advanced metastatic breast cancer [130]. Cobleigh et al. reported on an open label trial in 222 patients with advanced metastatic breast cancer receiving trastuzumab monotherapy (Table 2) [131]. The overall response rate was 22%, with a median duration of response of 9.1 months and median survival of 13 months.

The method by which HER2/neu over-expression is determined, either by immunohistochemistry (IHC) or fluorescent in-situ hybridization (FISH), plays a significant role in the response to trastuzumab. Vogel et al. studied HER2/neu over-expression by FISH among 114 breast cancer patients with either 2+ or 3+ over-expression by IHC that were treated with trastuzumab.[130] The overall response rate was 26%. Response rates in 111 assessable patients with 3+ and 2+ HER2 over-expression by IHC were 35% and none, respectively. The response rates in 108 assessable patients with and without HER2 gene amplification by FISH analysis were 34% and 7%, respectively.

In vitro data demonstrated a synergistic decrease in cell growth when anti-HER2/neu mAb and chemotherapy (*e.g.*, cisplatin, paclitaxel) were used in combination [132]. Numerous combinations of trastuzumab with chemotherapeutic agents have been reported [133–137]. Slamon et al. reported on the results of a multicenter randomized controlled clinical trial of trastuzumab that included 469 breast cancer patients whose tumors over-expressed HER2 at the 2+ or 3+ level by IHC [137]. Patients with no prior anthracycline exposure received AC alone or in combination with trastuzumab. Patients who had been previously treated with anthracyclines received paclitaxel alone or in combination with trastuzumab. After a 14-month follow-up, the addition of trastuzumab to chemotherapy led to a significantly improved time to disease progression (7.8 months vs. 4.6 months, $p = 0.0001$), overall response rate (50% vs. 32%, $p < 0.0001$), and higher median response duration (9.1 vs. 6.1 months, $p = 0.0002$). After a 29-month follow-up the overall survival remained significantly increased, 25.4 months versus 20.3 months ($p < 0.025$).

Table 2. Selected trials of monoclonal antibody therapy for solid malignancies

Monoclonal Antibody	Indication	Trial Design	Patient Number	Response	Response Duration	Overall Survival	Reference Number
Traztuzumab	Advanced, previously treated, HER2-expressing, metastatic breast cancer	Single arm, Phase II trial of Traztuzumab at loading dose of 4 mg/kg , followed by a 2-mg/kg maintenance dose at weekly intervals	222	ORR = 15%, CR = 4%	Median duration of response = 9.1 months	Median survival = 13.0 months	131
Traztuzumab	Previously treated and untreated HER-2 expressing metastatic breast cancer	Randomized, Phase III trial of trastuzumab plus chemotherapy (*) vs. chemotherapy alone (*)	469	Traztuzumab plus chemotherapy arm (n = 235): ORR = 50%, CR = 8% vs. Chemotherapy arm (n = 234): ORR = 32%, CR = 3%	Traztuzumab plus chemotherapy arm: TTP = 7.4 months vs. Chemotherapy arm : TTP = 4.6 months	Traztuzumab plus chemotherapy arm = 25.4 months vs.Chemotherapy arm = 20.3 months	137
Bevacizumab	Previously untreated metastatic colorectal cancer	Randomized, Phase III trial of irinotecan, fluorouracil, and leucovorin (IFL) plus bevacizumab (5 mg/kg every two weeks) vs. IFL plus placebo	813	IFL plus bevacizumab arm (n = 412): ORR = 44.8% vs. IFL plus placebo arm (n = 411): ORR = 34.8%	IFL plus bevacizumab arm: PFS = 10.6 months vs. IFL plus placebo arm: PFS = 6.2 months	IFL plus bevacizumab arm = 20.3 months vs.IFL plus placebo arm = 15.6 months	141

Bevacizumab	Previously treated metastatic, clear cell renal cell carcinoma	Randomized, double-blind, Phase II trial of bevacizumab (at doses of 3 and 10 mg/kg given every two weeks) vs. Placebo	116	Bevacizumab 3 mg/kg arm (n = 37): ORR = 0 vs. bevacizumab 10 mg/kg arm (n = 39): ORR = 10% vs. Placebo arm (n = 40): ORR = 0	Bevacizumab 3 mg/kg arm: TTP = 3.0 months vs. bevacizumab 10 mg/kg arm: TTP = 4.8 months vs. Placebo arm: TTP = 2.5 months	Not reported. No statistical difference in survival between the three arms.	146
Cetuximab	Metastatic colorectal cancer refractory to treatment with irinotecan	Randomized Phase III trial cetuximab (initial dose of 400 mg/m^2 followed by weekly dose of 250 mg/m^2) plus irinotecan vs. cetuximab monotherapy	329	Cetuximab plus irinotecan arm (n = 218): ORR = 22.9% vs. cetuximab monotherapy (n = 111): ORR = 10.8%	Cetuximab plus irinotecan arm: TTP = 4.1 months vs. cetuximab monotherapy: TTP = 1.5 months	Cetuximab plus irinotecan arm = 8.6 months vs. cetuximab monotherapy = 6.9 months	152
Edrecolomab	Untreated, resected stage III colon cancer	Randomized, Phase III trial of edrecolomab (initial dose of 500 mg followed by 4 doses of 100 mg every 4 weeks), plus fluorouracil-folinic acid (F-FA) vs. F-FA alone vs. edrecolomab monotherapy as adjuvant therapy	2671	Not applicable.	Edrecolomab plus F-FA arm (n = 912): DFS = 63.8% at 3 years vs. F-FA alone arm (n = 927): DFS = 65.5% at 3 years vs. edrecolomab monotherapy arm (n=922): DFS = 53.0% at 3 years	Edrecolomab plus F-FA arm = 74.4% at 3 years vs. F-FA alone arm = 76.1% at 3 years vs. edrecolomab monotherapy arm = 70.1% at 3 years	158

ORR = overall response rate; CR = complete response; (*) = Patients who had not previously received adjuvant (postoperative) therapy with an anthracycline were treated with doxorubicin or epirubicin and cyclophosphamide. Patients who had previously received adjuvant anthracycline were treated with paclitaxel; TTP = time to progression; DFS = disease-free survival.

The combination of weekly paclitaxel and trastuzumab was examined in 94 metastatic breast cancer patients whose disease did or did not over-express HER2/neu by IHC [134]. The intent-to-treat response rate for all 95 patients enrolled was 56.8%. In patients with HER2-overexpressing tumors, overall response rates ranged from 67% to 81% compared with 41% to 46% in patients with HER2-normal expression. Esteva and colleagues reported response rates of 67% for FISH positive patients treated with the combination of weekly docetaxel and trastuzumab [135]. Burstein et al. studied the clinical efficacy and side effect profile of vinorelbine and trastuzumab; an overall response rates of 75% were observed [136]. The use of trastuzumab as part of adjuvant therapy for breast cancer is under current clinical investigation [138]. The National Surgical Adjuvant Breast and Bowel Project and United States Inter-Group are using sequential doxorubicin and cyclophosphamide followed by paclitaxel and either concomitant or delayed trastuzumab. The Breast Cancer International Research Group is also investigating adjuvant therapy with traztuzumab in combination with docetaxel and carboplatin.

Bevacizumab (Avastin™)

Bevacizumab is a recombinant humanized mAb (IgG1) with selectivity against VEGF, which is expressed in colorectal, breast, ovarian and non-small cell lung cancer [139]. The mAb is able to inhibit endothelial cell mitogenic activity, vascular permeability enhancing activity, and angiogenic properties.

Kabbinavar et al. reported on a phase II randomized trial comparing bevacizumab combined with 5-fluoruracil (5FU) and leucovorin (LV) as compared with 5FU/LV alone in patients with advanced metastatic colorectal cancer [140]. The arms containing bevacizumab were associated with superior response rates, longer median time to disease progression, and longer median survival. These studies led to the development of the phase III study of bevacizumab plus irinotecan, 5FU and LV (IFL) versus IFL alone as first-line treatment of metastatic colorectal cancer [141]. As compared with IFL alone, the combination of bevacizumab and IFL increased the overall response rate from 34.8% to 44.8% and increased the median duration of response from 7.1 to 10.4 months. The addition of bevacizumab to IFL also resulted in a significant improvement in overall survival (20.3 months vs. 15.6 months, $p < 0.0001$). Hurwitz et al. subsequently reported on a third patient cohort of the above-described trial, who received bevacizumab combined with 5FU/LV, and compared them with results for concurrently enrolled patients who received IFL [142]. A total of 923 patients were randomly assigned to receive IFL plus placebo, IFL plus bevacizumab, or 5FU/LV plus bevacizumab. After an interim analysis confirmed acceptable safety for IFL plus bevacizumab, further accrual to the 5FU/LV plus bevacizumab arm was discontinued. Overall response rates were 40.0% and 37.0%, and median response durations were 8.5 and 7.2 months, for 5FU/LV plus bevacizumab arm ($n = 110$) and IFL/placebo arm ($n = 100$), respectively. Median progression-free survival rates were 8.8 and 6.8 months, respectively; the median overall survival rates were 18.3 and 15.1 months, respectively. The investigators concluded that 5FU/LV plus bevacizumab was as active as IFL plus bevacizumab, and was an acceptable treatment alternative for patients with previously untreated metastatic colorectal cancer.

E3200, an Eastern Cooperative Oncology Group (ECOG) study, is a randomized phase III trial that evaluated bevacizumab alone versus bevacizumab plus oxaliplatin, LV, and 5FU (FOLFOX4) versus FOLFOX4 alone in previously treated advanced colorectal cancer. The clinical outcomes of E3200 were reported on 829 patients at the 2005 Annual Meeting of American Society of Clinical Oncology [143]. Bowel perforation was infrequent (1.1%), but it occurred only in patients treated with bevacizumab. The overall survival rates for bevacizumab alone, bevacizumab plus FOLFOX4, and FOLFOX4 alone were 10.2 months, 12.5 months, and 10.7 months ($p = 0.0024$), respectively. Progression-free survival rates were 5.5 months, 7.4 months, and 5.5 months ($p = 0.0003$) for the three arms, respectively.

Bevacizumab was investigated in a randomized phase II trial of paclitaxel and carboplatin (PC) with or without bevacizumab in advanced non-small cell lung cancer (NSCLC) [144]. Treatment with PC plus bevacizumab resulted in a higher response rate (31.5% vs. 18.8%), longer median time to progression (7.4 vs. 4.2 months), and a slight increase in survival (17.7 vs. 14.9 months), as compared with PC alone. Based on these results ECOG conducted a randomized, phase II/III trial of PC with or without bevacizumab (E4599) in 842 patients with advanced NSCLC [145]. Results from E4599 were presented at 2005 Annual Meeting of American Society of Clinical Oncology. The overall response rates were 10% and 27% ($p < 0.0001$) and progression-free survival rates were 4.5 months and 6.4 months ($p < 0.0001$) for the PC alone and PC plus bevacizumab arms, respectively. The median overall survival rates were 10.2 months and 12.5 months ($p = 0.0075$) for the two arms, respectively. Based on these results PC plus bevacizumab has become new treatment standard in advanced NSCLC for ECOG.

In a randomized, double-blind, phase II trial, bevacizumab was compared to placebo in the treatment of metastatic renal cell carcinoma [146]. The trial was stopped after the interim analysis met the criteria for early stopping. One hundred and sixteen patients randomly assigned to receive placebo ($n= 40$), low-dose bevacizumab ($n = 37$), or high-dose bevacizumab ($n= 39$). There was a significant prolongation of the time to progression of disease in the high-dose bevacizumab group as compared with the placebo group ($p < 0.001$). There was a small difference, of borderline significance ($p = 0.053$), between the time to progression of disease in the low-dose bevacizumab group and that in the placebo group. However, bevacizumab did not result in any significant survival advantage.

Cetuximab (Erbitux™)

Cetuximab is a chimeric IgG1 mAb that binds to the extracellular domain of epidermal growth factor receptor (EGFR) competitively inhibiting EGF binding and thus its action [147]. Activation of EGFR leads to a cascade of functions such as proliferation, differentiation, survival and angiogenesis. Over-expression of EGFR is frequently identified in solid tumors, such as colorectal, breast, lung, head and neck, glioblastoma, bladder, ovarian cancer and many more and is generally associated with a poor prognosis [148]. Blockade of EGFR by cetuximab has been shown to inhibit the growth of colon cancer cell lines *in vitro* and of xenografts by disrupting the EGFR mediated signal transduction both as a single agent and in combination with chemotherapy [16, 149]. Cetuximab is generally very well tolerated with allergic reactions, acne type skin rashes, abdominal pain, nausea, vomiting and asthenia being the most common adverse events [150]. Anaphylactic reactions have been noted in a small percentage of patients.

In a phase II, open-label trial, 57 patients with EGFR-expressing tumors that had failed prior therapy with irinotecan, received weekly cetuximab alone [151]. Five patients achieved a partial response; 21 additional patients had stable disease or minor responses. The median survival was 6.4 months. Cunningham and colleagues studied the efficacy of cetuximab in combination with irinotecan as compared to cetuximab alone in 329 patients with metastatic colorectal cancer, whose cancer was refractory to treatment with irinotecan [152]. The rate of response in the cituximab plus irinotecan group was significantly higher than that in the monotherapy group (22.9% vs. 10.8%). The median time to progression was significantly greater in the combination-therapy group (4.1 vs. 1.5 months), and there was a trend towards improved survival time (8.6 months vs. 6.9 months), but it did not reach statistical significance. Results were presented at the 2005 Annual Meeting of American Society of Clinical Oncology on a phase II trial cetuximab in combination with the FOLFOX-4 regimen as first-line treatment of 42 patients with EGFR-expressing metastatic colorectal cancer that resulted in an overall response rate of 72% [153]. Cetuximab has demonstrated activity in other solid tumors such as renal cell carcinoma and pancreatic cancer [154, 155].

Edrecolomab (Panorex, 17-1A)

Edrocolomab is a murine-derived mAb that recognizes the human tumor-associated antigen Ep-CAM (otherwise known as 17-1A) [156]. It is being studied as part of adjuvant treatment of colorectal cancer. In a study of 189 patients with resected stage III colorectal cancer, treatment with edrecolomab resulted in a 32% increase in overall survival compared with no treatment ($p < 0.01$) and decreased the tumor recurrence rate by 23% ($p < 0.04$) [157]. Based on these data edrecolomab was investigated as adjuvant therapy in patients with resected stage III colon cancer as part of a randomized, multi-national trial [158]. Following surgery, 2761 patients were randomly assigned to edrecolomab plus 5FU-folinic acid, 5FU-folinic acid alone, or edrecolomab alone. At a median follow-up time of 26 months, there was no difference in the 3-year overall survival (74.7% vs. 76.1%, $p=0.53$) between the edrecolomab plus 5FU-folinic acid arm and the 5FU-folinic acid alone arm. The disease-free survival was significantly lower on the edrecolomab alone arm than on chemotherapy alone arm (53.0% vs. 65.5%).

SUMMARY

Improved understanding of tumor biology has allowed the development of targeted therapy including mAbs. Although many of the clinically available mAbs have activity by themselves, their efficacy is significantly improved when combined with conventional therapies, particularly cytotoxic chemotherapy. Clinical trials of combinations of mAbs with conventional chemotherapy have demonstrated significant responses and improvement in overall survival for a variety of malignancies including a number of advanced solid tumors in which there had not been significant clinical advancements for several years. These agents have significantly altered clinical care and established new standards for several diseases. Ongoing clinical trials are now investigating these combinations earlier in the disease course as part of first-line and adjuvant therapies where it is anticipated that they will result in significant improvement in these settings.

REFERENCES

1. Werner RG. Economic aspects of commercial manufacture of biopharmaceuticals. J Biotechnol. 2004;113:171–182.
2. Lin MZ, Teitell MA, Schiller GJ. The evolution of antibodies into versatile tumor-targeting agents. Clin Cancer Res. 2005;11:129–138.
3. Carter P. Improving the efficacy of antibody-based cancer therapies. Nat Rev Cancer. 2001;1:118–129.
4. Hunkapiller T, Goverman J, Koop BF, Hood L. Implications of the diversity of the immunoglobulin gene superfamily. Cold Spring Harb Symp Quant Biol. 1989;54 Pt 1:15–29.
5. Tonegawa S. Somatic generation of antibody diversity. Nature. 1983;302:575–581.
6. Presta L. Antibody engineering for therapeutics. Curr Opin Struct Biol. 2003;13:519–525.
7. Hudson PJ, Souriau C. Engineered antibodies. Nat Med. 2003;9:129–134.
8. Cao Y, Lam L. Bispecific antibody conjugates in therapeutics. Adv Drug Deliv Rev. 2003;55:171–197.
9. Kufer P, Lutterbuse R, Baeuerle PA. A revival of bispecific antibodies. Trends Biotechnol. 2004;22:238–244.
10. Scott AM, Welt S. Antibody-based immunological therapies. Curr Opin Immunol. 1997;9:717–722.
11. Ranson M, Sliwkowski MX. Perspectives on anti-HER monoclonal antibodies. Oncology. 2002;63 Suppl 1:17–24.
12. Gerber HP, Ferrara N. Pharmacology and pharmacodynamics of bevacizumab as monotherapy or in combination with cytotoxic therapy in preclinical studies. Cancer Res. 2005;65:671–680.
13. Tarli L, Balza E, Viti F, et al. A high-affinity human antibody that targets tumoral blood vessels. Blood. 1999;94:192–198.
14. Davis TA, Maloney DG, Czerwinski DK, Liles TM, Levy R. Anti-idiotype antibodies can induce long-term complete remissions in non-Hodgkin's lymphoma without eradicating the malignant clone. Blood. 1998;92:1184–1190.
15. Cragg MS, French RR, Glennie MJ. Signaling antibodies in cancer therapy. Curr Opin Immunol. 1999;11:541–547.
16. Grunwald V, Hidalgo M. Developing inhibitors of the epidermal growth factor receptor for cancer treatment. J Natl Cancer Inst. 2003;95:851–867.
17. Besnault L, Schrantz N, Auffredou MT, Leca G, Bourgeade MF, Vazquez A. B cell receptor cross-linking triggers a caspase-8-dependent apoptotic pathway that is independent of the death effector domain of Fas-associated death domain protein. J Immunol. 2001;167:733–740.

18. Clynes RA, Towers TL, Presta LG, Ravetch JV. Inhibitory Fc receptors modulate in vivo cytoxicity against tumor targets. Nat Med. 2000;6:443–446.
19. Treon SP, Hansen M, Branagan AR, et al. Polymorphisms in FcgammaRIIIA (CD16) receptor expression are associated with clinical response to rituximab in Waldenstrom's macroglobulinemia. J Clin Oncol. 2005;23:474–481.
20. Cragg MS, Glennie MJ. Antibody specificity controls in vivo effector mechanisms of anti-CD20 reagents. Blood. 2004;103:2738–2743.
21. King DM, Albertini MR, Schalch H, et al. Phase I clinical trial of the immunocytokine EMD 273063 in melanoma patients. J Clin Oncol. 2004;22:4463–4473.
22. Pastan II, Kreitman RJ. Immunotoxins for targeted cancer therapy. Adv Drug Deliv Rev. 1998;31:53–88.
23. Kreitman RJ, Wilson WH, Bergeron K, et al. Efficacy of the anti-CD22 recombinant immunotoxin BL22 in chemotherapy-resistant hairy-cell leukemia. N Engl J Med. 2001;345:241–247.
24. Bagshawe KD, Sharma SK, Begent RH. Antibody-directed enzyme prodrug therapy (ADEPT) for cancer. Expert Opin Biol Ther. 2004;4:1777–1789.
25. Rader C. Antibody libraries in drug and target discovery. Drug Discov Today. 2001;6:36–43.
26. Kohler G, Milstein C. Continuous cultures of fused cells secreting antibody of predefined specificity. Nature. 1975;256:495–497.
27. Bain B, Brazil M. Adalimumab. Nat Rev Drug Discov. 2003;2:693–694.
28. Smith GP. Filamentous fusion phage: novel expression vectors that display cloned antigens on the virion surface. Science. 1985;228:1315–1317.
29. Burton DR, Barbas CF, 3rd. Human antibodies from combinatorial libraries. Adv Immunol. 1994;57:191–280.
30. Winter G, Griffiths AD, Hawkins RE, Hoogenboom HR. Making antibodies by phage display technology. Annu Rev Immunol. 1994;12:433–455.
31. Lipovsek D, Pluckthun A. In-vitro protein evolution by ribosome display and mRNA display. J Immunol Methods. 2004;290:51–67.
32. Feldhaus MJ, Siegel RW. Yeast display of antibody fragments: a discovery and characterization platform. J Immunol Methods. 2004;290:69–80.
33. Spieker-Polet H, Sethupathi P, Yam PC, Knight KL. Rabbit monoclonal antibodies: generating a fusion partner to produce rabbit-rabbit hybridomas. Proc Natl Acad Sci U S A. 1995;92:9348–9352.
34. Rader C, Barbas CF, 3rd. Phage display of combinatorial antibody libraries. Curr Opin Biotechnol. 1997;8:503–508.
35. Fellouse FA, Wiesmann C, Sidhu SS. Synthetic antibodies from a four-amino-acid code: a dominant role for tyrosine in antigen recognition. Proc Natl Acad Sci U S A. 2004;101:12467–12472.
36. Knappik A, Ge L, Honegger A, et al. Fully synthetic human combinatorial antibody libraries (HuCAL) based on modular consensus frameworks and CDRs randomized with trinucleotides. J Mol Biol. 2000;296:57–86.
37. Vaughan TJ, Williams AJ, Pritchard K, et al. Human antibodies with sub-nanomolar affinities isolated from a large non-immunized phage display library. Nat Biotechnol. 1996;14:309–314.
38. Rader C, Ritter G, Nathan S, et al. The rabbit antibody repertoire as a novel source for the generation of therapeutic human antibodies. J Biol Chem. 2000;275:13668–13676.
39. Tsurushita N, Park M, Pakabunto K, et al. Humanization of a chicken anti-IL-12 monoclonal antibody. J Immunol Methods. 2004;295:9–19.
40. Kellermann SA, Green LL. Antibody discovery: the use of transgenic mice to generate human monoclonal antibodies for therapeutics. Curr Opin Biotechnol. 2002;13:593–597.
41. Reisner Y, Dagan S. The Trimera mouse: generating human monoclonal antibodies and an animal model for human diseases. Trends Biotechnol. 1998;16:242–246.
42. Pasqualini R, Arap W. Hybridoma-free generation of monoclonal antibodies. Proc Natl Acad Sci U S A. 2004;101:257–259.
43. Teeling JL, French RR, Cragg MS, et al. Characterization of new human CD20 monoclonal antibodies with potent cytolytic activity against non-Hodgkin lymphomas. Blood. 2004;104:1793–1800.

44. Tsurushita N, Hinton PR, Kumar S. Design of humanized antibodies: From anti-Tac to Zenapax. Methods. 2005;36:69–83.
45. Morrison SL, Johnson MJ, Herzenberg LA, Oi VT. Chimeric human antibody molecules: mouse antigen-binding domains with human constant region domains. Proc Natl Acad Sci U S A. 1984;81:6851–6855.
46. Riechmann L, Clark M, Waldmann H, Winter G. Reshaping human antibodies for therapy. Nature. 1988;332:323–327.
47. Holmes MA, Buss TN, Foote J. Conformational correction mechanisms aiding antigen recognition by a humanized antibody. J Exp Med. 1998;187:479–485.
48. Foote J, Winter G. Antibody framework residues affecting the conformation of the hypervariable loops. J Mol Biol. 1992;224:487–499.
49. Wedemayer GJ, Patten PA, Wang LH, Schultz PG, Stevens RC. Structural insights into the evolution of an antibody combining site. Science. 1997;276:1665–1669.
50. Rosok MJ, Yelton DE, Harris LJ, et al. A combinatorial library strategy for the rapid humanization of anticarcinoma BR96 Fab. J Biol Chem. 1996;271:22611–22618.
51. Baca M, Presta LG, O'Connor SJ, Wells JA. Antibody humanization using monovalent phage display. J Biol Chem. 1997;272:10678–10684.
52. Jespers LS, Roberts A, Mahler SM, Winter G, Hoogenboom HR. Guiding the selection of human antibodies from phage display repertoires to a single epitope of an antigen. Biotechnology (N Y). 1994;12:899–903.
53. Osbourn J, Groves M, Vaughan T. From rodent reagents to human therapeutics using antibody guided selection. Methods. 2005;36:61–68.
54. Rader C, Cheresh DA, Barbas CF, 3rd. A phage display approach for rapid antibody humanization: designed combinatorial V gene libraries. Proc Natl Acad Sci U S A. 1998;95:8910–8915.
55. Ritter G, Cohen LS, Williams C, Jr., Richards EC, Old LJ, Welt S. Serological analysis of human anti-human antibody responses in colon cancer patients treated with repeated doses of humanized monoclonal antibody A33. Cancer Res. 2001;61:6851–6859.
56. Clark M. Antibody humanization: a case of the 'Emperor's new clothes'? Immunol Today. 2000;21:397–402.
57. Barbas CF, 3rd, Burton DR. Selection and evolution of high-affinity human anti-viral antibodies. Trends Biotechnol. 1996;14:230–234.
58. Rajewsky K. Clonal selection and learning in the antibody system. Nature. 1996;381:751–758.
59. Barbas CF, 3rd, Hu D, Dunlop N, et al. In vitro evolution of a neutralizing human antibody to human immunodeficiency virus type 1 to enhance affinity and broaden strain cross-reactivity. Proc Natl Acad Sci U S A. 1994;91:3809–3813.
60. Chowdhury PS, Pastan I. Improving antibody affinity by mimicking somatic hypermutation in vitro. Nat Biotechnol. 1999;17:568–572.
61. Ho M, Kreitman RJ, Onda M, Pastan I. In vitro antibody evolution targeting germline hot spots to increase activity of an anti-CD22 immunotoxin. J Biol Chem. 2005;280:607–617.
62. Yang WP, Green K, Pinz-Sweeney S, Briones AT, Burton DR, Barbas CF, 3rd. CDR walking mutagenesis for the affinity maturation of a potent human anti-HIV-1 antibody into the picomolar range. J Mol Biol. 1995;254:392–403.
63. Schier R, McCall A, Adams GP, et al. Isolation of picomolar affinity anti-c-erbB-2 single-chain Fv by molecular evolution of the complementarity determining regions in the center of the antibody binding site. J Mol Biol. 1996;263:551–567.
64. Rader C, Popkov M, Neves JA, Barbas CF, 3rd. Integrin alpha(v)beta3 targeted therapy for Kaposi's sarcoma with an in vitro evolved antibody. Faseb J. 2002;16:2000–2002.
65. Adams GP, Schier R. Generating improved single-chain Fv molecules for tumor targeting. J Immunol Methods. 1999;231:249–260.
66. Roopenian DC, Christianson GJ, Sproule TJ, et al. The MHC class I-like IgG receptor controls perinatal IgG transport, IgG homeostasis, and fate of IgG-Fc-coupled drugs. J Immunol. 2003;170:3528–3533.

67. Shields RL, Namenuk AK, Hong K, et al. High resolution mapping of the binding site on human IgG1 for Fc gamma RI, Fc gamma RII, Fc gamma RIII, and FcRn and design of IgG1 variants with improved binding to the Fc gamma R. J Biol Chem. 2001;276:6591–6604.
68. Boye J, Elter T, Engert A. An overview of the current clinical use of the anti-CD20 monoclonal antibody rituximab. Ann Oncol. 2003;14:520–535.
69. Demidem A, Lam T, Alas S, Hariharan K, Hanna N, Bonavida B. Chimeric anti-CD20 (IDEC-C2B8) monoclonal antibody sensitizes a B cell lymphoma cell line to cell killing by cytotoxic drugs. Cancer Biother Radiopharm. 1997;12:177–186.
70. Golay J, Zaffaroni L, Vaccari T, et al. Biologic response of B lymphoma cells to anti-CD20 monoclonal antibody rituximab in vitro: CD55 and CD59 regulate complement-mediated cell lysis. Blood. 2000;95:3900–3908.
71. Tedder TF, Forsgren A, Boyd AW, Nadler LM, Schlossman SF. Antibodies reactive with the B1 molecule inhibit cell cycle progression but not activation of human B lymphocytes. Eur J Immunol. 1986;16:881–887.
72. Maloney DG, Liles TM, Czerwinski DK, et al. Phase I clinical trial using escalating single-dose infusion of chimeric anti-CD20 monoclonal antibody (IDEC-C2B8) in patients with recurrent B-cell lymphoma. Blood. 1994;84:2457–2466.
73. Maloney DG, Grillo-Lopez AJ, White CA, et al. IDEC-C2B8 (Rituximab) anti-CD20 monoclonal antibody therapy in patients with relapsed low-grade non-Hodgkin's lymphoma. Blood. 1997;90:2188–2195.
74. McLaughlin P, Grillo-Lopez AJ, Link BK, et al. Rituximab chimeric anti-CD20 monoclonal antibody therapy for relapsed indolent lymphoma: half of patients respond to a four-dose treatment program. J Clin Oncol. 1998;16:2825–2833.
75. Cheson BD, Horning SJ, Coiffier B, et al. Report of an international workshop to standardize response criteria for non-Hodgkin's lymphomas. NCI Sponsored International Working Group. J Clin Oncol. 1999;17:1244.
76. Berinstein NL, Grillo-Lopez AJ, White CA, et al. Association of serum Rituximab (IDEC-C2B8) concentration and anti-tumor response in the treatment of recurrent low-grade or follicular non-Hodgkin's lymphoma. Ann Oncol. 1998;9:995–1001.
77. Davis TA, Grillo-Lopez AJ, White CA, et al. Rituximab anti-CD20 monoclonal antibody therapy in non-Hodgkin's lymphoma: safety and efficacy of re-treatment. J Clin Oncol. 2000;18:3135–3143.
78. Hainsworth JD, Litchy S, Burris HA, 3rd, et al. Rituximab as first-line and maintenance therapy for patients with indolent non-hodgkin's lymphoma. J Clin Oncol. 2002;20:4261–4267.
79. Witzig TE, Vukov AM, Habermann TM, et al. Rituximab therapy for patients with newly diagnosed, advanced-stage, follicular grade I non-Hodgkin's lymphoma: a phase II trial in the North Central Cancer Treatment Group. J Clin Oncol. 2005;23:1103–1108.
80. Ghielmini M, Schmitz SF, Cogliatti SB, et al. Prolonged treatment with rituximab in patients with follicular lymphoma significantly increases event-free survival and response duration compared with the standard weekly x 4 schedule. Blood. 2004;103:4416–4423.
81. Czuczman MS, Grillo-Lopez AJ, White CA, et al. Treatment of patients with low-grade B-cell lymphoma with the combination of chimeric anti-CD20 monoclonal antibody and CHOP chemotherapy. J Clin Oncol. 1999;17:268–276.
82. Czuczman MS, Koryzna A, Mohr A, et al. Rituximab in combination with fludarabine chemotherapy in low-grade or follicular lymphoma. J Clin Oncol. 2005;23:694–704.
83. McLaughlin P, Hagemeister FB, Rodriguez MA, et al. Safety of fludarabine, mitoxantrone, and dexamethasone combined with rituximab in the treatment of stage IV indolent lymphoma. Semin Oncol. 2000;27:37–41.
84. Vose JM, Link BK, Grossbard ML, et al. Phase II study of rituximab in combination with chop chemotherapy in patients with previously untreated, aggressive non-Hodgkin's lymphoma. J Clin Oncol. 2001;19:389–397.
85. Coiffier B, Lepage E, Briere J, et al. CHOP chemotherapy plus rituximab compared with CHOP alone in elderly patients with diffuse large-B-cell lymphoma. N Engl J Med. 2002;346:235–242.

86. Feugier P, Van Hoof A, Sebban C, et al. Long-Term Results of the R-CHOP Study in the Treatment of Elderly Patients With Diffuse Large B-Cell Lymphoma: A Study by the Groupe d'Etude des Lymphomes de l'Adulte. J Clin Oncol. 2005;23:4117–4126.
87. Coiffier B, Haioun C, Ketterer N, et al. Rituximab (anti-CD20 monoclonal antibody) for the treatment of patients with relapsing or refractory aggressive lymphoma: a multicenter phase II study. Blood. 1998;92:1927–1932.
88. Hainsworth JD, Litchy S, Barton JH, et al. Single-agent rituximab as first-line and maintenance treatment for patients with chronic lymphocytic leukemia or small lymphocytic lymphoma: a phase II trial of the Minnie Pearl Cancer Research Network. J Clin Oncol. 2003;21:1746–1751.
89. Schulz H, Klein SK, Rehwald U, et al. Phase 2 study of a combined immunochemotherapy using rituximab and fludarabine in patients with chronic lymphocytic leukemia. Blood. 2002;100:3115–3120.
90. Byrd JC, Rai K, Peterson BL, et al. Addition of rituximab to fludarabine may prolong progression-free survival and overall survival in patients with previously untreated chronic lymphocytic leukemia: an updated retrospective comparative analysis of CALGB 9712 and CALGB 9011. Blood. 2005;105:49–53.
91. Milenic DE, Brechbiel MW. Targeting of radio-isotopes for cancer therapy. Cancer Biol Ther. 2004;3:361–370.
92. Witzig TE. Efficacy and safety of 90Y ibritumomab tiuxetan (Zevalin) radioimmunotherapy for non-Hodgkin's lymphoma. Semin Oncol. 2003;30:11–16.
93. Wiseman GA, White CA, Stabin M, et al. Phase I/II 90Y-Zevalin (yttrium-90 ibritumomab tiuxetan, IDEC-Y2B8) radioimmunotherapy dosimetry results in relapsed or refractory non-Hodgkin's lymphoma. Eur J Nucl Med. 2000;27:766–777.
94. Witzig TE, White CA, Gordon LI, et al. Safety of yttrium-90 ibritumomab tiuxetan radioimmunotherapy for relapsed low-grade, follicular, or transformed non-hodgkin's lymphoma. J Clin Oncol. 2003;21:1263–1270.
95. Witzig TE, White CA, Wiseman GA, et al. Phase I/II trial of IDEC-Y2B8 radioimmunotherapy for treatment of relapsed or refractory CD20(+) B-cell non-Hodgkin's lymphoma. J Clin Oncol. 1999;17:3793–3803.
96. Gordon LI, Molina A, Witzig T, et al. Durable responses after ibritumomab tiuxetan radioimmunotherapy for CD20+ B-cell lymphoma: long-term follow-up of a phase 1/2 study. Blood. 2004;103:4429–4431.
97. Witzig TE, Flinn IW, Gordon LI, et al. Treatment with ibritumomab tiuxetan radioimmunotherapy in patients with rituximab-refractory follicular non-Hodgkin's lymphoma. J Clin Oncol. 2002;20:3262–3269.
98. Witzig TE, Gordon LI, Cabanillas F, et al. Randomized controlled trial of yttrium-90-labeled ibritumomab tiuxetan radioimmunotherapy versus rituximab immunotherapy for patients with relapsed or refractory low-grade, follicular, or transformed B-cell non-Hodgkin's lymphoma. J Clin Oncol. 2002;20:2453–2463.
99. Kaminski MS, Estes J, Zasadny KR, et al. Radioimmunotherapy with iodine (131)I tositumomab for relapsed or refractory B-cell non-Hodgkin lymphoma: updated results and long-term follow-up of the University of Michigan experience. Blood. 2000;96:1259–1266.
100. Vose JM, Wahl RL, Saleh M, et al. Multicenter phase II study of iodine-131 tositumomab for chemotherapy-relapsed/refractory low-grade and transformed low-grade B-cell non-Hodgkin's lymphomas. J Clin Oncol. 2000;18:1316–1323.
101. Kaminski MS, Tuck M, Estes J, et al. 131I-tositumomab therapy as initial treatment for follicular lymphoma. N Engl J Med. 2005;352:441–449.
102. Horning SJ, Younes A, Jain V, et al. Efficacy and safety of tositumomab and iodine-131 tositumomab (Bexxar) in B-cell lymphoma, progressive after rituximab. J Clin Oncol. 2005;23:712–719.
103. Gopal AK, Gooley TA, Maloney DG, et al. High-dose radioimmunotherapy versus conventional high-dose therapy and autologous hematopoietic stem cell transplantation for relapsed follicular non-Hodgkin lymphoma: a multivariable cohort analysis. Blood. 2003;102:2351–2357.

104. Wellhausen SR, Peiper SC. CD33: biochemical and biological characterization and evaluation of clinical relevance. J Biol Regul Homeost Agents. 2002;16:139–143.
105. Giles FJ. Gemtuzumab ozogamicin: promise and challenge in patients with acute myeloid leukemia. Expert Rev Anticancer Ther. 2002;2:630–640.
106. van Der Velden VH, te Marvelde JG, Hoogeveen PG, et al. Targeting of the CD33-calicheamicin immunoconjugate Mylotarg (CMA-676) in acute myeloid leukemia: in vivo and in vitro saturation and internalization by leukemic and normal myeloid cells. Blood. 2001;97:3197–3204.
107. Amico D, Barbui AM, Erba E, Rambaldi A, Introna M, Golay J. Differential response of human acute myeloid leukemia cells to gemtuzumab ozogamicin in vitro: role of Chk1 and Chk2 phosphorylation and caspase 3. Blood. 2003;101:4589–4597.
108. Sievers EL, Larson RA, Stadtmauer EA, et al. Efficacy and safety of gemtuzumab ozogamicin in patients with CD33-positive acute myeloid leukemia in first relapse. J Clin Oncol. 2001;19:3244–3254.
109. Wadleigh M, Richardson PG, Zahrieh D, et al. Prior gemtuzumab ozogamicin exposure significantly increases the risk of veno-occlusive disease in patients who undergo myeloablative allogeneic stem cell transplantation. Blood. 2003;102:1578–1582.
110. Bross PF, Beitz J, Chen G, et al. Approval summary: gemtuzumab ozogamicin in relapsed acute myeloid leukemia. Clin Cancer Res. 2001;7:1490–1496.
111. Alvarado Y, Tsimberidou A, Kantarjian H, et al. Pilot study of Mylotarg, idarubicin and cytarabine combination regimen in patients with primary resistant or relapsed acute myeloid leukemia. Cancer Chemother Pharmacol. 2003;51:87–90.
112. Cortes J, Tsimberidou AM, Alvarez R, et al. Mylotarg combined with topotecan and cytarabine in patients with refractory acute myelogenous leukemia. Cancer Chemother Pharmacol. 2002;50:497–500.
113. Estey EH, Giles FJ, Beran M, et al. Experience with gemtuzumab ozogamycin ("mylotarg") and all-trans retinoic acid in untreated acute promyelocytic leukemia. Blood. 2002;99:4222–4224.
114. Dyer MJ, Hale G, Hayhoe FG, Waldmann H. Effects of CAMPATH-1 antibodies in vivo in patients with lymphoid malignancies: influence of antibody isotype. Blood. 1989;73:1431–1439.
115. Rowan W, Tite J, Topley P, Brett SJ. Cross-linking of the CAMPATH-1 antigen (CD52) mediates growth inhibition in human B- and T-lymphoma cell lines, and subsequent emergence of CD52-deficient cells. Immunology. 1998;95:427–436.
116. Lundin J, Osterborg A, Brittinger G, et al. CAMPATH-1H monoclonal antibody in therapy for previously treated low-grade non-Hodgkin's lymphomas: a phase II multicenter study. European Study Group of CAMPATH-1H Treatment in Low-Grade Non-Hodgkin's Lymphoma. J Clin Oncol. 1998;16:3257–3263.
117. Nguyen DD, Cao TM, Dugan K, Starcher SA, Fechter RL, Coutre SE. Cytomegalovirus viremia during Campath-1H therapy for relapsed and refractory chronic lymphocytic leukemia and prolymphocytic leukemia. Clin Lymphoma. 2002;3:105–110.
118. Rai KR, Freter CE, Mercier RJ, et al. Alemtuzumab in previously treated chronic lymphocytic leukemia patients who also had received fludarabine. J Clin Oncol. 2002;20:3891–3897.
119. Keating MJ, Flinn I, Jain V, et al. Therapeutic role of alemtuzumab (Campath-1H) in patients who have failed fludarabine: results of a large international study. Blood. 2002;99:3554–3561.
120. Osterborg A, Fassas AS, Anagnostopoulos A, Dyer MJ, Catovsky D, Mellstedt H. Humanized CD52 monoclonal antibody Campath-1H as first-line treatment in chronic lymphocytic leukaemia. Br J Haematol. 1996;93:151–153.
121. Keating MJ, Cazin B, Coutre S, et al. Campath-1H treatment of T-cell prolymphocytic leukemia in patients for whom at least one prior chemotherapy regimen has failed. J Clin Oncol. 2002;20:205–213.
122. Uppenkamp M, Engert A, Diehl V, Bunjes D, Huhn D, Brittinger G. Monoclonal antibody therapy with CAMPATH-1H in patients with relapsed high- and low-grade non-Hodgkin's lymphomas: a multicenter phase I/II study. Ann Hematol. 2002;81:26–32.
123. Faderl S, Thomas DA, O'Brien S, et al. Experience with alemtuzumab plus rituximab in patients with relapsed and refractory lymphoid malignancies. Blood. 2003;101:3413–3415.

124. Kennedy B, Rawstron A, Carter C, et al. Campath-1H and fludarabine in combination are highly active in refractory chronic lymphocytic leukemia. Blood. 2002;99:2245–2247.
125. Kottaridis PD, Milligan DW, Chopra R, et al. In vivo CAMPATH-1H prevents graft-versus-host disease following nonmyeloablative stem cell transplantation. Blood. 2000;96:2419–2425.
126. Slamon DJ, Godolphin W, Jones LA, et al. Studies of the HER-2/neu proto-oncogene in human breast and ovarian cancer. Science. 1989;244:707–712.
127. Slamon DJ, Clark GM, Wong SG, Levin WJ, Ullrich A, McGuire WL. Human breast cancer: correlation of relapse and survival with amplification of the HER-2/neu oncogene. Science. 1987;235:177–182.
128. McKenzie SJ, Marks PJ, Lam T, et al. Generation and characterization of monoclonal antibodies specific for the human neu oncogene product, p185. Oncogene. 1989;4:543–548.
129. Hancock MC, Langton BC, Chan T, et al. A monoclonal antibody against the c-erbB-2 protein enhances the cytotoxicity of cis-diamminedichloroplatinum against human breast and ovarian tumor cell lines. Cancer Res. 1991;51:4575–4580.
130. Vogel CL, Cobleigh MA, Tripathy D, et al. Efficacy and safety of trastuzumab as a single agent in first-line treatment of HER2-overexpressing metastatic breast cancer. J Clin Oncol. 2002;20:719–726.
131. Cobleigh MA, Vogel CL, Tripathy D, et al. Multinational study of the efficacy and safety of humanized anti-HER2 monoclonal antibody in women who have HER2-overexpressing metastatic breast cancer that has progressed after chemotherapy for metastatic disease. J Clin Oncol. 1999;17:2639–2648.
132. Pietras RJ, Fendly BM, Chazin VR, Pegram MD, Howell SB, Slamon DJ. Antibody to HER-2/neu receptor blocks DNA repair after cisplatin in human breast and ovarian cancer cells. Oncogene. 1994;9:1829–1838.
133. Pegram MD, Lipton A, Hayes DF, et al. Phase II study of receptor-enhanced chemosensitivity using recombinant humanized anti-p185HER2/neu monoclonal antibody plus cisplatin in patients with HER2/neu-overexpressing metastatic breast cancer refractory to chemotherapy treatment. J Clin Oncol. 1998;16:2659–2671.
134. Seidman AD, Fornier MN, Esteva FJ, et al. Weekly trastuzumab and paclitaxel therapy for metastatic breast cancer with analysis of efficacy by HER2 immunophenotype and gene amplification. J Clin Oncol. 2001;19:2587–2595.
135. Esteva FJ, Valero V, Booser D, et al. Phase II study of weekly docetaxel and trastuzumab for patients with HER-2-overexpressing metastatic breast cancer. J Clin Oncol. 2002;20:1800–1808.
136. Burstein HJ, Kuter I, Campos SM, et al. Clinical activity of trastuzumab and vinorelbine in women with HER2-overexpressing metastatic breast cancer. J Clin Oncol. 2001;19:2722–2730.
137. Slamon DJ, Leyland-Jones B, Shak S, et al. Use of chemotherapy plus a monoclonal antibody against HER2 for metastatic breast cancer that overexpresses HER2. N Engl J Med. 2001;344:783–792.
138. Baselga J, Gianni L, Geyer C, Perez EA, Riva A, Jackisch C. Future options with trastuzumab for primary systemic and adjuvant therapy. Semin Oncol. 2004;31:51–57.
139. Lee JC, Chow NH, Wang ST, Huang SM. Prognostic value of vascular endothelial growth factor expression in colorectal cancer patients. Eur J Cancer. 2000;36:748–753.
140. Kabbinavar F, Hurwitz HI, Fehrenbacher L, et al. Phase II, randomized trial comparing bevacizumab plus fluorouracil (FU)/leucovorin (LV) with FU/LV alone in patients with metastatic colorectal cancer. J Clin Oncol. 2003;21:60–65.
141. Hurwitz H, Fehrenbacher L, Novotny W, et al. Bevacizumab plus irinotecan, fluorouracil, and leucovorin for metastatic colorectal cancer. N Engl J Med. 2004;350:2335–2342.
142. Hurwitz HI, Fehrenbacher L, Hainsworth JD, et al. Bevacizumab in combination with fluorouracil and leucovorin: an active regimen for first-line metastatic colorectal cancer. J Clin Oncol. 2005;23:3502–3508.
143. Giantonio BJ PC, NJ Meropol, PJ O'Dwyer, EP Mitchell, SR Alberts, MA Schwartz, AB Benson. High-dose bevacizumab improves survival when combined with FOLFOX4 in previously treated

advanced colorectal cancer: Results from the Eastern Cooperative Oncology Group (ECOG) study E3200. Proc Am Soc Clin Oncol Abstract #2; 2005.
144. Johnson DH, Fehrenbacher L, Novotny WF, et al. Randomized phase II trial comparing bevacizumab plus carboplatin and paclitaxel with carboplatin and paclitaxel alone in previously untreated locally advanced or metastatic non-small-cell lung cancer. J Clin Oncol. 2004;22:2184–2191.
145. Sandler AB RG, J Brahmer, A Dowlati, JH Schiller, MC Perry, DH Johnson. Randomized phase II/III Trial of paclitaxel (P) plus carboplatin (C) with or without bevacizumab (NSC # 704865) in patients with advanced non-squamous non-small cell lung cancer (NSCLC): An Eastern Cooperative Oncology Group (ECOG) Trial - E4599. Proc Am Soc Clin Onc (Abstract No: LBA4); 2005.
146. Yang JC, Haworth L, Sherry RM, et al. A randomized trial of bevacizumab, an anti-vascular endothelial growth factor antibody, for metastatic renal cancer. N Engl J Med. 2003;349:427–434.
147. Ciardiello F, Tortora G. Anti-epidermal growth factor receptor drugs in cancer therapy. Expert Opin Investig Drugs. 2002;11:755–768.
148. Nicholson RI, Gee JM, Harper ME. EGFR and cancer prognosis. Eur J Cancer. 2001;37 Suppl 4:S9–15.
149. Ciardiello F, Bianco R, Damiano V, et al. Antitumor activity of sequential treatment with topotecan and anti-epidermal growth factor receptor monoclonal antibody C225. Clin Cancer Res. 1999;5:909–916.
150. Robert F, Ezekiel MP, Spencer SA, et al. Phase I study of anti–epidermal growth factor receptor antibody cetuximab in combination with radiation therapy in patients with advanced head and neck cancer. J Clin Oncol. 2001;19:3234–3243.
151. Saltz LB, Meropol NJ, Loehrer PJ, Sr., Needle MN, Kopit J, Mayer RJ. Phase II trial of cetuximab in patients with refractory colorectal cancer that expresses the epidermal growth factor receptor. J Clin Oncol. 2004;22:1201–1208.
152. Cunningham D, Humblet Y, Siena S, et al. Cetuximab monotherapy and cetuximab plus irinotecan in irinotecan-refractory metastatic colorectal cancer. N Engl J Med. 2004;351:337–345.
153. Díaz Rubio E JT, E van Cutsem, A Cervantes, T André, Y Humblet, P Soulié, S Corretgé, O Kisker, A de Gramont. Cetuximab in combination with oxaliplatin/5-fluorouracil (5-FU)/folinic acid (FA) (FOLFOX-4) in the first-line treatment of patients with epidermal growth factor receptor (EGFR)-expressing metastatic colorectal cancer: An international phase II study. Am Soc Clin Oncol (Abstract No: 3535); 2005.
154. Motzer RJ, Amato R, Todd M, et al. Phase II trial of antiepidermal growth factor receptor antibody C225 in patients with advanced renal cell carcinoma. Invest New Drugs. 2003;21:99–101.
155. Xiong HQ, Rosenberg A, LoBuglio A, et al. Cetuximab, a monoclonal antibody targeting the epidermal growth factor receptor, in combination with gemcitabine for advanced pancreatic cancer: a multicenter phase II Trial. J Clin Oncol. 2004;22:2610–2616.
156. Adkins JC, Spencer CM. Edrecolomab (monoclonal antibody 17–1A). Drugs. 1998;56:619–626; discussion 627–618.
157. Riethmuller G, Holz E, Schlimok G, et al. Monoclonal antibody therapy for resected Dukes' C colorectal cancer: seven-year outcome of a multicenter randomized trial. J Clin Oncol. 1998;16:1788–1794.
158. Punt CJ, Nagy A, Douillard JY, et al. Edrecolomab alone or in combination with fluorouracil and folinic acid in the adjuvant treatment of stage III colon cancer: a randomised study. Lancet. 2002;360:671–677.

CHAPTER 21

UNMASKING TUMOR CELL IMMUNOGENICITY BY CHEMOTHERAPY: IMPLICATIONS FOR THERAPY

IRMA LARMA, ROBBERT G. VAN DER MOST, AND RICHARD A. LAKE
National Research Centre for Asbestos-related Diseases, UWA Departmant of Medicine, Sir Charles Gairdner Hospital, 4th floor G Block, Nedlands, Perth, Western Australia 6009

Keywords: Immunogenicity, NKG2D, TRAIL, chemotherapy, immunotherapy, danger signals

INTRODUCTION

Cytotoxic drugs are widely used for the treatment of most tumors. In many cases, however, chemotherapy as a sole anti-tumour therapy fails to achieve curative responses. Dose-limiting collateral damage is one of the main problems: cytotoxic drugs not only kill tumor cells but also normal cells. Because of the way that most chemotherapy agents work, rapidly dividing normal cells are targeted, and hair loss, lymphopenia and mucositis are common side effects. Combining chemotherapy with immunotherapy is attractive as these therapies could potentially synergize to control tumor growth. However, chemotherapy-induced lymphopenia has been a major stumbling block in the further development of such combination therapy. Now, with our growing understanding of the immune response and anti-tumor immunity, immunotherapy is considered to be a viable and promising option to enhance the anti-tumor effects of chemotherapy.

Cytotoxic drugs commonly kill cells by interfering with DNA synthesis or by deregulating specific metabolic pathways, usually those that are linked to DNA synthesis. In most cases, this results in a form of programmed cell death or apoptosis (Table 1). However, it is clear that different drugs use different routes to reach that point (Table 1).

Successful chemotherapy will result in massive tumor cell death and the subsequent release of large amounts of tumor antigens. One of the key questions is how does the immune system respond to this surge of antigens. We know that chemotherapy

H.L. Kaufman and J.D. Wolchok (eds.), General Principles of Tumor Immunotherapy, 485–498.

Table 1. Common cytotoxic drugs and their mechanism of action

Name	Class	Target pathway	Cell death
Gemcitabine	DNA chain terminator	DNA synthesis	Apoptosis
Doxorubicin	DNA cross-linker /Topoisomerase inhibitor	DNA synthesis	Apoptosis
Cisplatin	DNA cross-linker	DNA synthesis	Apoptosis
Temozolomide	DNA alkylating	DNA synthesis	Apoptosis
Vincristine	Vince alkaloid	Prevent microtubule formation	Apoptosis
Cyclophosphamide	DNA alkylating	DNA synthesis	Apoptosis
Taxol	Tubulin interaction	Prevents microtubule depolymerisation	Apoptosis
Fludaribine	Nucleoside analogue	DNA synthesis	Apoptosis
Coramsine	Plant extract	Membrane integrity	Necrosis
PEP	Plant extract	Membrane integrity	Necrosis

changes both the immunogenic *context* of the antigen and the amount being presented to antigen presenting cells. Here, we will discuss how different chemotherapies can alter the immunogenic status of tumor, i.e. how tumor antigens can be perceived as immunogenic. We will also discuss how this *context* could be useful in enhancing the efficacy of immunotherapy.

TUMOUR ANTIGENS AND CHEMOTHERAPY

Successful anti-tumor immunity requires presentation of the tumor antigen to anti-tumor T cells by professional antigen presenting cells (APC), most importantly dendritic cells (DC). Although many cell types are important in generating anti-tumor immune responses, $CD8^+$ T cells are seen as the key effectors, so we will primarily discuss the recruitment and activation of these cells. Cells known to play important roles include other lymphocytes such as $CD4^+$ T cells, NK cells and NKT cells and macrophages. It is now clear that the response of our major player, the CD8+ T cell is orchestrated by DC according to *context*.

After DC pick up antigen from tumor cells, they travel to the lymph nodes where they present the antigen to $CD8^+$ T cells. This process is called 'cross-presentation': exogenous antigens 'cross' into the MHC class I presentation route that is normally reserved for endogenous antigens. The ensuing response can be either immunogenic or tolerogenic, depending on the activation state of the presenting DC. Antigen presentation may result in $CD8^+$ T cell proliferation but not necessarily T cell activation, as shown by Sherman and colleagues [1]. In the activating scenario, $CD8^+$ T cells differentiate into cytotoxic T lymphocytes (CTL) that acquire the capacity to kill antigen-positive tumor cells. These CTL can travel through the circulatory system to the tumor site [2].

Source of Antigen

Most cells express MHC class I molecules and process and present endogenous antigens that can be recognized by $CD8^+$ T cells. Tumor cells usually lack co-stimulatory molecules and, therefore, do not directly activate $CD8^+$ T cells. Thus, the generation of an anti-tumor response depends on antigen cross-presentation, and a particular subset of DC, characterized by the expression of CD11c and CD8, is very efficient at presenting exogenous antigens. Although several mechanisms by which $CD8^+$ DC present antigen have been described [3], the precise way in which these DC acquire antigen is still unclear. The most widely held hypotheses are: (i) phagocytosis of dying cells and cellular debris; (ii) "nibbling" peptides from live cells by DC [4]; (iii) transfer of peptides via heat shock proteins (Hsp) [5]. Clearly, dying (apoptotic/necrotic) cells are rapidly ingested by phagocytes (DC and macrophages), including the cells that are involved in cross-presentation. However, not all apoptosis is equal and, as such, not all cross-presented antigens will induce an immune response. Cross-presentation is involved both in induction of immunity as well as in the maintenance of tolerance. So how does the APC decide whether the antigen is presented in immunogenic or tolerogenic context?

Immunogenic vs. Tolerogenic Apoptosis

Before we look at the effects of chemotherapy on antigen cross-presentation, we need to discuss what happens in a non-drug induced setting. Apoptotic cells translocate phosphatidylserine (PS) to the outer leaflet of the membrane, acting like a 'signal flag' for APC. Most dying cells are probably taken up by macrophages rather than DC, and stimulate the production of anti-inflammatory signals (IL-10, TGF-β). These cytokines act on immature DC and can suppress DC maturation as well as the production of inflammatory signals. On the other hand, apoptosis of infected cells is associated with immunogenic cross-presentation and depends on the presence of inflammatory and co-stimulatory signals. Pathogen-associated molecular patterns (PAMP), which include double-stranded RNA, lipopolysaccharides and unmethylated CpG oligodeoxynucleotides are recognized by Toll-like receptors (TLR). Through these receptors, PAMPs activate DC and promote an immune response [6]. Production of type I interferons, which have been involved in the generation of $CD8^+$ T cell responses against cross-presenting antigens [7], is a critical component of this response. The essential role of TLR ligation and type-I IFN production in the generation of productive immune responses may suggest that the default action of cross-presenting DC is to maintain tolerance. Without immuno-stimulatory signals, tumors are perceived as normal cells and cross-presented tumor antigens should be tolerogenic. Hernandez *et al.* [1] have shown that in the absence of pro-inflammatory (IL-12) and co-stimulatory (anti-CD40 antibody) signals, cross-presented antigens in the Islets of Langerhans fail to induce an immune response, i.e. they are tolerogenic. However, in the presence of anti-CD40 antibody and IL-12, specific $CD8^+$ T cell responses against cross-presented antigens were observed.

TUMOUR ANTIGEN IMMUNOGENICITY

Tumor antigens are cross-presented and their immunogenicity can range from tolerogenic [8] to weakly immunogenic [9]. The amount of tumor antigen that is presented may be a factor that influences immunogenicity. Chemotherapy has a clear capacity to increase antigen load and this may be sufficient to turn tolerogenic antigen into immunogenic antigen. Chemotherapy-induced apoptotic tumor cells provide a good source of cross-presented antigens that may invoke effector function [10]. Successful chemotherapy results in massive tumour cell death, and subsequent release of antigens. This overall increase in the total amount of tumor antigen available for cross-presentation by APC could mean that more potential tumor antigens reach a threshold for immune recognition. Thus, tumor cell death alters the repertoire of cross-presented antigens and has the capacity to create *neo*-tumor antigens.

There is more to this process than antigen load. Apoptotic cell death provides a context to the cross-presented antigens, and it is increasingly clear that not all apoptosis is equal. Whereas all chemotherapies result in some type of cell death, not all have capacity to make tolerogenic tumour antigens immunogenic. This was clearly shown in a groundbreaking study by Casares and co-workers [11]. Tumor cells that had been killed with the anthracyclin doxorubicin provided protective immunity upon injection into mice, whereas mitomycin C killed cells did not do so. Furthermore, treatment of established tumors with doxorubicin resulted in regression, which was not seen in mitomycin treated mice, although both chemotherapies induced tumor cell death. A potential explanation was provided by the observation that doxorubicin killed cells, but not mitomycin C killed cells, were taken up by DC. Thus, it seems likely that doxorubicin-triggered apoptosis is associated with a unique 'flag'. Puzzling, however, gemcitabine-killed tumour cells are also taken up by DCs, and promote tumour antigen cross-presentation, but do not result in as strong an anti-tumour immune response as seen with doxorubicin. This leaves us to question the nature of pro-inflammatory or "danger" signals that are associated with chemotherapy induced cell death.

Danger Signals

As discussed above, simple uptake of dying cells by DC does not guarantee strong anti-tumor immune responses. Other signals are required to instruct the immune system of the immunogenicity of cellular death. A *Danger* model proposed by Matzinger [12, 13] suggests that dying cells may provide a signal to the immune system, alerting it to important contextual information. A series of experiments by Shi *et al.* [14] have shown that cells contain in their cytoplasm endogenous adjuvants, which, acting as danger signals, can promote generation of $CD8^+$ T cell responses to particulate antigens. These adjuvants are increased in the cytosol of injured cells or in cells undergoing apoptosis. Furthermore, these endogenous adjuvants are released from injured and dying cells and act on APCs, stimulating antigen internalization, maturation and migration to draining lymph nodes. In addition, released adjuvants stimulate both $CD4^+$ and $CD8^+$ T cell responses [15]. These endogenous adjuvants include, amongst others, uric acid, damaged DNA, heat shock proteins and cytokines. Here we will discuss uric acid and DNA damage.

Uric acid

Uric acid is an end product of purine metabolism. Purine is one of the building blocks of nucleic acid (DNA and RNA). When cells die, their nucleic acid is degraded, resulting in the release of purine. Purine is then metabolized into uric acid, which is removed from the system without any harm. However, with massive cell death, concentrations of uric acid are significantly increased. Shi *et al.* [16] identified uric acid as one of the endogenous adjuvants released from injured and dying cells. They showed that uric acid can stimulate dendritic cell maturation, increase expression of the co-stimulatory molecules CD80 and CD86, and, when injected with a particulate antigen into mice, enhanced the generation of $CD8^+$ T cell responses. Interestingly, the concentration of uric acid required to elicit the adjuvant effect was exactly that concentration at which uric acid precipitates. Subsequent experiments showed that crystalline, but not soluble, uric acid, was highly stimulatory. The role of uric acid in innate immunity is also supported by a study of its role in anti-tumor response [17]. It was found that chemotherapy-induced apoptosis of tumor cells was accompanied by increased levels of uric acid, which in turn led to tumor rejection. Furthermore, these authors found that injection of crystalline uric acid accelerated rejection and that tumor regression was delayed by uricase treatment. Taken together, these data suggest that the increased cell death induced by chemotherapy has the potential to release uric acid, which could act as a danger signal to alert the immune system. In normal cell death, levels of uric acid will be low and will not result in crystallization. However, with massive chemotherapy-induced cell death, the amount of uric acid release may reach the crystallization point, resulting in the induction of an immune response.

DNA damage

Particular forms of nucleic acids can be immuno-stimulatory. In the case of viral or bacterial infection, pathogen-derived DNA or RNA can induce an immune response through ligation of Toll-like receptors (TLR). Four TLR are involved in the recognition of foreign nucleic acid; TLR-3 recognizes double-stranded (viral) RNA, TLR-9 recognizes unmethylated CpG-containing oligodeoxynucleotides (bacterial and herpes virus DNA), and TLR-7 and –8 recognize some virus associated single-stranded RNA. All nucleic acid recognizing TLR are located in the endosome, suggesting that endosomal presence of nucleic acids is the key to their immuno-stimulatory effects. Indeed, double-stranded viral RNA from phagocytosed cells ends up in the endosomes of the phagocytosing cells where it activates TLR-3 [18]. Intriguingly, a recent study has shown that cross-linked DNA may also act as a *danger signal*, converting a tolerogenic response into an immunogenic one [19]. This effect was associated with the drugs chlorambucil and melphalan, both nitrogen mustards, which induce apoptosis by cross-linking DNA. Note that these alkylating agents are chemically related to cyclophosphamide, a drug that has long been known for its immuno-potentiating capacity. In these studies, UV irradiation, which also cross-links DNA led to immuno-stimulatory cell death. It is unclear how cross-linked DNA activates DC, but an intriguing clue was suggested by the finding that failure of phagocytosing cells to rapidly degrade DNA in their lysosomes (by inactivating DNaseII) led to IFN-β and IFN-γ production [20].

NKG2D GENOTOXIC STRESS LIGANDS

Cellular detection of DNA damage leads to the activation of a genotoxic stress-response pathway, or DNA damage response. This results in p53-dependent cell cycle arrest or apoptosis, depending on the extent of damage. If damage is 'manageable', cell cycle arrest and DNA repair functions are induced. However, if damage is too extensive, apoptosis is induced. The DNA damage response is also associated with up-regulation of the cell surface ligands for the NK cell activating receptor NKG2D [21]. In this sense, genotoxic stress has the capacity to alert the immune system to danger. Upregulation of NKG2D ligands may play a role in the immunosurveillance of tumors as tumor cells and transformed cells are usually under chronic genotoxic stress.

NKG2D is an activation receptor expressed on all human and mouse natural killer (NK) cells, and on all human γδ T-cells and $CD8^+$ αβ T cells. In mice, this receptor is expressed on activated $CD8^+$ αβT cells and is constitutively expressed on γδT cells and natural killer T (NKT) cells [22]. Recently, expression of NKG2D was also described on newly discovered interferon-producing killer dendritic cells (IKDC) [23]. Ligation of NKG2D activates NK cells, stimulating IFN-γ production and NK mediated cell lysis, and may provide a CD28-like co-stimulatory signal for $CD8^+$ T cells [24], although this latter notion is somewhat controversial. Two families of NKG2D ligands have been distinguished, the MIC family (MICA and MICB genes) expressed in humans and RAET1 family (H60, Rae1 and Mult 1 genes), expressed in both mice and humans.

How could this mechanism affect recognition of tumor cells after chemotherapy? Normal cells do not express NKG2D ligands, whereas they are highly expressed on tumor cells and on infected cells. Thus, such cells could be prime targets for NK-mediated lysis. Interestingly, transformed cells that do not constitutively over-express NGG2D ligands will up-regulate the expression of these molecules after exposure to chemotherapeutic DNA damaging drugs [25]. Thus, chemotherapy could potentially unmask NKG2D-mediated immune recognition. The matter is complicated because many tumor cells constitutively express NKG2D ligands. Since engagement of NKG2D may result in an immune response, this leads to the question how tumor cells that constitutively express NKG2D ligands evade NKG2D-mediated tumour surveillance? In humans, elevated levels of soluble MICA (sMICA) and ULBP2 (sULBP2) have been reported in many cancer patients [26, 27]. These soluble proteins could act as decoys for NKG2D receptor binding. Furthermore, persistent expression of NKG2D ligands have been associated with down regulation of NKG2D expression and impaired activation of NK cells and $CD8^+$ T cells [28]. The reciprocal effect may also occur: at least some experimental tumors in mice downregulate H60 expression *in vivo* [29].

Selective expression of NKG2D ligands by tumor cells makes it an attractive target for anti-tumor therapy. In fact, DNA damaging agents, such as chemotherapy or radiation, have been shown to induce the expression of ligands for NKG2D. Upregulation of NKG2D ligands on tumor cells by chemotherapy agents may provide alternative routes to cell death, one which is NK-mediated and one through enhancement of T-cell responses. An intriguing possibility is that apoptotic tumor cells could activate the newly discovered IKDC through NKG2D ligation. Clearly, a better understanding of NKG2D ligand expression and NKG2D-mediated immune activation may allow the rational design of chemotherapies that specifically enhance the immunogenicity of otherwise tolerogenic tumor cells.

TUMOUR NECROSIS FACTOR-RELATED APOPTOSIS INDUCING LIGAND (TRAIL)

The main immune effector cells that kill tumor cells are $CD8^+$ T cells and NK cells. These cell types use two main mechanisms to destroy tumor cells: i) by releasing perforin and granzyme and ii) by expression of death ligands such as Fas ligand (FasL). Death ligands bind to specific receptors on target cells to induce apoptosis.

One of these death receptors is tumor necrosis factor–related apoptosis inducing ligand (TRAIL), also known as Apo2L. TRAIL is a member of transmembrane family of proteins with sequence homology to FasL and Tumour Necrosis Factor (TNF). TRAIL ligation signals apoptosis in similar way to Fas [30]. Although the exact biological role of TRAIL is not fully understood, there is evidence of a role for TRAIL in the regulation of autoimmunity as well as in tumor immunosurveillance. Experiments in TRAIL-deficient mice have shown impaired anti-tumor surveillance by the immune cells [31, 32] and high sensitivity to experimental autoimmune diseases [33].

Unlike other TNF family members, which display tightly regulated expression patterns on activated cells, TRAIL mRNA is constitutively expressed in a wide variety of normal tissue cells [34]. However, the expression of functional TRAIL seems to be restricted to activated immune cells, including T cells [35], NK cells [36], monocytes [37], DC [38], IKDC [23] and neutrophils [39]. TRAIL exerts its effect on target cells by engaging its receptors, DR4, KILLER/DR5, DcR1/TRAIL-R3, DcR2/TRAIL-R4 and recently discovered receptor called osteoprotegin (OPG). DR5 and to a lesser extent DR4 are death receptors that trigger caspase-mediated apoptosis. The other three receptors do not induce apoptosis but act as decoy receptors protecting cells from TRAIL-mediated cell death. DR4 and DR5 mRNA can be detected in a wide variety of normal tissue and tumors, but expression of the proteins is more limited. In fact, cell surface expression of DR5, and in some cases DR4, has been broadly found on TRAIL-sensitive tumor cell lines and in primary tumors, and is absent in most normal tissue. Moreover, the abundance of decoy receptors in the normal tissue may explain their resistance to TRAIL-mediated apoptosis.

Importantly, chemotherapeutic drugs, as well as radiation, can modify TRAIL resistance. Doxorubicin can sensitize TRAIL-resistant prostate cancer cells, by down-regulating cFLIP [40]. In addition, doxorubicin, etoposide and cisplatin up-regulate DR4 and DR5 cell surface receptors, reversing the TRAIL-resistance in a number of tumors [41]. Furthermore, radiation and chemotherapy, such as cisplatinum, can up-regulate the DR5 expression in a p53 dependent manner. Finally, the proteasome inhibitor bortezomib has been shown to sensitize tumors to TRAIL-mediated lysis [42].

The fact that different chemotherapeutic drugs can sensitive tumor cells to TRAIL-mediated lysis has been successfully exploited and recombinant TRAIL, as well as anti-DR4 and DR5 antibodies have been developed. However, NK cells and IKDC also kill cells through TRAIL and chemotherapy-induced TRAIL sensitivity could therefore synergize with NK cell based therapies.

CHEMOTHERAPEUTIC DRUGS INTERACT WITH NON-TUMOR CELLS: TUMOR STROMA AND THE IMMUNE SYSTEM

Stroma Interactions

Chemotherapeutic drugs do not only kill tumor cells but also affect normal cells. As discussed above, this is one of the reasons that cytostatics can cause severe side-effects. However, there are now several examples illustrating the potential of chemotherapeutic drugs to positively influence anti-tumor T cell responses by targeting the tumor stroma. In this discussion we have chosen to operationally define stroma as the non-tumor cell material that is associated with the tumor mass. As a first example, cyclophosphamide has been shown to change the phenotype of tumor-infiltrating macrophages from IL-10 secreting M2 cells to IFN-γ secreting M1 cells, in a T cell dependent fashion [43]. Paclitaxel enhances IL-12 production of tumor-infiltrating macrophages [44]. Several drugs, including cyclophosphamide and paclitaxel have been shown to induce production of the anti-angiogenic protein thrombospondin-1 in endothelial cells [45]. Finally, the anti-vascular drug MDXAA [46] has been found to trigger anti-tumor $CD8^+$ T cell responses. These examples illustrate that the tumor stroma can be successfully modified to induce anti-tumor immunity.

Lymphocyte Depletion

Cytotoxic drugs generally deplete lymphocytes, resulting in a profound lymphopenia. Although lymphocyte depletion has long been considered a major stumbling block for anti-tumor immunotherapy, recent developments have changed this view [47]. First, lymphodepletion includes depletion of regulatory $CD4^+$ $CD25^+$

T cells [48]. As these cells have been shown to actively suppress T cell and NK cell responses against the tumor, their transient absence may facilitate immunotherapy. The immuno-potentiating effects of cyclophosphamide have been attributed to the depletion or inactivation of regulatory T cells [49]. Furthermore, lymphodepletion triggers a phase of T cell regeneration called homeostatic proliferation which is driven by cytokines such as IL-7 and IL-15. Homeostatically proliferating T cells appear to be more sensitive to self antigens and may provide a suitable target for immunotherapy. IL-21 could be potentially important cytokine to amplify this process [47].

CHEMOTHERAPY ENHANCES THE EFFECT OF IMMUNOTHERAPY

In summary, chemotherapy increases antigen cross-presentation, exposing *neo*-antigens, and may provide immunostimulatory signals. These signals include uric acid, heat shock proteins, and damaged DNA. Genotoxic stress may also lead to the upregulation of NKG2D ligands. Finally, chemotherapeutic drugs can sensitize cells to TRAIL-mediated lysis. On the other hand, chemotherapy often induces severe lymphopenia, depleting both effector cells and regulatory $CD4^+$ $CD25^+$ T cells. Thus, chemotherapy may expose tumor antigens and activate DC, but a lack of effector cells could still limit successful responses. This state of affairs may explain why the immune effects of conventional chemotherapy are limited. However, our increased understanding of apoptotic cell death and endogenous danger signals may help us to design immunotherapeutic strategies that complement chemotherapeutic drugs. There are several conceivable strategies.

1. A conceptually straightforward approach is to provide an immunostimulatory context to the increased levels of post-chemotherapy tumor antigen presentation. This can be done using TLR ligands (poly-I:C, CpG-containing oligo-deoxynucleotides) or immune activating agonistic antibodies. Agonistic anti-CD40 antibody has received considerable attention. Post-chemotherapy treatment with anti-CD40 dramatically increased curative responses in a mouse model of mesothelioma [50], and such combination therapies are currently being considered for clinical trials.
2. The absence of effector cells, resulting from drug-induced lymphopenia, may limit the potential immune stimulatory effects of chemotherapeutic cell death. Thus, attempts to accelerate immune system recovery after chemotherapy may be fruitful. Cytokines such as interleukin-2 (IL-2), IL-7, IL-15 and IL-21 may play a role in this process as they drive homeostatic T cell proliferation. This may have the added benefit that IL-7 and IL-15, but not IL-2 [51], may favor the expansion of $CD8^+$ T cells as compared to regulatory $CD4^+$ $CD25^+$ T cells [52]. IL-15 is an attractive cytokine for therapy as it also activates DC [53] and rescues tolerized $CD8^+$ T cells [54]. IL-21 is involved in homeostatic T cell proliferation and also stimulates NK cells and may therefore synergize with

chemotherapies that upregulate NKG2D ligands or sensitize tumor cells for TRAIL-mediated lysis [55].

3. Vaccination with tumor antigens has been widely evaluated but has met with limited success. Combination with chemotherapy could enhance the efficacy of vaccination [56]. For cyclophosphamide, it has been shown that the induced anti-tumor $CD8^+$ T cell responses depend on anti-tumor effector cells that were activated *before* chemotherapy [57]. In fact, the efficacy of cyclophosphamide has been directly correlated with the immunogenicity of the tumor [58]. Thus, treatment of non-immunogenic tumors may benefit from vaccination prior to chemotherapy to create a pool of tumor-specific memory T cells that can be mobilized post chemotherapy. This has the added benefit that memory cells appear to survive better then naïve T cells during chemotherapy. Vaccination after chemotherapy could also be successful as it could skew the regenerating T cell repertoire towards tumor antigens. One of the more successful vaccine types comprise irradiated or killed tumor cells that express co-stimulatory molecules (e.g. B7-family members), cytokines or GM-CSF [56].
4. Passive immunotherapy in the form of adoptive transfer of activated tumor-specific $CD8^+$ T cells has received considerable attention after groundbreaking work from Belldegrun and coworkers [59]. These investigators cultured patient T cells in the presence of high concentrations of IL-2, which promoted differentiation of T cells in LAK (lymphokine activated killer) cells. These cells were then transferred back into patients after lymphodepleting chemotherapy. This approach has met some spectacular successes in melanoma patients [60]. Replacement of IL-2 by IL-15 may further optimize this strategy [54]. An interesting approach is to genetically engineer the transferred T cells to lower their activation threshold. A general feature of adoptive T cell transfer approaches is that they work better in a lymphopenic host, exposing the potential synergy between chemo- and immunotherapy.

CONCLUDING REMARKS

Our thinking on the relationship between chemotherapy and the immune system has radically changed during the last decade. Once considered incompatible, chemo- and immuno-therapy are now seen as a practical partnership. The massive tumor cell apoptosis that follows successful chemotherapy increases the amount of cross-presented antigen, may expose *neo*-tumor antigens and provides a variety of immuno-stimulatory signals. This could present the ideal staging ground for immunotherapy. Mild lymphopenia is not necessarily a negative factor for immunotherapy as regulatory T cells are depleted and homeostatic T cell proliferation can be exploited. Cytokines such as IL-7 and IL-15 could be critically important in this respect. Finally, both chemotherapy and the tumor itself could negatively affect DC function, in which case DC stimulatory protocols such as GM-CSF, flt3L or passive DC transfer/vaccination may need to be part of a combined immunotherapy strategy.

REFERENCES

1. Hernandez, J., Aung, S., Marquardt, K., and Sherman, L.A., 2002, Uncoupling of proliferate potential and gain of effector function by $CD8^+$ T cells responding to self-antigens, *J. Exp. Med.* 196:323–333.
2. Lake, R.A., and Robinson, B.W.S., 2005, Immunotherapy and chemotherapy – a practical partnership, *Nat. Rev. Cancer.* 5:397–405.
3. Rock, K.L., and Shen, L., 2005, Cross-presentation: underlying mechanism and role in immune surveillance, *Immunol. Rev.* 207:166–183.
4. Harshyne, L.A., Watkins, S.C., Gambotto, A., and Barrat-Boyes, S.M., 2001, Dendritic cells acquire antigens from live cells for cross-presentation to CTL, *J. Immunol.* 166:3717–3723.
5. Radons, J., and Multhoff, G., 2005, Immunostimulatory functions of membrane-bound and exported heat shock protein 70, *Exerc. Immunol. Rev.* 11:17–33.
6. Reis e Sousa, C., 2004, Toll-like receptors and dendritic cells: for whom the bug tolls, *Semin. Immunol.* 16(1):27–34.
7. Le Bon, A., Etchart, N., Rossmann, C., Ashton, M., Hou, S., Gewert, D., Borrow, P., and Tough. D.F., 2003, Cross-priming of $CD8^+$ T cells stimulated by virus-induced type I interferon, *Nat. Immunol.* 4:1009–1015.
8. Lyman, M.A., Aung, S., Biggs, J.A., and Sherman, L.A., 2004, A spontaneously arising pancreatic tumor does not promote the differentiation of naive CD8+ T lymphocytes into effector CTL, *J.* Immunol. 172:6558–6567.
9. Marzo, A.L., Lake, R.A., Lo, D., Sherman, L, McWilliam, A., Nelson, D., Bruce W. S. Robinson, B.W.S., and Scott, B., 1999, Tumor antigens are constitutively presented in the draining lymph nodes, *J. Immunol.* 162:5838–5845.
10. Nowak, A.K., Lake, R.A., Marzo, A.L., Scott, B., Heath, W.R., Collins, E.J., Frelinger, J.A., and Robinson, B.W.S., 2003a, Induction of tumour cell apoptosis in vivo increases tumour antigen cross-presentation, cross-priming rather than cross-tolerating tumour specific CD8 T cells, *J Immunol.* 170:4905–4913.
11. Casares, N., Pequignot, M.O., Tesniere, A., Ghiringhelli, F., Roux, S., Chaput, N., Schmitt, E., Hamai, A., Hervas-Stubbs, S., Obeid, M., Countant, F., Metivier, D., Pichard, E., Aucouturier, P., Pierron, G., Garrido, C., Zitvogel, L., and Kroemer, G., 2005, Caspase-dependent immunogenicity of doxorubicin-induced tumour cell death, *J. Exp. Med.* 202:1691–1701.
12. Matzinger, P., 1994, Tolerance, danger and the extended family, *Annu. Rev. Immunol.* 12:991–1045.
13. Matzinger, P., 1998, An innate sense of danger, *Semin. Immunol.* 10:399–415.
14. Shi, Y., Zheng, W., and Rock, K.L., 2000, Cell injury releases endogenous adjuvants that stimulate cytotoxic T-cell responses, *Proc Natl. Acad. Sci. USA.* 97:14590–14595.
15. Shi, Y., and Rock, K.L., 2002, Cell death releases endogenous adjuvants that selectively enhance immune surveillance of particulate antigens, *Eur. J. Immunol.* 32:155–162.
16. Shi, Y., Evans, J.E., and Rock, K.L., 2003, Molecular identification of a danger signal that alerts the immune system to dying cells, *Nature.* 425: 516–521.
17. Hu, D.E., Moore, A.M., Thomsen, L.L., and Brindle, K.M., 2004, Uric acid promotes tumour immune rejection, *Cancer Res.* 64:5059–5062.
18. Schulz, O., Diebold, S.S., Chen, M., Naslund, T.I., Nolte, M.A., Alexopoulou, L., Azuma, Y.T., Flavell, R.A., Liljestrom, P., and Reis e Sousa, C., 2005, Toll-like receptor3 promotes cross-priming to virus-infected cells, *Nature.* 433(7028):887–892.
19. Rad, A.N., Pollara, G., Sohaib, S.M.A., Chiang, C., Chain, B.M., and Katz, D.R., 2003, The different influence of allogeneic tumour cell death via DNA damage on dendritic cell maturation and antigen presentation, *Cancer Res.* 63:5143–5150.
20. Okabe, Y., Kawane, K., Akira, S., Taniguchi, T., and Nagata, S., 2005, Toll-like receptor-independent gene induction program activated by mammalian DNA escaped from apoptotic DNA degradation, *J. Exp. Med.* 202(10):1333–1339.
21. Gasser, S., and Raulet, D.H., 2006, The DNA damage response aroused the immune system, *Cancer Res.* 66:3959–3962.

22. Vivier, E., Tomasello, E., and Paul, P., 2002, Lymphocyte activation via NKG2D: towards a new paradigm in immune recognition?, *Curr. Opin. Immunol.* 14:306–311.
23. Chan, C.W., Crafton, E., Fan, H.N., Flook, J., Yoshimura, K., Skarica, M., Brockstedt, D., Dubensky, T.W., Stins, M.F., Lanier, L.L., Pardoll, D.M., and Housseau, F., 2006, Interferon-producing killer cells provide a link between innate and adaptive immunity, *Nat. Med.* 12: 207–213.
24. Markiewicz, M.A., Carayannopoulos L.N., Naidenko, O.V., Matsui, K., Burack, W.R., Wise, E.L., Fremont, D.H., Allen, P.M., Yokoyama, W.M., Colonna, M., and Shaw, A.S., 2005, Costimulation through NKG2D enhances murine $CD8^{+}$CTL function: similarities and differences between NKG2D and CD28 costimulation, *J. Immunol.* 175:2825–2833.
25. Gasser, S., Orsulic, S., Brown, E.J., and Raulet, D.H., 2005, The DNA damage pathway regulates innate immune system ligands of the NKG2D receptor, *Nature.* 436:1186–1190.
26. Waldhauer, I., and Steinle, A., 2006, Proteolytic release of soluble UL16-binding protein 2 from tumour cells, *Cancer Res.* 66:2520–2526.
27. Groh, V., Wu, J., Yee, C., and Spies, T., 2002, Tumour-derived soluble MIC ligands impair expression of NKG2D and T-cell activation, *Nature.* 419:734–738.
28. Wiemann, K., Mittrucker, H., Feger, U., Welte, S.A. Yokoyama, W.M., Spies, T, Rammensee, H.G., and Steinle, A., 2005, Systemic NKG2D down-regulation impairs NK and CD8 T cell responses in vivo, *J. Immunol.* 175:720–729.
29. Bui, J.D., Carayannopoulos, L.N., Lanier, L.L., Yokoyama, W.M., and Screiber, R.D., 2006, IFN-dependent down-regulation of the NKG2D ligand H60 on tumors, *J. Immunol.* 176:905–913.
30. Wang, S., and El-Deiry, W.S., 2003, TRAIL and apoptosis induction by TNF-family death receptors, *Oncogene.* 22:8628–2633.
31. Cretney, E., Takeda, K., Yagita, H., Glaccum M., Peschon, J.J., and Smyth, M.J., 2002, Increased susceptibility to tumour initiation and metastasis in TNF-related apoptosis-inducing ligand-deficient mice, *J. Immunol.* 168(3):1356–1361.
32. Smyth, M.J., Takeda, K., Hayakawa, Y., Peschon, J.J., vad den Brink, M.R., and Yagita, H., 2003, Nature's TRAIL-on a path to cancer immunotherapy, *Immunity.* 18(1):1–6.
33. Lamhamedi-Cherradi, S.E., Zheng, S.J., Maguschak, K.A., Peschon, J., and Chen, Y.H., 2003, Defective thymocyte apoptosis and accelerated autoimmune diseases in TRAIL-/- mice, *Nat. Immunol.* 4(3):255–260.
34. Wiley, S.R., Schooley, K., Smolak, P.J., Din, W.S., Huang, C.P., Nicholl, J.K., Sutherland, G.R., Smith, T.D., Rauch, C., and Smith, C.A., 1995, Identification and characterisation of a new member of the TNF family that induces apoptosis, *Immunity.* 3(6):673–682.
35. Kayagaki, N., Yamaguchi, N., Nakayama, M., Kawasaki, A., Akiba, H., Okumura, K., and Yagita, H., 1999a, Involvement of TNF-related apoptosis-inducing ligand in human CD4+ T cell-mediated cytotoxicity. *J. Immunol.* 162(5):2639–2647.
36. Kayagaki, N., Yamaguchi, N., Nakayama, M., Takeda, K., Akiba, H., Tsutsui, H., Okamura, H., Nakanishi, K., Okumura, K., and Yagita, H., 1999b, Expression and function of TNF-related apoptosis-inducing ligand on murine activated NK cells. *J. Immunol.* 163(4):1906–1913.
37. Griffith, T.S., Wiley, S.R., Kubin, M.Z., Sedger, L.M., Maliszewski, C.R., and Fanger, N.A., 1999, Monocyte-mediated tumouricidal activity via the tumour necrosis factor-related cytokine, TRAIL, *J. Exp. Med.* 189(8):1343–1354.
38. Fanger, N.A., Maliszewski, C.R., Schooley, K., and Griffuth, T.S., 1999, Human dendritic cells mediate cellular apoptosis via tumour necrosis factor-related apoptosis-inducing ligand (TRAIL), *J. Exp. Med.* 190(8):1155–1164.
39. Koga, Y., Matsuzaki, A., Suminoe, A., Hattori, H and Hara, T., 2004, Neutrophil-derived TNF-related apoptosis-inducing ligand (TRAIL): a novel mechanism of antitumor effect by neutrophils, *Cancer Res.* 64(3):1037–1043.
40. Kelly, M.M., Hoel, B.D., and Voelkel-Johnson, C., 2002, Doxorubicin pretreatmant sensitizes prostate cancer cell lines to TRAIL induced apoptosis which correlates with the loss of c-FLIP expression, *Cancer Bio. Ther.* y1(5)yy:520–527.

41. Mattarollo, S.R. Kenna, T., Nieda, M., and Nicol, A.J., 2006, Chemotherapy pretreatmant sensitizes solid tumour-derived cell line to $V\alpha24^{+}$ NKT cell-mediated cytotoxicity, *Int. J. Cancer.* y119: 1630–1637.
42. Lundqvist, A. Abrams, S.I., Schrump, D.S., Alvarez, G., Suffredini, D., Berg, M., and Childs, R., 2006, Bortezomib and depsipeptide sensitize tumors to tumor necrosis factor-related apoptosis-inducing ligand: a novel method to potentiate natural killer cell tumor cytotoxicity, *Cancer Res.* y66(14)y:7317–7325.
43. Ibe, S., Qin, Z., Schuler, T., Preiss, S., and Blankenstein, T., 2001, Tumour rejection by disturbing tumour stroma cell interactions, *J. Exp. Med.* yy194(11)y:1549–1559.
44. Mullins, D.W., Burger, C.J., and Elgert, K.D., 1999, Paclitaxel enhgances macrophage IL-12 production in tumour-bearing hosts through nitric oxide, *J. Immunol.* y162:6811–6818.
45. Bocci, G., Francia, G., Man, S., Lawler, J., and Kerbel, R.S., 2003, Thrombospodin 1, a mediator of the antiangiogenic effects of low-dose metronomic chemotherapy, *Proc. Natl. Acad. Sci. U S A.* y100(22)yy:12917–12922.
46. Jassar, A.S., Suzuki, E., Kapoor, V., Sun, J., Silverberg, M.B., Cheung, L., Burdick, M.D., Strieter, R.M., Ching, L., Kaiser, L.R., and Albelds, S.M., 2005, Activation of tumour-associated macrophages by the vascular disrupting angent 5,6-dimethylxanthenone-4-acetic acid induces an effective $CD8^{+}$T-cell-mediated antitumour immune response in murine models of lung cancer and mesothelioma, *Cancer Res.* yy64(24)y:11752–11761.
47. Krupica, T., Fry, T.J., and Mackall, C.L., 2006, Autoimmunity during lymphopenia: a two-hit model, *Clin. Immunol.* y120:121–128.
48. Beyer, M., Kochanek, M., Darabi, K., Popov, A., Jensen, M., Endl, E., Knolle, P.A., Thomas, R.K., von Bergwelt-Bailon, M., Debey, S., Hallek, M., and Schultze, J.L., 2005, Reduced frequencies and suppressive function of $CD4^{+}CD25^{hi}$ regulatory T cells in patients with chronic lymphocytic leukemia after therapy with fludarabine, *Blood.* yy106(6)yy:2018–1025.
49. Lutsiak, M.E.C., Semnani, R.T., De Pascalis, R., Kashmiri, S.V.S., Schlom, J., and Sabzevari, H., 2005, Inhibition of $CD4^{+}CD25^{+}$T regulatory cell function implicated in enhanced immune response by low-dose cyclophosphamide, *Blood.* y105(7)y:2862–2868.
50. Nowak, A.K., Robinson, B.W., Lake, R.A., 2003b, Synergy between chemotherapy and immunotherapy in the treatment of established murine solid tumours, *Cancer Res.* yy63(15)yy: 4490–4496.
51. Zhang, H., Chua, K.S., Guimond, M., Kapoor, V., Brown, M.V., Fleisher, T.A., Long, L.M., Bernstein, D., Hill, B.J., Douek, D.C., Berzofsky, J.A., Carrter, C.S., Read, E.J., Helman, L.J., and Mackall, C.L., 2005, Lymphopenia and interleukin-2 therapy alter homeostasis of $CD4^{+}CD25^{+}$ regulatory T cells, *Nat. Med.* y11(11)yy:1238–1243.
52. Rosenberg, S.A., Sportes, C., Ahmadzadeh, M., Fry, T.J., Ngo, L.T., Schwarz, S.L., Stetler-Stevenson, M., Morton, K.E., Mavroukakis, S.A., Morre, M., Buffet, R., Mackall, C.L., and Gress, R.E., 2006, IL-17 administration to humans leads to expansion of $CD8^{+}$ and $CD4^{+}$cells but a relative decreas of $CD4^{+}$ T-regulatory cells, *J. Immunother.* yy29(3)y:313–319.
53. Kuwajima, S., Sato, T., Ishida, K., Tada, H., Tezuka, H., and Ohteki, T., 2006, Interleukin 15-dependent crosstalk between conventional and plasmacytoid dendritic cells is essential for CpG-induced immune activation, *Nature Immunol.* y7(7)yy:740–746.
54. Teague, R.M., Sther, B.D., Sacks, J.A., Huang, M.Z., Dossett, M.L., Morimoto, J., Tan, X., Sutton, S.E., Cooke, M.P., Ohlen, C., and Greenberg, P.D., 2006, Interleukin-15 rescues tolerant $CD8^{+}$T cells for use in adaptive immunotherapy of established tumors, *Nat. Med.* yy12(3)y:335–341.
55. Smyth, M.J., Hayakawa, Y., Cretney, E., Zerafa, N., Sivakumar, P., Yagita, H., and Takeda, K., 2006, IL-21 enhances tumour-specific CTL induction by anti-DR5 antibody therapy, *J.Immunol.* y176:6347–6355.
56. Emens, L.A., and Jaffee, E.M., 2005, Leveraging the activity of tumour vaccines with cytotoxic chemotherapy, *Cancer Res.* yy65(18)y:8059–8064.
57. Ercolini, A.M., Ladle, B.H., Manning, E.A., Pfannenstiel, L.W., Armstrong, T.D., Machiels, J.H., Bieler, J.G., Emans, L.A., Reilly, R.T., and Jaffee, E.M., 2005, Recruitment of latent pools of high-avidity $CD8^{+}$T cells to the antitumour immune response, *J. Exp. Med.* yy201(10)y:1591–1602.

58. Le, H.N., Lee, N.C., Tsung, K., and Norton, J.A., 2001, Pre-existing tumour-sensitized T cells are essential for eradication of established tumours by IL-12 and cyclophosphamide plus IL-12, *J Immunol.* y167:6765–6772.
59. Belldegrun, A., Uppenkamp, I., and Rosenberg, S.A., 1988, Anti-tumour reactivity of human lymphokine activated killer (LAK) cells after fresh and cultured preparations of renal cell cancers, *J. Urol.* y139(1)yy:150–155.
60. Dudley, M.E., Wunderlich, J.R., Robbins, P.F., Yang, J.C., Hwu, P., Schwartzentruber, D.J., Topalian, S.L., Sherry, R., Restifo, N.P., Hubicki, A.M., Robinson, M.R., Raffeld, M., Duray, P., Seipp, C.A., Rogers-Freezer, L., Morton, K.E., Mavroukakis, S.A. White, D.E. and Rosenberg, S.A., 2002, Cancer regression and autoimmunity in patients after clonal repopulation with antitumour lymphocytes, *Science.* y298(5594)yy:850–854.

INDEX